Learning and Memory
in Normal Aging

◆

Learning and Memory in Normal Aging

◆

Donald H. Kausler

Department of Psychology
University of Missouri
Columbia, Missouri 65211

Academic Press

A Division of Harcourt Brace & Company

San Diego   New York   Boston   London   Sydney   Tokyo   Toronto

Copyright © 1994 by ACADEMIC PRESS, INC.

All Rights Reserved.
No part of this publication may be reproduced or transmitted in any form or by any
means, electronic or mechanical, including photocopy, recording, or any information
storage and retrieval system, without permission in writing from the publisher.

Academic Press, Inc.
525 B Street, Suite 1900, San Diego, California 92101-4495

United Kingdom Edition published by
Academic Press Limited
24–28 Oval Road, London NW1 7DX

Library of Congress Cataloging-in-Publication Data

Kausler, Donald H.
    Learning and memory in normal aging / Donald H. Kausler.
        p.   cm.
    Includes index.
    ISBN 0-12-402655-9
    1. Memory in old age. 2. Learning, Psychology of, in old age.
    I. Title.
    BF724.85.M45K38   1994
    155.67--dc20   93-43189
                                                                              CIP

PRINTED IN THE UNITED STATES OF AMERICA
94 95 96 97 98 99   BC   9 8 7 6 5 4 3 2 1

CONTENTS

PREFACE   xiii

CHAPTER · 1   Conditioning and Instrumental Learning

Introduction   1

Learning or Memory?   3

Adult Age Differences in Conditioning   4

Classical Conditioning   7

Operant Conditioning   14

Adult Age Differences in Instrumental Learning   18

Maze Learning   18

Explanation of Age Differences in Maze Learning   20

Spatial Learning and Spatial Cognition   21

CHAPTER · 2   Skill Learning and Procedural Learning

Adult Age Differences in Motor-Skill Learning   26

Attributes of Motor Behaviors   28

Laboratory Studies: Real-World Motor-Learning Tasks   32

Laboratory Studies: Controlled Motor-Learning Tasks   34

Expertise and Maintenance of Motor Skills   41

Learning Theory and Explanation of Adult Age Differences in
Motor-Skill Learning   44

Adult Age Differences in Perceptual Learning   46

Target Detection   47

Stimulus Discrimination   47

Pattern-Recognition Learning   53

Attentional Learning   54

Expertise and Maintenance of a Perceptual Skill   56

Adult Age Differences in Learning Mental Skills   57

Adult Age Differences in Procedural Learning   57

Dissociation and Procedural Learning   57

Evidence for Procedural Learning in Late Adulthood   63

CHAPTER · 3   Verbal Learning

Introduction   66

Adult Age Differences in Paired-Associate Learning   66

Historical Perspective: Early Studies   67

Historical Perspective: Methodological Problems and Issues   69

Stage Analysis of Potential Age-Sensitive Processes   77

Research with Manipulable Independent Variables: Preexperimental
    Associative Strength   84

Research with Manipulable Independent Variables: Rate of Item Presentation   86

Research with Manipulable Independent Variables: Mediational Instructions
    and Materials   91

Research with Manipulable Independent Variables: Intentional versus
    Incidental Learning   97

Comments   98

Adult Age Differences in Serial Learning   98

Historical Perspective   98

Research with Manipulable Independent Variables   99

Analysis of Age-Sensitive Processes   102

CHAPTER · 4   Mnemonics and Transfer

Mnemonics   105

Pegword Method   106

Method of Loci   106

Keyword Method   108

Supplementary Procedures   110

Individual Differences Variables   111

Alternative Methods of Mnemonic Training   113

Adult Age Differences in Transfer   117

Specific versus Nonspecific Transfer: Implications for Adult Age Differences   117

Laboratory Studies of Nonspecific Transfer   120

Laboratory Studies of Specific Transfer   122

Comments   129

CHAPTER · 5   Sensory Memory and Short-Term/ Primary Memory

Introduction   131

Overview of the Human Memory System   134

Adult Age Differences in Sensory Memory   135

Iconic Memory   135

Echoic Memory   141

Other Senses   149

Adult Age Differences in Short-Term/Primary Memory   149

Primary Memory: STS Capacity and Memory Span   151

Primary Memory: STS Capacity and the Recency Effect   157

Primary Memory: Flexibility of Representation   160

Primary Memory: Rate of Loss of Information   162

Primary Memory: Search of Content   168

CHAPTER · 6   Models of Long-Term Episodic Memory

Introduction   175

Dual-Store Models   175

Nature of Dual-Store Models   175

Explanation of Age Differences in Secondary Memory   176

Levels-of-Processing Model   181

Nature of the Levels-of-Processing Model   181

Orienting Tasks and Variation in Depth of Processing   183

Noncued Recall versus Cued Recall: Encoding or Retrieval as the Locus of Age
   Differences in Episodic Memory   187

Elaboration as the Locus of Age Differences in Episodic Memory   190

Cognitive Resources and Cognitive Support   193

Trace Distinctiveness as the Locus of Age Differences in Episodic Memory   193

Primary Memory and the Recency Effect Reconsidered   196

Comments   199

General Resources   201

Overview   201

Processing Rate and Working-Memory Models   203

Inhibition Model   207

Network Theory   207

Processing Rate and Adult Age Differences in Episodic
   Long-Term Memory   208

Working Memory and Adult Age Differences in Episodic
   Long-Term Memory   212

Inhibition and Adult Age Differences in Episodic
   Long-Term Memory   220

Generality of Resource Decrements   223

CHAPTER · 7   Long-Term Episodic Memory:
Effortful Phenomena

Introduction   229

Adult Age Differences in Organizational Processes   229

Categorical Organization   230

Other Forms of Intrinsic Organization   238

Subjective Organization   240

Multitrial Free Recall   243

Generation Effect   244

Encoding Variability and the Lag Effect   246

Recognition Memory   249

Single Item Recognition Memory   249

Recognition versus Recall   253

Adult Age Difference in Picture and Face Memory   254

Picture Memory   255

Face Memory   259

Adult Age Differences in Retrieval   261

Encoding Specificity   261

Output Interference   267

Effects of Prior Retrieval on Later Retrieval   268

Cued Recall and Indirect Retrieval   269

Fan Effect   270

Adult Age Differences in Prospective Memory   271

CHAPTER · 8   Long-Term Episodic Memory: Discourse

Introduction   276

Adult Age Differences in Sentence Memory   277

Syntactic and Semantic Constraints   277

Normal Sentence Recall   279

Adult Age Differences in Paragraph Memory   281

Recall of Ideas   281

Modality of Presentation   282

Attributes of the Text   283

Comprehension of Content   283

Medical Information   289

Adult Age Differences in Memory for Longer Discourses   289

Schema Abstraction   290

Levels of Propositions   292

Qualitative and Quantitative Age Differences in Discourse Memory   294

Procedural Variables   295

Attributes of the Discourse   298

Prior Knowledge   299

Individual Differences Variables   303

CHAPTER · 9   Long-Term Episodic Memory: Automaticity and Rehearsal Independence

Introduction   306

Adult Age Differences in Memory for Noncontent Attributes of
    Episodic Events   307

Frequency-of-Occurrence Memory   307

Temporal Memory   312

Spatial Memory   315

Source Memory   321

Other Noncontent Attributes   323

Adult Age Differences in Memory for Activities and Actions   326

Memory for the Content of Activities and Actions   327

Encoding of Activity and Action Information   335

Memory for Noncontent Attributes   339

Reality Monitoring and Source Memory   342

Adult Age Differences in Other Forms of Rehearsal-
    Independent Memory   343

CHAPTER · 10   Long-Term Episodic Memory: Retention and Forgetting

Introduction   346

Adult Age Differences in Real-Life Forgetting   346

Impersonal Events   346

Personal Idiosyncratic Events: Autobiographical Memory   352

Why Forgetting?   354

Proactive and Retroactive Interference   354

Interference Proneness   355

Problems in Testing the Interference Proneness Hypothesis   355

Laboratory Studies: Retention of Successive Lists   357

Laboratory Studies: Single-List Retention   362

Laboratory Studies: Retention of Activities and Actions   367

Laboratory Studies: Retention of Noncontent Attributes   369

CHAPTER · 11   Long-Term Episodic Memory: Implicit Memory

Nature of Implicit Memory   370
Adult Age Differences in Implicit Memory   374
Why Age Sensitivity on Some Tasks and Not Other Tasks?   382
Conscious Recollection versus Automaticity   383
Future Research   385

CHAPTER · 12   Generic (Semantic) Memory and Metamemory

Introduction   387
Adult Age Differences in the Internal Lexicon   388
Age Differences in Structure   388
Age Differences in Lexical Access for Words   395
Stimulus Degradation and Lexical Access   402
Verbal Fluency   404
Age Differences in Lexical Access for Categorical Information   404
Separate Memory Systems?   409
When Lexical Access Fails   412
Adult Age Differences in the Use of Syntax   414
Adult Age Differences in Metamemory   415
Age Differences in Off-Line Evaluation of Episodic Memory   416
Age Differences in On-Line Evaluation of Episodic Memory   424
Age Differences in Episodic Memory Monitoring Skills   428
Age Differences in Self-Evaluation of Factual Memory Proficiency   431

REFERENCES   433
AUTHOR INDEX   513
SUBJECT INDEX   533

Producing this book occurred early in my retirement from the University of Missouri. Many experts in cognitive aging firmly believe that intensive mental activity is essential for slowing down whatever adverse effects aging has on mental functioning. If this belief is true, I should be able to function well for some time to come.

Some readers may be familiar with my earlier work *Experimental Psychology, Cognition, and Human Aging* (Springer-Verlag, 1991). The motivation for the present work came from comments made by Dr. Patrick Rabbitt, in a review of this earlier work. He noted that my coverage of learning and memory constituted a book within a book, and from those comments came the notion of doing a more comprehensive work devoted fully to this subject.

The past three years have offered a wealth of new information on learning and memory. There have been exciting new developments in such areas as mnemonic training, general resource models, prospective memory, implicit memory, meta-memory, and so on. Writing this book gave me the opportunity to discuss more thoroughly earlier research on a number of topics, such as paired-associate learning and short-term memory. In common with my efforts in the 1991 book, I have continued in my attempt to provide introductions to the basic concepts and theories indigenous to specific areas of research. I did not follow Dr. Rabbitt's suggestion that my writings on learning and memory should include more information on neuropsychology and memory performance. I am well aware of my own limitations, and I leave this writing to others who are much better informed in this area than I am.

I am most grateful for the excellent support provided by the editorial and production staffs of Academic Press, especially to Nikki Fine, Diane Scott, and Michael Early. Less direct, but just as important, support was given by my wife Marty. Despite several serious physical health problems, she persisted in encouraging me to complete this project. Finally, we both benefited greatly from the periods of relaxation provided by frequent interactions with our grandchildren, Neil and Tara Ratna, Rose, Paige, and Donald, III, Kausler, and Rebecca and Daniel Krupsaw.

DONALD H. KAUSLER

CHAPTER 1

Conditioning and Instrumental Learning

Introduction

Imagine what life would be like if all learning suddenly stopped at some point in late adulthood. Knowledge, of course, would be frozen. That is, there would be no further additions to knowledge—no updating of information concerning, for example, local, national, and international events. The names of a new mayor, a new senator, and a new prime minister for a foreign country would all be perceived, but they would be unfamiliar every time they were encountered. An elderly person planning a trip to a foreign country would find nothing but frustration in trying to acquire a working vocabulary for traveling in that country. Attendance at adult education classes would be a wasted effort.

Knowledge is far from being the only aspect of human behavior to suffer if all learning suddenly ceased. There would be no hope of elderly people acquiring new recreational skills. Golf and bridge would be impossible, unless they had been mastered before the void in new learning occurred (even if they had been learned before, there would be no hope of further improvement in skill). Suppose illness forced confinement to a wheelchair. There would be no chance of ever mastering the maneuverability of the wheelchair. Conditioning therapies of either physical or psychological illness could not possibly be successful. Movement to a new apartment in a new neighborhood would be chaotic and most likely disastrous. The operation of a tricky new lock on the front door would have to be rediscovered by trial and error every time the lock was used. Each day's outing to a new supermarket would be a brand new adventure, requiring assistance each time from some good Samaritan to find the way to and from home. A loose step would be a hazard every time the staircase was ascended or descended. New neighbors would stay strangers forever—there would be no way of associating their names with their faces.

There is a brighter side, however. Without new learning, attitudes would also remain frozen, as would fears and hates. There could be no additions to the prejudices and fears people possess.

1

Learning is obviously critical for adaptation to our environments. It is little wonder that it has long been an area of great importance in psychology. From our analysis of a world without learning for elderly people, it should be apparent that learning is just as important for elderly adults as it is for younger adults. Fortunately, learning has no age barrier. Given normal aging, elderly people remain highly active learners. They acquire new information, they learn new recreational skills, they learn to operate new gadgets and devices, they learn their way around new neighborhoods, they learn to avoid hazardous obstacles, they learn to relate new names to new faces, and they also learn new prejudices and fears. Of course, to say that learning occurs in late adulthood is not to say that it occurs without losses in proficiency relative to the proficiency manifested earlier in life. The critical importance of learning to human adaptability makes it essential that we discover the extent to which learning proficiency is affected by human aging and that we understand the reasons why it is so affected.

Adult age differences in learning are usually interpreted from the perspective of stimulus–response (S-R) psychology and associationism, both in its classical form and in the form of stage analysis. In this chapter and in Chapters 2, 3, and 4, our task is to review the many studies that have been concerned with adult age differences in learning. Our review will also cover the closely related areas of transfer and mnemonics. Transfer refers to the effects of learning one task on the subsequent acquisition of a new task. Transfer phenomena have also been interpreted largely from the perspective of S-R psychology and associationism. A mnemonic is basically a form of transfer in which indivduals are taught a device of some kind to help them acquire new material at a faster rate.

Our review of experimental aging studies on learning is complicated by the tremendous diversity of learning activities. This diversity should have been apparent in the sample of activities missing in a life without learning. Reflecting this diversity, the psychology of learning along with its extension to the experimental psychology of aging is commonly divided into five areas. The areas clearly differ in terms of the task structures and complexities they represent. But do the areas differ in the nature of the processes postulated to mediate learning or in the products postulated to result from learning? To associationists, the answer is no— all learning involves contiguity between S and R elements and the products of all learning are S-R associations. This monistic concept of learning (i.e., only one kind of learning), however, has been challenged by a number of learning psychologists who view learning pluralistically. That is, they believe that there are truly different kinds of learning, both in terms of mediating processes and in terms of what the products of learning are.

The five areas are conditioning, instrumental learning, skill learning, procedural learning, and verbal learning. According to some psychologists, learning fears and prejudices are examples of conditioning. To these same psychologists, learning to avoid a hazardous step is also an example of conditioning, but conditioning of a different kind than the conditioning entering into the acquisition of a fear or prejudice. Learning one's way around a neighborhood or apartment is an example of instrumental learning, whereas learning to maneuver a wheelchair and to play golf are examples of one form of skill learning, namely motor-skill learning. Learning to interpret the blips that appear on a radar screen and learning to play bridge are examples of other forms of skill learning, namely perceptual and mental, respectively. Procedural learning, however, is not task bound. It cuts across such diverse tasks as classical conditioning, motor-skill learning, and reading, and it is in reference to a dissociation between the acquisition of a skill of some kind and memory for events surrounding that acquisition. Learning title-name and face-name associations are examples of verbal learning. In verbal learning, linguistic elements (e.g., words or letters) always serve as sources of response elements, whereas either linguistic elements or pictorial and graphic elements (e.g., pictures of faces) serve as stimulus elements. Our review will cover all five areas. The impact of associationism has been especially great on verbal learning research. Accordingly, associationism will be especially stressed in our coverage of verbal learning and transfer research. We will take a somewhat more flexible approach in covering aging research on conditioning, instrumental learning, and motor-skill learning. Surprisingly, it is in these areas that alternatives to associationism have often been proposed.

Nonverbal learning as it involves conditioning, instrumental learning, skill learning, and procedural learning will be covered in Chapters 1 and 2. Verbal learning will be reviewed in Chapter 3, and its extensions to transfer and mnemonics will be reviewed in Chapter 4.

Learning or Memory?

In later chapters we will review research on adult age differences in memory. The concepts of learning and memory are obviously related, and they are difficult to distinguish. Learning usually connotes rote practice on a task in which proficiency of performance improves progressively with practice. This connotation fits nicely, for example, the events that took place when you *learned* to ride a bicycle—you had the intent to master the skill and you practiced long and hard. But it does not fit the *memory* you still have of the first bad spill you had while learning. That memory required neither intent to remember nor practice (one trial was sufficient). Similarly, you learn with repetition of the task to respond with a conditioned response to a conditioned stimulus, to make a left turn at this corner and a right turn at the next corner, and to respond with a specific name to a specific face, just as you have memory of some of the words in a list presented only once. The "progressive increments in performance with practice" distinction becomes blurred, however, when the list of words is presented several more times.

As you increase the number of words recalled after each trial, is it because you have "learned" more words or because you have improved your memory for which words were in the list? Perhaps the best way to distinguish between learning and memory is in terms of the conceptual framework guiding the research on specific tasks. Craik (1977) has made a valiant effort to clarify the distinction between learning and memory in these terms. His effort is well worth repeating here:

> Running parallel to the change in emphasis from S-R to information processing theories, there has been a change in emphasis from studies of learning to studies of memory. Within the general framework of S-R theories, human learning and retention have been described and analyzed in terms of interference theory (e.g., Postman, 1961; Postman & Underwood, 1973); this theory focuses attention on the hypothesized association between stimuli and responses (or, at least, between their internal representations). Thus, empirical work in this tradition has been directed toward elucidating the factors relevant to the acquisition and breakdown of the associative bond; 'learning' is the formation of new associations and 'forgetting' is their loss or inhibition. In human learning, much of the experimental work has used the paired-associate paradigm in which stimuli and responses are verbal units—numbers, letters, words, or nonsense syllables; short lists of such stimulus-response pairs are typically presented for several learning trials and this acquisition phase is then followed by a task to measure retention or transfer. By way of contrast, information processing studies of memory have more often involved situations in which the material to be learned is presented for one trial only—the focus has thus been on factors which affect the subject's *memory* for the once-presented events: factors concerned with registration, storage, and retrieval of the events (pp. 384–385).

We will follow Craik's (1977) distinction in the remainder of this book. Most research on the tasks to be covered in Chapters 1–4 was initiated from the perspective of S-R psychology and associationism. This is certainly true, for example, with the paired-associate learning task, long a favorite of associationists. At the same time, however, we recognize the fact that a single paired associate could be viewed as being composed of a to-be-remembered item (the response element) and a cue (the stimulus item) for its later recall. Similarly, memory for the words in a free-recall task (a favorite task employed by memory researchers working within the information processing framework) may be viewed in terms of the learning of associations among items and between each item as a response element and the laboratory context as a broad stimulus element (see Kausler, 1974). Our distinction between learning and memory is obviously arbitrary and imperfect, but, hopefully, you will learn to live with it, just as learning and memory researchers have.

Adult Age Differences in Conditioning

Conditioning is generally considered to be the simplest kind of learning. Simplicity in this context refers to the fact that single response elements are involved in learning—not to any allusion that the mechanisms underlying learning are simple and fully comprehended.

Actually, the existence of two kinds of conditioning has long been recognized by learning psychologists: *classical* or *Pavlovian conditioning* and *operant conditioning*. They differ procedurally in a fundamental way. In classical conditioning, a response—the unconditioned response (UCR)—is naturally (i.e., reflexively) elicited by a particular stimulus—the unconditioned stimulus (UCS). For example, an eyeblink is the UCR elicited by a puff of air to the eye as the UCS. The objective of conditioning is to transfer control of the response's elicitation to another stimulus element—the conditioned stimulus (CS)—an element that at the start of conditioning bears no relationship to the response (i.e., it is neutral). For the eyeblink response the CS is likely to be either a change in brightness of a glass disk facing the subjects or a tone. To accomplish this objective, conditioning trials are initiated in which the CS just precedes (and also overlaps) the UCS. There are alternative procedures for promoting the acquisition of a new response similar to the UCR—the conditioned response (CR)—but the procedure described here (the delay procedure) has been the one employed in most aging studies of conditioning. For example, the CS may have its onset 500 ms before the onset of the UCS. On early trials the response in question (e.g., an eyeblink) will be elicited only by the UCS. However, eventually the response, now the CR, will occur in the interval prior to the occurrence of the UCS. This sequence of events for the conditioning of an eyeblink is summarized in the Part A of Figure 1.1.

In operant conditioning the to-be-modified response is emitted by the subject. Procedurally, the critical element is the stimulus event that follows emission of the response. In some cases, the stimulus event is designed to increase the rate of emitting the response in question. In other cases, it is some other attribute of a response, such as its speed, that is to be altered by making receipt of the stimulus event contingent on whether or not the response displayed the appropriate attribute. One way of accomplishing this objective is through the use of positive reinforcement whereby the subject's response is followed by an event that is attractive to the subject (a positive reinforcer, such as a piece of candy, beer, praise, or whatever else works with the subject at hand). Alternatively, negative reinforcement may be employed, whereby the subject's response is followed by the termination of some aversive or obnoxious stimulus (e.g., an electric shock). In other cases, the stimulus event is designed to to decrease the rate of emitting the response in question. This may be accomplished by means of punishment, that is, following each occurrence of the response with an aversive stimulus event (e.g., an electric shock, an insult, or whatever else is deemed appropriate for the subject at hand). An alternative form of punishment is to follow the response with the taking away of something that is attractive to the subject (e.g., use of the family car). The sequence of events for both positive reinforcement (S$^+$) and punishment (S$^-$) are summarized in Part B of Figure 1.1.

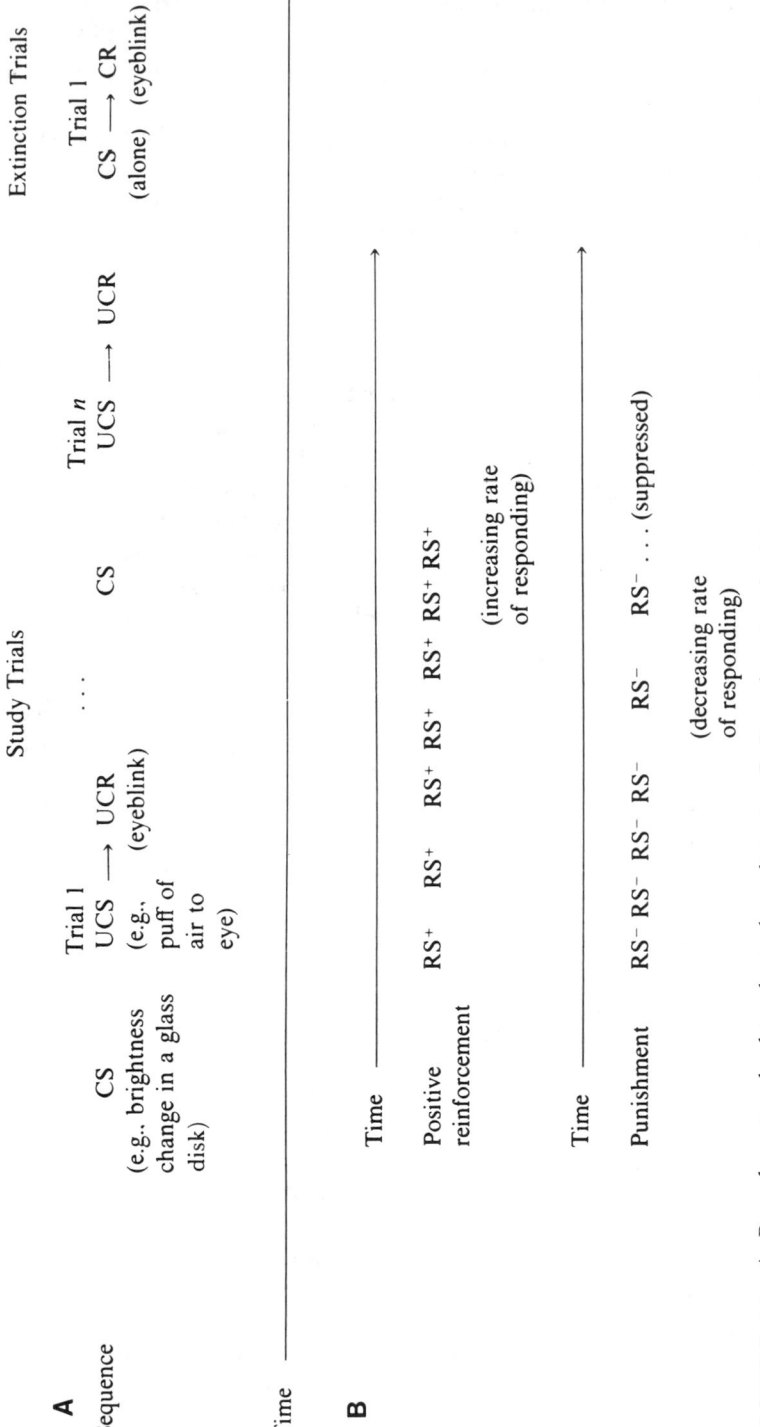

FIGURE 1.1 A: Procedures involved in classical conditioning. B: Procedures involved in positive reinforcement and punishment (operant training).

Classical Conditioning

To those of you who think of classical conditioning only in terms of training a dog to salivate when a bell is sounded, the existence of an age deficit in classical conditioning is likely to be a stimulus for eliciting a yawn and a "so what" response. Actually, classical conditioning is a learning phenomenon of considerable practical importance. For example, the therapies mentioned earlier in this chapter are attempts to modify behavior by means of the application of classical conditioning training. Systolic blood pressure is an example of a "behavior" that seemingly can be so modified (Whitehead, Lurie, & Blackwell, 1976). The treatment calls for the establishment of a UCS that elicits the lowering of the blood pressure (the UCR). To produce this natural stimulus, the patient is tilted head down through an arc of 15°. As the body moves through the arc, a bell (the CS) is sounded. Amazingly, in some case, the bell becomes associated with a lowering of blood pressure, and it therefore serves as a psychological control over heightened pressure. Alcoholism is another behavior that that has been successfully treated, at least in some cases, by means of classical conditioning. The treatment, known as aversive therapy, will not be described in detail here (see Sherman, 1973, for elaboration). Briefly, it consists of pairing the taste of an alcoholic beverage as the CS with either electric shock or a nausea-producing drug as the UCS. The unpleasant biological state elicited by the UCS is the UCR, and a modified form of this state eventually becomes the CR elicited by the taste of the alcoholic beverage. If elderly people are indeed more difficult to condition than younger people, then there is good reason to question the effectiveness of these therapeutic methods beyond middle adulthood. This highly significant ecological issue has received surprisingly little attention in the gerontological literature.

The importance of classical conditioning goes well beyond its practical use in therapy. For many years, classical conditioning has served as a kind of model for conceptualizing and, therefore, explaining how a number of specific human behaviors are acquired. Included are many fears, phobias, attitudes, and prejudices (Baron & Byrne, 1977; Staats & Staats, 1958). For example, a phobia is viewed in terms of the phobic object being a CS that is associated with fear (or conditioned pain) as the CR. Presumably, the conditioning occurred because the CS was innocently present at the time the victim experienced a painful, or noxious, stimulus (the UCS). Pain itself is, therefore, the UCR elicited by the UCS. Pain, however, is a complex physiological response that has many components, only some of which are conditionable in the sense of becoming part of the CR elicited by the CS. Those components make up the experience of fear or anxiety that is felt on subsequent encounters with the CS, or phobic object. Our awareness of age-related deficits in classical conditioning should make us wonder about the extent of acquiring new fears or phobias during late adulthood—or, for that matter, new prejudices, attitudes, and any other behavior presumed learned through classical conditioning. We may also wonder about the extent to which behaviors that are successfully learned through conditioning by elderly people can be eliminated through extinction training (i.e., through repeated presentations of the CS without further occurrences of the UCS). Again, these important ecological issues have received little attention in the gerontological literature.

Our speculation that elderly people are less conditionable than younger people in the real world of therapy, phobias, and prejudices is based on laboratory studies of adult age differences in classical conditioning. The tasks employed in these studies, on the surface, seem far removed from real-world examples of conditioning. Nevertheless, these tasks capture the essence of the procedures and processes of classical conditioning wherever they take place. Moreover, laboratory studies permit the analysis of adult age differences in conditionability under carefully controlled conditions. As a result, there is good reason for our confidence in the generalizability of these laboratory-based results to age differences in real-world conditionability (i.e., their external or ecological validity).

The task most frequently employed in studying adult age differences in rate of classical conditioning is the eyeblink conditioning task described earlier. Apparently, the first study to report the very slow acquisition of a conditioned eyeblink by elderly subjects was by Gakkel and Zinna (1953; cited in Jerome, 1959) with an auditory CS. However, elderly nursing home residents served as the subjects in this study, and there were no comparison groups of young adults and normally aging elderly adults. Other early researchers (Braun & Geiselhart (1959); Kimble and Pennypacker, 1963; Solyom and Barik, 1965) did compare elderly adults with young adults in their rates of acquiring a conditioned eyeblink response, and without exception did find the rate to be much slower for elderly adults than for young adults (see Botwinick, 1970, for further review).

Representative of the results obtained in these early studies are those of Braun and Geiselhart (1959). They are plotted in Figure 1.2 in terms of the percentage of trials in blocks of 10 trials in which the CR occurred to the CS (an increase in brightness of a glass disk) during the delay preceding the UCS. Their subjects included children (average age, 9.4 yr) as well as young adults and elderly adults (average age, 70.5 yr). Note that their elderly subjects showed very little sign of conditioning (or learning). By contrast, their young adult subjects showed considerable learning and the negatively accelerated learning curve (diminishing increments in performance scores with increasing trials; see Figure 1.2) characteristic of many learning tasks. (For some tasks, the learning curve tends to be positively accelerated—increasing increments in performance scores with increasing trials). Although others (e.g., Kimble & Pennypacker, 1963) also found considerably faster conditioning for young adults than for elderly adults, they reported somewhat greater learning for their elderly subjects than that reported by Braun and Geiselhart (1959).

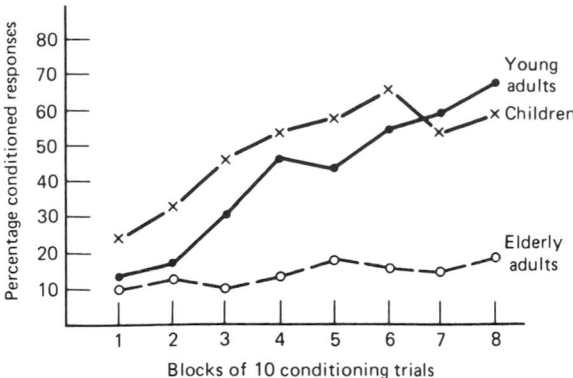

FIGURE 1.2 Age differences in rate of classical conditioning (eyeblink response). (Adapted from Braun & Geiselhart, 1959, Figure 1.)

The age difference in conditioning rate favoring young adults was found in several other early studies using other kinds of tasks. For one of these tasks (Botwinick & Kornetsky, 1960; Shmavonian, Miller, & Cohen, 1968, 1970), the UCR is a change in the galvanic skin response (GSR) produced by an electric shock as the UCS. The CS is a tone that precedes the shock, and the CR is a change in the GSR elicited by the CS. For another task (Marinesco & Kreindler, 1934), the UCR is a reflexive retraction of the hand produced by an electric current as the UCS. The CS is a colored light, and the CR is a withdrawal of the hand as elicited by the CS. Not only did Marinesco and Kriendler's (1934) elderly subjects require twice as many trials as their young subjects to acquire the conditioned response, but they also extinguished considerably more slowly once they had acquired the response. By contrast, other investigators (Braun & Geiselhart, 1959; Botwinick & Kornetsky, 1960) reported that their elderly subjects extinguished more rapidly than young adults. Interestingly, Botwinick (1970) has speculated that the disparity in age differences for rate of extinction may be due to the different kinds of responses used in these studies. He noted that the hand withdrawal response employed by Marinesco and Kreindler (1934) is completely voluntary, while the eyeblink response employed by Braun and Geiselhart (1959) is only partially voluntary and the GSR response employed by Botwinick and Kornetsky (1960) is completely involuntary.

Marinesco and Kriendler (1934) also discovered that their elderly subjects had considerably greater difficulty in establishing differentiation, or discrimination, than did their young subjects. Differentiation means distinguishing between the actual CS and other neutral stimuli (symbolized as CS') that bear some form of relatedness to the CS. In the laboratory, the CS may be a red light and the CS' a yellow light; in the real world, a phobic CS may be a horse and the CS' a pony.

Differentiation in the laboratory is accomplished by having two kinds of trials that are intermingled: (1) those in which the CS is presented and then followed by the UCS and (2) those in which the CS' is presented without the UCS following it.

The results from these early studies imply that elderly adults are "slower learners" (i.e., they condition at a slower rate than young adults). There is a problem, however, in accepting this implication. The age difference in conditioning rate may be attributable to age-related deficits in nonlearning or nonassociative factors that adversely affect conditioning rather than to an age-related deficit in learning per se. One possibility is that the age difference simply reflects a motivational difference produced by the greater anxiety experienced by young adults than by elderly adults during conditioning trials. According to Spence (1958), high drive from a high level of anxiety should result in greater energization of a gradually accruing habit (the Habit × Drive concept of Hull's, 1943, learning theory) than low drive from a low level of anxiety, and therefore should lead to a higher level of performance even if habit strength is equivalent for high-drive and low-drive subjects. Anxiety may be considered to be a source of drive—but are elderly adults likely to be *less* anxious than young adults? In his review of the research dealing with adult age differences in anxiety, Kausler (1990a) concluded that there is no reason to believe that there are major age differences in either state or trait anxiety levels.

There are, however, a number of other nonlearning factors that conceivably could account for the pronounced age difference in the rate of conditioning, at least for the eyeblink response. For example, the latency of the CR to the CS may be much longer for elderly subjects than for young adult subjects. If true, the delay separating the onset of the CS and the onset of the UCS may be too brief for elderly subjects to avoid the CR from being masked by the UCR. A number of these nonlearning factors were carefully examined in studies by Woodruff-Pak and Thompson (1988) and Solomon, Pomerleau, Bennett, James, and Morse (1989). In addition, both teams of investigators included subjects at various age levels between early and late adulthood. If conditioning rate is indeed slower in late adulthood than in early adulthood, then a question of further interest is when in the adult life span the decline in rate becomes apparent. With such animals as the rabbit as subjects, there is convincing evidence that the decline begins in the animal's "middle age" (e.g., Powell, Buchanan, & Hernandez, 1981; Woodruff-Pak, Lavond, Logan, & Thompson, 1987).

In their first experiment, Woodruff-Pak and Thompson (1988) compared the conditioning rates of subjects in the age ranges of 18 to 27 yr (mean age = 20.2 yr), 40 to 49 yr (mean age = 44.9 yr), 50 to 59 yr (mean age = 52.8 yr), and 60 to 83 yr (mean age = 73.1 yr). The delay conditioning procedure was employed with an eyeblink as the UCR and the CR and an airpuff and a tone as the UCS and the CS. In the delay procedure the CS is initiated before the onset of the

UCS, and the CS remains on at least until the onset of the UCS. The interval separating the onset of the CS and the onset of the UCS on each trial (the interstimulus interval or ISI) was 400 ms. The percentage of CRs for each of 12 blocks of 8 trials per block are shown in part A of Figure 1.3 for each age group. Note the pronounced slow rate of conditioning for the two older groups of subjects (their rates did not differ). Even in the last block of trials the subjects at these age levels were eliciting CRs for fewer than half of the trials. The difference in rate of acquisition did not differ significantly for the two younger groups, both of which acquired the CR at a significantly faster rate than the two older groups. In their second experiment, Woodruff-Pak and Thompson (1988) compared conditioning rates for subjects in the age ranges of 18 to 22 yr and 28 to 39 yr and found virtually identical fast rates of acquisition. The subjects in Solomon et al.'s

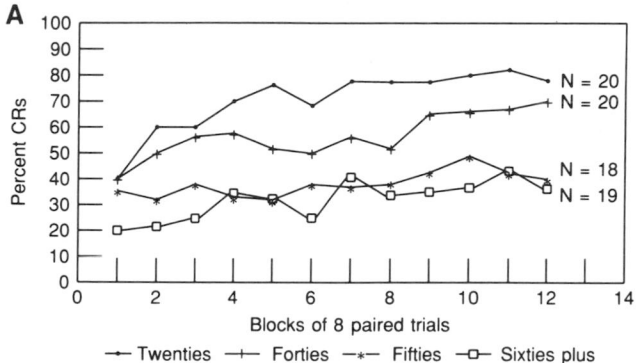

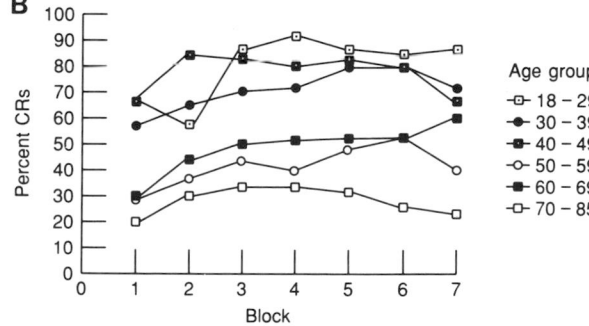

FIGURE 1.3 Mean percentage of conditioned eyeblink responses (CR) over blocks of trials for adults of varying ages. (A: Reprinted from Woodruff-Pak & Thompson, 1988, Figure 1; copyright 1988 by the American Psychological Association; B: Reprinted from Solomon, Pomerleau, Bennett, James, & Morse, 1989, Figure 2. Copyright 1989 by the American Psychological Association.)

(1989) study were in the age ranges of 18 to 29 yr, 30 to 39 yr, 40 to 49 yr, 50 to 59 yr, 60 to 69 yr, and 70 to 85 yr. The task itself was very comparable to that of Woodruff-Pak and Thompson. The percentage of CRs for each of 7 blocks of 9 trials per block are shown in part B of Figure 1.3. Note again that an age-related deficit in acquisition rate was not apparent until subjects were in their 50s, in striking agreement with the results obtained by Woodruff-Pak and Thompson (1988). Note further for both studies the negatively accelerated learning curves (i.e., large increments in scores early in practice, followed by progressively slower increments) for younger adults and the nearly flat learning curves for older adults.

In combination, these two studies ruled out a number of nonassociative factors as being responsible for the slower conditioning rates manifested by subjects over age 50. The most important of these factors is the longer latency of a conditioned eyeblink to occur for elderly adults than for young adults. In Woodruff-Pak and Thompson's (1988) study there were only 400 ms separating the onset of the CS and the onset of the UCS. This may be too little time for a conditioned eyeblink to be elicited for elderly subjects, but sufficient time for young subjects. However, a longer latency of the CR to the UCS by older subjects (and the resulting masking of the CR by the UCR) does not fully account for the pronounced slower rate of acquisition by older subjects. In both Woodruff-Pak and Thompson's (1988) study and Solomon et al.'s (1989) study, the percentage of CRs to the CS for each age group on probe trials in which the CS occurred alone (i.e., no UCS followed) was nearly identical to the percentage manifested on CS-UCS trials. For these probe trials, there was no opportunity for the CR to be masked by the UCR. On the other hand, it does appear that the magnitude of the age difference in rate of eyeblink conditioning is somewhat exaggerated by the use of a brief ISI (e.g., 400 ms). This possibility was suggested in a study by Solomon, Blanchard, Levine, Velazquez and Groccia-Ellison (1991) in which only young and elderly subjects were compared in eyeblink conditioning rates with the delay procedure. They employed ISIs of 400 ms, 650 ms, and 900 ms. The rate of acquisition for their young subjects to attain a criterion of 8 CRs in any block of 9 trials was largely unaffected by the variation in the ISI. By contrast, the rate of acquisition for their elderly subjects was much faster with the longer ISIs. Consequently, the age-related deficit in rate was greatly diminished with longer ISIs, but, nevertheless, remained rather pronounced.

Other negligible nonassociative factors appear to be an age difference in blink rate, an age difference in sensitivity to the airpuff, and an age difference in habituation of the UCR. Habituation refers to a decline in the amplitude of the UCR with repeated presentations of the UCS. Kimble and Pennypacker (1963) had earlier reported greater habituation for their elderly subjects than for their young subjects, an age difference that could contribute to the slower acquisition of the CR by elderly subjects. However, Solomon et al. (1989) found no age difference in habituation during the conditioning trials. The amplitude of the

UCR did decline with repeated presentations over trials of the UCS, but no more for their elderly subjects than for their young subjects.

Nor is the slower rate of conditioning by elderly subjects restricted to the delay conditioning procedure. Finkbinder and Woodruff-Pak (1991) found age differences in conditioning with the trace conditioning procedure to be much like those found with the delay procedure. In the trace procedure there is a blank interval that separates the offset of the CS and the onset of the UCS. In their study that interval was 1800 ms. Their subjects were adults ranging in age from 17 to 81 yr. As in studies with the delay procedure, there was little difference in conditioning rates between young adults and middle-aged adults, and a much slower rate with elderly adults than with younger adults.

What then is responsible for the conditioning/learning deficit experienced by individuals beyond age 50? To attempt an answer to this question, we must first ask what subjects are learning during the course of classical conditioning. To associationists, classical conditioning is simply another form of learning in which an S-R association is acquired through contiguous occurrences of the association's S and R elements. This account of classical conditioning has met considerable opposition over the years for reasons that are beyond the scope of our review (see Anderson and Borkowski, 1978, for an excellent analysis of theoretical issues involving classical conditioning). Contemporary theorists have stressed, instead, the cognitive nature of classical conditioning. According to one view (e.g., Logan, 1977), subjects being conditioned learn an association between two stimulus elements (i.e., the CS and the UCS) rather than an association between stimulus and response elements.

According to another view (e.g., Rescorla, 1972), one that is highly consonant with information processing psychology, subjects being conditioned simply learn the informational value of the CS, namely the fact that its onset reliably predicts the forthcoming occurrence of the UCS. The CS then serves to prepare the subject for the arrival of the UCS. For example, blinking to the CS protects the eye from the seemingly inevitable puff of air (UCS).

The age-related deficit in conditioning rate is difficult to explain from any of these theoretical perspectives. The to-be-learned response element is not rehearsed in the traditional sense of rote rehearsal. Consequently, less rehearsal per trial by elderly subjects than by young subjects, the standard associative explanation of a learning deficit, does not apply. Moreover, to hypothesize that healthy, cognitively alert elderly people (Solomon et al., 1989, for example, administered cognitive tests to their elderly subjects to assure that no one suspected of dementia was included in their study) are less capable than younger adults of learning the informational value of the CS and the nature of the CS-UCS contingency seems far-fetched. Nevertheless, this hypothesis has been, in fact, defended by some psychologists (e.g., Birren, 1964), and there is actually recent support for it. Durkin et al. (in preparation) found pronounced age-related deficits in both eyeblink conditioning and heart rate conditioning (with the deficits appearing in each case earlier than the 50s). However, only eyeblink conditioning scores correlated significantly with scores on several cognitively demanding verbal memory tasks. The implication is that eyeblink conditioning involves conscious awareness of the CS-UCS contingency, and it is therefore affected adversely by the reduced cognitive resources of many older adults. By contrast, heart rate conditioning occurs without awareness, and it is therefore unaffected by reductions in cognitive resources with normal aging. (see Dawson & Schell, 1987, for a discussion of the role played by awareness in classical conditioning.)

A remaining explanation is a biological one. Animal research has clearly revealed that the cerebellum plays a critical role in the conditioning of the eyeblink response (e.g., Thompson, 1986). Woodruff-Pak and Sheffield (1987) demonstrated that the correlation between the age of rabbits and the number of Purkinje cells in the cerebellum is strikingly high ($r = -.77$). Other investigators have demonstrated that there is a major loss of these cells in the human cerebellum with normal aging (e.g., Hall, Miller, & Corsellis, 1975). It is difficult not to accept Woodruff-Pak and Thompson's conclusion that "age differences in conditionability are likely to be a consequence of the documented loss of Purkinje cells and other changes in the cerebellum" (1988, p. 228).

Operant Conditioning

The use of positive reinforcement to increase the rate of responding of some desired response has been employed either with elderly subjects from some special population or with rats as subjects. There have been studies indicating that elderly psychotic patients (e.g., Ayllon & Azrin, 1965), patients diagnosed as having senile dementia (e.g., Ankus & Quarrington, 1972; D. J. Mueller & Atlas, 1972), and nursing home residents (e.g., Baltes & Zerbe, 1976) are amenable to behavior modification through the use of positive reinforcements. The responses modified in rate are usually those relevant to the caretaking needs of the patients. There have been a scattering of studies contrasting young and old rats in the effects of positive reinforcement on the rate of bar pressing (see Jakubczak, 1973, for a general review of these studies). Unfortunately, these studies have yielded highly conflicting results. For example, Goodrick found greater responding for young rats than old rats in one study (1965), greater responding for old rats than for young rats in a second study (1969), and no age difference in a third study (1970).

When operant methodology has been applied with normally aging individuals, it has usually been in the context of enhancing speed of responding by elderly subjects. One such study is by Grant, Storandt, and Botwinick (1978). Their young adult and elderly subjects received 20 trials on the Digit-Symbol subtest of the Wechsler Adult Intelligence Scale (WAIS; Wechsler, 1958) either with or without reinforcement following each trial. The offering of money for each digit substitution on later trials that exceeded the number of substitutions on the first trial may be viewed as positive reinforcement, and the taking away of money when the number of substitutions fell below the number on the first trial may be viewed as punishment. The reinforced subjects received both the positive rein-forcement and the punishment, and the nonreinforced subjects received neither. As may be seen in Figure 1.4, the combined reinforcement resulted in faster performance over trials (as measured by the increase in number of substitutions per trial) for both the young and the elderly subjects, but especially for the elderly subjects, relative to nonreinforcement. A similar outcome was reported by F. W. Hoyer, Hoyer, Treat, and Baltes (1978) for performance on a letter-cancellation task when S & H green stamps served as the source of positive reinforcement. In several later studies, Perone and Baron (1982, 1983a, 1983b) found a comparable benefit from combined reinforcement and punishment on response speed when elderly subjects had to acquire a complex sequence of responses. Money was given whenever a response in the sequence was executed within some designated time limit and a mild punishment (turning off the apparatus) whenever a response omission occurred. Reinforcement contingent on the speed of responding was also found by Baron, Menich, and Perone (1983) and Baron and Menich (1985)

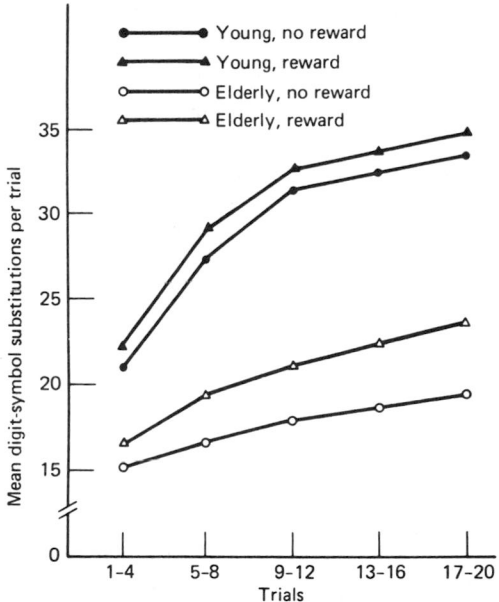

FIGURE 1.4 Mean number of digit-symbol substitutions completed per trial for groups of young and elderly subjects receiving either no monetary reward or a monetary reward. (Adapted from Grant, Storandt, & Botwinick, 1978, Table 1.)

to increase response speed on a matching-to-sample task (subjects are first given a stimulus, in this case a symbol, followed by a pair of stimuli, and they are asked to identify which member of the pair matches the prior stimulus), and by Menich and Baron (1990) with a memory scanning task (see Chapter 5, pp. 168–172) for elaboration).

The most intriguing use of positive reinforcement has been in the attempt to increase the frequencies of elderly adults' alpha brain waves by means of biofeedback as the source of reinforcement (Woodruff, 1975; Woodruff, 1982; Woodruff & Birren, 1972; Woodruff & Kramer, 1979) (see Woodruff-Pak, 1988, for further review). With normal aging, there is a slowing of alpha waves, a slowing that has been argued by Surwillo (1963, 1968) to lead to the slower reaction times of elderly adults, relative to younger adults, on many tasks (a principle known as gating theory). If this is the case, then training elderly adults to increase the frequency of their alpha waves could conceivably increase their response speed on many tasks. The training procedure consists of first establishing the baseline alpha wave frequency for a subject, and then following each increase in that frequency with feedback in the form of a sensory stimulus (e.g., a tone) as the reinforcement. Some elderly adults have been found to modify their frequency through this training procedure to the point where it is equal to that of young adults, and some of them may show faster reaction times as a result. However, even after such training their reaction times remain much slower than those of young adults.

Another variation of operant training, with a more complicated kind of reinforcement, should be of great interest to gerontological psychologists, but, apparently, it has not been. It is avoidance learning. In active-avoidance learning, a response is emitted that enables the organism to avoid receipt of a noxious stimulus. Learning to move cautiously around a loose step to avoid a painful fall is an example of such learning. Buying fire or automobile insurance to avoid the painful experience produced by loss or damage of property is another example. The processes of active-avoidance learning are complex and not fully comprehended. One popular conceptualization, but one with many opponents as well, is that of two-factor theory (see Bolles, 1979, for elaboration). The theory views the learning as progressing through two stages. The nature of this progression is illustrated in Figure 1.5 with respect to the loose step situation. In the first stage, fear is learned by means of classical conditioning. Falling on the step is the UCS for producing pain as the UCR. Because falling is preceded by the sight of the step itself, such sight meets the criterion for serving as a CS, one that becomes associated with conditioned pain, or fear, as the CR. In the second stage, the response of circumventing the loose step (the avoidance behavior) is positively reinforced. The positive reinforcement results from the alleviation of the fear elicited by the sight of the step (out of sight, out of fear). An obvious reason for having a gerontological interest in avoidance learning is the presumed involvement, at

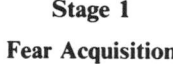

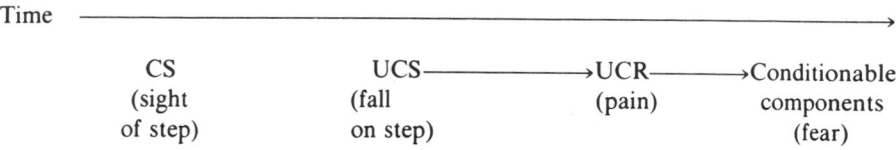

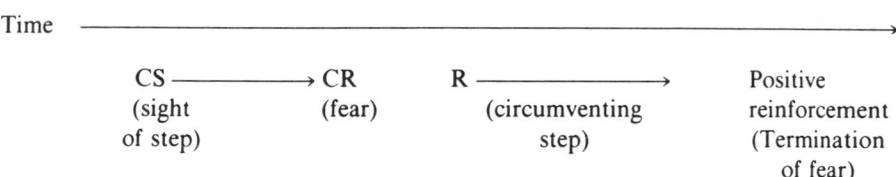

FIGURE 1.5   Schematic representation of the two-factor theory of avoidance learning as applied to learning to avoid a loose step.

least according to the two-factor theory, of age-sensitive classical conditioning in the total learning activity. If elderly adults are slower in fear acquisition, then they should also be slower in overall avoidance learning. The fact that elderly adults may differ from young adults in pain threshold adds further to our conjecture about possible age differences in avoidance learning as well as all other pain-derived fear acquisition.

What is actually known about age differences in active avoidance learning is, unfortunately, based solely on animal research (see Woodruff-Pak, 1990, for further review). Most of these animal aging studies were conducted by Doty (1966a, 1966b; Doty & Doty, 1964; Doty & Johnston, 1966). In general, they indicate poorer avoidance learning by old rats than by young rats. However, the extent of the age-related deficit seems to depend on the complexity of the avoidance task—the greater the complexity, the greater the age-related deficit. Interestingly, Doty and Johnston (1966) also found that the avoidance-learning proficiency of old rats is greatly improved by the administration of certain drugs (e.g., eserine) that may affect fear acquisition. The effect of age on the acquisition of a passive-avoidance response (i.e., inhibiting a response in order to avoid an aversive stimulus—for example, learning *not* to enter a box where an electric shock is given) is less certain. Gold, McGaugh, Hankins, Rose, and Vasquez (1982) found little in the way of an age difference in acquisition by their young and old rats. However, they did find that long-term retention of the passive avoidance response was far greater in young than in old rats. Generalization from the rat to the human avoidance learner is certainly tenuous. But there really is not much choice. Conducting avoidance learning research with elderly human subjects may certainly be questioned on ethical grounds. Perhaps generalization from animal to human subjects is not as risky as it may appear to be. There are areas of research in which considerable commonality has been found between studies with animal subjects and studies with human subjects. For example, the substantial age deficit in spatial memory found for rats (Wallace, Krauter, & Campbell, 1980) closely parallels the age deficit found for human subjects (see Chapter 9, pp. 315–321), and the slight age deficit found for rats (Wallace et al., 1980) on a task involving short-term memory parallels that found for human subjects on somewhat comparable tasks (see Chapter 5, pp. 151–157).

Adult Age Differences in Instrumental Learning

The traditional apparatus for studying instrumental learning is the familiar multiple-choice-point maze. The learner's task is to learn the correct path leading from a starting point to some goal at the end of the maze. (The learner's behavior is instrumental for reaching the goal, thus the name for this kind of task.) For example, there might be five left-right choice-points, with the correct path being left-left-right-left-right-goal. Instrumental learning is seemingly more complex than classical conditioning, but the distinction between instrumental learning and operant conditioning is often a matter of choice of terminology. For example, maze learning involves the acquisition of "an arrangement of responses" (Anderson & Borkowski, 1978, p. 337), whereas operant conditioning may involve the acquisition of a "chain" of responses (as in the studies by Perone and Baron, 1982, 1983a, 1983b, cited earlier). At any rate, the maze-learning task was employed in psychological research long before operant methodology was introduced, and it has served for many years to be the standard one for investigating instrumental learning. With human subjects, the maze is usually a paper one for which subjects see only one choice-point at a time, and they respond verbally by saying left or right at each choice-point. With animal subjects, the maze is a spatial one through which the subjects move their entire bodies.

Maze Learning

There has been little research on maze learning by noncollege-aged subjects, especially research in which normally aging elderly subjects have been contrasted with young adults. An early study by Husband (1930) compared undergraduate students as subjects with older subjects. Although the older subjects averaged only 36.7 yr of age, they were, nevertheless, poorer maze learners than the undergraduates. Their inferior performance, however, was relatively slight with respect to the number of trials needed to learn the maze (about 25% more trials) but quite large with respect to total time taken in learning the maze (about 80% more time). A later study by von Wright (1957) contrasted young adults with somewhat older adults (median age = 50 yr). Older subjects were again less proficient than young adults, with the deficit in trials-to-learn being more pronounced than in Husband's study (nearly 50% more trials). There have been studies in which older adults have been included as age-matched control subjects for comparison with either Korsakoff's Disease subjects (e.g., Brooks & Baddeley, 1976; Cermak, Lewis, Butters, & Goodglass, 1973) or Senile Dementia of the Alzheimer's Type (SDAT) subjects (Martin, 1987). Unfortunately, these studies rarely include both young adult and normally aging subjects. In the study by Brooks and Baddeley (1976), however, there were small groups of late adolescent control subjects and middle-aged subjects, both of which received 10 trials on the Porteus Maze Test (Porteus, 1959), a paper-and-pencil maze in which subjects trace their way through a Hampton Court-like labyrinth of passageways. The middle-aged subjects were characterized by many more errors in learning the maze than were the younger subjects.

By contrast, aging research on maze learning by rats and mice has been quite popular for many years, beginning with pioneering studies by Hubbert (1915) and Stone (1929). These earlier studies (see Jerome, 1959, for a detailed review) revealed little difference in maze-learning proficiency between young-mature and old rats. More recent studies (e.g., Goodrick, 1968, 1972; see Arenberg and Robertson-Tchabo, 1977, and Woodruff-Pak, 1990, for detailed reviews), however, have indicated that old rats are slower maze learners than young rats, but only when the task itself is a complex one. Complexity of a maze is defined in terms of the number of choice-points intervening between the start and goal components. With only one choice-point, age differences are negligible or nonexistent. This seems to be true for maze learning for young and old mice as well (Spangler & Ingram, 1986). With 4 choice-points, age differences are modest, and, with 14 choice-points, they become pronounced. Such age deficits with complex mazes are also apparent for mice (J. M. Warren, 1986). Interestingly, these studies indicate further that the age deficit largely disappears, even with a highly complex maze, when the old learner is guided through the maze. Guidance simply means that cul-de-sacs (blind alleys) are closed off during study trials, thus avoiding errors (i.e., wrong turns) while practicing the maze. The cul-de-sacs are open, of course, during the test trials to permit comparisons in learning scores (e.g., number of errors) among age groups. Even more interesting is the finding with both rats (Goodrick, 1984) and mice (Ingram, Weindruch, Spangler, Freeman, & Walford, 1987) of a greatly reduced age-related deficit in learning even complex mazes when the old subjects had been raised on a restricted diet. It is again risky to generalize to human beings, but it is tempting to speculate about the implications of this evidence for our generally overweight population.

Explanation of Age Differences in Maze Learning

Explanation of age differences in maze learning, whether for human or animal subjects, like explanation of age differences for any kind of learning, depends on one's broader perspective regarding what is being learned and how it is being learned during practice on the task at hand. To associationists (e.g., Hull, 1943), what is acquired during practice on a maze is a chain of S-R associations. Each link of the chain involves one of the choice-points. The R element of a given link is the correct turning response at that choice-point (i.e., either left or right), and the S element is some unspecified distinctive cue present at the choice-point. Age deficits in human maze learning may then be accounted for in terms of a rehearsal-deficit principle. Rehearsal in this case refers to the verbal representation of a correct turning response. Thus, if that turn is left, the subject is assumed to say left over and over—but to a smaller degree by older subjects.

For many years, cognitively oriented learning theorists have rebelled against this response-centered explanation of maze learning. The pioneer in this rebellion was Tolman (1932). Tolman argued that even rats (and certainly human beings) learn environmental information during their exposure to a maze. In effect, the learner acquires a cognitive map, a map that relates representations of stimuli in the maze to one another. Thus, a perception-centered explanation replaces the response-centered explanation of associationists. Turning responses at choice-points remain important in this cognitive explanation, but only for performance on the maze. Explanation of age deficits from this cognitive perspective follows an interesting course. Elderly learners may be assumed to be distracted by irrelevant stimuli in the maze environment, at least to a greater extent than young learners, thereby delaying their acquisition of truly relevant environmental information. This explanation is consonant with what we will discover later about age differences on a memory task that does involve discrimination between relevant and irrelevant information (see Chapter 6, pp. 220–221). We now need to argue that elderly rats or mice, like elderly human beings, are especially susceptible to distraction by irrelevant stimuli. Interestingly, we discovered earlier that the age-related deficit in animal maze learning disappears when subjects are guided through the maze. Such guidance should prohibit attention directed at irrelevant stimuli present in cul-de-sacs. Of course, guidance also prohibits making erroneous turning responses, and its effects on age differences in learning could, therefore, be explained associatively.

Maze learning is sufficiently complex that it is likely to be affected by the limited capacity of one's cognitive resources, a capacity that seemingly declines from early to late adulthood. There is, in fact, evidence from an intriguing study by Crossley and Hiscock (1992) to indicate that this is the case. Their young adult, middle-aged, and elderly subjects performed on what they termed easy and difficult mazes. Easy mazes simply required subjects to follow a red line that traced the pathway through a maze, while difficult mazes required them to navigate through them without aid. Most important, both easy and difficult mazes were performed under a dual-task condition in which the other task was finger tapping. The finger tapping task was also performed alone. This procedure enabled the investigators to determine the mean percentage decrement in tapping rate under the dual-task condition relative to tapping rate when performed alone. For their young subjects, that decrement was about 6% while performing on the easy mazes and about 10% while performing on the difficult mazes. For their elderly subjects, the comparable decrements were about 18% and 27%. The disportionate effect of the more difficult mazes for the elderly subjects presumably reflects the diminished cognitive resources they have for maze learning relative to young subjects.

Spatial Learning and Spatial Cognition

Knowing how people learn to navigate about a strange environment is undoubtedly an important objective of learning theory and research. The importance was stated nicely by G. L. Allen, Siegel, and Rosinski:

> An important issue in the study of spatial cognition concerns the representation of spatial information in memory. Of particular interest is the representation of information from a geographic area that cannot be perceived simultaneously. A traveler in a large-scale environment, such as a city, typically cannot see his destination from his starting point. Thus, he must rely on his ability to interpret perceptual information accompanying his own movement in order to reach his destination successfully. Occlusion, parallax, expansion, and other perceptual cues indicating motion, orientation, and velocity form the visual context of the traveler's movement, and it is this context that is structured as spatial knowledge. Recognizing the contextual features (i.e., the unique perceptual characteristics) of a spatial event is the difference between finding one's way and getting lost (1978, p. 617).

They were talking about a cognitive map that represents a novel environment, such as a strange city, a new apartment in an already-familiar neighborhood, and, perhaps, most important, a new institutional residence. The ability to acquire representations of these kinds of environments is essential for unrestrained mobility, which, in turn, is essential for the overall adaptability of the organism. Mastery of a novel environment's spatial features is here considered to be a learning phenomenon, somewhat related to the acquisition of a cognitive map of a complex maze. Many trials through the novel environment are likely to be needed before full mastery occurs. Spatial cognition of this kind is to be distinguished from spatial memory of the kind that will be discussed in Chapter 9. Spatial memory refers to memory for the locations of objects or events, such as memory for where in your friends' new apartment they placed the vase you gave them as a wedding gift, usually after a single exposure to the location.

An awareness of the problems elderly people face in acquiring cognitive maps of their own physical environments is needed to be in the position to enhance their adaptability and to reduce the stress produced by getting lost. Planning environments that aid spatial cognition and accelerate the rate of acquiring cognitive maps of their environments is a likely consequence of this awareness. The fact that problems do exist in the spatial learning of elderly people is dramatically illustrated in a study by Weber, Brown, and Weldon (1978). Their primary subjects were residents, ranging in age from 72 to 93 yr, of a nursing home, all of whom were ambulatory, had adequate vision, and were cognitively alert, as indicated by their highly effective communicative skills. Cognitive maps of their residential environment were evaluated by an intriguing procedure that was used originally to assess recognizability of locations in a city (Milgram, Greenwald, Kessler, McKenna, & Walters, 1972). The procedure consisted of showing slides from various areas of both the interior and the exterior of the nursing home. For each slide, a subject attempted to identify on a map of the total area where the depicted scene was located. The results, expressed in percentages of correct identifications, are shown in Table 1.1 for four different residential halls and several other areas. Note that the halls were especially poorly identified correctly and that even presumably distinctive areas, such as the dining room and the nursing station, were identified correctly by relatively small percentages of the residents. Weber et al. (1978) also found that accuracy in identification correlated nega-

TABLE 1.1

Accuracy of Identifying Scenes in a Nursing Home for Elderly Residents of That Home and Undergraduates Who Had Visited the Home[a]

| | Mean of correct identification (%) | |
Area	Elderly residents	Students
Hall 1	12.7	47.5
Hall 2	5.0	27.8
Hall 3	3.9	19.8
Hall 4	13.2	33.3
Dining room/living room	60.5	80.8
Nursing station/front lobby	51.7	85.2
Exterior	32.5	48.2

[a] Adapted from Weber, Brown, & Weldon, 1978, table 2. (Copyright 1978 by Beech Hill Enterprises, Inc. Used by permission of the publisher and the author.)

tively (and statistically significantly) with age (in general, the older the resident, the poorer the accuracy), but, surprisingly, they failed to find a significant correlation between accuracy and duration of residence in the home (a positive correlation was expected). These results were replicated by Herman and Bruce (1981), who also found that accuracy was no greater for ambulatory residents than for residents confined to a wheelchair.

For comparisons sake, Weber et al. (1978) included a small group of undergraduates as part of their study. As a course assignment, they toured the home, spending about 40 min spread equally over all of the areas. After the tour, they were tested unexpectedly in the same manner as the residents. Their strikingly superior identification scores are also given in Table 1.1. There is one obvious conclusion from these results—the design of a nursing home, in general, fails to provide distinctive and attractive stimuli that prod interest among the residents in exploring their environment and becoming comfortably familiar with that environment. Hopefully, designers of such homes will be more cognizant of these problems in the future.

Contemporary psychologists have introduced new and highly innovative procedures for studying the acquisition of spatial cognitive maps, procedures that appear to have considerably greater ecological validity than the older maze-learning procedure (see Anderson, 1980, for a detailed review of these procedures, and Kirasic, 1989, for further review of aging research). For example, G. L. Allen et al. (1978) had their young adult subjects take a walk through a novel environment. The walk was simulated by means of a series of slides showing various scenes and locations in a community. The subjects were then tested for their ability to recognize not only previously exposed scenes but also other scenes that were not actually seen but could be inferred to be in the environment covered by the walk.

This procedure, or some variation of it, has been applied in several studies with normally aging adults (Kirasic, Allen, & Haggerty, 1992; Kirasic & Bernicki, 1990; Lipman, 1991; Lipman & Caplan, 1992); Ohta, 1981; S. L. Simon, Walsh, Regnier, & Krauss, 1992). Moreover, M. E. Hunt and Roll (1987) found that a simple way of simulating familiarization with a novel building by means of drawings and pictures of key locations in the building was as effective in acquiring knowledge of the building by elderly subjects as was an actual tour of the building.

Not surprisingly, elderly adults have been demonstrated to acquire considerably less knowledge about a novel environment with such simulations than do younger adults (see Hartley, Harker, and Walsh, 1980; Kirasic and Allen, 1985; and Ohta, 1981, for further discussion). Especially important are the studies by Lipman (Lipman, 1991; Lipman & Caplan, 1992). Her results indicate that two types of information are acquired during a simulated trip through a novel neighborhood. The first consists of knowledge about landmarks in the neighborhood and the second of route knowledge (e.g., turns along the route). The two types

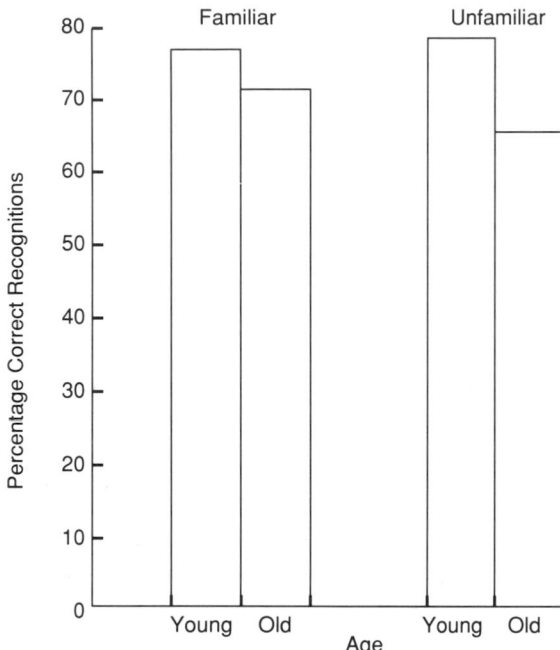

FIGURE 1.6 Percentages of correct recognitions of pictures of familiar and unfamiliar supermarkets. (Adapted from data in Kirasic, 1991).

appear to be differentially age sensitive, with landmark acquisition being less impaired in late adulthood than route acquisition. Proficiency in acquiring information about a novel environment has been found by S. L. Simon et al. (1992) to be related positively to the use elderly adults make of their own neighborhood (e.g., the number of services used within the neighborhood). In fact, the scores earned by their elderly subjects on a simulated trip proved to be a better predictor of neighborhood use than either the number of years they lived in the neighborhood or their mobility.

Elderly adults have also been found to learn less about a novel supermarket and other novel buildings than do younger adults following exploratory trips through the buildings (Kirasic, 1981, as cited in Kirasic & Allen, 1985; Kirasic, 1991). For example, Kirasic (1991) gave her young adult and elderly subjects a shopping list for purchases to be made in both a familiar supermarket and an unfamiliar supermarket. The subjects were then given a recognition memory test consisting of 25 pictures from the store actually visited and 25 pictures from a different store (i.e., foils or distractors). The percentage of correct recognitions are given in Figure 1.6. The main effect for age was statistically significant. Although the age-related deficit was somewhat greater for the unfamiliar market than for the familiar market, the Age × Familiarity interaction did not attain statistical significance.

Retention tests of the area in which subjects live have also been given in several studies (Evans, Brennan, Skorpanich, & Held, 1984; Walsh, Krauss, & Regnier, 1981). Especially informative is the study by Evans et al. (1984). Their young and elderly adult subjects were asked to recall as many buildings as possible in a familiar downtown area and to locate familiar buildings on a grid map. Here too elderly adults were far less knowledgeable than young adults in both building recall and building location. Both the ability to acquire novel spatial information and the ability to retain long-standing spatial information appear to be highly age-sensitive processes.

CHAPTER 2

Skill Learning and Procedural Learning

Adult Age Differences in Motor-Skill Learning

Motor-skill learning refers to any learning in which an individual must acquire one or more precise motor responses (i.e., bodily movements of some kind). Usually these responses must be closely coordinated with the perception of a sequence of stimuli (for this reason, this kind of learning is often referred to as perceptual-motor learning). As stimuli change, the sequence of responses must change accordingly. In some instances, there is little, if any, stimulus change involved, and the underlying motor-skill learning is relatively easy. This is the case in learning to operate a lock or the ignition of a car. In other cases, there is a great deal of stimulus change involved, and motor-skill learning increases greatly in complexity as a result. Consider as an example the complexity involved in learning to hit a fastball or a curveball thrown by a major league pitcher. Here tracking the trajectory of the ball must be coordinated with a number of bodily movements. Programming a computer to accomplish this hitting task is at least as complicated as programming a computer to play chess (Fitts, 1964).

The importance of motor-skill learning to human adaptability is indicated in the following remarks by Fitts: "Living, moving, and behavior are almost synonymous terms. Thus the study of motor and perceptual-motor skill learning is in a very real sense the study of a large segment of the field of psychology" (1964, p. 243).

Attesting to the importance of motor-skill learning is the virtually endless list of everyday activities that are the products of our motor-skill learning; brushing our teeth in the way dentists recommend, tying our shoes, driving a car, starting a power mower, typing a letter, playing the piano, and so on. These are motor skills that once acquired in childhood or early adulthood become highly overlearned and largely automatized. As a result, they are usually maintained throughout the adult life span (although the speed of performance may slow down for some behaviors in late adulthood), unless, of course, they are decimated by a

crippling illness or accident. Witness the many great performances by Pablo Ca-
sals and Arthur Rubenstein at very advanced ages. Claudio Arrau, the great
Chilean pianist, celebrated his 75th birthday with a recital in which he played
faultlessly the technically strenuous Sonata No. 3 in F Minor by Brahms. While
he was in his 60s, Ted Williams could probably have hit a major league fastball at
least as well as most current major league players. In his 40s (and even somewhat
in his 50s), Jack Nicklaus displayed the same great stroke he had years earlier as
a young professional golfer—still great enough to continue to win major golf
championships.

We do not have to turn to aging virtuosos or Hall of Famers to demonstrate
the overall stability of many motor skills during middle and late adulthood. Analysis of industrial accidents (Dillingham, 1981; McFarland & O'Doherty, 1959;
Root, 1981; see Sterns, Barrett, & Alexander, 1985, for a detailed review) reveals
an interesting pattern. The frequency of workplace accidents, in contrast to automobile accidents, decreases with increasing age. For example, Birren (1964)
reported that pilots between age 40 and age 60 have, if anything, fewer accidents
than younger pilots. The absence of an age effect, at least through age 60, cannot
be attributed solely to the greater experience of the older pilot. Even when years
of experience is held constant for all ages, there is a slight decline in accident
rate (again, through age 60). There is further evidence to indicate that older
pilots (from 30 to 50 yr of age) retain their routine flying skills (e.g., rudder
control) fairly well, relative to pilots in their 20s, although the communication
skills of older pilots do show some age-related decline (Morrow, Leirer, & Yesavage, 1990; Morrow, Yesavage, Leirer, & Tinklenberg, 1993). Communication
skills are more likely to be affected adversely by age-related declines in working-
memory capacity than are routine flying skills. However, the severity of injury is
greatest for older workers. Accidents occurring to older workers are often attributable to slower responses. This may be seen in an analysis of agricultural accidents (King, 1955). Accidents that result from being hit by a falling or moving
object (i.e., accidents produced often by failure to respond fast enough) increase
slowly but progressively from early to late adulthood. On the other hand, agricultural accidents that are seemingly unaffected by speed, such as being injured by a
frequently used tool, decrease slowly but progressively with increasing age.

Our main concern, however, is with adult age differences in new motor-skill
learning. As with other kinds of learning, there are no age limits regarding the
necessity of, or the desire for, participating in new motor-skill learning. Adults of
all ages may have to learn to master a wheelchair, to drive a stick-shift car after
years of driving with automatic transmission, to eat with chopsticks, to play golf,
to operate a complicated piece of machinery, and so on. What happens to proficiency in skill learning over the adult life span is obviously a question of great
practical importance. Before we review studies on age differences in motor-skill
learning there is a preliminary topic that requires our consideration, namely adult

age differences in several basic characteristics or attributes of motor behaviors. Age differences in these attributes are likely to be important determiners of age-related deficits in the acquisition of new motor behaviors.

Attributes of Motor Behaviors

Perhaps the most frequently replicated finding in the experimental psychology of aging is the slower responding to stimuli by older adults than by younger adults (see Salthouse, 1985a; Spirduso and MacRae, 1990; and Welford, 1977, 1984a, 1987, for further reviews). The range of motor responses and stimuli that has been investigated has been immense, ranging from pressing a button on a simple-reaction-time task to dialing a telephone (see Mortimer, Pirozzolo, and Maletta, 1982, for an overview of the aging motor system). Numerous investigators have found simple reaction time to a single stimulus to correlate moderately and positively with age (e.g., Borkan & Norris, 1980; Botwinick, 1971; Robertson-Tchabo & Arenberg, 1976). For example, the correlation coefficient in Borkan and Norris's (1980) study was .29 for 687 individuals ranging in age from 17 to 102 years, and it was .41 in Robertson-Tchabo and Arenberg's (1976) study for 90 individuals ranging in age from 20 to 80 yr. That is, speed of responding (e.g., pressing a button) to the onset of a stimulus (e.g., a tone) decreases monotonically as age increases from early to late adulthood. The degree of correlation is as great or perhaps even greater with a choice-reaction-time task (e.g., Borkan & Norris, 1980; Botwinick, Brinley, & Robbin, 1959; Goldfarb, 1941; Robertson-Tchabo & Arenberg, 1976). On a choice-reaction-time task one response (e.g., pressing Button A) is made to Stimulus 1 (e.g., a tone of a given frequency), and a different response (e.g., pressing Button B) is made to Stimulus 2 (a tone of a different frequency). Elderly adults have also been found to be much slower than younger adults in such behaviors as movement of the hand toward a target (Hodgkins, 1962), movement of a lever from side to side (Singleton, 1955), tapping alternately between targets (Welford, Norris, & Shock, 1969), writing words and digits (Birren & Botwinick, 1951), sorting cards (Botwinick & Birren, 1965; Botwinick, Robbin, & Brinley, 1960; Crossman & Szafran, 1956), dialing a telephone (Potvin et al., 1973), performing on a serial reaction-time task (Leonard, 1953), adjusting a dial (Simon, 1960), naming objects in pictures (Thomas, Fozard, & Waugh, 1977) along with many other behaviors (see Welford, 1977, for a description of these other behaviors). For example, Birren and Botwinick (1951) had subjects in their 20s through their 80s write a series of words and found that the mean time increased by over 100% from the 20s through the 60s.

In general, elderly adults become disproportionately slower than young adults as the complexity of the responses to be performed increases (Griew, 1959; Jordan & Rabbitt, 1977; W. R. Miles, 1931a, 1931b: K. Light & Spirduso, 1990). Illustrative of this disportionately are the results obtained by W. R. Miles (1931a,

1931b) and K. E. Light and Spirduso (1990). Miles' subjects (1931a, 1931b) ranged in age from their 20s to their 60s. For simply releasing a key, the subjects in their 60s were about 9.5% slower than the subjects in their 20s. However, for the more complex response of pressing a key the subjects in their 60s were 22% slower. Light and Spirduso's (1990) subjects performed on a choice-reaction time in which subjects made different kinds of microswitch press movements to red and yellow lights. The age difference in reaction time increased as the complexity of the movements increased.

Normally aging individuals also appear to resemble brain-damaged older individuals in their speeded-response characteristics more closely than normal young adults resemble brain-damaged young adults (Goldstein & Shelly, 1975). Response speed, however, does increase for normally aging individuals with extended practice on reaction-time tasks, but so does the speed of younger adults (Noble, Baker, & Jones, 1964) (see also p. 48). The result is that age differences in response speed persist even after extensive practice.

The locus of the slowing of motor responses has been the subject of numerous investigations, especially with reaction-time tasks (e.g., Birren & Botwinick, 1955; Birren, Riegel, & Morrison, 1962; Botwinick, 1971; Botwinick & Thompson, 1966; Brinley, 1965; Gottsdanker, 1980a; Weiss, 1965; see Goggin & Stelmach, 1990, for further review). In general, the strategy has been to fractionate reaction time into a premotor and a motor component by means of electromyographic recordings of muscle-action potentials. The premotor time is the time between presentation of the stimulus and the activation of the forearm muscle for the arm making the response to the stimulus. The motor time is the time between this muscle activation and the actual movement of the hand in executing the response. The evidence has indicated that it is the longer premotor time of elderly adults, relative to younger adults, that contributes the major share to the slower response by elderly adults. Included in premotor time are central processes that program the response to be selected for performance (Welford, 1984b). As described by Clark, Lanphear, and Riddick:

> Response selection is a memory-dependent process in which the response appropriate or paired with a stimulus must be retrieved from memory (Kerr, 1978; Sternberg, 1969a; Theios, 1975). For example, in typing the letter *f*, the typist must retrieve from memory the response (depress the left index finger) appropriate to the identified stimulus, *f*. Response selection is seen as the translation stage between the stimulus identification stage of processing and the stage, response programming, where the actual commands to execute the response are processed (1987, p. 82).

The problem elderly adults have with response selection presumably accounts for the disportionate slowing they display on a choice-reaction-time task, relative to a simple reaction-time task and to young adult performers, in which on some trials the stimuli and responses are compatible (e.g., left light on, press the left button; right light on, press the right button) and on other trials they are incompatible (e.g., left light on, press the right button; right light on, press the left button) (e.g., Simon, 1967). Thus subjects have to select which response to execute on any given trial, namely one that is either compatible or incompatible with the presented stimulus. Clark et al. (1987) demonstrated that response selection by elderly adults could be facilitated by appropriate training. Their training program for an experimental group of elderly subjects consisted of playing a video game for 2 hr per week over 7 wk. They reasoned that practice on a video game would facilitate response selection because playing the game successfully requires speeded response selection. Their control group of subjects received no training on the video game. Mean adjusted (for pretraining group differences in reaction times) posttraining choice-reaction times are plotted in Figure 2.1. It may be seen that the training procedure was especially effective in facilitating reaction times under the condition of stimulus–response (S-R) incompatability. Experimental subjects were actually faster on incompatible trials than on compatible trials. By contrast, control subjects were considerably slower on incompatible trials than on compatible trials. They reasoned that video game playing altered the strategy used by their elderly subjects in speeded tasks in general, namely the strategy of transmitting S-R information into a short-term-memory buffer in preparation for performance. Of course, it seems likely that young adults may have similarly improved their response-selection process by a comparable training experience.

Preparation for an impending response may also be an age-sensitive process. (Salthouse, 1985a, however, has argued that the evidence is not very conclusive.) Here a warning signal precedes the onset of a stimulus, with the response to the

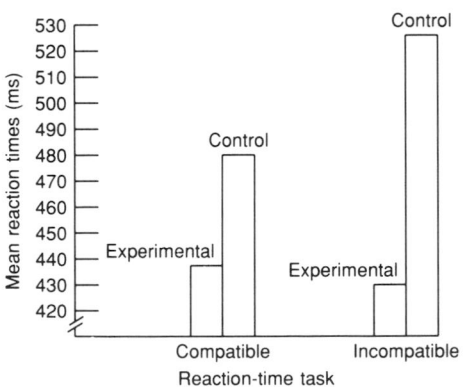

FIGURE 2.1 Mean posttraining reaction times for elderly trained (experimental) and not trained (control) subjects on a video game. (Adapted from Clark, Lanphear, & Riddick, 1987, Table 2.)

signal to be made as quickly as possible. Reaction times of elderly subjects tend to increase to a greater extent than those of younger subjects as the time separating the warning signal and the stimulus increases (e.g., Botwinick et al., 1959; Gottsdanker, 1980b; Loveless & Sanford, 1974). Apparently, elderly subjects are less capable than younger subjects of maintaining control of their preparation or "set" to respond (Gottsdanker, 1989b; Loveless & Sanford, 1974).

Another problem confronting elderly subjects is their diminished proficiency, relative to young subjects, in the use of advance information, or cues, as to what response to expect to select for execution (Rabbitt & Birren, 1967; Gottsdanker, 1980a; Waugh & Vyas, 1980). For example, a cue may signal, with a high probability of being correct, the next stimulus to appear in an incompatible-choice-reaction-time task. However, elderly adults are certainly capable of using advance information to facilitate their responding. The utilization by elderly subjects of precues for preparing response selection may be seen in the results obtained by Larish and Stelmach (1982) and Stelmach, Goggin, and Garcia-Colera (1987). For example, Stelmach et al. (1987) had their young adult, middle-aged, and elderly subjects perform simple-movement responses that varied over trials in terms of which arm to move, the direction of movement, and the extent of movement. Precues varied in the amount of information they conveyed. On some trials, no precues were given to signal the movement requested. On other trials, only one precue (e.g., which arm to move) was given; on still other trials, two precues were given (e.g., which arm and which direction to move); and on the remaining trials all three dimensions (arm, direction, and extent) were precued. As may be seen in Figure 2.2, the reaction-times-to-initiate-movements of subjects of all ages were markedly facilitated as the uncertainty of what movement to make decreased (0 uncertainty means all three precues were given; 3 uncertainty means the absence of precues). Also apparent is the disportionate slowing of movement for elderly subjects, relative to younger subjects, when no advance information was given. Stelmach, Goggin, and Amrhein (1988) discovered further that the movement responses of elderly subjects are disrupted more than the movement responses of young adult subjects when the precues are invalid and subjects have to restructure their motor program for, say, which arm to move or which direction to move.

Apparent adult age differences in four other attributes of motor responses should be noted. Stelmach, Amrhein, and Goggin (1988) discovered that elderly subjects have greater difficulty than young adults in coordinating bimanual movements, that is, movements of the two hands. On some trials, each hand was signaled to move the same distance; on other trials, they were signaled to move different distances. The second attribute is called coincidence–anticipation accuracy. Here subjects are required to make a response when a moving target stimulus (e.g., a light) reaches its destination. Haywood (1980) found that elderly subjects are less accurate in timing the arrival than are young adult subjects. The

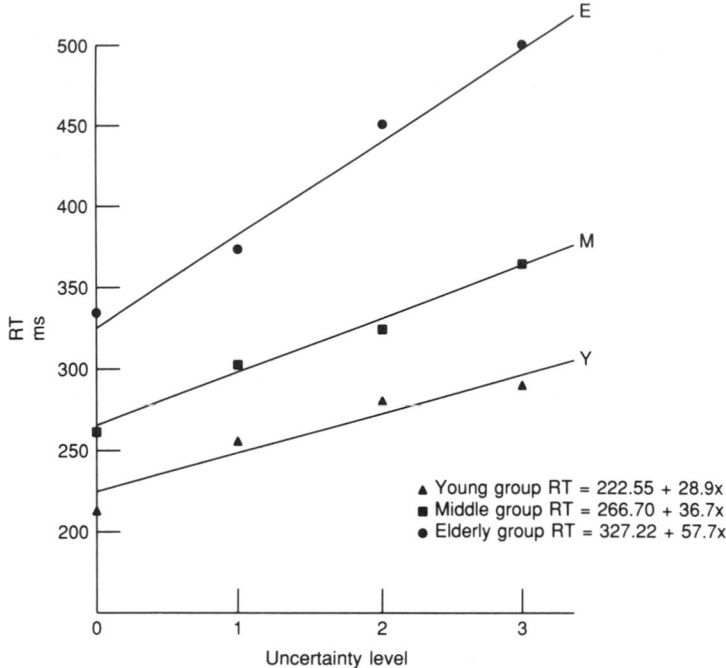

FIGURE 2.2 Reaction time (RT) plotted as a function of uncertainty. (Reproduced from Stelmach, Goggin, & Garcia-Colera, 1987, Figure 3; © Beech Hill Publishing Company.)

third attribute is preparing a new plan for a change in direction of a movement. When a change in direction other than the one originally planned is called for, elderly subjects were found to perform as if the original plan had never been prepared (Amrhein, Stelmach, & Goggin, 1991; Amrhein, Von Dras, & Anderson, 1993), a factor that is likely to contribute to the greater incidence of serious falls among elderly adults than among younger adults (Amrhein & Morris, 1989). The fourth attribute consists of mental blocks, apparently attributable to lapses in concentration, while performing a response repeatedly. These blocks result in exceptionally slow responses relative to responses without blocks. For male subjects only, Bunce, Warr, and Cochrane (1993) found a linear increase with age in the number of mental blocks occurring during continuous performance on a choice-reaction-time task. Moreover, the rate of the increase with age was much greater for men of low physical fitness than for men of high physical fitness.

Laboratory Studies: Real-World Motor-Learning Tasks

Research on adult age differences in motor-skill learning was off to a rousing start. Early studies employed a number of tasks carried over from the real world, including learning archery (Lashley, 1915), shooting a basketball (Noble, 1922), and learning to use chopsticks (Tachibana, 1927). Although these studies provided contrasts between young and older subjects, they also suffered from a number of methodological deficiencies (see Ruch, 1933, for a thorough analysis). In a number of them, the investigator was simply curious to see if learning continues beyond the teens and early 20s. Thus, Lashley's (1915) oldest archery subject was only 36 yr old, and Noble's (1922) oldest shooting subject only 32. This is not a problem in Tachibana's (1927) chopsticks study. But there is a different kind of problem. Only two subjects were employed—a 21-yr-old woman (who learned readily) and an 89-yr-old woman (who did not learn at all). The sample size was not much larger in Noble's (1922) basketball study—there were only three 20-yr-old and three 32-yr-old shooters. There is another, more insidious problem inherent in this type of study, namely, control over prior experience with the task at hand and other related tasks. The standard control, as applied by Lashley (1915) in the archery study, is to use only naive subjects, that is, subjects who report having had no formal contact with the particular task. However, an investigator cannot have complete faith in the reliability of a subject's self-reported past history. At any rate, Lashley (1915) found very little age decline in learning archery (again through age 36), and Noble (1922) found that his older subjects (again only age 32) learned basketball shooting more readily than his younger subjects.

Many of these methodological problems even enter into what gerontological psychologists generally consider to be the best of these early real-world studies, those of Thorndike, Bregman, Tilton, and Woodyard (1928). In one of their studies, young subjects, 20 to 25 yr, and older subjects, 35 to 57 yr, were given 15 hr of practice writing left-handed (all of the subjects, of course, were right-handed). There was little effect of age variation on the degree to which the quality of writing improved over the lengthy, and surely tortuous, practice sessions. However, a pronounced age difference was found in the degree to which speed of writing increased with practice. Not surprisingly, the young subjects increased their speed considerably more than did the older subjects. In another of their studies, Thorndike et al. (1928) had a group of five subjects, ranging in age from 23 to 38 yr, practice typewriting. Although the subjects made considerable progress, it is difficult to determine with so few subjects and such a limited range of age what effect, if any, age variation had on mastering the typing skill. More subjects were employed in a later typing study by Leonard and Newman (1965). After several hours of practice in typing their young and elderly subjects both improved their typing speeds considerably and by about the same amounts (with the young subjects typing faster than the elderly subjects throughout practice).

In contemporary research, the emphasis on real-world tasks has shifted from training typing skills to training word-processing skills or computer software skills (Charness, Schumann, & Boritz, in press; Czaja, Hammond, Blascovich, &

Swede, 1989; Egan & Gomez, 1985; Elias, Elias, Robbins, & Gage, 1987; Gist, Rosen, & Schwoerer, 1988; Hartley, Hartley, & Johnson, 1984; Krauss, Florini, & Bellos, 1985; Zandri & Charness, 1989). These studies have revealed that elderly adults can learn to use computers but that the rate of acquisition is indeed slower than it is for young adults, and the number of errors made while learning is greater for older than younger adults (Czaja & Sharit, 1993). As noted by Czaja and Sharit (1993), the difficulty older people have in acquiring computer skills has important implications for their placement in a work world that increasingly relies on the use of computers. Elias et al. (1987) discovered further that there is little difference in rate of acquisition of word-processing skills between middle-aged and young adult subjects.

Laboratory Studies: Controlled Motor-Learning Tasks

Assurance of age equality in prior experience and familiarity can best be accomplished by the use of artificial laboratory tasks, tasks that represent novel experiences for subjects of all ages. In using such tasks, investigators risk concerns about the degree of external validity and ecological validity inherent in their results. The hope, however, is that these tasks, like the laboratory tasks employed in other areas of learning, do gain access to the basic processes that enter into real-world activities. A number of them have been introduced over the years into basic research on motor-skill learning, and many of them eventually entered into experimental aging research on motor-skill learning. The pioneers in this component of the experimental psychology of aging were Snoddy (1926) and Ruch (1934), Snoddy with research on mirror-vision tracing of a figure and Ruch with research on the pursuit-rotor task. A number of excellent aging studies on motor-skill learning have appeared since 1934. Our review will examine only a few representative studies (for more comprehensive reviews of studies through the early 1970s see Welford, 1958, 1959, 1977). In our review we will be guided by the distinction made by researchers in motor-skill learning between tasks that involve *discrete responses* and tasks that involve *continuous responses* (Ellis, 1978).

Among the real-world tasks involving a discrete response are kicking a football and turning the ignition of a car. A laboratory task that approximates these kinds of activities must require a movement of some specified distance, amplitude, or direction. The classic variant is to have subjects draw a line having a specified length, such as 6 in. (Thorndike et al., 1928). Subjects practice on this line-drawing task either with or without knowledge of results. Knowledge of results consists of feedback concerning the amount of error present in a just-drawn line (i.e., information regarding how far off it is from the specified distance). As you might expect, accuracy improves steadily with knowledge of results but not without it. A modification of the line-drawing task has been used in aging studies by Szafran (1953, as reported in Welford, 1959) and Anshel (1978). In Szafran's study, subjects in three age groups (18–29, 30–49, and 50–69) attempted to move a hand sideways a set distance with and without knowledge of results regarding accuracy. Age differences in mean errors (inches) averaged over trials were pronounced with knowledge of results but not without knowledge of results. With little learning occurring without knowledge of results, there is no reason to expect age differences to appear. However, with knowledge of results, the oldest subjects were decidedly poorer in performance than the young and middle-aged subjects (who did not differ from one another). Most important, both young and middle-aged subjects benefited greatly from knowledge of results, whereas the oldest subjects benefited only slightly. As noted by Welford (1959), younger subjects seem to find the translation from vision to kinesthesis easier to accomplish than do older subjects. That is, for visual feedback to be effective in improving performance on this kind of task, it has to be converted somehow into kinesthetic cues (i.e., stimuli produced by muscle movements) that signal when to stop movement.

The later study by Anshel (1978) employed only a knowledge-of-results condition. Young and elderly subjects were required to move a cylinder 80° from a resting point. Overall, the young subjects were superior to the elderly subjects in terms of the mean error averaged over 20 trials. However, the improvement in accuracy from the first to last trial was as great for the elderly subjects as it was for the young. Thus, the poorer performance of the elderly subjects resulted from their initially poor performance level rather than from their inability to utilize knowledge of results. Elderly subjects have also been found to be less accurate than young adult subjects in judging which of two successive self-movements of a hand matched a previously established criterion distance of movement (Marshall, Elias, & Wright, 1985). However, Marshall et al. (1985) did discover that accuracy for their elderly subjects, as well as their young subjects, increased monotonically as the difference between the noncriterion movement and the prior criterion increased. Other researchers (Jordan, 1978; Warabi, Noda, & Kato, 1986; Winchester & Roy, 1991) have also discovered the difficulty older adults have, relative to younger adults, in correcting aiming errors when required to make a rapid movement.

Why elderly subjects have difficulty in producing an accurate movement of specified dimensions may be the consequence of their poor retention of kinesthetic memory traces (Toole, Pyne, & McTarsney, 1984). Consider a relatively accurate movement that is confirmed as such by feedback given to the subject. Reproducing that same movement on the next trial should be contingent on the short-term memory for the kinesthetic cues produced by the prior movement. If the memory trace of those cues has been lost, then the next trial would find the subject with no available information to signal when to stop the movement. Toole et al. (1984) compared young adult, middle-aged, and elderly subjects in their ability to remember kinesthetic information by having them move a linear slide several different distances and then having them reproduce the series of movements. In effect, the subjects received a serial learning task in which movements rather than words served as items. They found no significant age-related deficits in reproducing the movements for shorter series (1, 3, or 6 separate movements). The absence of age differences here is surprising from the perspective of the stimulus-persistence principle, a principle that stresses longer lasting neural traces of stimuli for elderly adults than for younger adults (Axelrod, 1963; see Botwinick, 1978, and Kausler, 1991, for elaboration). The traces of proprioceptive stimuli would be expected to last longer for elderly subjects than for younger subjects, and they would therefore be more likely to serve as a source of interference for the elderly subjects in their memory of the proprioceptive stimuli for the next movement in the series. Dick, Kean, and Sands (1988) also reported no age-related deficit in memory for only a single movement. It seems unlikely therefore that a more rapid loss of kinesthetic memory traces by elderly subjects than by young adult subjects accounts for the poor performance of elderly subjects in Szafran's (1953; in Welford, 1959) or Anshel's (1978) studies. In fact, the results obtained by Toole et al. (1984) and Dick et al. (1988) make the poor acquisition of a single-movement response by elderly subjects in the earlier studies difficult to explain. However, Toole et al. (1984) did find a significant age-related deficit in the serial acquisition of movements when longer series were required (9 or 12 movements).

Driving a car through traffic and running with a football while dodging tacklers are examples of real-world tasks involving continuous responses. In each case, the proficiency of motor performance is greatly dependent on the ability to coordinate movements with rapidly changing visual-stimulus inputs. One of the standard laboratory tasks that simulates the kind of learning involved in such activities requires subjects to trace a figure while looking at it in a mirror. This is a difficult task at all ages, but it is especially difficult for elderly subjects. This differential difficulty was demonstrated in Snoddy's (1926) pioneering research, and it was confirmed in a more recent study by Wright and Payne (1985). In Snoddy's (1926) study, young and elderly subjects received many trials tracing with a stylus a six-pointed star cut through a metal plate. The early stages of practice were particularly difficult for the elderly subjects. It is here that the novel input provided by a reverse, or mirror-image, display is highly disruptive. Eventually, even the elderly subjects learned to adapt to this novel input, and they began to improve both their accuracy and time scores in tracing this figure. In Wright and Paynes's (1985) study, young and elderly subjects tracked a small, silver target as it moved clockwise through a narrow star-shaped pathway. They received three 90-s trials, with each trial analyzed in terms of time on target for consecutive 30-s periods (making 9 trials overall). Shown in Figure 2.3 are mean times on target (reported separately for men and women) over the 9 trials. It is clear that the elderly subjects performed well below the level of the young subjects and that the age-related deficit increased as practice progressed.

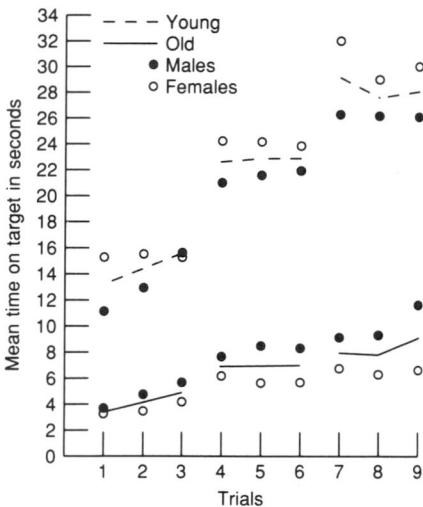

FIGURE 2.3 Performance in mirror tracking as a function of age and amount of practice. (Adapted from B. M. Wright & Payne, 1985, Figure 1.)

A similar result was obtained by Ruch (1934), this time with a pursuit-rotor task. For this task, subjects attempt to hold a stylus on a small button located on a disk that revolves rapidly. In one of Ruch's conditions, subjects were allowed to view the apparatus directly while holding the stylus; in a second condition, they could see the apparatus only in a mirror. The results for three age groups under both conditions are plotted in Figure 2.4. The scores are the mean number of revolutions produced over 25 trials of 30 s each (the disk revolved only when the stylus was on target, and the subject attempted to keep it revolving). It may be seen that an age-related deficit existed under each condition. However, expressed relatively, the deficit was especially pronounced in the mirror-vision condition (B, Figure 2.4), with elderly subjects averaging a score that was about 55% of that earned by middle-aged subjects. By contrast, in the direct vision condition (A, Figure 2.6), the elderly subjects earned a score that was about 82% of that earned by middle-aged subjects. A number of other studies reviewed by Welford (1959) reveal further the considerable difficulty encountered by elderly people in mastering a task with mirror-image visual inputs. The difficulty persists when the mirror image is imaginary rather than real. That is, subjects are required to draw a figure the way it would look if seen in a mirror without actually seeing the mirror image. As noted by Welford:

> The subject is required in a mirror task to, as it were, turn the display around mentally or to employ some rule of procedure. The mirror does, in short, require that some additional stage or process be inserted in the translation from display to

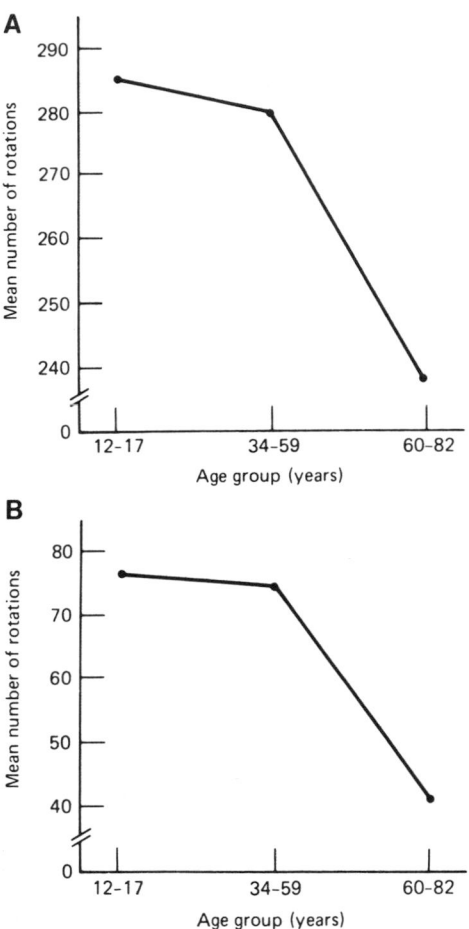

FIGURE 2.4   Age differences in pursuit-rotor performance under direct vision (A) and mirror vision (B). (Adapted from data in Ruch, 1934.)

action, and the fundamental question would seem to be why such an extra stage causes difficulty for older people and whether some types of stage cause more difficulty than others (1959, pp. 595–596).

The question of age differences in the ability to rotate figures mentally has been an important one in recent years with a task other than a mirror-image motor task. That task is the mental rotation task introduced some years ago by Shepard and Metzler (1971). Subjects are presented with a standard visual pattern or configuration, and they are then tested with another pattern or configuration that either conforms or doesn't conform to the standard if the standard were rotated a number of degrees. Determining whether or not the test stimulus matches the standard stimulus requires a subject to rotate the test stimulus mentally (i.e., by means of imagery). A number of studies (e.g., Gaylord & Marsh, 1975; see Kausler, 1991, for further review) have reported that elderly adults are considerably slower than young adults in making such mental rotations. The difficulty elderly adults have with such mental rotations bears some relevance to the existence of age differences in the ability to translate mirror image inputs into a format suitable for coordinating with movements.

More generally, the mirror-image research suggests that age deficits in motor-skill learning are likely to increase as the involvement of cognitive processes intervening between visual input and motor responding increases. Performing on a mirror-image task is, in effect, performing under dual-task conditions. The subject must translate the visual information presented while performing the motor response concurrently. Conceivably, an age-related reduction in cognitive resources makes performance especially difficult for elderly subjects under these conditions. The reduction in resources may be the consequence of deterioration with aging of visuospatial centers in the right cerebral hemisphere (Lapidot, 1987).

The translation of mirror images is only one possible age-sensitive process adversely affecting motor-skill learning by elderly adults. Problem solving is another potential intervening response for affecting adult age differences in motor-skill learning, as may be seen in studies by Kay (1954, 1955). Subjects of various ages performed on a task in which they pressed keys continuously as lights above the keys went on. There were 12 keys and 12 corresponding lights. In one condition, the keys corresponded directly to the lights. That is, there was complete S-R compatability (the key on the far left was pressed when the light on the far left went on, and so on). In a second S-R incompatability condition, a translation process was required to press the correct key. For example, the key on the far left might correspond to the fifth light from the left, and so on. Age differences were slight in the direct correspondence condition, where the demand on cognitive resources was minimal, and quite pronounced in the translation condition, where the demand on limited cognitive resources was likely to strain the reduced capacity of elderly subjects.

Two-hand coordination is another process that seems to be highly age sensitive. In a large-scale study conducted around 1950, Pacaud (as edited by Welford, 1989) tested over 4000 French railway workers, ranging in age from their 20s to their 50s, on a number of tasks. One of these tasks required the manipulation of two controls, one with each hand, to trace over a design. There was a pronounced decline in performance over the age decades, as measured both by the time to complete the tracing and errors made in tracing (i.e., traces falling outside of a designated tolerance level).

On the other hand, the ability to utilize knowledge of results seems to be age insensitive for a task involving continuous responses. Swanson and Lee (1992) had their subjects perform three movements, each to a barrier in a specified time. The time allotments were well within the times needed to perform each movement by their elderly subjects. Thus, the subject's goal was not to move as rapidly as possible, but rather to time each movement as accurately as possible. Subjects performed under two conditions that varied the way in which knowledge of results (verbal feedback of the actual time of a specific movement) was combined with movement components. In a blocked condition, subjects received knowledge of results for only one of the three movements for the first 30 trials, knowledge of results for only the second of the three movements for the next 30 trials, and knowledge of results for only the third movement on the remaining 30 trials. In a random condition, subjects also received knowledge of results for only one movement on each trial, but the specific movement varied in a quasi-random order over the 90 trials assuring that each of the three movements received knowledge of results for 30 trials. In addition, each subject performed the same task for 6 more trials after a retention interval of 10 min. Mean constant errors (a measure of timing accuracy) are shown in Figure 2.5 for blocks of 6 trials. Clearly, the subjects in both age groups improved in accuracy with practice. That is, a standard negatively accelerated learning curve was exhibited for both age groups. However, neither the interaction between age and blocks nor the interaction

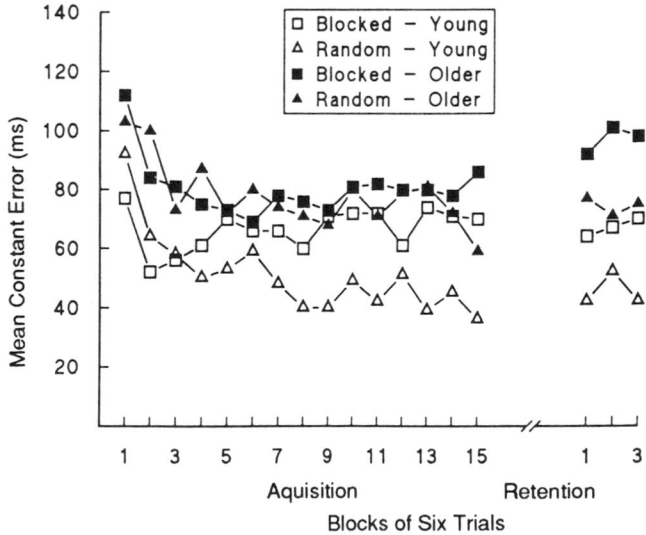

FIGURE 2.5   Mean constant errors for movements (timing accuracy) with practice as a function of knowledge of results. (Adapted from Swanson & Lee, 1992, Figure 1.)

between age and condition of knowledge of results attained statistical significance. A further analysis of constant error scores for subjects in the blocked condition revealed that accuracy of movement improved within a specific block only for the movement receiving knowledge of results. This was equally true for young and elderly subjects. From this pattern of results, Swanson and Lee (1992) concluded that their elderly subjects were as proficient as their young subjects in processing and using knowledge of results and that the age-related deficit in accuracy simply reflected the better timing ability of younger adults overall.

Finally, the pursuit-rotor task has figured in research on age differences in *motor reminiscence.* Reminiscence here refers to an increment in performance on a motor task following a rest break. That is, performance, defined, for example, as contact time with the target area on the revolving disk, is greater following a rest than preceding the rest, even though there has been no further practice. Reminiscence obviously conflicts with forgetting (which predicts poorer performance following the rest than preceding it). Its presence is presumably due to the recovery during the rest break from various negative performance factors, particularly fatigue. In early studies, Thumin (1962) and Gutman (1965) found that reminiscence did occur for elderly subjects as well as for young adult subjects. However, the amount of reminiscence (i.e., postrest gain in performance) was greater for the young subjects than for the elderly subjects. As may be seen in Figure 2.3, Wright and Payne (1985) also found greater reminiscence for young than for elderly subjects. Their subjects received 40-s rests between Trials 3 and 4 and between Trials 6 and 7. Note, for example, the far greater increment in time on target from Trial 3 to Trial 4 for the young subjects than for the elderly subjects. This outcome is somewhat surprising in that fatigue, a likely major contributor to reminiscence (through its dissipation during the rest break), is likely to accumulate at a faster rate for elderly subjects than for young subjects.

From Figure 2.3, it may also be seen that elderly adults differed from young adults not only in overall performance levels, but also in the rate of improving performance with practice on the task. That is, acceleration of the learning curve was greater for the young subjects than for the elderly subjects. An overall performance decrement was also reported by Durkin et al. (in preparation). However, in this case, the rate of improvement in performance with practice was equal for young adult and elderly subjects.

Expertise and Maintenance of Motor Skills

Earlier we argued that motor programs remain largely intact during adulthood. Once established, adults maintain the ability to speak fluently (a programmed motor skill), ride a bicycle, play difficult musical compositions on the piano, and type skillfully. Our earlier comments were based on anecdotal evidence, such as that provided by Claudio Arrau. A study by Hill (1957) provides more objective confirmation of our point, even though the study is a real-world one and has many methodological complications (e.g., only one subject provided longitudinal data). Hill, the single subject, mastered typewriting at age 30. At the time of mastery, he typed the same 100-word passage many times and had maintained records of his performance on this passage. At age 55 and again at age 80, Hill returned to the keyboard and again practiced typewriting. According to his own account, there had been very little practice during the many intervening years. At age 80, his first typing of the 100-word passage was at the level he had attained after 8 days of typing at age 30. After approximately 30 days, he attained the level that had taken 126 days of practice to reach at age 30. This is a truly remarkable savings, one indicating that the motor program for typing had suffered little damage over 50 yr, years filled with little additional practice.

Hill, of course, was not an expert typist. An important further question concerns what effect aging has on those individuals who are expert typists or are experts in any other motor skill. The issue of expertise in typing was confronted directly by Salthouse (1984). In one of his studies, the subjects were skilled typists between the ages of 20 and 72 years. Of interest is the extent to which typing speed slows down with aging, as would be expected from the overall slower motor responses of older adults relative to younger adults. The subjects typed a lengthy passage displayed on a computer screen with their interkey intervals between strokes recorded. The mean interval score, as an index of typing speed, for each subject is shown in Figure 2.6.

It may be seen by the flat regression line relating age to typing rate that speed of typing was unrelated to age. That is, the older expert typists were as rapid in their typing as the younger experts. However, in a later study by Bosman (1993), older skilled typists were found to have some age-related deficit in the translation phase of typing (i.e., translating textual characteristics into a motor program) but not in the execution phase (i.e., striking the appropriate keys). Salthouse's (1984) subjects also performed on a serial-choice-reaction-time task in which they received uppercase and lowercase versions of the letters "L" and "R," and they pressed different keys for the different versions of these letters. Also shown in Figure 2.6 are the mean interkey intervals for each subject and the best fitting regression line relating age to response rate. Here the slowing down in response rate with aging is clearly apparent. The lack of an aging effect for typing was obviously an exception to the otherwise general slowing down with aging of motor responses, an exception attributable to the expertise of the older typists. Why the exception? Through a series of ingenious variations in the presentation of the to-be-typed material, Salthouse (1984) was able to answer this important question. He discovered an apparent compensatory process present in the older typists, that is, a process that compensated for their slower movements, namely, their greater sensitivity, relative to younger typists, to characters farther in ad-

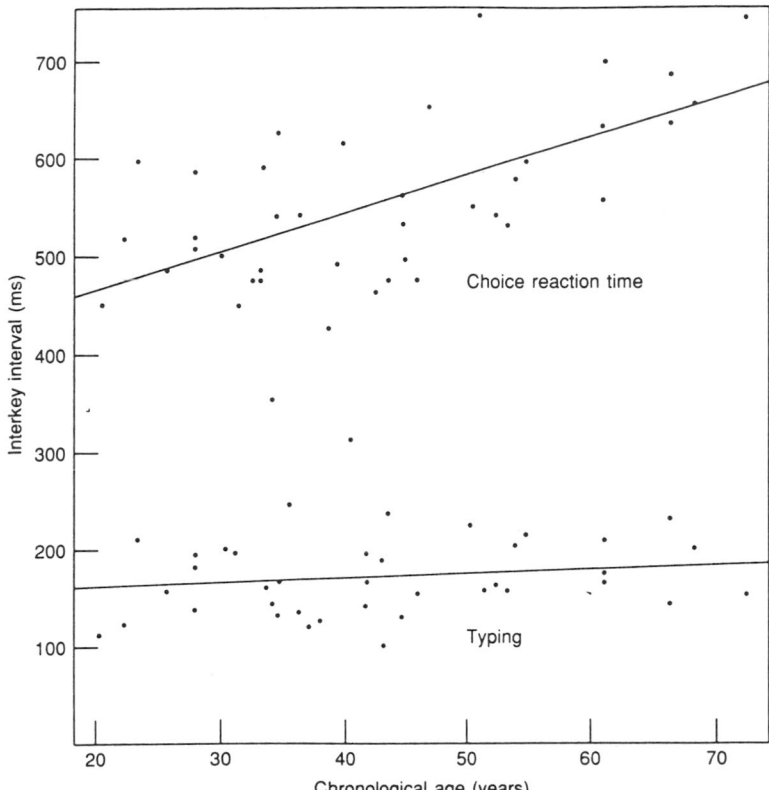

FIGURE 2.6 Median interkey interval in milliseconds for the normal typing and choice-reaction-time tasks as a function of typist age in Study 2. (Each point represents a single typist, and the solid lines illustrate the regression equations relating interkey interval to age). (Reprinted from Salthouse, 1984, Figure 2. Copyright 1984 by the American Psychological Association.)

vance of the currently typed characters (a discovery later replicated by Bosman, 1993).

The role that expertise seemingly has in compensating for the slowing down of perceptual-motor behaviors has been demonstrated for skills other than typing, such as that possessed by skilled musicians (e.g., Clifton, 1986) and skilled athletes (Allard & Burnett, 1985; see Charness, 1989, for further review). Of great interest will be future research directed at other exceptions to the slowing down of motor behaviors with aging when expertise is present. If other exceptions are found, a topic of further interest will be the discovery of the compensatory processes that develop with expertise (see Charness, 1989; Rybash, Hoyer, & Roodin, 1986; and Salthouse, 1990, for further discussion).

The expert typists in Salthouse's (1984) study were performing under conditions in which there were no distracting irrelevant stimuli. Would older expert typists be able to apply their compensatory process when such irrelevant stimuli are present? There is ample evidence (e.g., Rabbitt, 1965, see Chapter 6, p. 207 for review) to indicate that the screening out of irrelevant stimuli is a highly age-sensitive process that interferes with performance on the task at hand more for older subjects than for younger subjects. This may well be the case for older expert typists who would find the cognitive resources needed to apply the compensatory process diminished by their efforts to avoid attention to the irrelevant stimuli. That experts of different ages may be differentially affected in their performances by irrelevant stimuli was nicely demonstrated in a study by Molander and Bäckman (1990). Rather than expert typists, expert miniature golfers were employed in their study. Younger (19–36 yr) and older (49–59 yr) experts played a round of miniature golf while sounds could be heard in the background. The sounds were either those of tape-recorded traffic noises or those of a radio broadcast of a soccer game (soccer is very big in Sweden where this study was conducted). The younger players averaged about the same score playing in the soccer broadcast condition (mean = 39.8 shots) as in the traffic noise condition (mean = 39.0 shots). By contrast, the older players performed much more poorly in the soccer condition (mean = 53.2 shots) than in the traffic noise condition (mean = 47.1 shots). The difficulty the older players had in screening out the more meaningful soccer game seemingly diminished the cognitive resources they needed to play golf at their optimal level.

Learning Theory and Explanation of Adult Age Differences in Motor-Skill Learning

To associationists, motor-skill learning has been traditionally viewed as being essentially equivalent to instrumental learning. As in maze learning, a subject needs to acquire a sequence of responses. It is the nature of the stimuli associated with these responses that offers the primary distinction between the two kinds of learning. For maze learning, the stimuli are largely external cues present in the environment. For motor-skill learning, the stimuli are proprioceptive, or kinesthetic, cues produced by the organism's own movements. A given response in a series of motor responses is presumed to be linked associatively to the stimuli generated by the prior response in the series. Age differences in motor-skill learning for some tasks may be accounted for nicely from this perspective in terms of the stimulus-persistence concept. The trace of proprioceptive stimuli from any response in a chain of responses may be postulated to persist longer for elderly subjects than for young adult subjects. These persisting stimuli should interfere with the elicitation of later responses in the chain that are temporally far removed from the source of the persisting stimuli (but see p. 36 for conflicting evidence).

For other tasks, such as those involving mirror vision, there is another form of interference that must be considered. The visual stimuli relevant to the task (i.e., the stimuli from mirror vision) are related to stimuli (i.e., the stimuli as they would appear in normal vision) that are associated with familiar responses that conflict with the responses needed to perform the task at hand (e.g., moving a stylus through a star-shaped pattern viewed in a mirror). These well-established responses must be inhibited in order to make the novel task-relevant responses. In effect, these competing responses create interference. A familiar argument in the experimental psychology of aging is that elderly adults are more "interference prone" than young adults. Tests of adult age differences in susceptibility to interference effects have usually been made with lists of paired associates. We will discover in Chapters 4 and 10 that there is little evidence to support the interference-proneness position. However, this evidence is for verbal associations, not associations involving highly overlearned motor responses. Here an adult age difference in interference proneness remains an untested and still viable possibility.

This conceptualization of motor-skill learning emphasizes the operation of what is commonly referred to as an *open-loop system*. An open-loop system has to rely on trial and error for the organism to hit upon, eventually, appropriate response elements in the chain. Neoassociationists (e.g., J.A. Adams, 1971), however, have proposed a vastly different alternative to the open-loop view. The alternative emphasizes the operation of a *closed-loop system*. The basic component of this system is a feedback loop, much like that of a thermostat (Ellis, 1978). A thermostat is set at some specific temperature. When the actual temperature dips below this set value, the disparity is detected and the heating unit is activated. Thus, the system allows for the detection *and* the correction of an error (i.e., disparity from a set value). In motor-skill learning, information provided by feedback of some kind, such as knowledge of results, enables an individual to acquire gradually a perceptual trace, or image, of what task movements should be like. This trace functions like the standard temperature on a thermostat. If feedback for a given movement fails to match this standard, then an adjustment in movement toward the standard is made on the next trial. Thus, an attempt is made to correct an error, just as a heating system corrects an error. From this perspective, motor-skill learning is largely a problem-solving task. That is, the organism attempts to solve the problem created by an error, defined, in this case, as a disparity from some standard value. Accordingly, we could argue that age deficits in motor-skill learning result from the less proficient problem-solving ability of elderly adults relative to young adults (see also p. 39). Specifically, elderly adults may have greater difficulty in abstracting proprioceptive traces to serve as standards, or prototypes, for evaluating the accuracy of subsequent responses. If true, the age-related deficit in the abstraction process would be one that is not generally found when the abstraction needed to form a prototype is derived from visual information, such as geometric patterns (Hess & Slaughter, 1986a, 1986b). There is an important difference, however, between the two situations. With geometric patterns, only one prototype is required; with many motor tasks involving multiple movements, a number of different prototypes may be required. We discovered earlier that age-related deficits are especially pronounced when subjects have to retain information about a lengthy series of movements, each movement presumably involving its own abstracted prototype.

Both open-loop and closed-loop theories of motor-skill learning have met serious opposition over the years, at least for explaining highly skilled motor operations, such as typing and playing the piano (e.g., Lashley, 1951). Responses in a complex chain are believed to unfold too rapidly to serve effectively as the source of proprioceptive stimuli for subsequent responses in the chain. That is, continuous interchanges between stimuli and responses would slow down performance to the point where highly skilled high-speed levels would be impossible. To explain rapid, errorless, complex sequences of motor responses, many psychologists (e.g., Keele, 1968) have argued for the acquisition of a motor program with extensive practice on a task. Such a program is viewed as being a cognitive structure that, once acquired, may be subsequently activated and translated into a flow of movements that progress automatically and without interruption.

Consider, for example, the operations of skilled typists (Salthouse, 1984; Shaffer, 1973). Their typing, having become programmed and, therefore, automatic, makes virtually no demands on their processing capacities. Moreover, as we discovered earlier, changes can be made in the program by expert typists to compensate for age-related deficits in the slowing down of the finger movements that represent the end products of the program's operation.

Adult Age Differences in Perceptual Learning

As defined by Ellis, a noted authority in the area, "Perceptual learning refers to any modification of perception which can be attributed to learning" (Ellis, 1972, p. 157). Ellis (1972) gave a number of everyday examples of perceptual learning. They include learning to read maps, learning to identify objects seen under a microscope, learning to adjust to bifocal glasses, and learning to recognize a particular symphony whether it is played by an orchestra or a rock band. Like other forms of skill learning, the need for new perceptual learning continues throughout the life span. Our interest rests in age differences in the proficiency of perceptual learning. There have been a number of aging studies that seemingly apply to perceptual learning, even though reference to perceptual learning for the task at hand is rarely made. There have been several studies that have dealt with the acquisition of what are likely to be novel skills for adults of all ages. One of these skills is mirror-reading of sentences or words. This skill is usually referred to as involving procedural learning, and it will be discussed in a later section of this chapter. We should note here, however, that the rate of learning this skill seems to be about the same for elderly adults as for young adults. Another of these skills is the identification of words when only fragments of those words may be seen. Hashtroudi, Chrosniak, and Schwartz (1991; Experiment 2) discovered that their young subjects became increasingly better at this task as practice progresses. By contrast, their elderly subjects showed little improvement in the skill from the early trials to the late trials. In a somewhat similar study, but with inconspicuous words rather than word fragments, Kline, Culler, and Sucec (1977) also found a practice effect for the reading skill with their young subjects but no practice effect for either their middle-aged or elderly subjects.

Target Detection

The focus of most studies on perceptual learning has been on the improvement of a preexisting skill with practice rather than on the acquisition of a task that requires a novel skill. One such skill is the detection of the presence of a briefly exposed target stimulus. In a study by Salthouse and Somberg (1982), young adult and elderly subjects received a large number of trials in which on each trial a target stimulus (a configuration of 5 dots within a larger pattern of 60 dots) was either present or absent and the subjects responded by pressing different keys for present and absent. Both the young and elderly subjects displayed pronounced negatively accelerated learning curves (i.e., especially large increments in performance early in practice). Although the elderly subjects clearly demonstrated their ability to improve their detection skill with practice, they, nevertheless, performed well below the level of the young subjects throughout the learning trials.

Stimulus Discrimination

Another skill that improves with practice is discriminating between stimuli in order to associate a different response with each stimulus. There are several laboratory tasks that involve discrimination learning and that, hopefully, simulate the kinds of processes entering into everyday discrimination learning. One of these tasks, namely, stimulus differentiation, was discussed earlier in conjunction with classical conditioning (see p. 9) Here subjects learn to discriminate between the CS and a CS' (a stimulus similar to the CS such that the CR is eventually given to the CS but not to the CS'). There we discovered that elderly subjects find it much more difficult to accomplish stimulus differentiation than do young adult subjects (Marinesco & Kreindler, 1934). To a certain degree, a choice-reaction-time task has a discrimination-learning component to it. That is, subjects make one response to one stimulus (e.g., a red light) and a different response to a second stimulus (e.g., a yellow light). There is no doubt that both young adults and elderly adults improve their performance with extended practice on this kind of task (Noble, Baker, & Jones, 1964; Poon et al. 1976). Improvement is measured here by faster reaction times with practice on the task. For example, Poon et al. (1976) found that their elderly subjects actually reduced their reaction times with practice to a greater degree than their young subjects, although the young subjects responded considerably faster than the elderly subjects even at the end of practice. In a well-known study, Murrell (1970) discovered that the reaction time of a single older subject (a 57-yr-old woman) reached the performance level of his two young subjects after thousands of trials. However, it is seems likely that little of the performance gain with practice on a choice-reaction-time task is attributable to discrimination learning per se. Surely it is not difficult for adult subjects of any age to discriminate between two distinctive stimuli throughout a lengthy practice session. The increments in response speed with practice are more likely to be simply in the motor components of the task.

A more difficult visual discrimination learning task that involved stimuli more complex than colored lights was employed by Salthouse and Somberg (1982). Accuracy scores clearly increased with practice for both their young adult and elderly subjects, with both age groups showing negatively accelerated curves. Elderly adults can indeed learn more difficult visual discrimination tasks. However, even at the end of many trials, the elderly subjects were performing at an accuracy level well below that of the young adult subjects.

Discrimination learning of a still more complex form enters into what is called *solution shift* tasks (Kendler & Kendler, 1962). The traditional forms of these tasks are illustrated in Figure 2.7. Subjects perform on an original task involving a discrimination between two stimuli and then receive a transfer task that requires either a *reversal shift* of the solution or a *nonreversal shift* of the solution. On the original task, one requiring four successively presented stimuli of the kind shown in the top part of Figure 2.7, subjects acquire a single-dimension concept that usually involves only a bilevel relevant stimulus dimension and a bilevel irrelevant dimension. For the problem shown in Figure 2.7 the relevant and irrelevant dimensions are form (square = +; triangle = −) and brightness (black and white) respectively. After the solution of this problem is attained, subjects are shifted unexpectedly and without interruption to either the reversal-shift problem or the nonreversal-shift problem, both of which are illustrated in the bottom part of Figure 2.12. The transfer problem in both cases involves the same stimuli presented on the original task (top part of Figure 2.7). However, in the reversal-shift condition, form remains the relevant stimulus dimension, but triangle becomes the positive value and square the negative value, whereas in the nonreversal-shift condition, brightness becomes the relevant stimulus dimension (e.g., with black designated the positive value) and form the irrelevant stimulus dimension.

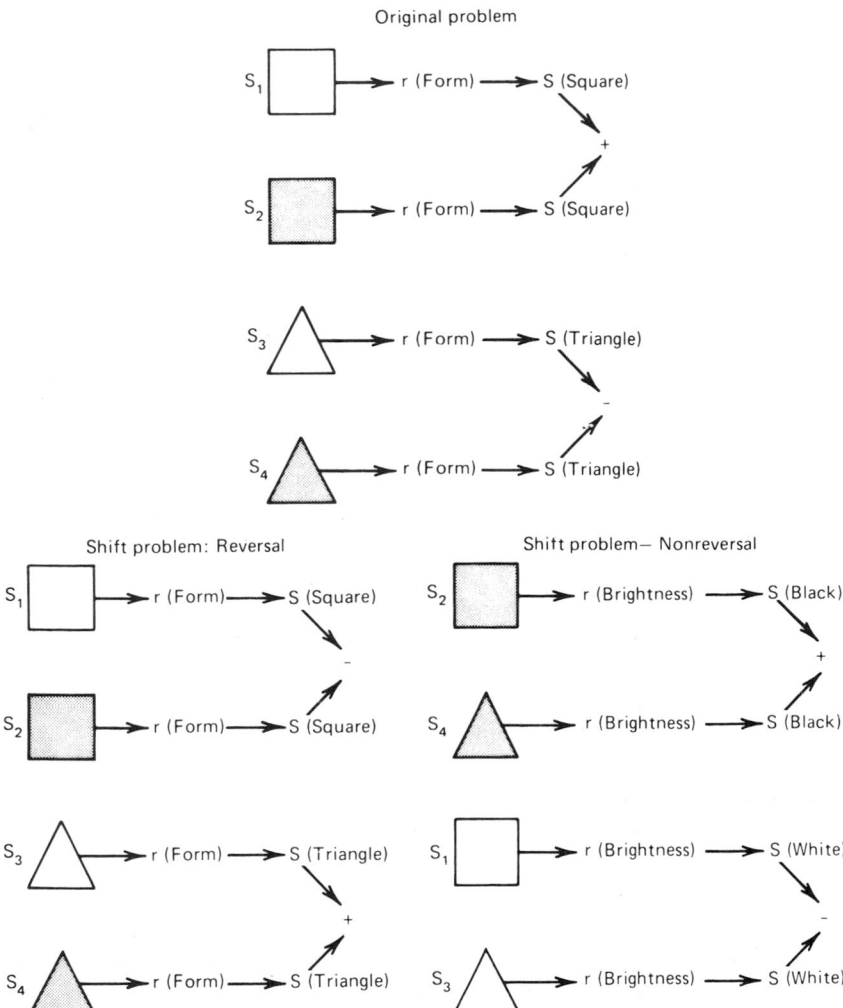

FIGURE 2.7 Representative objects and conditions for introducing reversal and nonreversal shift.

The contrast between the two shift conditions is of great interest to associationists. From the perspective of classical associationism, a nonreversal-shift solution should be easier to accomplish than a reversal-shift solution. Note that one of the two positive instances following a nonreversal shift (the black square) had also been a positive instance on the original task (i.e., it possesses both the positive feature, squareness, of the original task and the positive feature, blackness, of the transfer task). Therefore, a "yes" response to this stimulus (S_2 in Figure 2.7) has already accrued considerable associative strength prior to the shift, strength that should carry over to the new task. As a result, subjects need learn only to give a "yes" response to the other stimulus object (S_4 in Figure 2.7) to solve the transfer problem. By contrast, neither of the positive instances (S_3 and S_4) following a reversal shift had been a positive instance on the original task. Therefore, there is no previously accrued associative strength to transfer to the new task, and the "yes" response to each new positive instance must start from scratch. Again, the net effect should be to make a nonreversal shift easier than a reversal shift.

A very different outcome is expected, however, from the perspective of stage analysis and its emphasis on mediation as a means of connecting S and R elements (see Chapter 3, pp. 82–84). Exposure to the instances of the original task results in a mediating verbal chain that begins with the response that names the relevant dimension (form in Figure 2.7). This response produces its own stimulus consequences, the words *square* and *triangle*, that, in turn, become associated with positive ("yes" response) and negative ("no" response) values (*top*, Figure 2.7) On the reversal-transfer problem, there is no need to unlearn, or inhibit, the mediating verbal response of form—it still identifies the relevant stimulus dimension. All a subject has to do is reverse the positive and negative values for the two stimulus consequences of this mediating response (*bottom left*, Figure 2.7). This is not the case for a subject confronted by a nonreversal shift. Now the original mediating response is no longer appropriate, and it must be extinguished or actively inhibited. At the same time, a new mediating response, one that names brightness as the relevant dimension, must be established, and its stimulus consequences must be differentially associated with positive and negative values (*bottom right*, Figure 2.7). The net effect is the prediction that a reversal shift should be easier to master than a nonreversal shift.

A number of studies have revealed that older children and young adults solve reversal-shift problems faster than nonreversal-shift problems, whereas the opposite is true for young children (Kendler & Kendler, 1962). The implication is quite clear. Older children and young adults engage in the higher order process of mediation during performance on a solution-shift task, whereas young children engage in the lower order process of rote rehearsal. What about elderly adults? If they regress to the processes characteristic of early childhood, then they would be expected to relinquish the use of mediation and to revert to the rote acquisition of a solution-shift task. The advantage of a reversal shift over a nonreversal shift would, therefore, be expected to disappear. Unfortunately, the only study that provided a direct contrast between reversal- and nonreversal-shift proficiency for elderly subjects yielded inconclusive results. Rogers, Keyes, and Fuller (1976) found both kinds of shift problems to be very difficult for their elderly subjects—40% failed to solve the reversal-shift problem and 53% the nonreversal-shift problem. For the few remaining subjects who did attain shift solutions, the reversal shift was easier for some kinds of stimulus materials and the nonreversal shift for other kinds.

There have been several aging studies, however, that have made effective use of modified versions of the traditional reversal- and nonreversal-shift conditions. The modification of the reversal shift results in what is called an *intradimensional-shift* problem. Here, the relevant and irrelevant dimensions from the original task are unaltered on the transfer task (as is also true for the reversal shift per se), but the attribute values from the original task are replaced by new attribute values on the transfer task. For example, consider an original task in which form is the relevant dimension, with square and triangle the positive and negative values respectively, and color is the irrelevant dimension, with red and green as the attribute values. On the transfer task, form remains the relevant stimulus dimension but with new attribute values, say circle (+) and diamond (−). Color remains the irrelevant stimulus dimension but also with new attribute values, say blue and yellow. The modification of the nonreversal shift results in what is called an *extradimensional shift*. As in a traditional nonreversal shift, the previous relevant stimulus dimension becomes irrelevant, whereas the previous irrelevant dimension becomes relevant. However, the attributes of the original task are replaced by new attribute values on the transfer task, as in an intradimensional shift. Thus, color would become the relevant dimension, with blue (+) and yellow (−) as new attribute values; form would become the irrelevant dimension, with circle and diamond as new attribute values. The predictions regarding these modified transfer tasks parallel those for the traditional tasks from which they are derived. Most important, young adults are expected to master an intradimensional shift more easily than an extradimensional shift. The mediating verbal response (e.g., form) remains operative in an intradimensional shift, but it must be extinguished or inhibited and replaced by a new mediating response (e.g., color) in an extradimensional shift. This expectancy has been confirmed in a number of studies (e.g., P. J. Johnson, 1967).

The transition to modified shift tasks is an important step to be taken in experimental aging research. The traditional shift tasks are likely to be especially confusing to many elderly subjects through their continued use of the same instances employed in the original acquisition task, but with new decisions to be made for those old instances. Such confusion is avoided in the modified task conditions through the use of new instances that are quite distinctive from the old instances. Nevertheless, the studies employing these modified shift tasks have demonstrated convincingly that elderly subjects find an intradimensional shift to be no easier to make than an extradimensional shift (Coppinger & Nehrke, 1972; Nehrke, 1973; Nehrke & Coppinger, 1971). Moreover, the absence of an advantage for what should be a short-circuited condition (i.e., mediation) persists even after many overlearning trials on the original task (Nehrke & Sutterer, 1978). We will use as our representative example of research in this area an especially informative study by Witte (1971). His subjects were preschool children, young adults, "young" elderly adults (median age, 65 yr), and "old" elderly adults (median age, 74.5 yr). Subjects at each age level received, unexpectedly, new instances (e.g., a blue circle, a blue diamond, a yellow circle, and a yellow diamond) after attaining the solution to an original problem (e.g., with a red square, a red triangle, a green square, and a green triangle as instances). Of interest are the percentages of subjects, plotted in Figure 2.8), responding as if the new instances conformed to an intradimensional-shift condition. Note that the percentage of the "old" elderly subjects was well below that of both young adults and "young" elderly adults. In fact, the percentage approached that of presumably mediationally deficient preschool children.

The implication of these solution-shift studies is that many elderly people do experience a mediational deficit on a solution-shift task, just as they apparently do in paired-associate learning and transfer (see Chapter 3, pp. 91–97). A mediational deficit does not mean, of course, that new materials cannot be learned by most elderly people. It simply means that the rate of acquisition is likely to be slower than the rate characteristic of most young adults who do engage actively and spontaneously in mediation. Again, mediational activity is expected to short-circuit the slow process of learning any task by rote rehearsal. In addition, there remains the possibility that at least part of the loss of mediation with aging represents a production deficit that may be reversible with appropriate training and practice. We will discover in Chapter 3 that some success has occurred in

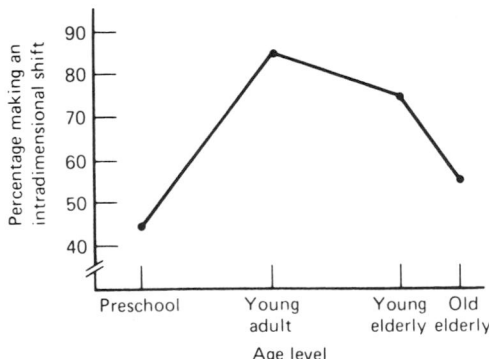

FIGURE 2.8 Age differences in the percentage of subjects manifesting an intradimensional shift. (Adapted from data in Witte, 1971.)

overcoming the age decrement commonly found for imaginal mediation in paired-associate learning.

Pattern-Recognition Learning

Yet another perceptual skill that improves with practice is pattern recognition. A pattern refers to a collection of stimulus elements that is recognized, or perceived, with respect to its representation in a class of objects. Thus, a specific automobile is recognized as such because its stimulus elements (four wheels, a hood, and so on) enable the perceiver to identify its membership in the "automobile" class of objects. Research on adult age differences in the proficiency of pattern recognition typically employs letters of the alphabet as the patterns to be recognized. The emphasis is on the time needed to process a single letter in order to identify the name of that letter. One methodology in this research is that of backward masking (see Kausler, 1991, for further review). A single letter is exposed briefly, and it is then followed, after a brief interval, by a masking stimulus that terminates the processing of the target letter. Processing time is assessed by determining the total time needed to permit identification of the target letter before masking occurs. This time is called the interstimulus interval (or ISI), and it is found by summing the time the target stimulus is exposed and the time between the offset of the target stimulus and the onset of the masking stimulus. Of course, there is no question of adults of all ages being able to recognize and identify letters of the alphabet. What is in question is the age difference in the minimal amount of time such identification requires. There is no doubt that elderly adults are somewhat slower than young adults in making these identifications. Our interest, however, rests in whether or not increases in the speed of pattern recognition can occur with practice for elderly adults as well as young adults. That is, can the speed of pattern recognition be increased by learning, and, if so, to the same amount for elderly adults as for young adults? The results obtained in a study by Hertzog, Williams, and Walsh (1976) suggest that the speed of letter identifications does increase equally with practice for young and elderly adults. Their subjects received many trials on each of five different days. Shown in Figure 2.9 are the reductions in the ISI over the five practice sessions. It may be seen that substantial increases in speed occurred with practice for both age groups and that the learning curves were essentially the same for young and elderly subjects (relatively constant increments from session to session rather than the standard negatively accelerated increments). Unfortunately, the age difference favoring the young adults was as pronounced at the end of practice as at its beginning.

An age-related deficit in pattern recognition learning was also found by Russo and Parkin (1993) for a different kind of material. In this case, subjects attempted to identify common objects when only fragments of those objects were exposed.

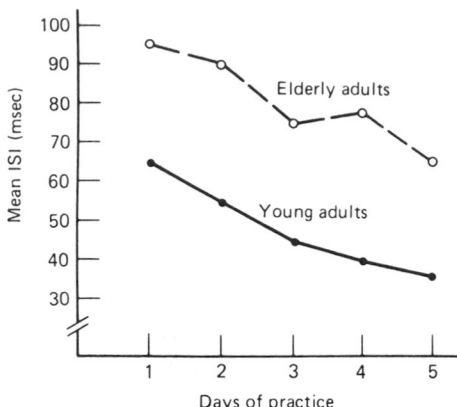

FIGURE 2.9 Effects of practice for both young and elderly subjects on central-processing time needed to avoid masking. ISI, interstimulus interval. (Adapted from Hertzog, Williams, & Walsh, 1976, Table 1.)

Attentional Learning

The final perceptual skill that improves with practice is attention. Attention in one form or another is a basic prerequisite for perception (or pattern recognition) to occur. One kind of attention is vigilance, that is, readiness for detecting a stimulus change in what otherwise is an invariant sequence of stimuli. Performance on a simple vigilance task does improve with practice for adults regardless of their ages. This was nicely demonstrated in a study by Parasuraman and Giambra (1991) in which the subjects were young adults, middle-aged adults, and elderly adults. For each of 20 sessions (30 min each) the subjects monitored a screen in which a square figure appeared. Occasionally, the figure in the center changed to a slightly larger square. We will consider only their high rate condition in which the changes occurred 40 times per min, with the subjects asked to signal each change. Increases in hit rates (i.e., correctly signaling a change) over the practice sessions clearly occurred for each age group. The three learning curves closely paralleled each other, and they all revealed the standard negatively accelerated form. Overall, hit rates were highest for the young adults and lowest for the elderly adults. Most important, the magnitudes of the age differences were about the same at the end of practice as at the beginning of practice.

Selective attention is another form of attention. Our limited processing capacity does not permit us to analyze fully all of the stimuli impinging on us at any one time. Consequently, our attention focuses on, or selects, some component of the complete array (the relevant stimulus or stimuli), whereas other components are presumably left unattended, or largely ignored (the irrelevant stimuli). Laboratory studies of age differences in selective attention commonly employ one set of letters as the relevant stimuli and a different set of letters as the irrelevant stimuli (see Kausler, 1991, for a detailed review of research on selective attention). The subject's task is to identify on each trial which of the relevant letters was displayed. A further variation is to have subjects perform under either consistent-mapping conditions or varied-mapping conditions. In the former, the same letters serve as targets (or relevant stimuli) across trials, and the same set of different letters serves as distractors (or irrelevant stimuli) across trials; in the latter, the target letters and distractor letters change across trials (with targets on some trials being distractors on other trials, and vice versa). There is ample evidence to show pronounced reductions in reaction times as practice progresses under both conditions (e.g., Plude et al., 1983). In effect, elderly adults seem to improve their performance with practice nearly as much as do young adults. However, not surprisingly, the reaction times of young adults remain much faster than those of elderly adults at all stages of practice.

A third form of attention is divided attention. It refers to the shared processing of multiple stimulus inputs, all of which are relevant to the ongoing activity of the organism. A familiar example is the automobile driver's division of attention between the visual stimuli inherent in the flow of traffic and the auditory stimuli provided by a passenger's conversation. As long as the traffic flow is slow and predictable, the driver manages with little effort to divide attention, or at least to alternate it rapidly, between the two inputs. However, as the traffic picks up in intensity, the driver is likely to tune out the chattering of the passenger.

Research on divided attention obviously calls for performance under dual-task conditions. In general, the evidence from a number of studies reveals that there is little in the way of an age-related deficit in the ability to divide attention as long as the tasks being performed are relatively undemanding ones (e.g., Somberg & Salthouse, 1982). However, when task demands are high, the cost of dividing attention is greater for elderly adults than for young adults (e.g., Salthouse, Rogan, & Prill, 1984; see Guttentag, 1989, and Kausler, 1991, for further review). Our interest is in the extent to which practice on dual tasks affects the magnitude of age-related deficits in the division of attention. In a study by McDowd (1986), her young and elderly subjects received six practice sessions spread over 6 wk. In each session, subjects received 15 trials on a visual-tracking task performed alone, 15 trials on a three-choice-tone-discrimination task performed alone, and 15 trials on the two tasks performed concurrently. The cost of divided attention was determined by a ratio scoring procedure in which performance on each task when performed alone is compared with performance when performed under dual-task conditions. Changes in these cost scores over the six practice sessions are shown in Figure 2.10. It may be seen that the cost was greater for her elderly subjects than for her young subjects in each practice session. More important, however, is the fact that her elderly subjects showed as much benefit from practice as her

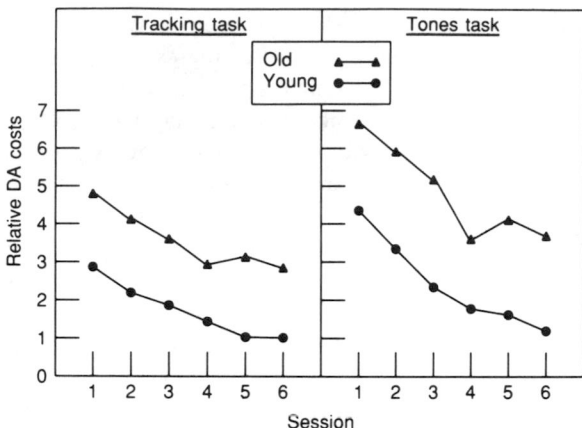

FIGURE 2.10 Relative divided-attention (DA) costs for old and young subjects across practice sessions for both the tones and the tracking tasks. (Adapted from McDowd, 1986, Figure 3.)

young subjects. For both groups, practice resulted in the standard negatively accelerated learning curve. Baron and Mattila (1989) also found improved ability to divide attention with practice for both young and elderly adults. Moreover, in their study, the age difference in the cost of divided attention actually decreased with practice. Elderly adults, like younger adults, have the capability of improving their skill in dividing attention through practice.

Expertise and Maintenance of a Perceptual Skill

Do years of use of a perceptual skill assure that the proficiency of that skill will be maintained at a high level during late adulthood? Research directed toward answering this question has been concerned primarily with selective attention. Are older medical technicians as proficient as younger technicians in searching displays to find the presence or absence of a designated-probe bacteria, when the technicians are equated in experience? This question is much like the one asked earlier about expertise in typing (see pp. 42–44). Clancy and Hoyer (1988) found only limited support for the critical role played by expertise in mitigating age-related declines in search proficiency. Middle-aged experts were no faster than middle-aged novices on a simple search task with bacteria shapes as probes and targets—and both groups were considerably slower than either young experts or young novices (who did not differ). However, only the middle-aged novices suffered pronounced performance decrements under a condition of divided attention (the secondary task consisted of tone detection). Overall, the results were not terribly supportive of experience playing a modulating role for age-related deficits on a selective attention task. On the other hand, Lewandowski, Kobus, Flood, and Hoyer (1988) did find that older, experienced sonar operators were as proficient as younger, experienced operators. Real-world expertise on this and other kinds of perceptual skills employed in various occupations is an area of research that merits considerably more investigation (see also Hoyer, 1985).

Adult Age Differences in Learning Mental Skills

Elderly adults who are aging normally are quite capable of learning such complex mental (or cognitive) skills as playing bridge and chess. Little, if anything, is known about age differences in the initial acquisition of such skills. An exception is the learning of word processing, a skill that is surely as much mental as it is motor. We discovered earlier (p. 34) that elderly adults can acquire this skill, but more slowly than younger adults do. However, it has been firmly established that older adults who have expertise in such higher mental skills as those involved in playing bridge and chess maintain them at a high level (Charness, 1981a, 1981b, 1981c, 1983, 1987). Considerable evidence suggests that less complex mental skills are clearly amenable to improved performance with practice for elderly adults as well as for younger adults. One such skill is the rapid scanning of the contents of information stored in short-term memory (see Chapter 1, p. 16, and also Salthouse and Somberg, 1982). Another is the skill (or skills) entering into performance on a digit-symbol test, a test often included as a component of an intelligence test. In a study by Beres and Baron (1981) young and elderly subjects received 100 trials spread over five days on a digit-symbol test. Shown in Figure 2.11 are the mean number of symbols completed on each of the 100 trials. Note the negatively accelerated learning curves for each age group. However, the young adults improved at a somewhat faster rate than the elderly adults. Consequently, the magnitude of the age difference favoring young adults was slightly greater at the end of practice than at the beginning. Nevertheless, the elderly subjects were performing at the end of practice at a level comparable to that of the young subjects at the beginning of practice. Finally, we will discover in Chapter 5 that practice on a digit-span task (a task requiring short-term memory) yields an increase in span length for both young adults and elderly adults. Like a digit-symbol test, a digit-span test is a common component of intelligence tests.

Adult Age Differences in Procedural Learning

Dissociation and Procedural Learning

One of psychology's most striking discoveries is the revelation that individuals suffering from organic amnesias, such as that resulting from Korsakoff's syndrome,

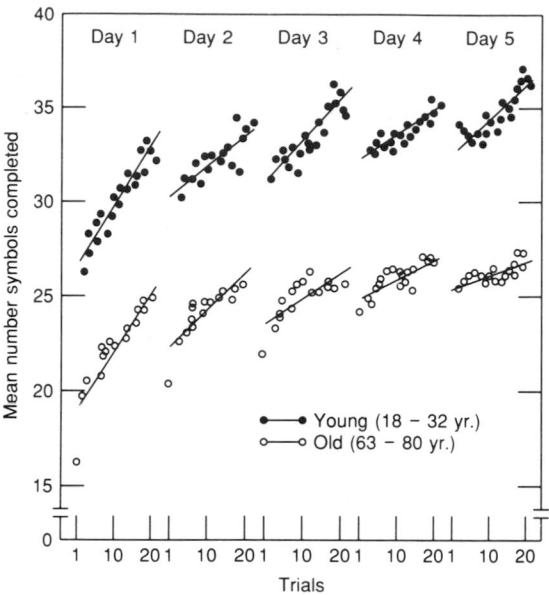

FIGURE 2.11 Points represent mean number of symbols completed by older and younger women on each of 100 training trials. Straight lines have been fitted to values for the 20 trials of each of the five training days. (Adapted from Beres & Baron, 1981, Figure 1.)

are able to acquire new skills but that they often have little recollection of having done so. The first anecdotal report of this dissociation between learning and episodic memory (i.e., memory for some personally experienced event; see Chapter 5, pp. 132–133) was by the Swiss psychiatrist Claparede (1911). While working with a Korsakoff's amnesic patient, Claparede pricked the patient's hand with a pin hidden in his hand. The patient subsequently withdrew her hand from Claparede but without knowing why she did so. She had acquired a conditioned-avoidance response without conscious recollection of the conditions producing the conditioning. Years later Weiskrantz and Warrington (1979) produced laboratory evidence for the existence of a similar dissociation between a classically conditioned eyeblink response and memory of having participated in the training situation. The two subjects were organic amnesics who did acquire the conditioned eyeblink to some degree in a single training session and manifested retention of the CR to the CS over a 24-hr interval. Even after only 10 min following the training session the patients did not remember what had happened during that session, and they expressed unfamiliarity with the conditioning equipment. Conditioning is clearly not the only form of learning entering into this kind of dissociation. For example, Milner (1962) reported that the famous amnesic patient H. M. was able to show considerable improvement in mirror-drawing proficiency over practice sessions spread over three days, but that he had no memory on each day of having practiced previously on the task. Other investigators have demonstrated a similar dissociation for a wide variety of other tasks, such as motor-skill learning (Corkin, 1968). Dissociations are also a characteristic of what has become known as implicit memory (see Chapter 11, p. 372).

In contemporary psychology, the acquisition of a skill per se is commonly referred to as *procedural learning* when there is a dissociation between it and episodic memory components of the task. The dissociation in memory-impaired individuals between procedural learning and its episodic-memory correlates has become a concept of growing interest in research on normally aging individuals. The question being asked is whether or not their age-related memory impairments are sufficiently similar to those of organic amnesics to produce a dissociation.

Before examining the limited evidence for dissociation in normally aging individuals, we need to point out that the episodic by-products of skill acquisition need not be limited to memory for participation in training and practice sessions. It seems highly unlikely that normally aging individuals will have a problem remembering such experiences as having their eyes blasted by an airpuff or having to struggle to learn mirror-drawing. However, there are more subtle memory by-products of the training experience for which memory may be impaired in late adulthood.

What we mean by by-products may be illustrated by reference to a study by N. J. Cohen and Squire (1980). They trained amnesic patients (including another famous patient, N. A.) and age-matched control subjects on a mirror-reading task, a task that involves the acquisition of a perceptual skill. The subjects saw a series of mirror reflections of word triads exposed by means of a tachistoscope. They read five blocks of 10 triads on each of three consecutive days, followed by a fourth block approximately 13 wk later. Within each block, half of the triads were common to all of the blocks (i.e., they were repeated in every block), and half were unique to that block (i.e., they were never repeated in other blocks). Shown in Figure 2.12 are the mean reading times per triad for N. A., a subgroup of Korsakoff's patients, and a subgroup of patients with amnesia induced by electroconvulsive therapy (or ECT), together with the mean reading times for the appropriate control groups. For the nonrepeated triads, note that the learning curves for the amnesic subjects and their control subjects were virtually indistinguishable. Thus, procedural learning (in this case, acquiring a pattern-recognition skill) was unaffected by the otherwise severe memory impairment. The outcome was quite different, however, for the repeated triads. For the control subjects, the speed of reading was greatly facilitated by remembering the words that had been read previously. The facilitation was much less for the amnesic subjects. Although

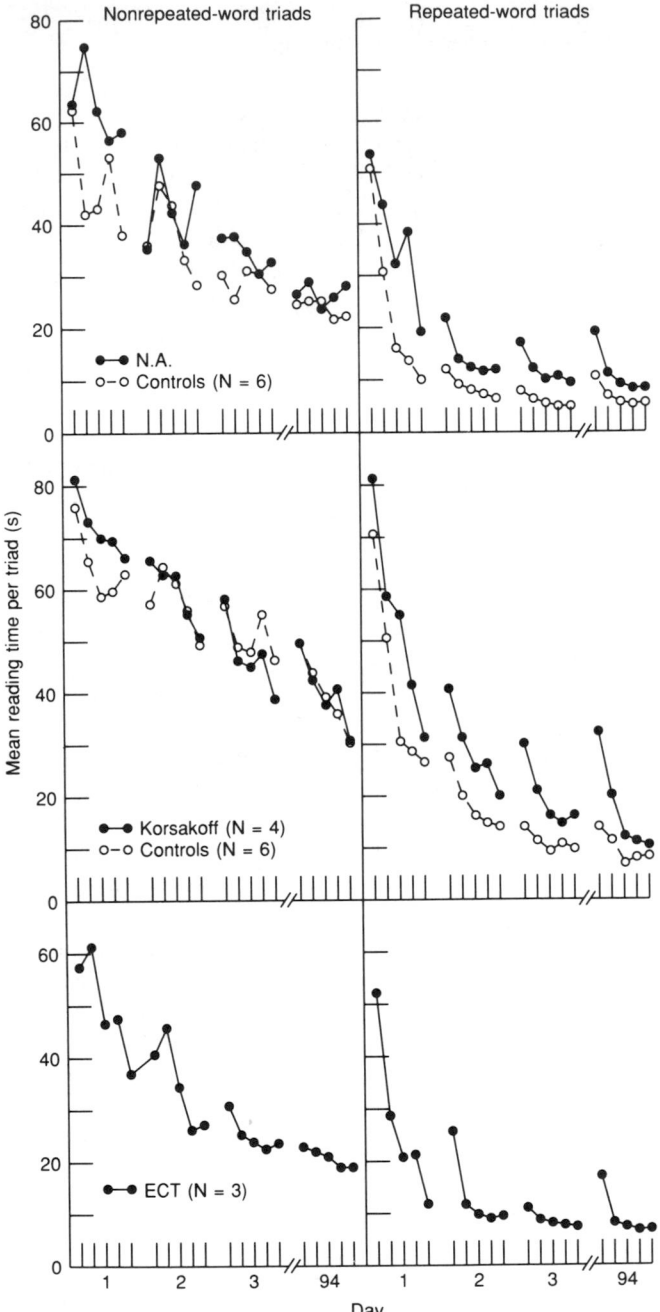

FIGURE 2.12 Acquisition of a mirror-reading skill during three daily sessions, and retention 3 ms later. The ability to mirror-read unique (nonrepeated) words was acquired at a normal rate by amnesic patients. The ability of amnesic patients to mirror read repeated words was inferior to the control rate because amnesic patients, unlike control subjects, could not remember the specific words that had been read. (Reprinted from Cohen & Squire, 1980, Figure 2. Copyright 1980 by the AAAS.)

they learned well to read mirror reflections of words as a general skill, they had difficulty remembering what words they had been reading.

Moscovitch, Winocur, and McLachlan (1986) employed a somewhat similar task with young adults and normally aging elderly adults as subjects (along with several other groups, including institutionalized elderly adults). They had their subjects read sentences in both normal script and geometrically transformed script (each letter was rotated 180° during an initial session and additional sessions 1 to 2 hr later and 2 wk later). Our interest is in the reading times for the transformed sentences. For the later reading sessions, some of the sentences were new ones that had not been encountered before, whereas others were repeated from the first reading session. Shown in part A of Figure 2.13 are mean reading times from session to session for the nonrepeated sentences. It is obvious that procedural learning, again in the form of acquiring a general pattern-recognition skill, occurred for both age groups and somewhat equivalently so for young and elderly subjects. That is, there was no apparent Age × Sessions interaction effect. Shown in part B of Figure 2.13 are the comparable mean reading times for repeated sentences. For both age groups there was clearly a savings from prior readings of the same sentences, and again to about the same degree for young and old subjects (i.e., no Age × Sessions interaction effect). This pattern clearly conflicts with that found by Cohen and Squire (1980) for amnesics and controls in reading times for repeated mirror-transformed words. Presumably, prior episodic content was as available for enhancing reading time for the elderly subjects as for the young subjects. That is, there was no dissociation present for the elderly subjects. Moscovitch et al. (1986) also asked their subjects after they had read each sentence in the delay sessions whether they were old (i.e., had been read before) or new (i.e., not read before). Here the age difference in hit rate for old sentences was roughly comparable to what is usually found on recognition-memory tests for verbal items. After 1 to 2 hr, the hit rates were 98% and 94% for young and old subjects, respectively; after 2 wk, they were 79% and 54%. Forgetting the content of the sentences was considerably greater for the elderly than for the young subjects. This evidence does suggest a dissociation for the elderly subjects when conscious recollection of the prior episodes is required. Nevertheless, there is no reason to believe that these results imply a dissociation between procedural learning and episodic memory that is anywhere near the magnitude found for severely memory-impaired amnesic patients. In fact, classification of mirror-reading as a procedural learning task for normally aging elderly adults is questionable.

This conclusion is supported by the results obtained by Hashtroudi, Chrosniak, and Schwartz (1991; Experiment 1). The task in their experiment was a variation of the mirror-reading task in which subjects read individual inverted words rather than sentences. Both new words and previously encountered words appeared over nine trials. Skill learning, defined here as the increment over trials

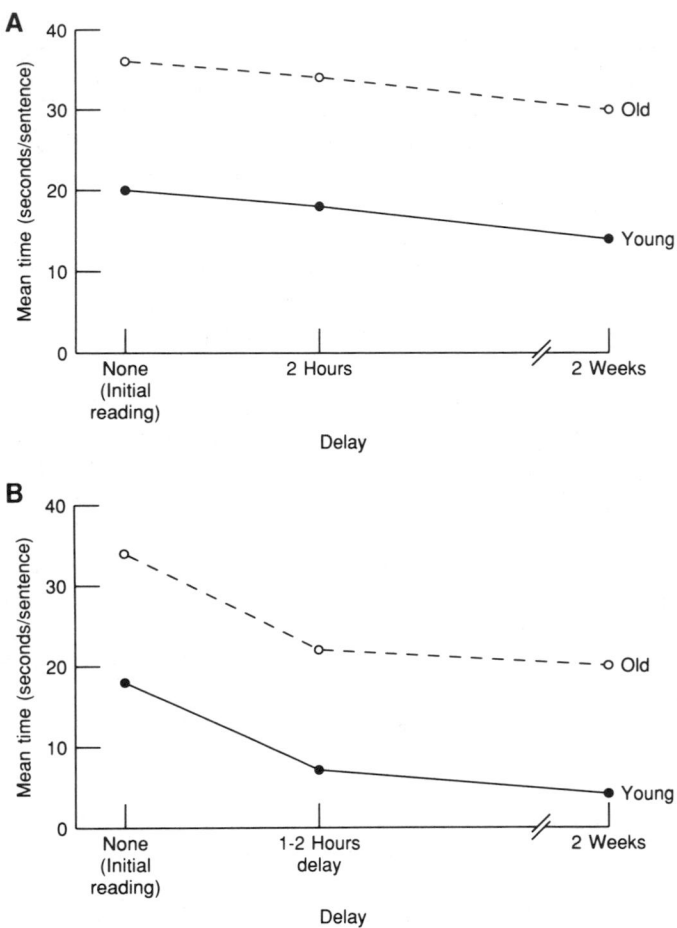

FIGURE 2.13 Reading times for geometrically transformed sentences. A: New sentences at each session. B: Repeated sentences. (Adapted from Moscovitch, Winocur, & McLachlan, 1986, Table 3.)

in the proportion of new words read correctly, increased more slowly for their elderly subjects than for their young subjects when each inverted word was presented for the same brief duration (450 ms) for every subject. However, this difference in learning rate disappeared when the exposure duration was increased (to 900 ms) for their elderly subjects. Most important, there was no age difference in the increased proportion of repeated words read correctly, relative to nonrepeated words, that occurred over trials. This suggests again the absence of a true dissociation in which an age-related deficit occurs for an episodic by-product of skill learning but not for learning the skill per se.

Evidence for Procedural Learning in Late Adulthood

A comparison of age differences for skill learning and for an episodic-memory by-product of that learning was also made by Howard and Howard (1989). Their preference, however, was to refer to indirect and direct tests of memory rather than to procedural learning and episodic memory tests. They employed a task patterned after one introduced by Nissen (Knopman & Nissen, 1987; Nissen & Bullemer, 1987). Subjects perform on a serial-reaction-time task in which an asterisk appears on a computer screen in one of four different spatial locations on each trial. The subject's task is to push one of four corresponding keys as each asterisk appears, with the same serial pattern of responding occurring repeatedly over many trials. Willingham, Nissen, and Bullemer (1989) demonstrated with young adult subjects that even those subjects who report no conscious awareness of the recurring pattern nevertheless show steady reductions in their reaction times per response unit. That is, they manifested skill or procedural learning without awareness of its occurrence.

In Howard and Howard's (1989) study, young adult and elderly subjects received four blocks of many trials in which there was either a 10-element or a 16-element pattern of responding that was repeated on each trial. As may be seen in Figure 2.14, both age groups "learned" the recurring pattern for both lengths of

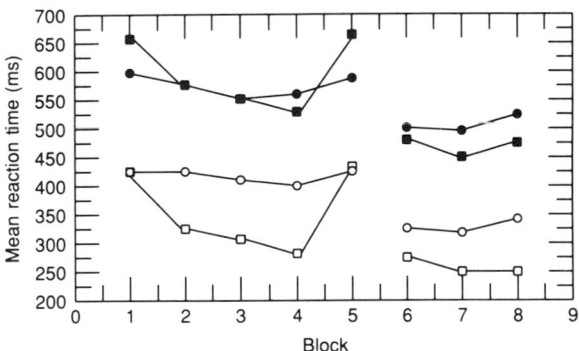

FIGURE 2.14 Mean of median response times in milliseconds as a function of block in the serial-reaction-time task. The two upper curves are for the older, and the lower curves for the younger participants. The short 10-element patterns are marked by squares and the long 16-element patterns by circles. ■, older subjects, short pattern; □, younger subjects, short pattern; ●, older subjects, long pattern; ○, younger subjects, long pattern. (Reprinted from Howard & Howard, 1989, Figure 1. Copyright 1989 by the American Psychological Association.)

series. That is, both age groups displayed a steady decrease in reaction time per response unit from the first through the fourth block of trials, and equivalently so, at least as indexed by the absence of a significant Age × Blocks interaction effect. The fourth block of trials was followed by a fifth block of trials in which the asterisks appeared in a different random order on each trial. The prior learning of a patterned sequence was irrelevant here, and accordingly reaction times increased for both age groups (see Figure 2.14). After a 30-min retention interval, the subjects returned to performance on the repeated sequences for three more blocks of trials, with further increments in speed of responding occurring over these blocks of trials (see Figure 2.14). Howard and Howard (1989) concluded from these results that there was no age difference in indirect learning, or skill/ procedural learning, in which conscious recollection of the pattern was not required (conscious recollection also plays an important role in research on implicit memory; see Chapter 11, pp. 383–385). This outcome could also be viewed as demonstrating preserved episodic memory for the content by both age groups, when recollection of that content is not required.

The situation is much like that for Moscovitch et al.'s (1986) elderly subjects who demonstrated a pronounced savings in reading transformed sentences that had been encountered previously. Procedural learning per se in Howard and Howard's (1989) study would be demonstrated by faster response times across trials when a new random pattern is presented on each trial, much like the new sentences in Moscovitch et al.'s (1986) study. That is, subjects would be demonstrating their mastery of the procedure required to translate each stimulus into a response as rapidly as possible, a phenomenon comparable to what is called nonspecific transfer with verbal learning materials (see Chapter 4, pp. 117–122). This condition was not included in Howard and Howard's (1989) study, making it impossible to determine if the age groups were comparable in procedural learning per se. The learning curves reported in their study may actually reflect the combined effects of procedural learning and memory for content without conscious recollection being required. However, this seems unlikely. In a later study, Howard and Howard (1992; Experiment 2) did include a condition in which each block of trials was a new random pattern as well as a condition in which the pattern was the same for each block of trials. For both young and elderly subjects, there was no significant change in response times from the first block of trials to the last block of trials in the random-pattern condition. By contrast, for both age groups, there was a significant decline in response times from the first to last blocks (and equally so for the two age groups) in the repeated pattern condition, thus replicating the outcome of their earlier (Howard & Howard, 1989) study. As noted by Howard and Howard, "This pattern suggests that general practice with the task (the random group) was having little effect on response time and that most of the improvement seen in the patterned groups was due to specific learning of the pattern" (1992, pp. 237–238).

Most important, Howard and Howard (1989) also gave their subjects a final block of trials in which conscious recollection of the episodic content of the repeated sequences was required—or direct memory, in their terms. Here subjects were asked to anticipate throughout each sequence of asterisks where the next one in the sequence would appear. There was a substantial age-related deficit in the accuracy of these anticipations, with the young and elderly subjects correctly anticipating 80% and 66%, respectively, on the short sequence and 58% and 41% on the long sequence. Howard and Howard concluded that "the dissociative effects of aging on direct versus indirect tests of memory that have been demonstrated for verbal materials also occur for a nonverbal serial sequence" (1989, p. 362). (The reference to verbal materials is in regard to tests of explicit and implicit memory for words in a list; see Chapter 11). Stated somewhat differently, what they demonstrated was an age-related deficit for the memory of a pattern of stimuli that was apparent only when a test requiring conscious recollection of that pattern was required. An age-related deficit on a comparable direct test, but not on a comparable indirect test, was also found in their later study (Howard & Howard, 1992). Thus, their normally aging subjects appeared to show a true dissociation.

Research on the "dissociative effects" of normal aging is still in its infancy. It is important to determine if the dissociative effects of the magnitude observed by Howard and Howard (1989) for procedural learning and the episodic by-products of that learning that require conscious recollection can be demonstrated for other tasks. A unique outcome in their study was the apparent equality in learning rate between young and elderly subjects on the procedural task. On many other learning tasks this probably would not be the case. The demonstration of a dissociation for elderly adults presumably requires the absence of an age-related deficit on the procedural task, combined with the presence of an age-related deficit on the episodic/recollection test. The generalizability of the outcome obtained by Howard and Howard (1989, 1992) to tasks other than their specific serial-reaction-time task must, unfortunately, be questioned by the results obtained by Harrington and Haaland (1992). Their young and elderly subjects performed on a serial-reaction-time task in which sequences of hand postures were either repeated over trials or were different sequences on each trial. In this case, performance over trials for their elderly subjects did not improve for either the random sequences or the repeated sequences. Consequently, procedural learning was apparent only for their young subjects. Thus, there was no dissociation—the elderly subjects were as impaired on the indirect test as they were on the direct test in which conscious recollection of the repeated sequence was required.

CHAPTER • 3

Verbal Learning

Introduction

Our emphasis shifts in this chapter from nonverbal learning to verbal learning. The traditional tasks employed in verbal learning research, both basic and gerontological, have been those of paired-associate learning and serial learning. In addition to reviewing aging research on these tasks, we will also review in Chapter 4 aging research in the related areas of transfer and mnemonics.

Adult Age Differences in Paired-Associate Learning

In many respects the paired-associate-learning task has been the prototypal one for investigating adult age differences in associative learning. The task is structured in terms of stimulus (S) and response (R) elements. Subjects receive a list to study in which there are multiple pairs of S and R elements (see, for example, the pairs listed in Table 3.1), with their task being to learn to respond with the R element of each pair when its S element is presented alone. Presumably, practice on the list assures the acquisition of an association between each pair of S and R elements. Acquisition of the list is complete when all of the R elements can be elicited by their S elements on a given trial without error. The importance of paired-associate learning is highlighted by the fact that much of real-life learning over the adult life span can be conceptualized in terms of learning associations between S and R elements (Belbin & Downs, 1965). Included are associations between faces as S elements and names as R elements, foreign-language words as S elements and their English translation as R elements, names of cities as S elements and names of their athletic teams in those cities as R elements, and so on. Learning of this kind takes place throughout the life span. We have good reason therefore to be interested in how aging affects paired-associate learning proficiency.

Historical Perspective: Early Studies

The broad scope of paired-associate learning is indicated further by the fact that many tasks, although not formally structured as paired associates (i.e., S and R elements are not identified as such to the learner), may, nevertheless, be conceptualized in terms of paired-associate learning. A digit-symbol test is such a task. Here subjects are given a coding system in which the digits 1 through 9 are each equated with an abstract symbol (e.g., $9 = >$). The code itself is in full view as subjects substitute symbols for the digits as they appear over and over in random order in a test booklet. In principle, each digit-symbol combination can be viewed as a paired associate (e.g., 9 as the S element for $>$ as the R element). Following performance on this task, subjects may be tested, unexpectedly, for the extent of paired-associate learning occurring during performance. This is accomplished by presenting the digits alone and asking subjects to reproduce for each one the symbol previously paired with it. It is exactly this procedure that provided what was probably the first evidence of adult age differences in paired-associate learning (Willoughby, 1927, 1929). In general, Willoughby found a trend toward lower symbol recall scores with increasing age over the adult life span. The fact that the subjects in this study were not informed in advance that their learning of digit-symbol pairs would eventually be assessed makes this a test of age differences in incidental learning. We will have more to say about age differences in incidental learning both later in this chapter and in following chapters.

The first study to examine adult age differences in paired-associate learning with truly elderly subjects included in the study and with formally structured S-and-R-paired elements and under intentional-learning conditions was that of Ruch (1934). (An earlier study by Thorndike et al., 1928, involved only young adult and middle-aged subjects). This is the same study that examined age differences in pursuit-rotor learning (Chapter 2, pp. 37–38); the same subjects served in both phases of the study. Interestingly, Ruch broadened the generalizability of his results by having all of his subjects practice on three different kinds of lists (see Table 3.1 for examples of pairs in each list).

One list consisted of word pairs in which the S and R elements were deliberately made to be logically related. The relationship was created by selecting R elements that were low word associates of their paired S elements (e.g., white and pink). Ruch (1934) believed that age differences in learning would be relatively slight for this kind of familiar material. Later investigators employing words as S and R elements have usually made sure that the paired words are associatively *unrelated* to each other at the start of practice, unless the effects of pre-experimental associative relatedness on rate of acquisition are of concern in their experiments (see pp. 84–86). A second list consisted of false equations of the kind shown in Table 3.1. Ruch (1934) believed that age differences, favoring younger subjects, would be especially pronounced for this kind of material. The reasoning was

TABLE 3.1

Sample Pairs Used in Three Lists[a]

		Type of list			
Word pairs		False equations		Nonsense equations	
S element	R element	S element	R element	S element	R element
Soft	Chair	3×3	4	$B \times D$	M
Nest	Owl	3×1	3	$A \times M$	B
Room	Light	5×5	11	$S \times Q$	H
White	Pink	6×3	5	$L \times B$	D

[a] From Ruch, 1934 and Korchin and Basowitz, 1957.

much like that given earlier for mirror-vision performance on the pursuit-rotor task. He assumed that the list material generated interference from past habits (e.g., the habit of responding "9" to 3×3, instead of responding "4," the R element actually paired with 3×3; see Table 3.1) and that this interference increases with increasing age. In effect, Ruch (1934) was studying negative transfer in which List 2 was the laboratory-acquired list and List 1 was a "list" acquired prior to entering the laboratory (to be discussed further when we examine transfer

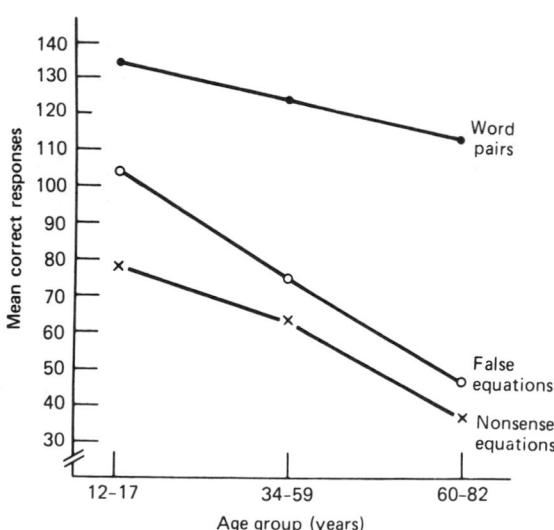

FIGURE 3.1 Age differences in paired-associate learning for three different kinds of material. (Adapted from data in Ruch, 1934.)

research in Chapter 4). The third list consisted of nonsense equations of the kind shown in Table 3.1. Age differences for this list were expected to fall in between those found for the other two lists. Ruch's predictions were fully confirmed, as can be seen in Figure 3.1 for the total number of correct responses (summed over the 15 trials given on each list; maximum score = 150 for each 10-pair list). From these results, Ruch concluded that there is an age-related deficit in paired-associate learning and that the magnitude of the deficit varies greatly with the attributes of the to-be-learned material.

Historical Perspective: Methodological Problems and Issues

Ruch (1934) was a pioneer, alas, in another way as well. His study was not only the first to report age-related deficits in formal paired-associate learning, but it was also the first to suffer many of the interpretative problems that long plagued aging research on verbal learning. The first problem in his study is the classic one of whether the reported age-related deficits resulted from a true ontogenetic change or from cohort differences. His older subjects obviously came from an earlier cohort or generation than his younger subjects, and the former may therefore have differed from the latter in their educational levels and other non-age variables, such as verbal ability, that differ among cohorts. It may be these differences rather than age per se that may have accounted for the slower learning by his older subjects (see Kausler, 1991, for a detailed discussion of cohort effects). Ruch's (1934) description of his age groups sheds little light on this issue. No information is given about non-age attributes of his subjects other than the brief notation that all of his subjects appeared to have a high socioeconomic background. This is a problem probably of greater magnitude than it was for the pursuit-rotor component of his study. That is, age differences in education and verbal ability are more likely to be confounding factors on a verbal-learning task than on a nonverbal-learning task. Pronounced age differences were also found by Pacaud in a study conducted around 1950 (as reported by Welford, 1989) for the recall of 25 pairs after a single study trial. The subjects were the same ones who performed on the motor-skills task described earlier (see p. 39). They were all French railway workers ranging in age from the 20s to the 50s. Although the subjects did have a common occupational tie, there is no assurance that those of different ages were equivalent in such non-age variables as educational level.

Fortunately, awareness of the importance of balancing age groups on critical non-age attributes had grown to the point that when Korchin and Basowitz (1957) replicated Ruch's (1934) study nearly 25 years later, they carefully matched their young (mean age, 26.8 years) and elderly (mean age, 78.1 years) with respect to scores on the Wechsler vocabulary test. Even with this matching, elderly subjects continued to have lower learning scores than young adult subjects on all three lists (now abbreviated to eight pairs and to six learning trials). As in

Ruch's (1934) study, the age difference favoring young adults was least for word pairs. Unlike Ruch's study, however, age differences were about the same for the false-equations list as for the nonsense-equations list. Of interest is the fact that Gladis and Braun (1958) and Arenberg (1967a) compared young adult and elderly subjects on the same paired-associate list (but with a different content than the content in Ruch's lists) and under almost identical practice conditions. The mean score did not change greatly from 1958 to 1967 for either age group. Consequently, the age-related deficit was about the same in 1967 as it was in 1957, despite the temporal separation of the two studies and the use of young adult and elderly subjects from different generations. These time-lag results (i.e., a comparison of subjects of the same age who were tested in widely separated years), combined with the results of later cross-sectional studies reporting comparable age-related deficits for age groups roughly comparable on such non-age attributes as educational level and verbal ability (e.g., Kausler & Puckett, 1980a; Salthouse, Kausler, & Saults, 1988a), make it highly likely that the age-related deficits are the products of ontogenetic change rather than cohort differences in learning proficiency. Especially important are the age differences reported by Salthouse et al. (1988a) with large samples of noncollege young adults (20–39 years of age), middle aged adults (40–59 years of age), and elderly adults (60–79 years of age), as well as college-student young adults. Actually, there were two independent studies, each with large samples. In each study subjects received two trials on an eight pair list composed of four-letter nouns as both S and R elements. Shown in Table 3.2 are the mean percentage of correct responses on Trial 2 for the age groups in each study. Note not only the presence of a pronounced age-related deficit for the elderly subjects in each study (relative to both college students and noncollege young adults) but also the fact that the deficit was already pronounced for the middle-aged subjects.

A remaining problem in accepting these age differences as resulting from a true age change in paired-associate learning ability is the likelihood that the health status of elderly subjects is poorer than that of younger adults. Diminished

TABLE 3.2
Percentage of Correct Responses on Trial 2 of a Paired-Associate-Learning Task[a]

Study	College students	Age group 20–39	40–59	60–79
Study 1	73.5	54.9	43.8	38.9
Study 2	66.0	61.8	45.3	33.8

[a] Salthouse, Kausler, & Saults, 1988a, Table 1. (Copyright 1988 by the American Psychological Association. Adapted by permission.)

physical health, rather than aging per se, could have produced the age differences reported by Salthouse et al. (1988a) and other earlier investigators employing the cross-sectional method of assessing age differences in paired-associate learning proficiency. This seems unlikely, however. Salthouse, Kausler, and Saults (1990) reanalyzed the learning scores from their earlier study by adjusting for several variables related to physical health status. As may be seen in Figure 3.2, the adjustment had virtually no effect on the pronounced negative linear relationship between age and learning scores.

Our conclusion regarding a true age change in paired-associate learning proficiency is strengthened by the longitudinal decrement in paired-associate learning scores reported by Gilbert (1935, 1973) and by Arenberg and Robertson-Tchabo (1977). Longitudinally tested subjects are obviously from the same cohort at each age they are tested. In Arenberg and Robertson-Tchabo's (1977) study the subjects were participants in the Baltimore Longitudinal Study. They were tested on alternate forms of the paired-associate-learning task to reduce the magnitude of progressive error. For one of the groups of subjects, the first list was acquired when they were around 40 yr of age and the second when they neared 50 yr of age. For another group, the lists were acquired when the subjects were around 55 yr of age and when they were in their early 60s. This procedure was repeated for a number of other age contrasts. The longitudinal decrements in performance, as expressed by mean errors made in learning the lists, may be seen in Figure 3.3 for subjects at age 40 and age 55 or so at the time of initial testing.

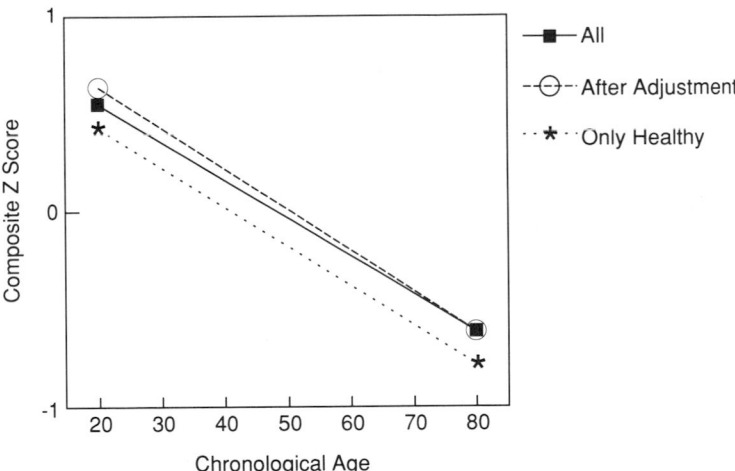

FIGURE 3.2 Relationship between age and paired-associate-learning scores as adjusted for health status. (Adapted from Salthouse, Kausler, & Saults, 1990, Figure 2.)

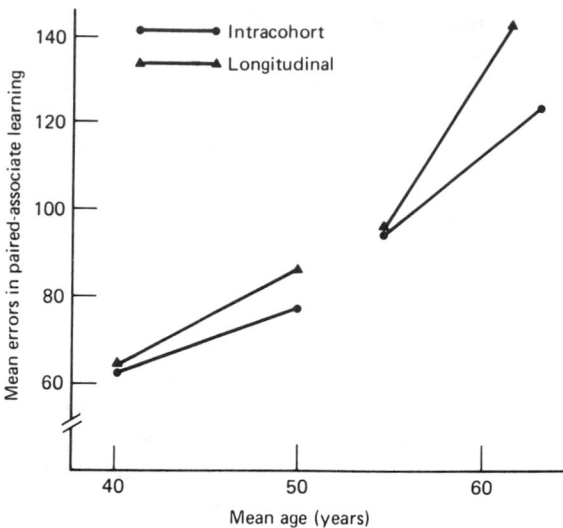

FIGURE 3.3 Age differences in paired-associate learning as assessed by two methods; intracohort cross-sectional and longitudinal. (Reprinted from Arenberg & Robertson-Tchabo, 1977, Figure 1. Copyright 1977 by Van Nostrand Reinhold Publishing.)

A related issue concerns the possibility of the age-related decline in paired-associate learning being greater for men than for women, and it may therefore be exaggerated in studies like that of Arenberg and Robertson-Tchabo (1977) in which only male subjects were involved. In general, women outperform men on a number of verbal learning tasks (e.g., Bolla-Wilson & Bleecker, 1986; Larrabee & Crook, 1993). Verbal learning is believed to involve a left-hemisphere function, and there is evidence suggesting that this function declines with normal aging to a greater degree for men than for women (Gur et al., 1991). It is therefore possible that the age-related decline in paired-associate learning proficiency may be greater for men than for women. However, Larrabee and Crook (1993), with a large sample ranging in age from 17 to 79 yr, failed to find a significant Age × Gender interaction in paired-associate learning scores. The implication is that the age-related decline in proficiency is no greater for men than for women, even though women do tend to outperform men overall.

A second problem inherent in Ruch's (1934) study is the difficulty of determining whether the age differences reported there represent true differences in learning ability or merely differences in performance. Ruch was well aware of the learning-performance distinction. In fact, he was quite concerned about the possibility that his older subjects could be less motivated and less involved with the task than his younger subjects. To enhance motivation, he paid his subjects for their participation. (An interesting pay scale was devised. Subjects received 2 cents per year of age for a 2-hr laboratory session. Thus a 60-year-old subject earned the grand sum of $1.20!). Moreover, Ruch (1934) observed that his oldest subjects gave every indication of being highly involved with the tasks. It does seem unlikely that extrinsic motivational factors alone could account for the pronounced age differences found in this study or in later studies reporting substantial age-related deficits in paired-associate learning. It could also be argued that the elderly subjects in Ruch's study, and in later studies as well, had a higher anxiety level than the young subjects and therefore had a higher drive level. High anxious subjects do perform more poorly than low anxious subjects on a paired-associate learning task (see Spence, 1958). However, as noted earlier (p. 10), it is unlikely that there is any pronounced age difference in anxiety level. A more serious problem is the possibility that age differences in fatigue contributed substantially to the age difference in learning scores (Jerome, 1959), as it may on an intelligence test (Furry & Baltes, 1973). The verbal learning tasks in Ruch's (1934) study were always given after the two practice sessions on the pursuit-rotor task (which can be a fatiguing experience). Of course, confounding by fatigue was an unlikely problem in Korchin and Basowitz's (1957) study, and pronounced age differences on the same task employed by Ruch (1934) remained.

The final problem is an important one that has received all too little attention by experimental aging psychologists. It concerns the nature of the dependent variable, or performance scores, employed by Ruch (1934), namely, total correct responses over a fixed number of trials. Do age differences on this overall score necessarily indicate age differences in learning when learning is defined in terms of the rate of acquiring new material (Jerome, 1959)? It is conceivable that elderly adults learn new material as rapidly as young adults—once the elderly adults get going on the task at hand. If true, the low overall score earned by the elderly subjects would be attributable entirely to their slow start. Beyond the first few trials, learning proficiency may be as great for elderly adults as for young adults.

Answers to questions about age differences in rate of learning require a finer grained analysis than the kind used by Ruch. What is needed is a trial-by-trial analysis of increments in scores on the learning task. This analysis yields what is called a *learning curve*. Our interest rests in age differences in paired-associate learning curves, differences that presumably reflect differences in rates of learning. Unfortunately, many of the aging studies on paired-associate learning that followed Ruch copied his mode of analysis and reported only total scores. There have been important exceptions, however. One of the first was in Korchin and Basowitz's (1957) replication study. They reported negatively accelerated learning curves for both age groups on all three of their lists. The curves for the word-pair list are shown in the part A of Figure 3.4. It may be seen that the age groups differed greatly in amount recalled after one study trial. Beyond that point, the two groups gained in amount recalled at approximately the same rate (by the

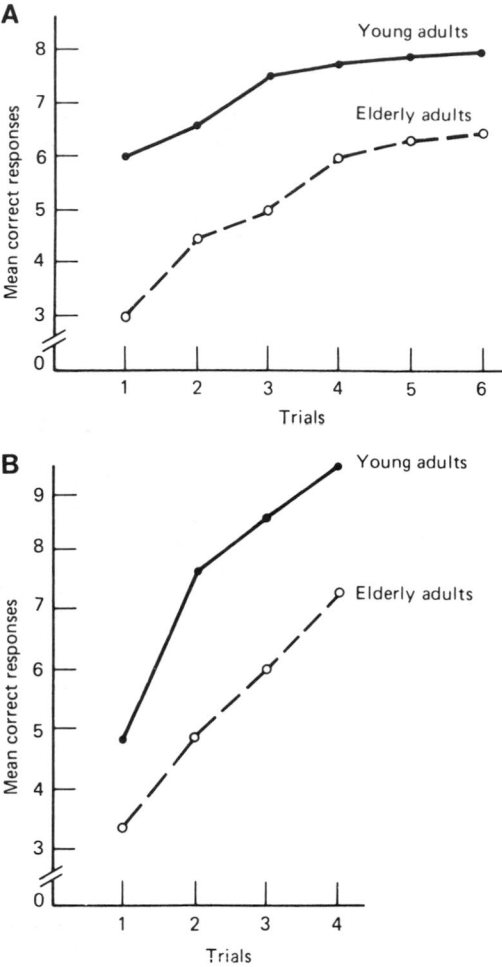

FIGURE 3.4 Learning curves for paired-associate learning by young and elderly subjects. (A: Adapted from Korchin & Basowitz, 1957, Figure 1. B: Adapted from data in Kausler & Puckett, 1980a.)

fourth trial, age comparisons are complicated by an obvious ceiling effect for young adults that was not present for elderly adults). The learning curves for the other two lists revealed very similar patterns. From this evidence, it could be argued that the elderly do have trouble activating their learning processes (a point we will return to in our later discussion of nonspecific transfer), but once these processes are activated, elderly subjects progress as well on a learning task as do young adult subjects.

Unfortunately, the results obtained by Korchin and Basowitz (1957) are more the exception than the rule. There have been several studies over the years for which trial-by-trial data are available. In general, these studies do indicate a slower rate of learning for elderly subjects than for young adult subjects. For example, Kausler and Puckett (1980a) gave their subjects four trials on their 10-pair list (nouns as both S and R elements). The mean number of correct anticipations of R elements over the four trials are shown in part B of Figure 3.4. Note the disparity on Trial 1 between age groups, but, more important, note the more rapid gain from Trial 1 to Trial 2 and from Trial 2 to Trial 3 for the young adults than for the elderly adults (by Trial 4, a ceiling effect is apparent for the young adults). Similar age differences in rate of learning are obvious in data reported by Monge (1971) and by Winn, Elias, and Marshall (1976). Their learning curves are expressed in a different format than that of a trial-by-trial analysis. The mean number of trials taken to reach successive criteria of mastery are determined for each age group. These successive criteria are one correct response, two correct responses, and so on, through N (the number of pairs in the list) correct responses. The list contained 10 word pairs in Monge's (1971) study and 7 nonsense-shape/nonsense-syllable (S-element/R-element) pairs in Winn et al.'s (1976) study. The curves found in Monge's study for subjects in their 20s and 50s are plotted in part A of Figure 3.5. It can be seen that the older subjects manifested a slower rate of mastery of the pairs than the younger subjects. An even greater disparity in rate of learning between young (mean age = 20 yr) and elderly (mean age = 65 yr) subjects is apparent in the results obtained by Winn et al. (1976) and plotted in part B of Figure 3.5. The greater disparity in learning rates found by Winn et al. (1976) than by Monge (1971) is probably the consequence of the greater difficulty of the learning materials entering into the former study. Leech and Witte (1971) did find that the rate of learning of elderly subjects could be accelerated by rewarding each correct response. Young adult subjects were not included in their study. However, it seems likely that their learning rate would also have been stimulated by rewards for correct responses, thus leaving the age difference in rate unaffected.

In summary, many laboratory studies have revealed that paired-associate learning proficiency is highly age sensitive. However, we need to recognize the strong possibility that these studies overestimate the extent of age-related deficits in everyday paired-associate learning. That is, the ecological validity (generalizability to the everyday world) of these studies is less than perfect. Laboratory studies typically employ a number of pairs (often as many as 12) within the to-be-learned list. In the everyday world, the "list" is likely to be much shorter. For example, elderly adults attending a social event may encounter one or two new face-name pairs they would like to learn—but not 10 or 12. Interpair interference tends to be generated when multiple pairs are to be acquired simultaneously (Battig, 1968). That is, there is the tendency for the R element of one pair to generalize

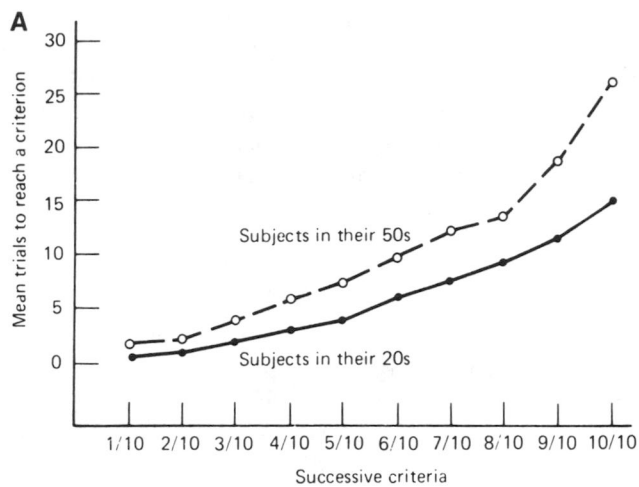

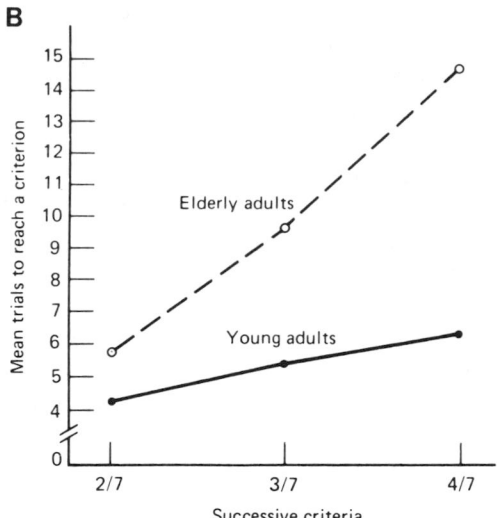

FIGURE 3.5 Learning curves for paired-associate learning by young and elderly subjects plotted as trials to attain successive criteria. (A: Adapted from data in Monge, 1971. B: Adapted from Winn, Elias, & Marshall, 1976, Table 2.)

erroneously to the S element of another pair. There is the definite possibility that the amount of interpair interference is greater for older adults than for younger adults (Kausler, 1989a). If true, then older adults are at a particular disadvantage in learning multiple paired associates. In addition, paired items in most laboratory studies are presented at a rapid rate (e.g., 2 or 3 s per pair) for study. In the everyday world, the study of paired items is likely to be self-paced. We will discover later (pp. 88–89) that the age-related deficit in learning even lengthy lists is greatly diminished with self-pacing. Finally, much of our everyday paired-associate learning occurs incidentally. Laboratory research, however, has focused on the intentional learning of paired associates. Age-related deficits in acquiring new information may be greater when that information is acquired intentionally than when it is acquired incidentally.

Stage Analysis of Potential Age-Sensitive Processes

Although expressed only vaguely, Ruch's (1934) theoretical orientation in his pioneering study was decidedly that of classical associationism. In classical associationism the major acquisition process is the accrual of S-to-R associative strength with rote rehearsal. Old habits, defined as associations learned prior to performance on the laboratory tasks, were expected to benefit elderly subjects in learning weakly related word pairs and to hinder them in learning false equations. Positive and negative effects were to be evaluated relative to the presumed neutral condition of learning nonsense equations. Here learning from scratch was demanded. That is, learning had to start from zero associative strength between S and R elements and build connections gradually by means of rehearsal responses. The age deficit manifested in this condition could, therefore, be viewed as evidence for decreasing associative-learning proficiency with increasing age. The adversity could either be diminished, as in the word-pairs condition, or increased, as in the false-equations condition, contingent on the kind and amount of transfer from past associative learning extant during practice on the task at hand.

This single-process view of age-related deficits in paired-associate learning remained dominant until the advent of stage analysis in the 1960s (Underwood & Schulz, 1960), in which paired-associate learning was conceptualized as undergoing four stages of acquisition, one of which of is the learning of S-to-R associations. The other three stages are response learning, stimulus learning, and R-to-S associative learning. There was, however, an interesting precursor to formal applications of stage analysis to age-related deficits in paired-associate learning. Korchin and Basowitz (1957) had the foresight to observe that one of the probable factors contributing to age-related deficits in their study is the fact that "the older person requires more time for the integration of a response" (p. 68). Just how age differences in response learning may have contributed to the age differences in total-learning learning scores is not very clear. It is possible that numbers, the R elements in their false-equation list (see Table 3.1), are easier to learn than are letters, the R elements in their nonsense-equations list. If true, the reduction in overall difficulty produced by easier response learning could compensate for the added difficulty produced by the interference present in the false-equations condition. The net effect would be lists that are roughly equal in the amount of age-related deficit they produce (as found in Korchin and Basowitz's, 1957 study).

There is evidence of a more direct nature to support the hypothesis that response learning is indeed an age-sensitive process. Response learning means that the R elements have become individually available to the subjects for associating with their paired S elements. One way of assuring that meaningful words have become available for entry into associations is to have subjects learn them prior to encountering them in a paired-associate list. To accomplish this objective, Canestrari (1964, as reported in Botwinick, 1967) had his experimental subjects, both young adult and elderly, learn a free-recall list composed of words prior to beginning practice on a paired-associate list (the free recall task itself will be discussed in our Memory chapters). It was these words that then served as the R elements of the paired-associate list. The paired-associate-learning scores for these experimental subjects were compared with those of control subjects, again both young adult and elderly, who practiced on the same paired-associate list but without the benefit of prior learning of the R elements. In effect, only the control subjects had to go through a response-learning stage in order to master the paired-associate list. The magnitude of the age-related deficit in paired-associate-learning scores was considerably less for experimental subjects than for control subjects. Thus, the savings produced by eliminating the age-sensitive, response-learning process for experimental subjects, or at least by greatly reducing its involvement, was sufficient to reduce the handicap elderly subjects face in paired-associate learning.

A different form of the deletion method was employed by Witte and Freund (1976) in their study, but the outcome was much the same. They compared paired-associate-learning scores for subjects who had to recall each R element as its S element was presented with scores for subjects who matched each S element with each R element from separate columns of randomly ordered elements. The matching method greatly reduced the necessity of learning each R element as a separate entity. The age-related deficit was again decreased greatly when the response-learning stage was largely eliminated (see Figure 3.6). However, in neither Canestrari's (1964) nor Witte and Freund's (1976) study did the age-related deficit disappear when the response learning stage was largely eliminated (see, for example, Figure 3.6), suggesting that there are other age-sensitive stages involved in paired-associate learning.

Indirect support for response learning's age sensitivity comes from the finding that the age-related deficit in rate of learning is especially large when nonsense syllables serve as the R elements of a paired-associate list. This was the case in the study by Winn et al. (1976) cited earlier (see Figure 3.5). Nonsense syllables are elements for which response learning is especially important when those

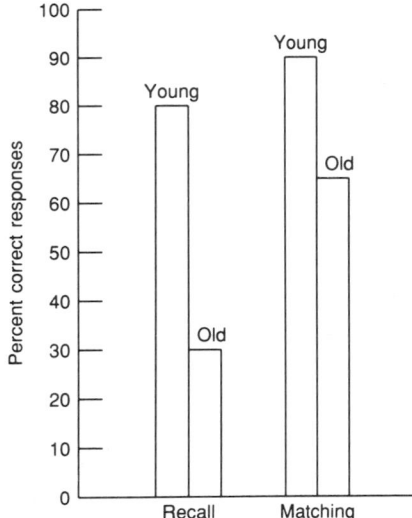

FIGURE 3.6 Age differences in correct responses on a paired-associate-learning task (Trial 3) under standard recall and matching conditions. (Adapted from Witte & Freund, 1976, Figure 1.)

elements function as responses in a paired-associate list. Syllables, such as *QOJ*, are unfamiliar to subjects prior to being encountered as the R elements of a learning list. Consequently, letters have to be integrated into novel sequences to become available as R elements for entry into S-R associations. This integrative form of response learning is generally accepted by stage analysts as being a special case of associative learning in which subjects learn associations between individual letters (see Kausler, 1974, pp. 122–130). The importance of the probable age sensitivity of this form of response learning should not be taken lightly. In real-life situations, response elements composed of unfamiliar letter sequences, such as *Ayatollah Khomeini*, are fairly common. Elderly people are likely to experience greater difficulty than young adults in integrating such sequences. Of course, the void in direct laboratory research on age differences in response integration as a form of response learning makes this conclusion quite tentative.

Another stage, or process, identified in stage analysis as being involved in paired-associate learning is that of R-S, or backward, associative learning. In effect, this process supplements S-R, or forward, associative learning. The existence of R-S associative learning becomes apparent when subjects are given an unexpected test after they have completed practice on a paired-associate list. On this test, they receive the R elements from the list, one at a time, and they are asked to recall the S element that had been paired with each R element. This test reverses the usual procedure, in which the S elements are presented and recall of the R elements is requested. It is not unusual to discover that a number of the S elements can be recalled when they are cued by their paired R elements. The process accounting for the learning of R-S associations offers no great mystery to stage analysts. They simply expand on the concept of rehearsal to include rehearsal responses directed at S elements as well as R elements. Connections in the backward direction are especially likely for subjects whose rehearsal is characterized by repeating the names of both elements of a pair throughout the pair's exposure during a study trial. For example, during exposure of the pair *apple-table*, the subject is assumed to be saying, covertly, "apple table apple table . . ." for as long as the pair is being shown. Note that *apple-table* are rehearsed contiguously but so are *table-apple*, thus promoting increments in the strength of both associations. Nevertheless, the flow of rehearsal is such that the two associations accrue strength asymmetrically, with the forward association gaining strength more rapidly than the backward association, as indicated in Figure 3.7. Consequently, more S-R associations than R-S associations should be recalled following a fixed number of trials on a paired-associate task. This expectancy has been confirmed in a number of studies (see Kausler, 1974, pp. 169–175).

The overall slower response rate of elderly adults, relative to younger adults, leads us to expect fewer rehearsal responses with increasing age and therefore fewer R-S associations that are acquired. With the free-recall task there is, in fact,

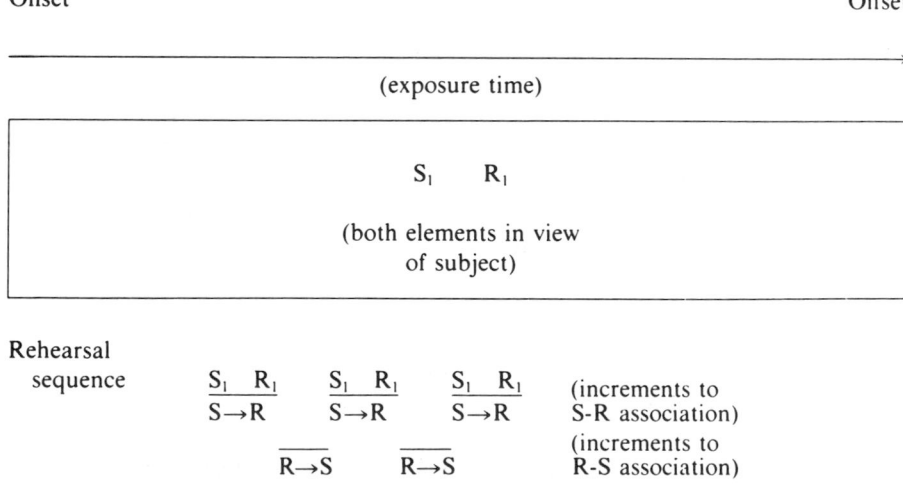

FIGURE 3.7 Schematic representation of rehearsal activity postulated to underlie the incidental learning of R-S, or backward, associations in addition to the intentional learning of S-R, or forward, associations.

evidence of fewer rehearsal responses by elderly subjects than by young subjects (see Chapter 6, pp. 177–179). In agreement with this hypothesis, Kausler and Lair (1965) found that their older subjects had a level of R-S recall that was about 71% of the amount of their S-R recall, whereas their younger subjects had a level that was about 85% of their S-R recall. Similar results were obtained later by Winn and Elias (1978). The age-related deficit found for R-S learning qualifies as an example of an age-related deficit in incidental learning. R-S learning, like the associative learning that occurs during practice on the digit–symbol test, is incidental in the sense that it occurs in the absence of intentionality to learn. However, from the perspective of stage analysis, there is nothing mysterious about either incidental learning per se or the existence of age-related deficits in incidental learning. The processes promoting the intentional learning of S-R associations are the same processes promoting the incidental learning of R-S associations. Consequently, if these processes themselves are age sensitive, whatever kinds of learning they produce should reflect that age sensitivity.

The bidirectional nature of associative learning has its real-life implications. Consider, for example, the postelection rehearsal of the list of new cabinet appointments. As subjects rehearse the fact that the new Secretary of State is Fillmore Jones, they are also rehearsing the fact that Fillmore Jones is the new Secretary of State. Thus, some learning of the R-to-S (name-to-position) association accompanies learning of the S-to-R (position-to-name) association. Our previous analysis suggests that elderly adults are likely to be less able than young adults to acquire the "Fillmore Jones is Secretary of State" association. This should be true even though the "Secretary of State is Fillmore Jones" association has been practiced enough at both age levels to reach a criterion of mastery. R-S associations also play an important role in determining transfer effects under certain conditions (to be discussed later in Chapter 4, pp. 127–128).

The third stage identified by stage analysts, that of *stimulus learning*, is a complex activity with several components. The only one we will consider, *stimulus selection*, is a further candidate for age sensitivity. Its operation focuses on the distinction between a nominal stimulus and a functional stimulus (Underwood, 1963). The distinction is probably uncalled for when a stimulus consists of a well-integrated element, such as a familiar word, as in our earlier *apple-table* example. It may be a different matter, however, when a stimulus consists of multiple components that are loosely related, if at all, to one another (e.g., the letters of a nonsense syllable, such as *JIX*). The separate components are likely to be redundant in the sense that any one alone would serve reliably as a cue for association with the response assigned to the total-stimulus element (i.e., the nominal, or experimenter-defined, stimulus). In stage analysis, the subject is viewed as being an active organism, rather than the passive being pictured by classical associationism. As an active organism, the subject may apply past habits to reduce the complexity of a current task. In this case, the past habit is our tendency to identify words largely in terms of their beginning and ending letters, while largely ignoring middle letters as being redundant sources of information. Transfer of this habit to such stimulus elements as *JIX*, means that either the initial letter or the terminal letter of the elements is likely to be selected as the effective, or functional, stimulus. Like other generalized habits, the stimulus-selection habit may decrease in its activation with increasing age, thus making stimulus selection an age-sensitive process. There are methods available for testing the operation of a selection habit (e.g., Postman & Greenbloom, 1967). Apparently, these methods have not been extended to use with elderly subjects. Consequently, nothing is known about the extent of an age-related deficit in the proficiency of this selection process.

There are many real-life situations in which opportunities for applying stimulus selection are rampant. For example, for many years Lincoln Continental automobiles contained two distinctive stimuli—a tire hump in the back and oval rear windows. These stimuli are redundant in the sense that either one, alone, may be noticed, or selected, and be associated reliably with the name of the car. Real-life exemplars of this kind offer intriguing possibilities for investigating age differences in stimulus selection under ecologically valid conditions.

The final stage is, of course, S-R associative learning. In agreement with classical associationists, stage analysts recognize that S-R associations may be acquired by rote-rehearsal activity. However, stage analysts also believe that S-R associations may be the product of mediation by an active subject who may construct, when the materials permit them, interacting images between S and R elements or sentences incorporating both S and R elements. As with the stimulus-selection process, mediation is viewed as the application of some general habit that transcends the specific elements entering into associations on the learning task in question (see Spiker, 1977). The habit was learned because its use was found in the subject's past history to facilitate learning of various tasks. Once learned, the habit, or generalized response, transfers to a new learning situation, and, once activated in the new situation, it is likely to be applied to all of the S-R components of the novel material.

The use of such mediators as imagery is assumed by stage analysts to be governed by a generalized response of the kind described above. Mediation consists of forming an interactive image that incorporates both the S element and the R element of a given pair. For example, with *apple-table* as a pair, a subject may construct an image of a huge red apple on a table that is breaking apart from the weight of the apple. Adult subjects are assumed to have learned the advantages of employing imagery to mediate associative learning long before they appear in the laboratory to master a list of paired associates. In effect, the skill of evoking images to represent linguistic events may be considered as an R element that is associated with a learning task as a broad, generic S element. Because even a novel learning task bears some degree of similarity to the many previous learning tasks encountered by a subject, it serves as an exemplar of the generic S element. Consequently, the very fact that a subject is confronted by that task serves to activate the use of imagery for mediating the specific S-R associations of the new task (Kausler, 1970). The nature of this exchange between the relevant generalized habit and the to-be-acquired novel associations is illustrated in Figure 3.8, where r_s is an internal response transforming a word to an image of that word.

The shift in perspective from that of classical associationism to that of stage analysis has important implications for the experimental psychology of aging. From the perspective of stage analysis, it is conceivable that age-related deficits occur in S-R associative learning because of the elderly individual's failure to use imagery for mediating S-to-R connections, in addition to, or instead of, the elderly individual's diminished amount of rote rehearsal activity. The use of imagery is expected to short-circuit the amount of practice needed to acquire an S-R association, relative to the amount needed for rote rehearsal. Thus, it may be a *qualitative change* in the nature of rehearsal activity (i.e., from mediated to rote) from early to late adulthood rather than a mere *quantitative change* in the amount of rote rehearsal (a change that should be readily compensated by allowing elderly adults additional rehearsal time), that accounts for age-related deficits in paired-

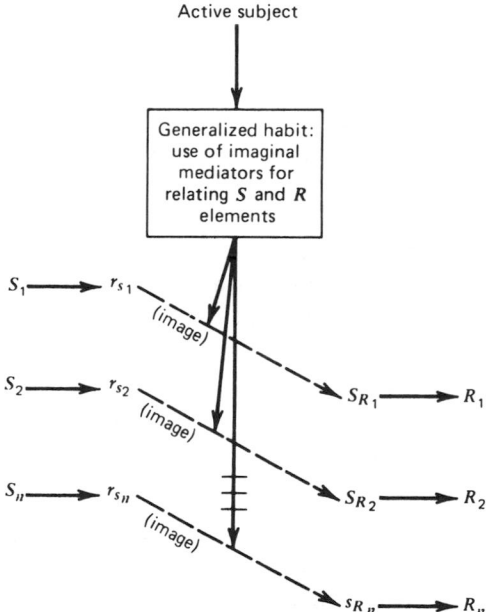

FIGURE 3.8 Conceptualization of the manner by which the generalized habit of using an imaginal mediator affects the learning of multiple S-R pairs in a learning list.

associate learning. Moreover, it is conceivable that rote rehearsal alone promotes little increments in the strengths of S-R associations. That is, additional activity by a learner, such as mediation, may be necessary to promote fully the acquisition of S-R associations. There is some evidence (Spear, Ekstrand, & Underwood, 1964) indicating that rote rehearsal does promote some degree of associative learning, but there is also ample evidence (e.g., Glenberg & Bradley, 1979) to indicate that the amount of learning may be quite modest.

Our preceding analysis suggests two possible reasons for a qualitative change in rehearsal activity with aging. One possibility is simply the failure of the generalized habit (Figure 3.8) to be activated by many elderly adults when they encounter novel learning tasks, such as a laboratory-based paired-associate task. The assumption here is that the basic ability to employ imagery and other forms of mediation is unaffected by aging—only the spontaneous activation of that ability is affected. In this case, the elderly adult would be regarded as experiencing a *production deficit*. The other possibility is an actual decline in the ability to employ mediation. In this case, elderly adults would be regarded as experiencing a true *mediational deficit*. In our review of aging research employing several different manipulable independent variables, we will attempt to evaluate the evidence favoring quantitative change or qualitative change and favoring a production deficit or a mediational deficit as determining factors for age-related deficits in paired-associate learning.

Finally, we should note that the involvement of interacting images to acquire S-R associations places a different perspective on the acquisition of R-S associations and the existence of age-related deficits in R-S learning. For those S-R associations learned via imagery, reinstatement of the R element on a test of R-S learning should serve to recover the interacting image, and thus enable a subject to name the S element that is an integral part of that image. That is, a form of redintegration may take place whereby a part of that which has been learned reinstates the entity that had been learned. If young adults acquire more S-R associations via the formation of interacting images than do elderly adults, they should also be expected to reinstate more S elements via redintegration when they are tested with R elements alone.

Research with Manipulable Independent Variables: Preexperimental Associative Strength

In the remainder of our review of paired-associate learning, we will consider those studies that have combined age variation with variation in a critical manipulable independent variable. Our objective is to evaluate further the evidence regarding the identification of age-sensitive processes. In this section, we will review studies that have varied the degree of preexperimental strength between S and R elements.

As we indicated earlier, associative strength need not be zero at the start of practice on a paired-associate task. Some degree of learning for S-R pairs may have already taken place through contiguous occurrences of elements in the subject's natural environment. Consequently, only a few rehearsal responses may be needed in the new (i.e., laboratory) context before their associative strengths exceed some threshold or minimal value for their activation in that context. In general, as the degree of preexperimental learning increases, the ease of learning a laboratory list should increase accordingly. Tests of this hypothesis require S and R elements that clearly vary in the strength of their preexperimental associations. Fortunately, there is a ready source of these elements, namely, word-association norms (e.g., Palermo & Jenkins, 1964). Although these norms were based on the responses of young adults, there is good reason to believe that word associations change relatively little from early to late adulthood (see Chapter 12, pp. 392–395). Word association norms permit selection of words in which the R element is a strong associate of the S element (e.g., *fast* as an associate of *slow*) as well as pairs in which the R element is a weak associate of the S element (e.g., *fly* as an associate of *eagle*). When transferred to paired-associate lists, *slow* and *eagle* become S elements paired with *fast* and *fly* as R elements.

Given lists of high- and low-associative strengths, we would clearly expect subjects to acquire the high-strength list in fewer trials than the low-strength list. More important, we would also expect the difference in trials to learn between young and elderly subjects to be less for a high-strength list than for a low-strength list. In fact, there is good reason to believe that age differences would all but disappear with pairs of high preexperimental associative strength. At this level, there should be little need for much rote rehearsal. Consequently, the contribution of this suspected age-sensitive process should be miniscule.

This predicted outcome has been found in several studies (Canestrari, 1966; Crossley & Hiscock, 1992; Kausler & Lair, 1966; Ross, 1968; Zaretsky & Halbertstam, 1968a, 1968b). Representative of the outcome is that obtained by Zaretsky and Halberstan (1968b). Both young (an age range of 20 to 45 yr) and elderly (an age range of 60 to 85 yr) subjects were hospital patients who received lists containing pairs of either high, medium, or low preexperimental associative strength (five pairs in each list). The age difference in trials to learn the list was virtually nonexistent with high-strength pairs (although it took a surprisingly large number of trials for both age groups to learn the list), modest with medium-strength pairs, and quite pronounced with low-strength pairs. Interestingly, nearly identical results were obtained with separate groups of brain-damaged young and elderly subjects. The replicability of these results for later cohorts of young and elderly adults is apparent from the results obtained by Crossley and Hiscock (1992). They gave their young adult, middle-aged, and elderly adult subjects pairs from the Wechsler Memory Scale (Wechsler, 1945, 1987). Both "easy" pairs (associatively related words, such as *baby-cries*) and "difficult" pairs (associatively unrelated words, such as *obey-inch*). A significant age difference in the number of responses recalled to stimulus elements was found only for the difficult pairs. Surprisingly, however, in their meta-analysis of paired-associate learning, Verhaeghen, Marcoen, and Goossens (1993) concluded that age-related deficits are as pronounced for highly related words as for lowly related words.

The pronounced age-related deficit for low-strength pairs is conceivably the result of either quantitative or qualitative changes in rehearsal activity from early to late adulthood. The differential age differences for high- and low-strength pairs is unlikely to be the consequence of poorer response learning by elderly subjects for the low-strength pairs than for the high-strength pairs. The response elements in the low-strength list were essentially equivalent to those in the high-strength list in terms of familiarity and meaningfulness. Nor is an age-related deficit in stimulus learning a likely contributor to the differential difficulty, given the use of highly integrated and familiar S elements in both lists.

Research with Manipulable Independent Variables: Rate of Item Presentation

Traditionally, basic research in paired-associate learning has been conducted with fairly rapid pacing conditions. That is, to-be-learned items are exposed, usually visually, at a rate varying across studies from 1 to 4 s per item. Extensions of this research to the study of adult age differences in paired-associate-learning proficiency have largely continued this tradition. For example, the age differences found by Korchin and Basowitz (1957) and Kausler and Lair (1965) were obtained with a 4-s rate, whereas those found by Kausler and Lair (1966) were obtained with a 3-s rate. Of great concern is the generalizability of these age differences, and those found in other, similar studies, to slower rates of presentation (and still faster rates, as well). Much of this concern follows from our knowledge of the general slowing down of responses in late adulthood. Conceivably, 3 or 4 s may not be enough time for many elderly subjects to give responses to S elements, even when the underlying associations have been fully learned. If true, then many age-related deficits in paired-associate-learning proficiency reported in the literature may represent performance decrements attributable to the slowness of responding by elderly subjects rather than decrements in learning ability per se. In support of a performance decrement is the fact that most errors made by elderly subjects during practice on a paired-associate list are errors of omission (i.e., failure to give any kind of response to S elements) rather than errors of commission (i.e., responding with an inappropriate R element) (Korchin & Basowitz, 1957).

Tests of the generalizability of age differences over varying rates of item presentation call for a factorial design in which the systematic variation of rate is combined with age variation. The earliest study to employ this design was by Canestrari (1963). Unfortunately, the results obtained are ambiguous (for further analysis of this and other studies that vary rate of presentation, see Witte, 1975). The source of the ambiguity is linked to the method used to present list materials to subjects, namely, the anticipation method. This is a frequently used method in paired-associate research (e.g., it was used by Korchin & Basowitz, 1957, and Kausler & Lair, 1965, 1966), but, as we will soon see, it is not the only method available. The nature of the anticipation method is illustrated in Figure 3.9 with reference to the rate conditions employed in Canestrari's (1963) study. Specifically, there were three levels of the rate variable: 1.5 s per item, 3 s per item, and self-pacing (i.e., subjects progress through the list at their own rate). For each

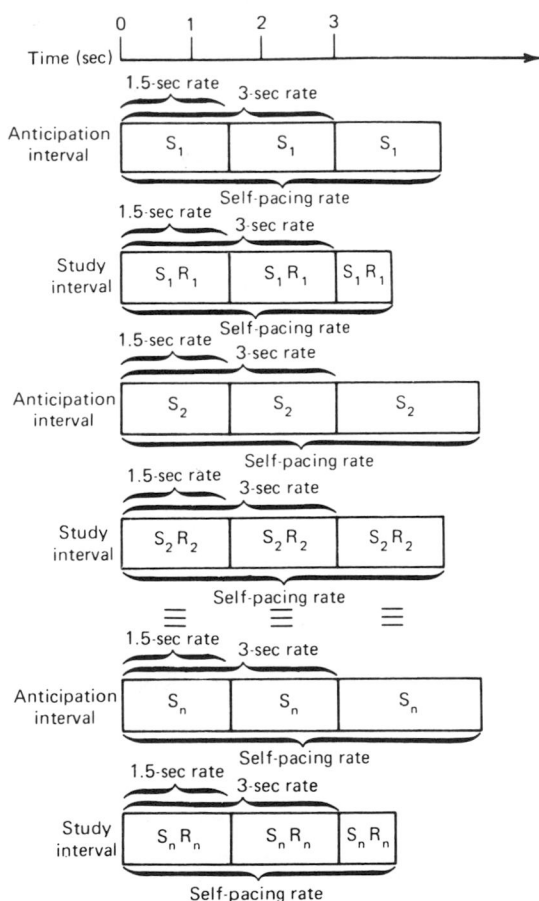

FIGURE 3.9 Schematic representation of the procedures used to vary duration of anticipation and study intervals in paired-associate learning. Durations are either 1.5 s, 3 s, or self-paced.

pacing condition, a trial consists of exposing first the S element of a pair, followed by exposure of both the S element and the R element. The first exposure is called the *anticipation interval*. During this interval, subjects attempt to respond with the R element that has been paired with the exposed S element. In Canestrari's (1963) study, the anticipation interval lasted either 1.5 s, 3 s, or an amount determined by each subject individually. The second exposure is called the *study interval*. During this interval, subjects have the opportunity to rehearse the S and R elements, thereby permitting learning of the response elements alone, selecting a functional stimulus when appropriate, and adding to the strengths of the S-R and R-S associations. The study interval in Canestrari's (1963) study also lasted either 1.5 s, 3 s, or an amount determined by each subject individually. Most important, the durations of the two intervals were yoked together. Thus, the 1.5-s anticipation interval was always accompanied by the 1.5-s study interval, the 3-s anticipation interval with the 3-s study interval, and the self-paced anticipation interval with the self-paced study interval. Consequently, the effect of varying rate on age differences in task proficiency could be due to either or both rate manipulations.

That effect is shown in Figure 3.10 for mean errors made in learning the list. The interaction apparent in this figure indicates a multiplicative relationship between age and rate. That is, the age-related deficit in proficiency decreased as overall performance improved across the levels of the rate variable for both age

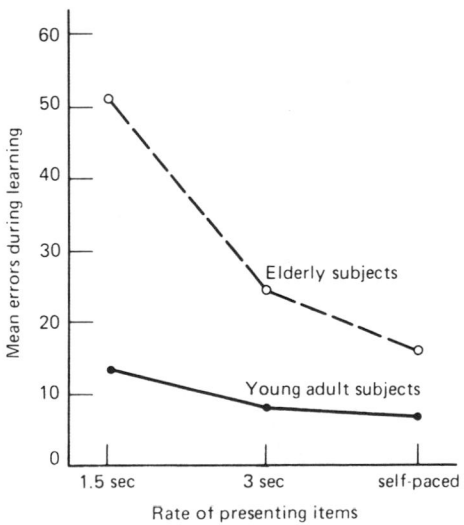

FIGURE 3.10   Age differences in paired-associate learning proficiency as affected by rate of presenting items. (Adapted from Canestrari, 1963, Table 2.)

groups. Our inference, therefore, is that the process altered by rate variation is age sensitive. That process could be the aforementioned speed of responding to S elements. The adverse effects of slower responding by elderly people simply become less pronounced as the duration of the anticipation interval increases. On the other hand, the age-sensitive process could be one that is affected by variation of the study interval. A possible candidate in this event is the rate of emitting rehearsal responses. According to this hypothesis, the slower rehearsal rate of elderly subjects is at least partially compensated for by lengthening the study interval, thereby giving them added time to rehearse S and R elements. Alternatively, elderly subjects may simply need more study time for evoking interacting images of S and R elements than do young subjects. The yoked nature of the variation in the two intervals makes it difficult to identify whatever the age-sensitive process is.

To untangle the confounding problems present in Canestrari's (1963) study, Monge and Hultsch (1971) wisely employed a factorial design in which duration of each interval was varied separately. There were three levels of each variable: 2.2 s, 4.4 s, and 6.6 s. Thus, nine groups were required at each age level—those receiving 2.2–2.2, 2.2–4.4, 2.2–6.6, 4.4–2.2, and so on combinations of anticipation-interval and study-interval durations. In agreement with the performance-deficit hypothesis, Monge and Hultsch (1971) found a significant interaction between age and duration of the anticipation interval, as illustrated in part A of Figure 3.11 (a similar outcome occurred in an earlier study by Arenberg [1965] in which duration of the anticipation interval was varied while the duration of the study interval was held constant). It may be seen that the age-related deficit was much greater with a fast rate (2.2 s) than with a slower rate (either 4.4 or 6.6 s). The resulting multiplicative relationship implies that an age-sensitive process is tapped by variation in the duration of the anticipation interval. The likely candidate, of course, seems to be speed of responding.

On the other hand, the interaction between age and duration of the study interval, shown in part B of Figure 3.11, did not attain statistical significance. In other words, the magnitude of the age-related deficit in learning proficiency was about as great with a brief study interval (2.2 s) as it was with longer intervals (4.4 or 6.6 s). The absence of an interaction between age and duration of study intervals was also found in a study by Hulicka, Sterns, and Grossman (1967). In their study, the anticipation method was replaced by a method (the recall method) in which study trials alternate with test trials. During each study trial, S-R pairs are presented successively for study with no performance being demanded of subjects. Each study trial is then followed by a test trial in which each S element is presented alone and subjects attempt to recall the R element paired with it. This method avoids the confusion, especially for elderly subjects (Kausler, 1963), created in the anticipation method by the constant alternation of performance (i.e., anticipation) and learning (i.e., study) periods. The absence of an

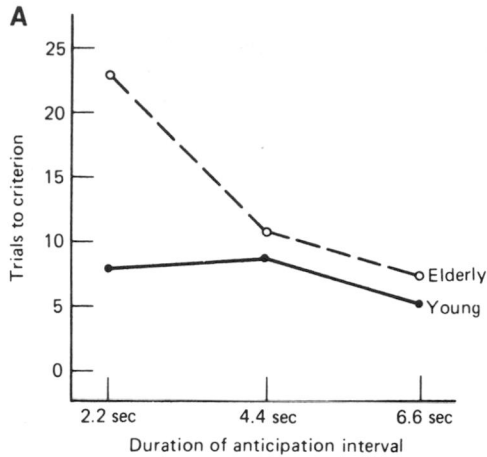

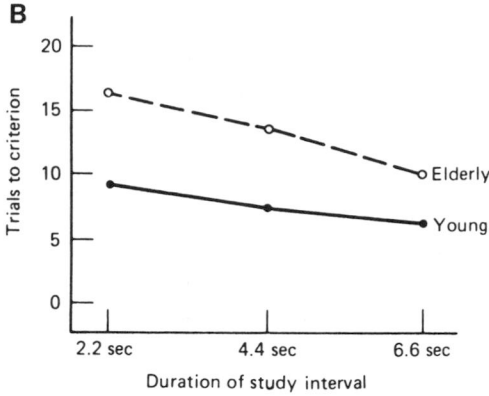

F I G U R E   3.11   Age differences in paired-associate-learning proficiency as affected separately by variation in duration of the anticipation interval (A) and study interval (B). (Adapted from data in Monge & Hultsch, 1971.)

interaction between age and study interval in both Monge and Hultsch's (1971) study and Hulicka et al.'s (1967) study indicates an additive relationship between age and duration of study intervals (but see Taub, 1967, for the presence of such an interaction). The implication is that the process altered by the manipulable independent variable is age insensitive. If that process is rote rehearsal activity, then it is unlikely that age differences in this process account for age differences in paired-associate-learning proficiency. At the same time, it is obvious that some process is altered, independently of age variation, by variation in the duration of study intervals. Note in the bottom half of Figure 3.11 that performance proficiency for both age groups improved progressively as duration increased, that is, there was a main effect for the variation of study intervals.

Our analysis does not rule out, however, the probable involvement of an age-sensitive process as a major factor contributing to adult age differences in paired-associate learning proficiency. It simply indicates that whatever that process is, it is not affected by the duration of study intervals. A strong candidate for age sensitivity is engagement in mediated rehearsal (e.g., the use of imagery to relate S and R elements together). Young adult subjects are more likely than elderly subjects to initiate mediated rehearsal regardless of the duration of the study interval. There is an alternative possibility, however, one that is yet to be tested for paired-associate learning. Free-recall research with young adult subjects has revealed that distributed rehearsal (i.e., rehearsal of a prior item at the time another item is presented) enhances the later recallability of the words in a list (see Chapter 6, p. 180), relative to rehearsal that involves only a currently present item. Distributed rehearsal is likely to occur for paired associates as well, and it is more likely for young adults than for elderly adults.

One other finding in this area of research is worth mentioning. Under complete self-pacing conditions, elderly subjects do take more total time to learn a list than do young adult subjects (Canestrari, 1963). Moreover, this disparity in total time remains about the same regardless of the specific pacing conditions that are introduced (Kinsbourne & Berryhill, 1972). For each age level, it takes about the same amount of total time to learn a list regardless of the specific pacing condition employed. For example, about three times as many trials are needed to learn a list with a 2-s rate of presentation than with a 6-s rate, but the total time involved stays invariant. This invariance is known as the total time principle, and it applies to elderly adults as well as young adults—the amount of total time is simply greater for the former, but it seems to be equally invariant regardless of age.

Research with Manipulable Independent Variables: Mediational Instructions and Materials

The use of mediators to relate S and R elements together is widely practiced by young adults during paired-associate learning. For example, Underwood and Schulz (1960) discovered that nearly 75% of the pairs learned by their young adult subjects were acquired through the use of a mediator of some kind. Our reference is to the spontaneous use of mediators, that is, use without any special prodding or instructions. Our discussion in the previous section implied that elderly adults are far less likely than young adults to use mediators spontaneously and that it is this age differential in spontaneous mediation that accounts for much of the age-related deficit found in paired-associate learning. An age difference in spontaneous mediation has indeed been found in several studies

(Hulicka, 1965a; Hulicka & Grossman, 1967). For example, Hulicka and Gross-man (1967) found that only 36% of their elderly subjects reported using media-tion during practice on a paired-associate list, compared to 68% of their young subjects. Moreover, young and elderly subjects also differ in the kinds of mediators they employ. Young adults are more likely to use imaginal mediators (i.e., con-structing interacting images of S and R elements) than verbal mediators (i.e., constructing phrases or sentences containing S and R elements), whereas elderly adults show the opposite pattern. This is another important factor contributing to age-related deficits in paired-associate learning. In general, imaginal mediators are more effective than verbal mediators in promoting paired-associate learning (Paivio, 1971). (An exception is the outcome reported by Knill, 1966, in which verbal mediators were as effective as imaginal mediators for both young adult and elderly adult subjects.) Interestingly, bizarre images may be no more effective as mediators than are common-event images, either for young adults (e.g., Nappe & Wollen, 1973) or elderly adults (Poon & Walsh-Sweeney, 1981). On the other hand, the complexity of mediators, once they are elicited, does not seem to differ greatly between young and elderly adults (Marshall et al., 1978).

The remaining issue is the extent to which the age difference in the sponta-neous use of mediators can be overcome by instructions and training. At stake is the important question of whether or not elderly adults have a true mediational deficiency relative to young adults, especially for imaginal mediators (Kausler, 1970). A true deficiency refers to the diminished ability to construct the images needed to relate S elements with R elements. The deficiency could be the con-sequence of biological degeneration. The right cerebral hemisphere is the locus of imaginal activity for most individuals. Conceivably, deterioration of the brain is asymmetrical, with atrophy occurring at a faster rate for the right hemisphere than for the left hemisphere. If true, it would account perhaps for the greater reliance on verbal mediators (a left hemisphere function) for most elderly adults. However, the evidence indicating such asymmetry in hemispheric deterioration is decidedly mixed, with some studies providing supporting evidence (e.g., Albert & Kaplan, 1980; Lapidot, 1987), others not (e.g., Borod & Goodglass, 1980; Byrd & Moscovitch, 1984). If a true deficiency does exist, then it is highly unlikely that any amount of instruction or training could restore mediational proficiency to the level characteristic of young adulthood.

Alternatively, elderly adults may be experiencing only a production deficiency, or performance decrement, brought about, most likely, by the lack of practice in mediation once they have left formal educational settings. If only a production deficiency is involved, the age-related deficit in paired-associate learning should be largely overcome through the effective use of instructions and training. There is, in fact, evidence (Treat, Poon, Fozard, & Popkin, 1978) indicating that elderly people do begin to use imaginal mediators spontaneously after practice on a number of paired-associate lists.

This issue has been examined in several additional studies employing instructions as an independent variable, beginning with a study by Hulicka and Grossman (1967). In their study, control groups of young adult and elderly adult subjects were given no special instructions as to how to learn pairs of S and R elements. By contrast, their experimental groups received training in the use of imaginal mediators and instructions as to the benefit of applying imaginal mediators in learning paired associates. Their results are shown in Figure 3.12. It may be seen that training improved the performance of elderly subjects by 18% (from 35% of the pairs recalled without special training to 53% with special training). The young adults also improved with special training, but to a smaller degree than the elderly adults (11%; from 70% to 81%). The resulting multiplicative relationship between age levels and training conditions implies that mediation, the process varied by training, is age sensitive. Subjects in the training condition were required to generate their own imaginal content linking together S and R elements. There were other training conditions involved in this study as well. In one, the investigators supplied both young and elderly subjects with a suggested content for each image. For example, with *army-bank* as a pair, the suggestion was to form an image of an army attacking a bank. Relative to the control, or noninstructed, condition, performance proficiency improved for both age groups (45%

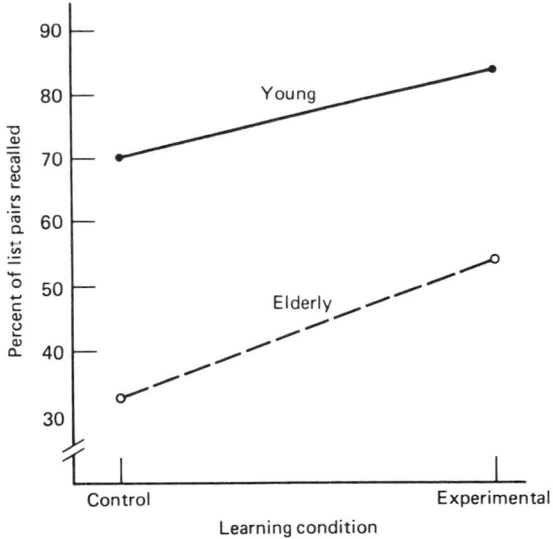

FIGURE 3.12 Age differences in paired-associate learning under neutral instructions (control) and experimental instructions (stressing the use of imagery to relate paired stimulus–response elements to one another). (Adapted from Hulicka & Grossman, 1967, Table 1.)

and 78% of the pairs being recalled by elderly and young subjects, respectively). Note, however, that the gain in proficiency was less pronounced than when subjects supplied their own imaginal content (10% gain for the elderly subjects, 8% for the young subjects). A final condition employed in this study consisted of training and instructions in the use of verbal mediators. Specifically, suggestions as to the content of connecting phrases were given (e.g., *army* attacks *bank*). Relative to the control condition, elderly subjects improved somewhat in proficiency of recall (a 12% gain; from 35% to 47%), whereas young subjects showed virtually no gain (1% from 70% to 71%).

A similar pattern of results was obtained by Canestrari (1968). There were three instructional conditions: (1) a control condition with no special instructions; (2) an experimental condition in which subjects were urged to use images corresponding to pictures shown that depicted interacting S and R elements; and (3) an experimental condition in which subjects were urged to use phrases corresponding to those given to them by the experimenter. The results, expressed as mean errors made in learning the list, are plotted in Figure 3.13 for both young adults (interestingly, male prisoners averaging 20.2 yr) and elderly adults (male residents of a Veterans Administration facility averaging 62.4 yr—the two age groups were comparable in educational levels, socioeconomic backgrounds, and vocabulary test scores). A multiplicative relationship may again be observed. In fact, the elderly subjects benefited more from both kinds of provided mediators than did the young subjects, although in this case the outcome is complicated by a possible ceiling effect for the young subjects. Knill (1966) also provided subjects with either imaginal or verbal mediators. Here too performance for elderly subjects benefited more than did performance for young adult subjects. Elderly sub-

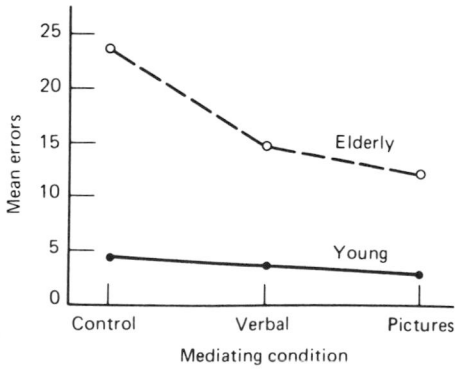

FIGURE 3.13   Age differences in paired-associate-learning proficiency as affected by variation in mediational instructions. (Adapted from Canestrari, 1968, Figure 1.)

jects clearly benefit from both verbal and imaginal instructions, but, as in Hulicka and Grossman's (1967) study, more so for the latter.

The improvement in performance for instructed elderly subjects clearly indicates that part of the age-related deficit in paired-associate learning proficiency is the consequence of a production deficit (or, perhaps more appropriately, a production inefficiency; Reese, 1976) that can be at least partially overcome by training and practice. However, it seems likely that some true loss of mediational ability in late adulthood is involved as well. Even with mediational prodding, paired-associate learning proficiency of elderly subjects remains well below the level of young adult subjects. Of course, it is conceivable that psychologists have yet to discover a fully effective means of overcoming production inefficiencies. Some hope of this possibility emerged in a complex study by Treat and Reese (1976). Imaginal mediational conditions were varied, together with several rate-of-presentation variables. With long anticipation intervals, their elderly subjects performed as well as their young adult subjects, but only when all of the subjects were encouraged to generate their own imagery content.

The issue of appropriate conditions for training in the use of imagery is a complex one (Poon, Walsh-Sweeney, & Fozard, 1980) that we will return to when we discuss mnemonics. The use of imagery is a major component of many mnemonic devices that have been introduced to enhance the ease of learning verbal materials.

Adult age differences in the use of imaginal mediators may also be investigated by varying the nature of the S and R elements. Considerable research with young adult subjects has indicated the greater involvement of imaginal mediation when concrete nouns (e.g., *apple*) serve as S and R elements than when abstract nouns (e.g., *mercy*) serve as elements. Concrete nouns are more readily "imaged" than are abstract nouns, as is reflected by the substantially higher ratings concrete nouns receive than abstract nouns from both young adult subjects (Paivio, Yuille, & Madigan, 1968) and elderly subjects (Kausler, 1980) when they are asked to rate the ease with which a word elicits an imaginal representation. Moreover, the ratings given individual words show a strikingly high correlation between young and elderly subjects (Kausler, 1980). Thus, it is not surprising that Rowe and Schnore (1971) found their elderly subjects, like their young adult subjects, to learn a paired-associate list composed of concrete nouns more readily than a list composed of abstract nouns. Their results, expressed as mean number of correct responses, are plotted in Figure 3.14. Note that the age-related deficit was much greater for abstract nouns than for concrete nouns. However, the age-related deficit did not disappear even with highly concrete nouns, again implying that imaginal mediational proficiency declines from early to late adulthood.

The major reason why mediational proficiency declines with normal aging appears to be the effortful nature of constructing images. As we observed in Chapter 2 (p. 39), the age-related decline in the construction of images is evident

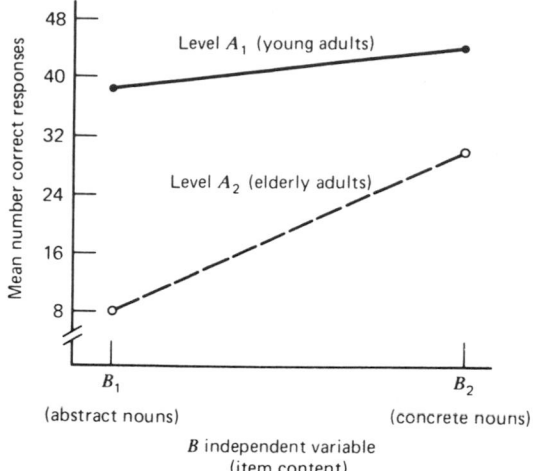

FIGURE 3.14 Multiplicative relationship for paired-associate learning yielded by the interaction between age variation and variation of items along the abstract-concrete dimension. (Adapted from Rowe & Schnore, 1971, Figure 1.)

for the mental rotation task, and it is also evident on other tasks, such as the paper-folding task, that require spatial visualization (see Salthouse, 1992a, for a review). Craik and Dirkx (1992) have given us direct evidence of the extent of the age-related deficit in the construction of images. Their young adult and elderly adult subjects performed on three different tests of imagery production, with scores on all three tests showing pronounced age differences. For example, one of these is the Clock Test (Paivio, 1978) in which subjects are given a series of times in digital form (e.g., 11:35) and are asked to tell if the hands on a regular clock would be at angle of greater or less than 90°. Solving such a problem clearly requires the production of an image of a regular clock with the hands in the designated positions. Of 36 such problems, their young subjects averaged 95% correct and their elderly subjects only 74% correct. Interestingly, elderly subjects seem to evaluate their imaginal ability unrealistically high. Pierce and Storandt (1987) found that their elderly subjects rated their imaginal ability as highly as their young adult subjects did in terms of the vividness of the images they experience and the control they have over those images.

As mentioned earlier (p. 92), there may be a biological reason for the difficulty elderly adults have in constructing images. A more cognitive explanation is also possible. An age-related decline in some cognitive resource may well underlie the difficulty elderly adults have in constructing images and therefore in the proficiency of paired-associate learning as a by-product. One possibility is an age-related decline in the rate of processing information, and another is an age-related decline in working memory's capacity (see Chapter 6, pp. 203–207). In agreement with this possibility are the results of a study by Salthouse (1992b). Statistical control of measures of cognitive speed of processing were found to attenuate significantly age differences on both a paper-folding task (a task involving imagery production) and a paired-associate-learning task (a task likely to involve imagery production).

Research with Manipulable Independent Variables:
Intentional versus Incidental Learning

As noted earlier, laboratory studies of age differences in paired-associate learning proficiency have ignored the fact that much of the everyday learning of verbal materials occurs incidentally rather than intentionally. For example, when you read that Joe Loser, the manager of your favorite baseball team, has been fired and replaced by new manager, John Hope, you are likely to learn the new *manager-Hope* association incidentally. That is, it is acquired without intentional rehearsal. (The new association is acquired despite the interference created by the previously learned *manager-Loser* association. This is an example of negative transfer—see Chapter 4, pp. 122–125).

The form of incidental learning identified in this example is called Type I incidental learning (Kausler & Trapp, 1960). When brought into the laboratory, Type I incidental learning is tested after drawing subjects attention to the to-be-learned material without specifically mentioning that a test of what has been learned will be given later. This is accomplished by the use of an orienting task that subjects perform on the material (see Chapter 6, p. 184). For example, word pairs may be presented, with subjects asked to rate (e.g., on a 1-to-5 scale) each pair in terms of the frequency they are likely to appear together in written sentences. At the end of the series of word pairs, subjects would be given the first word of each pair and asked to recall the word that had been paired with it. Scores for these incidental learning subjects could then be compared with those of intentional learning subjects who performed the same rating task but also knew in advance of the later recall test. This orienting-task procedure has been employed in a number of aging studies on memory (see Chapter 6, pp. 185–187) but not in aging studies on paired-associate learning. Consequently, there is a major gap in aging research on paired-associate learning.

There is another form of incidental learning as well—not surprisingly—called Type II incidental learning (Kausler & Trapp, 1960). Here material that is learned intentionally is accompanied by additional material that must be acquired incidentally, if at all. As noted earlier, learning R-S associations along with S-R associations may be viewed as being (Type II) incidental learning. We discovered then that older subjects are somewhat less proficient incidental learners than younger subjects. Further demonstration of this diminished proficiency was provided in a study by Crook, Larrabee, and Youngjohn (1993). Their procedure was patterned after one introduced years earlier by Hulicka (1965b). Their subjects were given a list of 14 face-name pairs to learn intentionally. On each of three study trials, a video display showed each face while the person depicted gave his/her first name. Each study trial was followed by a test trial in which each face reappeared while saying the name of the city where that person lived. On each test trial, subjects were asked to give the name to each face, with no reference given to the city. After a delay, the subjects were asked to recall the city associated with each face—a test of Type II incidental learning. For name recall (intentional learning), the young and elderly subjects averaged 12.67 and 7.38 names correctly recalled, respectively. This is an age-related loss of about 42%. On the test of incidental learning, the age groups averaged 5.02 and 2.37 cities recalled correctly. This is an age-related loss of about 53%. Thus, the decline from early to late adulthood appeared to be greater for the incidental material than for the intentionally learned material it accompanied. Surprisingly, however, Crook et al. (1993) concluded just the opposite. That is, they reasoned that the age-related decline was greater for intentional learning than for incidental learning. At any rate, the amount of incidental learning was quite low regardless of age.

Comments

From the foregoing review, it should be apparent that there has been relatively little research on adult age differences in paired-associate learning during the past 15 or so yr. However, this is not quite the whole story. Paired-associate learning has resurfaced in recent years in some disguised forms. For example, in Chapter 4 we will discover that the use of a mnemonic frequently calls upon a form of paired-associate learning. In Chapter 12 (pp. 410–411) we will encounter a phenomenon known as the episodic priming effect. The materials used to demonstrate the basic phenomenon, and the extent of adult age differences in the phenomenon, are paired-associate lists. In addition, the procedure used to test the principle of encoding specificity (Chapter 7, pp. 263–264) requires the use of what may be considered associatively related word pairs that form paired associates.

Adult Age Differences in Serial Learning

Historical Perspective

The psychology of verbal learning had its historical origin in research on serial learning. The originator was Herman Ebbinghaus (1885). He served as his own subject, learning list after list of nonsense syllables. The task he introduced was basically a form of serial learning in which a subject studies a series of items and then attempts to reproduce the series in the order the items were presented. What makes Ebbinghaus's research especially intriguing to us is the fact that, at age 33, the only subject (Ebbinghaus himself) was not exactly a young adult learner.

Despite this promising start, interest in serial learning by noncollege-aged subjects lagged well behind the intense interest found for other kinds of learning. Perhaps the first formal study of adult age differences in serial learning with verbal elements was that of Bromley (1958). By then, the task format preferred by investigators had shifted from that of serial reproduction (the entire series of items is presented for study, with subjects then trying to recall the items in the order presented) to that of serial anticipation. With this revised format, items, usually words, continue to be presented consecutively. However, as each item is exposed, subjects both study that item and anticipate what the next item in the series will be. Thus, each exposure of an item doubles as an anticipation interval as well as a study interval. This procedure continues for as many trials as needed until a subject attains some designated criterion of mastery, usually an errorless trial.

Bromley's (1958) study revealed cross-sectional age differences in serial-learning proficiency, favoring young adults. A number of subsequent cross-sectional studies (e.g., Eisdorfer & Service, 1967; Eisdorfer, Axelrod, & Wilkie, 1968) have replicated this finding. Typically, these studies employed young adult and elderly groups of subjects that were carefully matched with respect to educational levels and vocabulary test scores, thus making it unlikely that the age-related deficit in learning proficiency was attributable to cohort effects. Further support for this conclusion comes from the impressive longitudinal study by Arenberg and Robertson-Tchabo (1977). Their evidence indicating a true age change in serial-learning proficiency closely parallels the evidence found in the same study indicating a true age change in paired-associate-learning proficiency (see p. 71).

Research with Manipulable Independent Variables

Perhaps the most potent variable affecting rate of acquisition of items in a serial learning list is the position of those items in the list. With young adult subjects, many studies (see Kausler, 1974, pp. 276–288) have revealed that very few errors are made for the beginning items in the list and that only slightly more errors occur for the items at the end of the list. The highest concentration of errors occurs for those items embedded in the middle of the list, peaking at some point closer to the end of the list than to the beginning. This distribution of errors in a way that is both bowed and skewed (i.e., peak beyond midlist) is known as the *serial-position effect*. Bromley (1958) found that the serial-position effect is just as characteristic of elderly subjects as it is of young adult subjects—the total number of errors at each serial position is simply greater for the elderly subjects.

Other researchers (e.g., Eisdorfer et al., 1963) have also reported the age equivalence in overall serial-position effects. Many explanations of the serial-position effect have been offered over the years, none of which are completely satisfactory (see Kausler, 1974, pp. 276–288). An especially appealing one, however, argues that the distribution of errors simply reflects the order in which subjects learn ordinal placements of items in the list (Jensen, 1962a). That is, early items are learned first, then end items, and finally, midlist items. The absence of an age difference in the overall pattern of error distribution suggests that elderly adults apply the same basic strategy that young adults apply in learning a serial list.

An independent variable that has received considerable attention in aging research is the rate at which the list items are presented (Arenberg, 1967a; Eisdorfer, 1965; Eisdorfer et al., 1963; Wilkie & Eisdorfer, 1977). The differential effects of a fast rate versus a slow rate of item presentation may be seen in the results obtained by Eisdorfer and Service (1967). Their young adult and elderly subjects practiced on an eight-word serial list in which the words were presented at a rate of either 4 s per word or 10 s per word. Shown in part A of Figure 3.15 are the mean number of errors made in mastering the list under these two pacing conditions. The magnitude of the age difference favoring the young subjects was clearly less for the slower pacing condition. This pattern of decreasing age differences as the duration of item exposure increases has been found in other studies as well. For example, the results obtained by Arenberg (1967a) are plotted in part B of Figure 3.15. His procedure called for exposing each word of a 12-item list for 2 s, followed by a blank interval of either 1.8 s or 3.6 s. Thus, subjects at each of many age levels had a total time of either 3.8 s or 5.6 s to anticipate what the next word in the series would be. Note that age differences in mean trials to learn the list were considerably less pronounced with the slower pacing condition than with the faster pacing condition. Much of this decrease in the overall age-related deficit undoubtedly resulted from overcoming some of the adverse-performance effects experienced by elderly subjects under a fast-pacing condition. Strong support for this argument comes from the study by Eisdorfer et al. (1963). Some of their elderly subjects began practice on a serial list under a fast-pacing condition and were switched on later trials to a slower pacing condition. After the switch, their performance improved greatly, reaching the level of proficiency attained by other elderly subjects who received the slower rate throughout practice. If rate-of-presentation markedly affected the amount learned, then the subjects with the originally faster rate should have continued after the switch to lag behind the subjects with the originally slower rate.

There is one other variable that has been of concern in aging research on serial learning, namely the level of verbal ability of subjects as measured by a vocabulary test. In Eisdorfer and Service's (1967) study, half of the subjects at each age level were people having average vocabulary scores; the other half were people having above-average scores. Mean total errors are plotted in Figure 3.16.

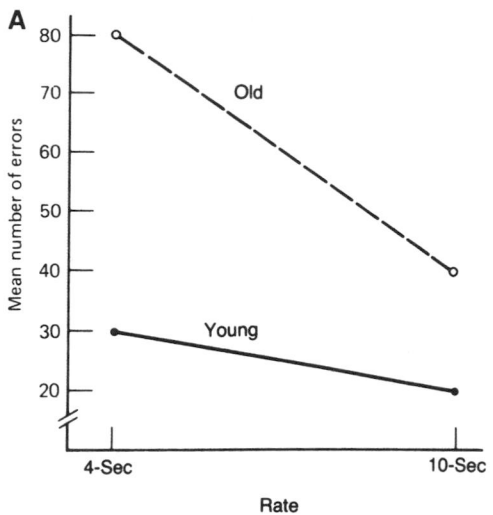

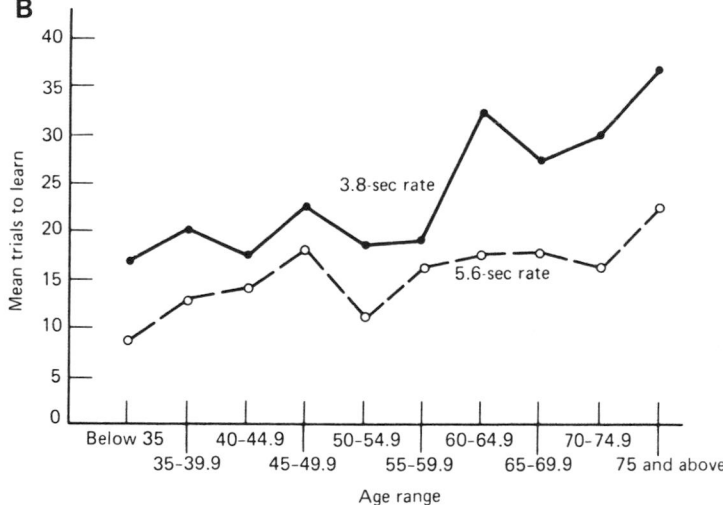

FIGURE 3.15 Age differences in serial-learning proficiency as affected by variation in duration of item exposure. (A: Adapted from Eisdorfer & Service, 1967, Figure 1. B: Adapted from Arenberg, 1967a, Table 2.)

Note that the elderly subjects of high verbal ability were clearly superior in learning proficiency with respect to elderly subjects of average verbal ability, but only under the fast rate of exposure. Under the slower rate, the two groups did not differ in learning proficiency (in fact, if anything, the elderly subjects of

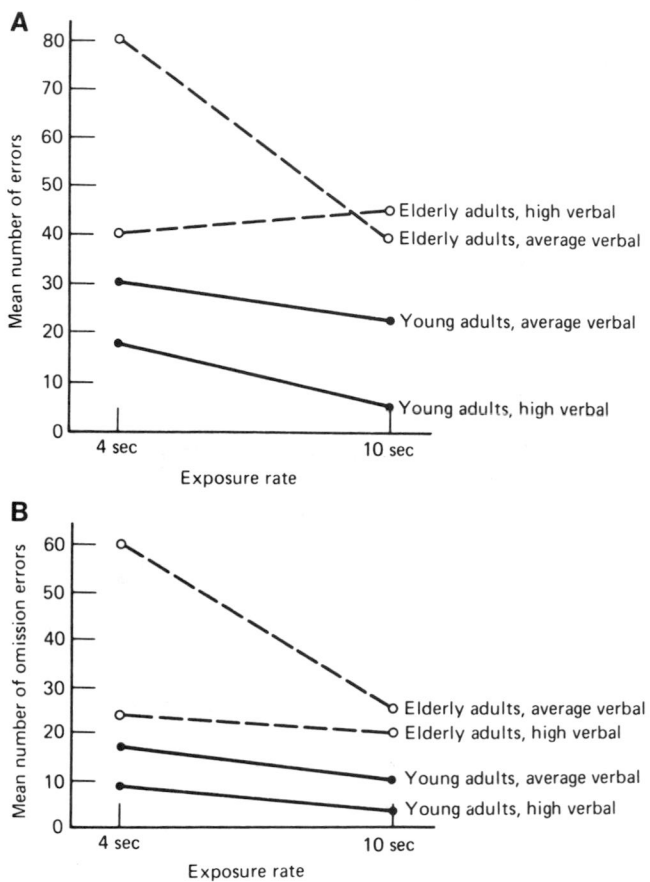

FIGURE 3.16   Age differences in total errors (A) and errors of omission (B) for young and elderly subjects of high and average verbal ability. (Adapted from Eisdorfer & Service, 1967, Figures 1, 2.)

average ability were slightly superior). By contrast, young adult subjects of high verbal ability were clearly superior in learning proficiency to their counterparts of average ability, regardless of rate of exposure.

Analysis of Age-Sensitive Processes

As in paired-associate learning, the presence of performance deficits does not rule out the existence of learning deficits as well. Even with a very slow rate of item presentation, such as the 10-s rate employed by Eisdorfer and Service

(1967), a sizable age deficit in serial-learning proficiency remains (see A, Figure 3.15). The specific age-sensitive process (or processes) remains unknown, however. The nature of serial learning per se is far from being understood. The position of associationists is that subjects acquire a series of S-R associations while learning a serial list. The response elements that would enter into these associations are clearly identified—they are the individual items of the serial list. What remains unidentified are the stimulus elements. There is evidence with young adult subjects to indicate that for some of the associations the functional stimulus is the item preceding an item serving as the response element. However, for other associations the functional stimulus appears to be the ordinality of the items—"first in the list" may be the stimulus for the first item, "second in the list" the stimulus for the second item, and so on (Young, 1962; see Kausler, 1974, pp. 267–274, for elaboration). If associations are indeed the product of serial learning, then the age-sensitive process may be one that is closely akin to the age-sensitive process entering into paired-associate learning. Indirect evidence in support of this hypothesis was provided in Arenberg's (1967a) study. His subjects learned a paired-associate list as well as a serial list. Of interest are the correlations between paired-associate learning scores and serial-learning scores. For each age range of subjects and for both fast- and slow-pacing conditions, the correlation coefficient was moderately high (r of about .60). It seems likely that learning processes shared by the two kinds of tasks at each age level account for much of the covariation between task proficiencies. A likely candidate for a shared process is mediated associative learning. We should note, however, that the correlation coefficients reported in Arenberg's (1967a) study are unusually high. Other investigators (e.g., Jensen, 1962b), working only with young adult subjects, have found the correlation to be considerably lower than .60.

There is an alternative way of conceptualizing serial learning. It may be viewed as involving two processes, acquiring the individual items per se and retaining the temporal order, or ordinal position, of those items (Crowder, 1976; Lee & Estes, 1977). The first process is basically equivalent to the response-learning stage of paired-associate learning. With highly familiar words and a short list (as in Eisdorfer and Service's, 1967, study), it seems unlikely that an age-related deficit in response learning would be a major contributor to the pronounced age-related deficit found for serial learning. The second process involves memory for the ordinal positions of the individual times, positions that reflect the temporal sequencing of the items. It has long been known that young adult subjects are fairly accurate in judging the ordinal positions for beginning and end items of a serial learning list but that they are less accurate in judging the positions for midlist items (Jahnke, Davis, & Bower, 1989; Schulz, 1955). In fact, the differential accuracy of ordinal and temporal information provides another, very viable explanation for serial-position effects in serial learning. That is, errors are most likely to occur for midlist items where there is little temporal discriminability among the items. There is good reason to believe that elderly adults would be much less accurate than young adults in similar judgments for all ordinal positions. Our reasoning is based on studies of age differences in temporal memory that will be reviewed in detail in Chapter 9 (pp. 312–315). Briefly, elderly subjects are much less accurate than young adults in reconstructing the temporal order in which a series of words was presented (e.g., Salthouse et al., 1988a). It is this age-related deficit in the ability to remember temporal information that probably accounts for much of the age-related deficit found for serial-learning proficiency.

Mnemonics and Transfer

Mnemonics

Of interest are the results of a survey of over 100 elderly adults conducted by Leirer, Morrow, Sheikh, and Pariante (1990). The subjects were asked to name the learning/memory skills they would like to improve. The most frequent skill listed was learning and remembering peoples' names. Learning names and associating them with the appropriate faces is a form of paired-associate learning. The second most frequent skill they named was learning and remembering dates. Such learning may be viewed as being a simple form of serial learning.

Given their diminished proficiency in verbal learning and their concern about it, elderly adults have become natural subjects for training in the use of a mnemonic technique of some kind. In effect, subjects are taught a means of enhancing the acquisition of to-be-learned material by applying some extrinsic aid that usually involves the use of imagery. Three such imaginal-based techniques have been of primary interest in aging research (see West, 1989, and Yesavage, Lapp, and Sheikh, 1989, for further review). They are the *pegword method*, the *method of loci*, and the *keyword method*. In general, training on the use of a mnemonic is a means of increasing the amount of nonspecific transfer (see pp. 119–120) subjects are expected to manifest following the completion of training. That is, subjects are taught the kinds of processes that should enhance the acquisition of new material of a kind similar in format to the training material, but differing in specific content. Without such training, subjects would have to discover on their own the kinds of processes that would improve their rate of acquisition for successive new lists of material. Instructing subjects to use interacting images to mediate the S and R elements of paired associates is a simple example of mnemonic training. As we discovered in Chapter 3, both young adult and elderly adult subjects benefit from such instruction. Our present interest is in more elaborate mnemonic techniques, techniques that usually require a lengthy training period to master and often make use of an extrinsic device of some kind.

Pegword Method

The pegword method is used to enhance the recall of items in a serial list. It calls for training subjects to use a plan, or strategy, while learning an ordered list of items. In effect, the plan provides a means of converting the serial list into the equivalent of a paired-associate list (Miller, Galanter, & Pribram, 1960). For this conversion, the to-be-learned serial items become R elements, each of which is associated with an S element inherent within the plan itself. The initial step taken by a subject is to learn fully a simple rhyme involving the numbers 1 through 10. Each number is associated with a word that may be readily transformed into a mental image. For example, the first line of the rhyme is "one is a bun." The user of the pegword system imagines a distinctive looking image of the first word in the series, one that is interacting with a "bun." If the first word is "car," the subject might create an image of a "Detroit sandwich" (or, perhaps, a "Japanese sandwich") in which a car is squeezed into a bun along with lettuce, mustard, and what have you. Each successive line of the rhyme serves a similar function; that is, it provides a pegword for constructing a compound image that includes a picture of a to-be-remembered item in the serial list. At recall, subjects then recite the lines to themselves. With "one is a bun," the appropriate image containing a car is recovered, thus identifying the first item in the list. This procedure continues until the last, "ten is a hen," is recited, and the tenth item of the list is recovered by means of its representation in an interaction with a hen.

Young adults who are taught to use this method learn 10-item serial lists much more readily than control subjects who are left to their own devices (e.g., Bugelski, Kidd, & Segmen, 1968). The effectiveness of the method with elderly subjects is questionable, however. Smith (1975a; Mason & Smith, 1977) found no gain in learning proficiency when it was applied by either middle-aged, or elderly subjects. On the other hand, young adult subjects in these studies manifested the expected benefit. A somewhat more promising outcome, however, was reported by Hellebusch (1976), who found elderly subjects as well as young subjects to benefit from the use of the method. However, the gain relative to control subjects was apparent only immediately after studying the list for the elderly subjects. By contrast, experimental young adult subjects continued to excel relative to control subjects, even after a 2-wk retention interval. An age-related deficit was also found to persist for proverbs learned with the pegword method (Wood & Pratt, 1987). Given these disappointing outcomes, it isn't surprising that there has been little recent interest in the pegword method by experimental aging researchers.

Method of Loci

The method of loci has been known for centuries to be a means of enhancing the acquisition of verbal material. For example, Cicero in his *De Oratore* described a remarkable feat by the Greek poet Simonides who had been present at a banquet attended by Romans. While he was outside of the building, it collapsed, crushing the attendants beyond recognition. However, Simondes was able to identify the bodies by their remembered locations (i.e., loci) in the building.

As with the pegword method, the method of loci transforms a serial list (e.g., the names of the people at the Roman banquet) into the equivalent of a paired-associate list. The serial learner is asked to imagine a trip through a familiar environs, such as the learner's own home (or the banquet area for Simonides). At successive distinctive locations in the environs, an image of successive words in the serial list is placed. Thus, if the first stop on the trip is a familiar chair in the living room, the learner might construct an image of a *car* (again, the first item in the serial list) seated comfortably with the front tires resting on an ottoman. To recover the words in the list, the subject travels the route again, this time naming the object found at each location. As with the pegword method, the method of loci promotes rapid serial learning by young adults (e.g., Bower, 1970).

As is also true with the pegword method, investigators have reported somewhat mixed results when the method of loci is used by elderly subjects. Robertson-Tchabo, Hausman, and Arenberg (1976) demonstrated that elderly subjects are able to apply the method successfully. However, they also discovered that their elderly subjects did not apply the newly learned method unless they were specifically instructed to do so. Rose and Yesavage (1983) also found that elderly subjects could use the method to enhance recall of items, relative to no training with the method, but the gain from the use of the method was less than that found for similarly trained, young adult subjects. Thus, as with the pegword method, the method of loci appears to be an even more effective mnemonic technique for younger adults than it is for elderly adults. Finkel and Yesavage (1989) discovered that the method of loci could be taught to elderly subjects by computer-aided instruction about as effectively as it could be taught by a human teacher (young adult subjects were not included in their study). That is, the gain from a pretest list of words (i.e., before mnemonic training) to a posttest list of words (i.e., after mnemonic training) was about the same for the two forms of instruction. Unfortunately, in their study there was no control group receiving only the two lists of words without interpolated mnemonic training. Consequently, it is possible that the gain from pretest to posttest simply resulted from the practice their subjects received on the first, or pretest, list. In other words, practice alone may have been sufficient to produce sufficient nonspecific transfer for yielding the gain in words recalled on the second, or posttest, list. In the absence of a control group receiving practice only, it is impossible to determine the effectiveness of the specific mnemonic training.

One of the more intriguing demonstrations of the potential effectiveness of the method for both young and elderly adults was given by Kliegl, Smith, and

Baltes (1989). Their training procedure permitted their subjects to expand the number of loci (familiar city landmarks) on the imagined trip as they became increasingly adept at employing the method. Eventually, subjects at both age levels were able to extend greatly the number of items that could be recalled as the number of loci expanded, but to a greater degree for the young adult subjects than for the elderly subjects. In a later study, Kliegl, Smith, and Baltes (1990) investigated the relationship between scores on a digit-symbol test and number of words from a lengthy list presumed learned with the aid of the method of loci. A moderately high positive correlation was found for their elderly subjects. Performance on a digit-symbol test is commonly used as an assessment of an individual's rate of processing information (see p. 210). The implication is that the efficacy of using the method of loci by elderly adults is affected adversely by their slower rate of processing information. Kliegl et al. (1990) offered an alternative explanation as well. Performance on a digit-symbol test may also be viewed as being an index of an individual's level of fluid intelligence. The efficacy of the use of the method of loci could therefore be limited by the reduced developmental capacity in fluid intelligence (see Baltes, 1987, for a discussion of fluid intelligence's developmental capacity). Of further interest is the finding that older adults who seemingly had expertise in the use of imagery (graphic designers) did attain higher levels of performance than other older adults without such expertise with the method employed earlier by Kliegl et al. (1989), but they, nevertheless, performed at a level below that of young adult subjects (Lindenberger, Kliegl, & Baltes, 1992).

Finally, Anschutz, Camp, Markley, and Kramer (1985) found that elderly adults could be trained to use the method of loci for improving their memory of shopping list items. However, many of the same subjects abandoned the use of the strategy when they were asked to learn new lists several weeks later, and many of them reported not using the method in their everyday lives when interviewed several years later (Anschutz, Camp, Markley, & Kramer, 1987).

Keyword Method

The keyword method was introduced by Atkinson and Raugh (1975) as a means of enhancing acquisition of a foreign language vocabulary. Consider, for example, the Russian word *gora* which means "mountain." Subjects are first instructed to find a "keyword," namely an English word that sounds as much as possible like a part (not necessarily all) of the foreign-language word and will lend itself to forming an interacting image with the English translation. In this case, the likely choice for the keyword is *garage*. A possible interacting image is that of a mountain squeezed tightly into a large garage. When encountering *gora* again, the recovered image should enable the subject to translate the word into "mountain." Atkinson and Raugh (1975) found their method, which is really a form of mediated paired-associate learning, to facilitate greatly the acquisition of a limited number of foreign-word-English-translation associations by young adults. The keyword method was later extended by McCarty (1980) as a means of facilitating face-name associations. It is this use of the keyword method that has found its way into a number of aging studies.

For face-name acquisition, subjects are trained to transform the person's name to a similar-sounding word that lends itself readily to an image. For example, for the name *Whalen*, the keyword is likely to be "whale." The next step is to identify a prominent feature of the person's face, such as a large mouth. A compound image is then constructed that incorporates both the facial feature and the key-word, such as a whale stuffed inside a large mouth. A future encounter with Whalen will, hopefully, activate the image and therefore the name. Here, too, the keyword method has been found to facilitate acquisition by young adults (McCarty, 1980).

Elderly adults have been found to use the keyword method rather effectively to learn face-name associations in the laboratory (Yesavage and Rose, 1984a). Yesavage and Rose employed young adult, middle-aged, and elderly subjects. Each subject received two lists each composed of 12 face-name pairs, the former component being a picture of a face. The first list was given as a pretest (i.e., before subjects received training on the use of the keyword method), and the second list was given as a posttest (i.e., after training). For the results shown in Figure 4.1, the experimenter provided the mnemonics, that is, the name transformation and the prominent facial feature to serve as mediators (somewhat comparable results

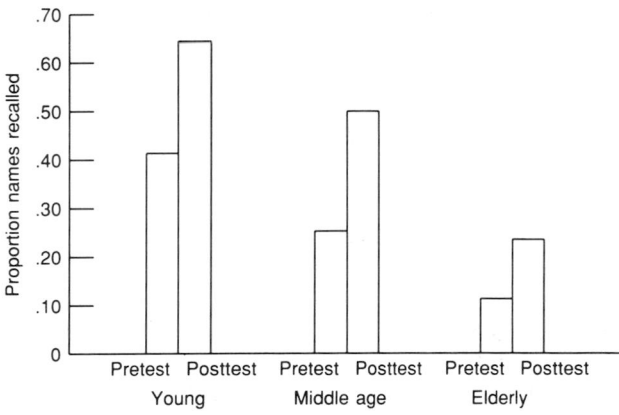

FIGURE 4.1 Proportion of names recalled to faces before (pretest) and after (posttest) training with the keyword method. (Adapted from Yesavage & Rose, 1984a, Table 1.)

were obtained when the subjects generated their own mnemonics). It may be seen that training with the keyword method was followed by a substantial increase in the proportion of names recalled to the face stimuli at all three age levels. However, even with the training, the elderly subjects still recalled only 24% of the names.

Supplementary Procedures

A potential means of enhancing the effectiveness of either the method of loci or the keyword method for elderly subjects is to have them make affective judgments for the images they have generated. The subjects in a study by Yesavage and Rose (1984b) received either training with the method of loci alone or training in which the method of loci was combined with an additional operation. Specifically, subjects in this second condition were required to judge the degree of pleasantness for each image involving a list item and its locus. Subjects in the locus only condition improved their proportion of items recalled from pretest (prior to training) to posttest (after training) by only .06. By contrast, subjects in the loci-plus-judgment condition improved their recall by .26. The investigators reasoned that the pleasantness judgment forced increased elaboration of item-loci compounded images, thus enhancing the durability of the images consistent with the levels-of-processing model of episodic memory; see Chapter 6, pp. 183–185). In agreement with this position, the loci-plus-judgment subjects showed no decline in proportion of items recalled after a 20-min delay, in contrast to the modest decline manifested by subjects in the loci-only condition. (According to the levels of processing model, elaboration serves to increase the durability of a memory trace over time; see Chapter 6, pp. 182–183). A similar outcome was obtained by Yesavage, Rose, and Bower (1983) with the keyword method. Elderly subjects who were required to make pleasantness ratings for each compound image of an object and a face they generated recalled more names than elderly subjects who generated the image without making a pleasantness judgment.

Another way of attempting to enhance the effectiveness of mnemonic training is to precede that training with a nonmnemonic training program that stresses some factor that is expected to facilitate the use of the mnemonic (Yesavage, 1983). These nonmnemonic programs include training elderly subjects in the use and value of imagery as a memory aid (Hill, Sheikh, & Yesavage, 1988) and training elderly subjects to relax (Yesavage & Jacob, 1984). Both of these nonmnemonic training conditions were included in a study by Gratzinger, Sheikh, Friedman, and Yesavage (1990), with subjects given mnemonic training with the keyword method. The gain from pretest to posttest recall scores for the two conditions did not differ significantly. Unfortunately, neither a control condition with practice only nor a condition with only mnemonic training were included in this study. Thus, it is impossible to separate the added benefit given by prior nonmnemonic training from the benefit given by mnemonic training alone. Interestingly, relaxation pretraining appears to improve learning proficiency for elderly subjects identified as being high in anxiety, but, strangely, it appears to hinder the learning proficiency of elderly subjects identified as being low in anxiety (Yesavage, Rose, & Spiegel, 1982). Anxiety remains a problem for elderly subjects even after they have completed a memory training program. Some time after training, Hill and Vandervoort (1992) had their subjects study and recall a lengthy list of new items, and they found a low, but statistically significant, correlation ($r = -.25$) between self-reported state anxiety scores and recall scores. Finally, Lachman, Weaver, Bandura, and Lewkowicz (1992) combined what they called a cognitive restructuring program with mnemonic training. Their elderly subjects viewed a videotape modeling adaptive response for dealing with laboratory and everyday learning tasks, and they then participated in group discussions stressing the controllability of learning by the learner. They found that the subjects in this group had a greater sense of their ability to improve their learning proficiency than did subjects in a control group. However, the two groups did not differ in their performance on a laboratory learning task.

Individual Differences Variables

The effectiveness of mnemonic training has been found to be correlated with several individual differences variables. Not surprisingly, one of these variables is age itself—the older the elderly adult, the less effective mnemonic training is likely to be (Verhaeghen, Marcoen, & Goossens, 1992). Yesavage, Sheikh, Friedman, and Tanke (1990) found the negative effect of age to be more pronounced with the complex method of loci than with the relatively simpler keyword method. The negative relationship with age, of course, limits the use of mnemonic training in that it is very old learners who are likely to experience the largest learning deficits and are therefore the most eligible candidates for mnemonic training. Closely related to age as a variable is the cognitive status of the learner as measured by the Mini-Mental State Examination (MMSE; Folstein, Folstein, & McHugh, 1975). Elderly adults who score relatively low on this test (but are still considered to be in the normal aging range) have greater difficulty with the more complex method of loci than with the simpler keyword method (Yesavage et al., 1990; see Figure 4.2). In fact, even elderly adults with minimal cognitive impairment, as measured by the MMSE, have difficulty benefiting from relatively complex mnemonic training (Hill, Yesavage, Sheikh, & Friedman, 1989). This is again unfortunate, in that the greater the impairment, the greater the need for mnemonic training. As observed by Yesavage et al. (1990), the cognitive status of an individual should be given heavy weight in deciding what kind of mnemonic training could benefit that person.

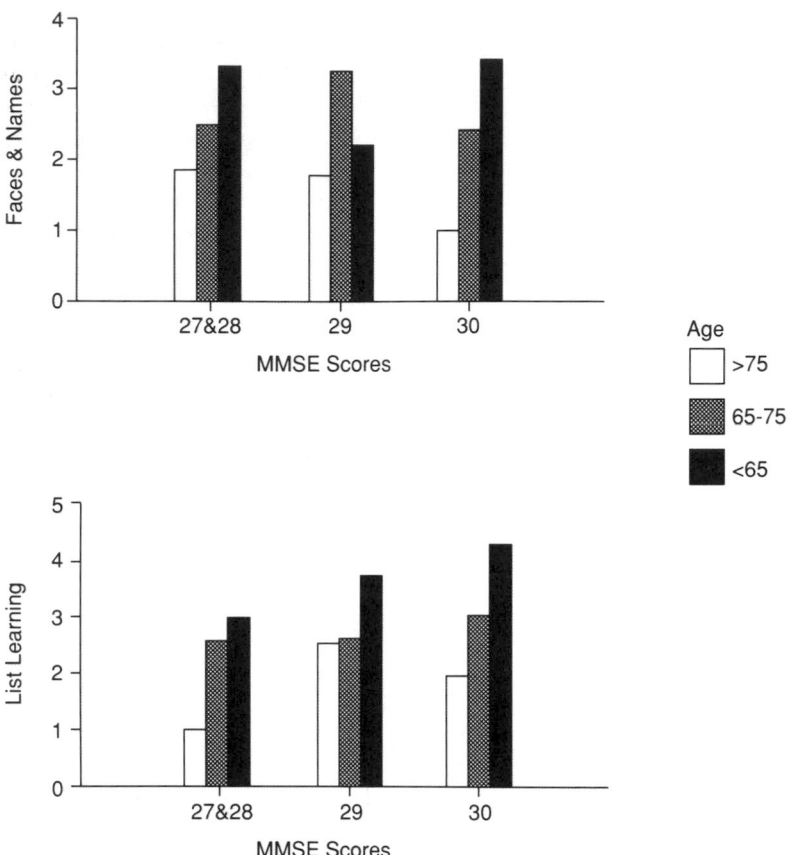

FIGURE 4.2   Improvement in face-name recall and list recall by age group and Mini-Mental State Examination (MMSE) score. (Adapted from Yesavage, Sheikh, Friedman, & Tanke, 1990, Figure 1.)

Young adult and elderly subjects appear to differ in their preference for the keyword strategy relative to an alternative strategy, at least for learning definitions of unfamiliar words (Brigham & Pressley, 1988). The alternative strategy in Brigham and Pressley's (1988) study was to incorporate each new word in a sentence. Before using either strategy, 65% of the young subjects and only 40% of the elderly subjects expressed a preference for the keyword strategy. After actually using each strategy, the preference for the keyword strategy increased to 98% for the young subjects but only to 42% for the elderly subjects. The keyword method is obviously not a favorite of older people. Zivian and Darjes (1983) asked their young adult and elderly subjects to rate 20 different memory strategies in terms of their usefulness in learning word lists. The correlation between the ratings for the two age groups was positive but rather low ($r = .29$). Again, there seems to be a pronounced age difference in the preference values of mnemonic strategies.

Elderly adults may be classified as being "complainers" or "noncomplainers" with respect to their perceived proficiency of their everyday learning and memory ability. It seems reasonable to assume that those people who feel their learning proficiency has diminished greatly would be the ones who would benefit the most from mnemonic training. Scogin, Storandt, and Lott (1985) found that laboratory mnemonic training improved the proficiency (i.e., a gain from pretest to posttest) for a group of elderly subjects who were classified as "complainers," relative to other "complainers" who did not receive mnemonic training, but that it had little effect on reducing the concerns these individuals had about their learning and memory functioning. Actually, their concerns were probably unwarranted in the first place, given the fact that the "complainers" performed as well as on various laboratory learning/memory tasks both before and after training as the "noncomplainers" included in the same study. Interestingly, Scogin and Bienias (1988) retested three years later a number of subjects included in Scogin et al.'s (1985) study. At that point, previously trained subjects did not differ in their laboratory performances from previously untrained subjects.

Elderly adults also differ in the degree of depression they have. Learning and memory concerns have been found to be especially prevalent in more severely depressed elderly adults (Kahn, Zarit, Hilbert, & Niederehe, 1975; Larrabee & Levin, 1986; Popkin, Gallagher, Thompson, & Moore, 1982). Zarit and his associates (Zarit, Cole, & Guider, 1981; Zarit, Gallagher, & Kramer, 1981) have discovered that mnemonic training does reduce memory concerns for these individuals and that it also seems to result in the reduction of depression as well.

Even a personality trait has been found to be related to the gain in scores from pretest to posttest for elderly subjects trained with the keyword method (Gratzinger et al., 1990). The trait is one called Openness (either open to experience or closed to experience; Costa & McCrae, 1988). Subjects who are more open to experience were found to have a moderately higher gain score than subjects less open to experience. By contrast, scores on neither the Neuroticism trait nor the Extraversion trait (Costa & McCrae, 1988) correlated significantly with gain scores (Gratzinger et al., 1990).

Alternative Methods of Mnemonic Training

Formal training with either the method of loci or the keyword method does seem to have a positive effect on the immediate learning proficiency of some elderly adults. In a meta-analysis of the studies employing these methods, Verhaeghen et al. (1992) concluded that the positive effect exceeds that obtained with either a practice alone control condition or a placebo control condition (i.e., a condition in which subjects receive training, but it is irrelevant to learning). However, they also concluded that the extent of the benefit depends, in part, on the duration of the training. Formal training needs to be both intensive and extensive, and it is therefore unlikely to attract many elderly adults to participate in it voluntarily. The advantage of intensive and extensive training was nicely demonstrated in studies by Swedish investigators (Neely & Bäckman, 1993a,b; Stigsdotter & Bäckman, 1989). Their elderly subjects received eight sessions of training spread over eight weeks. The sessions included training in the use of both interactive imagery and the method of loci. For some subjects, training in imagery was supplemented by training in attention and relaxation. The benefit of training in the use of imagery was demonstrated by the superior performance of the trained subjects over the control subjects on memory tests administered even as long as 3½ years after training. The benefit was especially pronounced for those subjects whose imagery training was supplemented by training in attention and relaxation.

Fortunately, these training methods need not be restricted to use in a laboratory setting. There are manuals available (e.g., Scogin & Flynn, 1986) that enable elderly subjects to teach themselves these method by means of descriptions of the methods and numerous practice exercises. However, Flynn and Storandt (1990) discovered that self-instruction on these mnemonics seems to be effective in improving learning proficiency only when it is supplemented by periodic group discussions. Imagery training and training with the method of loci were included in the manual for the elderly subjects in Scogin and Prohaska's (1992) study. However, following training, the self-trained subjects did not differ in word list recall from control subjects in a placebo condition, even though the trained subjects exceeded the placebo subjects in their subjective evaluations of their learning ability.

Mnemonic methods of the kind that involve the use of imagery have severe limitations in their likely everyday use by elderly people. In the first place, they are effortful to apply, and they require an imaginal ability that is likely to be difficult for many elderly adults to apply (see Chapter 3, pp. 92–97). Many elderly adults who learn a basic method, such as the keyword method, are likely to abandon its use soon after learning to use it, especially since they may find imagery difficult to use in the first place. Moreover, if used frequently, a method such as the keyword method is likely to engender more interference than facilitation. For example, a large mouth is surely characteristic of many new faces one encounters. How often can an image of a large mouth be incorporated with images of keywords without producing massive amounts of interference? What happens when one meets different individuals with the same surname? Conceivably, a different keyword could be found for each instance, but confusion is the likely result. Elderly adults aren't the only ones who are unlikely to use an imagery-based mnemonic in their everyday lives. Park, Smith, and Cavanaugh (1990) reported a survey of 69 memory researchers in which they rated on a five-point scale (1 = never use; 5 = use daily) the frequency with which they used mnemonics in their daily lives. The mean rating for these researchers were 1.20 for the pegword method, 1.39 for the method of loci, and 1.81 for the keyword method—all values that did not differ from those found for comparison groups of nonmemory psychologists and nonpsychology professors. Even the memory experts find little use for imagery-based mnemonics! Surely, their learning–memory proficiency could stand improvement. On the other hand, the keyword method could serve as a means of enhancing the acquisition of a limited foreign language vocabulary that elderly adults could use in visiting a foreign country. Here interference would surely be less than would be found in face-name learning. Unfortunately, as noted earlier, this use of the keyword method has apparently not been tested with elderly adults.

There is an option for a mnemonic device other than the use of imagery. We discovered in Chapter 3 that verbal mediators serve reasonably well as mediators for learning paired associates. Elderly adults may also be taught in a training program to use an organizational process (see Chapter 7, pp. 229–243, for a discussion of organizational processes) to enhance the recall of a lengthy serial-word list. Here subjects are taught to find relatedness among items within the list. Hill, Storandt, and Simeone (1990) found that instruction in the use of organization (by means of a take-home manual) resulted in a substantial gain from pretest to posttest, both for immediate recall and recall after 35 min, for their elderly subjects, relative to their placebo control subjects. Another promising verbal training procedure is to have subjects construct a story from the words in a list, with the words in the story being in the order they are in the list (Bellezza, 1981; Bower & Clark, 1969). It is known that when elderly subjects have no training prior to studying a lengthy serial-word list, a number of them report subsequently to having used a variety of mnemonics to learn the list (Camp, Markley, & Kramer, 1983; Hill, Allen, & Gregory, 1990). Hill et al. (1990) found that only about 12% of their elderly subjects reported the spontaneous use of the story mnemonic. Most important, however, this minority group recalled more of the words from the list than subjects using any other form of a mnemonic, and they recalled considerably more words than those subjects who relied only on rote repetition of the words. The story mnemonic, like the organizational mnemonic, can be made the focal point of a training program for elderly adults. When it is, it has been found to facilitate acquisition and retention over several days of a word list, relative to a placebo control group (Hill, Allen, & McWhorter, 1991). Drevenstedt and Bellezza (1993) discovered that the effectiveness of a story mnemonic varied greatly among three subgroups of elderly subjects that differed either in the narrative they constructed from the words or in the retrieval of the narrative they had constructed. The poorest word recall was found for those elderly subjects who constructed an impoverished narrative. These subjects also scored the lowest on measures of overall cognitive ability, such as a test of working memory capacity. Their elderly subjects who were highly proficient both in constructing a narrative and in recalling words from it recalled as many words as young adult subjects and scored the highest among the three subgroups in working memory and vocabulary test scores. Elderly subjects who encoded the words well into a continuous narrative but had later difficulty in retrieving those words fell between the other two subgroups both in word recall and in measures of cognitive ability.

One of the greatest problems in the use of mnemonics is the fact that the kinds of problems facing elderly adults in their everyday lives are usually not those involving intentional learning in which time is available for multiple trials and a mnemonic technique is relevant to the kind of material to be acquired. Instead, the problems are likely to involve information that is acquired incidentally and after only a single exposure to that information. Common examples are memory for the content of a conversation (e.g., with a physician), memory for an action performed at home (e.g., turning off the gas on the stove), and remembering to perform a needed action at the appropriate time (e.g., mailing a check to the utility company). Here the traditional mnemonic techniques have little applicability (Duke, Haley, & Bergquist, 1990).

Fortunately, for intentionally learned information, there is another mnemonic that doesn't involve the use of imagery and could readily be taught to elderly adults. It is a method that we will encounter later in our discussion of retrieval processes in memory (Chapter 7, pp. 268–269). There is no reason why it couldn't be applied in the acquisition of paired associates as well. It requires subjects to recall at short time intervals responses to stimuli for each subset of the total number of acquired paired associates. From the perspective of memory theory, the method focuses on retrieval processes rather than on the encoding processes that are the basic ingredients of standard mnemonic training methods, both imaginal and verbal in content. Consider, for example, attending a party where you meet six new people, all of whom you are likely to meet again. After the first two or three people have been introduced, say the name while viewing each face. Then a short time later, gaze at these faces again while forcing yourself to recall each name. Then go through the same steps for the next subset of people, and so on until all face-name associations have undergone a recall of the name at a short retention interval. Such short-term recall should serve to enhance long-term retention. Amazingly, through the use of this method, several researchers (Camp, 1989a; Hill, Evankovich, Sheikh, & Yesavage, 1987; see also Camp and McKitrick, 1992) have been able to have several SDAT subjects retain name-face associations for up to a week when previously they couldn't retain them for more than a few seconds. Unfortunately, others (Bäckman, Josephsson, Herlitz, Stigsdotter, & Vitanen, 1991) have not been as successful. The degree of severity of dementia is surely a critical factor in determining even limited success with any mnemonic training method applied to patients with senile dementia of the Alzheimer's type (SDAT). Even with information that is usually acquired incidentally and with limited opportunity for repetition or practice, a training program that stresses short-term retrieval may prove to be effective (e.g., repeating to oneself the instructions given by a physician) (Bergquist, Duke, & Davis, 1989).

Adult Age Differences in Transfer

In the real world, learning rarely occurs in a vacuum. Usually, learning of a particular task is affected by the learning of prior tasks. For some new tasks, prior learning hinders present learning, resulting in negative transfer, whereas for other tasks, prior learning facilitates present learning, resulting in positive transfer. Transfer varies not only in direction (i.e., positive versus negative) but also in amount for each direction. Our interest is mainly with the possibility of adult age differences in amount of transfer, whether positive or negative. However, we cannot ignore the possibility of age differences in direction of transfer for some kinds of transfer conditions.

Specific versus Nonspecific Transfer: Implications for Adult Age Differences

Tests of adult age differences in transfer effects are complicated by the existence of two distinctive sources of transfer—*specific* and *nonspecific*. Specific transfer results from a relationship of some kind between the S and R elements of the transfer task and the prior-learning task that affects acquisition of the transfer task. One form of relationship is one of particular relevance to the classical interference theory that was designed to explain both negative transfer and retroactive or proactive interference in retention (e.g., Melton & Irwin, 1940; Postman, 1961; Postman & Underwood, 1973; see Kausler, 1974, for a detailed review of interference theory and specific-transfer mechanisms). In it, the two tasks, or lists (usually paired-associate lists), have identical S elements and unrelated R elements. That is, the tasks form an A-B, A-C relationship (identical stimuli across lists, different responses) in which the A-C list forms the transfer task and the A-B list the prior learning task. With paired-associate lists, the first list pairs may be symbolized as A_1-B_1, A_2-B_2, and so on, and the second list pairs as A_1-C_1, A_2-C_2, and so on. For example, *apple-table* may be the A_1-B_1 pair of the first list and *apple-pencil* the A_1-C_1 pair of the second list. Interference generated by intruding A → B associations during practice on new A → C associations is expected to retard acquisition of the new associations. In principle, the previously learned A_1-B_1 association inhibits rehearsal of the A_1-C_1 association, the previously learned A_2-B_2 association inhibits rehearsal of the A_2-C_2 association, and so on. The net effect is negative specific transfer on the second list (although the negative effect is compensated for partly by the positive transfer from first-list stimulus learning to second-list stimulus learning—the stimuli are identical, meaning no new stimulus learning may be required in mastering the second list; see Chapter 3, pp. 81–82). Beginning with Ruch's (1934) pioneering research, elderly adults have long been viewed as being more interference prone than young adults and should therefore exhibit greater amounts of negative transfer. As noted in Chapter 3 (p. 75), interference may also occur among pairs when learning a single list, and perhaps to a greater degree for elderly subjects than for younger subjects.

Another form of interlist relationship of special interest to us is one in which successive lists continue to have identical S elements and different R elements, but this time the R elements of the two lists are related in some way. In transfer terminology, related R elements are symbolized as B and B'. With these symbols in mind, our new transfer condition may be identified as involving the learning of A-B, A-B' lists. As an example, consider *apple-table* as the A_1-B_1 pair (first list) and *apple-chair* as the A_2-B_2 pair (second, or transfer, list). Real-life A-B, A-B' sequences do exist. Owners of professional athletic teams seem to be especially fond of them. For example, the Milwaukee Bucks have existed for some years as a men's professional basketball team. When a women's professional basketball team was formed in Milwaukee, the owners, surely not coincidentally, named the team the Does. Note that Milwaukee → Bucks corresponds to an A→B association in a transfer sequence and Milwaukee → Does to an A→ B' association.

The relatedness between B and B' elements makes it possible to use the first-list association to mediate the learning of the new association in the transfer list. That is, intrusion of a B element during practice on the new list should enhance rather than hinder learning of the new set of associations. The net effect should be specific positive transfer, but only if mediation is indeed operating during learning of the transfer list's associations. It is this contingency that makes the A-B, A-B' transfer condition, or paradigm, intriguing to experimental aging psychologists (Kausler, 1970). Elderly subjects are less likely than young adult subjects to engage spontaneously in mediation during practice on A-B' pairs, and they should, therefore, be less likely to display specific positive transfer in this condition. There is, in fact, the possibility that related B and B' elements may be treated as if they are unrelated B and C elements. If true, the A-B, A-B' condition would become equivalent to an A-B, A-C condition. The consequence should then be specific negative transfer of the kind generated by an interference relationship.

Nonspecific transfer is always positive in direction. It occurs whenever successive tasks are of the same general format. For example, the tasks may all require paired-associate learning, or they may all require serial learning. In either case, prior learning of one task is expected to facilitate acquisition of subsequent tasks, even when the S and R elements of the successive tasks are unrelated to each other. The primary reason for this facilitation is the occurrence of what is called learning-to-learn (Goulet, 1972; Kausler, 1974; Postman, 1969). It is a general process that is independent of a task's specific content. During practice on the first task, subjects are learning not only the content of that task but also the kinds of skills demanded for proficient performance on it and other tasks. When the task format is that of paired-associate learning, one of these general skills is the use of mediation to link S and R elements together. The advantage gained by seeking out and utilizing mediators may not be discovered until a subject is deeply immersed in practice on the first paired-associate task. Once discovered, however, the skill should become operative immediately on all subsequent paired-associate tasks. These later lists should, therefore, be learned more easily than the initial list, thus yielding nonspecific positive transfer. Imaginal mnemonic training procedures, in fact, have as their objective the stimulation of learning-to-learn the use of imaginal mediators. Another reason for the presence of nonspecific positive transfer stems from the fact that it often takes subjects time to warm up to performing on a laboratory task, much the way it takes an athlete time to warm up before an athletic contest. Performance on a first task may be affected adversely by the failure of subjects to have warmed up sufficiently. This should not be true for subsequent tasks, thereby eliminating a potentially debilitating factor for performance on these later tasks.

The existence of nonspecific positive transfer complicates any attempt to evaluate the direction and magnitude of a specific transfer effect (i.e., an effect attributable to the relatedness of items across tasks). Consider, for example, transfer in the A-B, A-C condition. The hindrance in learning A-C pairs that is produced by negative specific transfer is compensated, at least in part, by the facilitation that is produced by nonspecific positive transfer from the first list (A-B) to the second list (A-C). The resultant is a reduction in the magnitude of the overall negative transfer that would otherwise be present in the absence of the positive contribution made by nonspecific transfer.

The standard means of assessing a specific-transfer effect at any age level calls for the use of experimental and control groups of subjects. The experimental group receives the list sequence defining the specific transfer condition, such as an A-B first list and an A-C second, or transfer, list. The control group receives a list sequence that permits an adjustment for the contribution made by nonspecific transfer to an overall transfer effect. That sequence consists of an A-B first list and a C-D transfer list. C and D in this context refer to the S and R elements of the transfer list, respectively. The letters symbolize the fact that these elements are unrelated to the S and R elements of the first list. For example, given *apple-table* as the A_1-B_1 pair of the first list, *book-jewel* could function as the C_1-D_1 pair of the transfer list.

With this design, experimental and control subjects have an equal opportunity to benefit from nonspecific positive transfer. That is, subjects in both groups should profit, and in approximately equal amounts, from the learning-to-learn and warm-up occurring during first-list practice. Whatever difference is then observed in second-list performance between the two groups must be attributable to the specific transfer present only in the experimental group. Inferior performance for the experimental group relative to the control group identifies the presence of negative specific transfer, whereas superior performance identifies the presence of positive specific transfer. In addition, the magnitude of the difference in performance between the two groups identifies the magnitude of the specific negative or positive transfer effect. These procedures are summarized in Figure 4.3 for both the A-B, A-C transfer condition and the A-B, A-B' condition. Our interest is primarily in age differences in specific transfer effects. From our preceding analyses, predictions are fairly straightforward—the amount of specific negative transfer (control group > experimental group; see part A, Figure 4.3) should be greater for elderly subjects than young adult subjects, whereas the amount of specific positive transfer (experimental group > control group; see part B, Figure 4.3) should be greater for young adult subjects.

Laboratory Studies of Nonspecific Transfer

Before turning to adult age differences in specific transfer, we will examine the limited information available about age differences in nonspecific transfer. We are mainly interested in adult age differences in nonspecific transfer on paired-associate-learning lists. However, the existence of nonspecific transfer is certainly not restricted to paired-associate learning. For example, even performance on a digit-span task shows pronounced increments in performance over a number of practice sessions for both young adults and elderly adults, although, as is true for most tasks, extensive practice seems to leave the magnitude of the age difference unaltered (Taub, 1973; Taub & Long, 1972). Both younger and older subjects also show nonspecific transfer on a free-recall task, with the magnitude of the age-related deficit being about the same on a second free-recall list as on a first list (Hultsch, 1974). Nonspecific transfer was also found for the transformed reading task described in Chapter 2 (pp. 61–63). Apparently, both young and elderly subjects acquired a pattern-recognition skill that facilitated reading times on later new transformed sentences or words, relative to reading times on earlier new sentences or words (i.e., learning-to-learn). Young adult subjects, but not elderly adult subjects, manifested nonspecific transfer for random sequences of hand postures, and neither young adult nor elderly adult subjects displayed nonspecific transfer for random sequences on a serial-reaction-time task involving responding to patterns of asterisks (see Chapter 2, pp. 64–65).

An early study by Monge (1969) indicated that elderly subjects may show less nonspecific transfer on paired-associate lists than do young adults. However, more recent studies by Treat, Poon, and Fozard (1981) and Erber, Abello, and Moninger (1988) imply that this may not be the case. Our interest is in the control

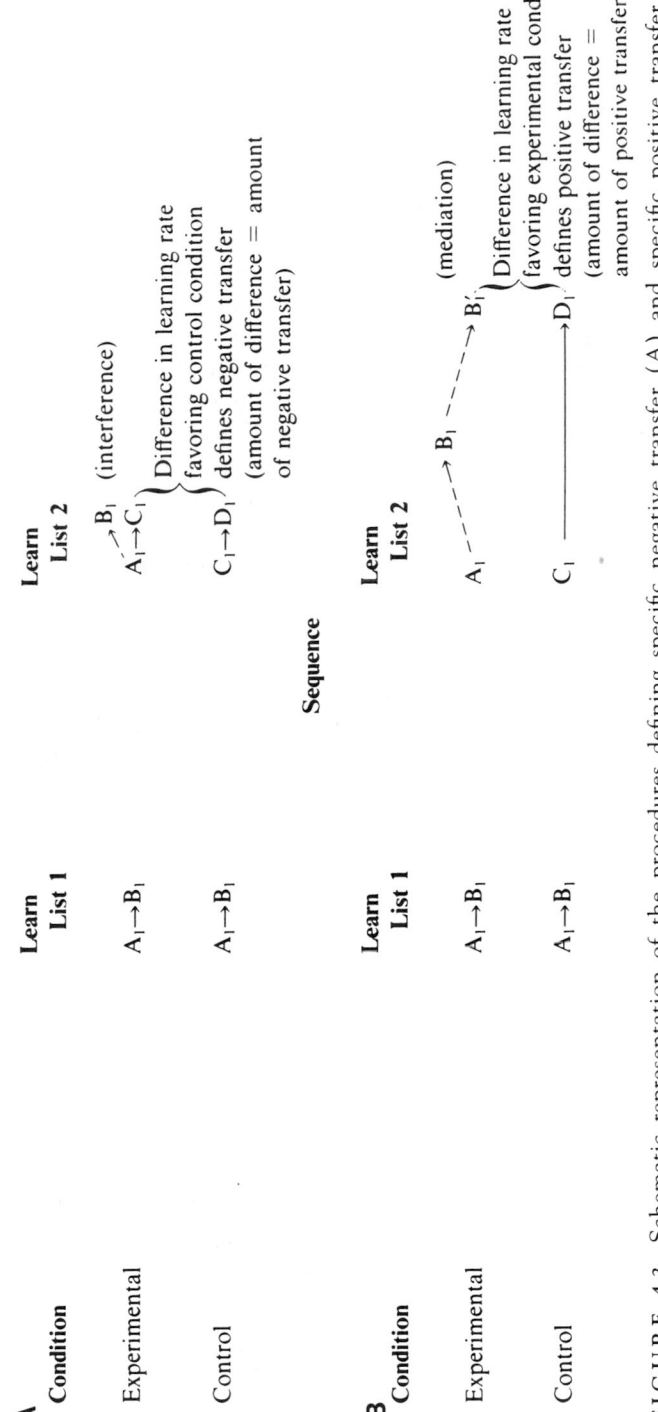

FIGURE 4.3 Schematic representation of the procedures defining specific negative transfer (A) and specific positive transfer (B panel).

condition in each study where subjects received no special instructions or train-ing as to how to acquire associations.

In Treat et al.'s (1981) study, both their young adult and elderly adult subjects received six paired-associate lists (10 pairs of concrete nouns per list; unrelated content across lists), each list practiced to a criterion of an errorless trial. The lists were spread over three sessions, 2 wk apart, with two lists received in each session. For the first list, the young and elderly subjects required averages of 4.80 and 14.67 trials, respectively, to attain the criterion. On the second list, the average number of trials was reduced by about one half for each age group (mean trials = 2.10 and 7.00). On the final list (the sixth one received), the means were reduced further to 1.80 and 4.78 for the young and elderly groups, respectively. It is apparent that pronounced nonspecific transfer occurred regardless of age, and to approximately equal degrees for the two age groups. In Erber et al.'s (1988) study, their young and elderly subjects received one study-test trial on three successive lists (unrelated content across list), each containing 14 word pairs. Shown in Figure 4.4 are recall scores on each list for each age group. From List 1 to List 3, recall scores increased by about 42% for the young subjects and about 30% for the elderly subjects, a relatively moderate age difference. On the other hand, it is also apparent that nonspecific transfer increased at a much faster rate for the young subjects. Their gain in recall scores from List 1 to List 2 was about 34%, while the gain was only about 12% for the elderly subjects. Of interest is the likely outcome if a fourth list had been tested. From Figure 4.4, it seems apparent that a plateau had already been reached by the third list for the young subjects, but not for the elderly subjects. Conceivably, the amount of nonspecific transfer for elderly subjects from the first to the fourth list would have approxi-mated that for young subjects.

Laboratory Studies of Specific Transfer

Studies of retroactive inhibition or interference that are directed at interfer-ence theory's account of forgetting (see Chapter 10 pp. 357–359) always include the appropriate group for evaluating specific negative transfer, namely, one re-ceiving an A-B, A-C list sequence. However, the single-list control group in these studies, although appropriate for assessing the effects of interference on retention, fails to provide a baseline for equating contributions from nonspecific transfer. Consequently, it is impossible to interpret age differences of the kind illustrated in Figure 4.5. Part A shows the mean number of trials to learn the A-B and A-C lists in Arenberg's (1967b) study, whereas the part B shows the comparable means in Hulicka's (1967a) study. In both studies, young adults improved in proficiency from the A-B list to the A-C list, whereas elderly subjects either showed no gain (part A) or a decrease in proficiency (part B). Thus, the age difference favoring

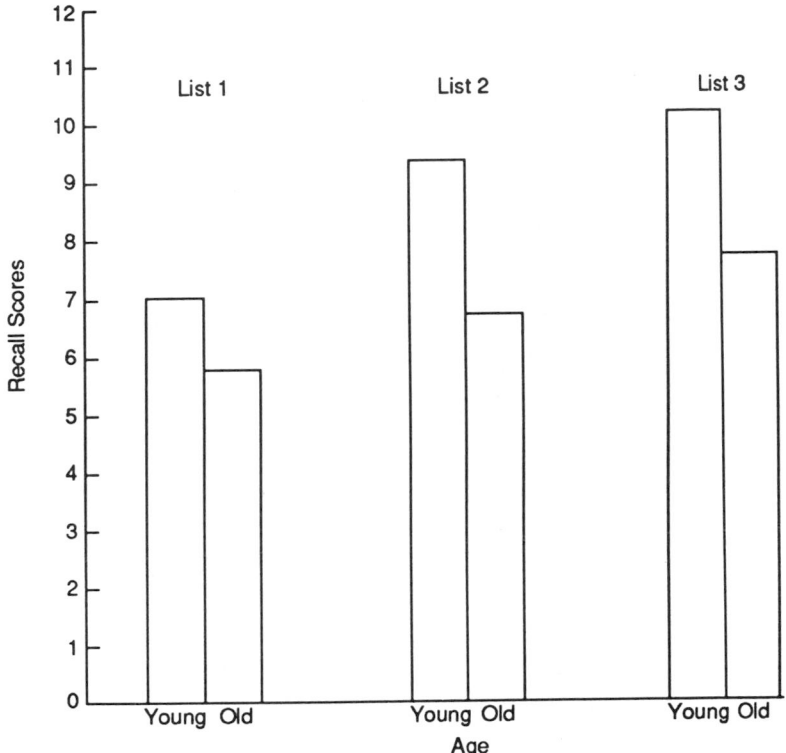

FIGURE 4.4 Nonspecific transfer as measured by recall scores on successive paired-associate lists. (Adapted from Erber, Abello, & Moninger, 1988, Table 2.)

young adults was greater in both studies for the A-C list than for the A-B list. Unfortunately, however, the obvious Age X List interaction effect could be due either to greater specific negative transfer for elderly subjects, in agreement with the possible age differential in interference proneness, or to greater nonspecific positive transfer for young subjects. The absence of an A-B, C-D control group for nonspecific transfer at each age level prohibits a distinction between these alternative explanations of the age difference.

The only study of age differences in specific negative transfer that did include the appropriate control groups appears to be that of Freund and Witte (1976). Rate of item presentation was also included as an independent variable in their study. We will consider only the results obtained with a moderately fast rate, a rate comparable to that used in most transfer studies with young adults. Both experimental and control groups learned the A-B list to a criterion of one error-

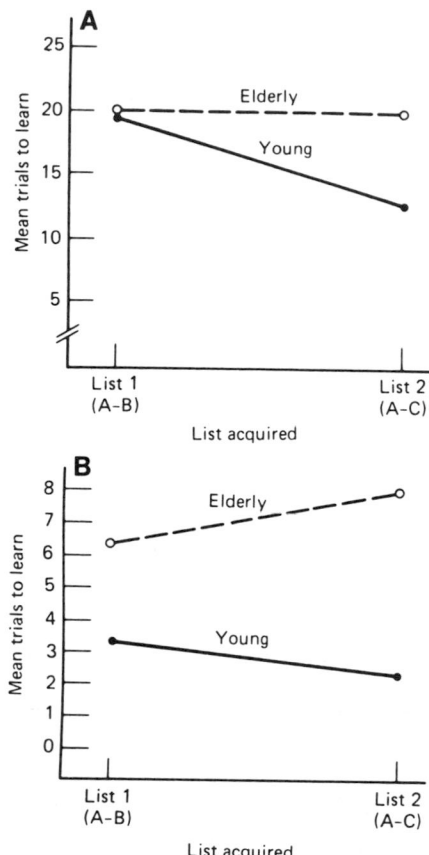

FIGURE 4.5   Age differences in trials to learn the first and second lists of an A-B, A-C sequence. (A: Adapted from Arenberg, 1967a, Table 1; B: Adapted from Hulicka, 1967b, Table 3.)

less trial. They then received four trials on the second list (A-C or C-D). The results, expressed in terms of mean number of correct responses on each trial of List 2 practice, are shown in Figure 4.6 (maximum score = 12 for young subjects, 6 for elderly subjects; list length was intentionally made shorter for the elderly subjects). Note that negative transfer did occur at both age levels on the early trials. That is, performance on the C-D list clearly exceeded performance on the A-C list at both age levels. Of greater importance to us, however, is the absence of any sign of more negative transfer for elderly subjects than for young adult subjects. This pattern conflicts with that expected if elderly subjects are indeed more interference prone than young adults. The absence of an age difference in

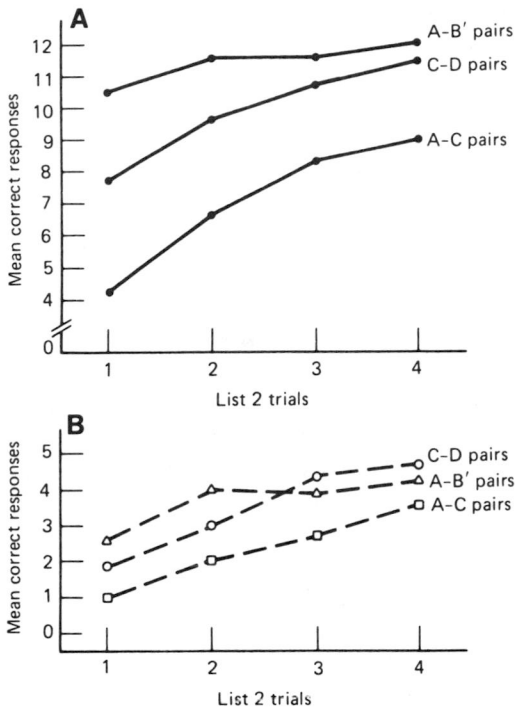

FIGURE 4.6 Correct responses by young adult (A) and elderly (B) subjects over trials on List 2 for various transfer conditions. (Reproduced from Freund & Witte, 1976, Figures 1, 2. Copyright 1976 by the University of Illinois Press.)

negative transfer is also in agreement with the absence of an age difference in the magnitude of retroactive inhibition (see Chapter 10, pp. 359–362). Here, too, an age differential in interference proneness leads us to expect more retroactive inhibition for elderly than for young adult subjects.

The possibility of an age differences in amount of specific negative transfer does not end with the A-B, A-C transfer condition. There are other transfer conditions that involve interference during practice on the transfer list. One of these conditions entered into a study by Lair, Moon, and Kausler (1969). Interference in this case was created by real-life associative learning. That is, the learning of the laboratory list was confronted by interference from preexperimental learning much the way it was in Ruch's (1934) list with false equations. The A-B list in Lair et al.'s study was a phantom one, in the sense that it really was not learned in the laboratory, as was also true for Ruch's (1934) false equation list. It consisted of word pairs, such as *table-chair*, that were strong word associates and, therefore, highly likely to have been well learned in the real world. Experimental subjects were then required to learn what is called an A-Br list. The A and B symbolize the fact that the S and R elements of the transfer list are the same elements contained in the first list; the r symbolizes the fact that these elements are re-paired on the transfer list. The nature of this re-pairing is illustrated in Table 4.1. Note that the experimental subjects must inhibit, or suppress, their prior *table → chair* association while acquiring the new *table → queen* association. Such suppression is made difficult by the presence of the word *chair* as the R element of another to-be-learned association in the laboratory list. Control subjects were required to learn a list containing the same R elements as the list learned by experimental subjects but with different S elements. The replacements were neutral with respect to prior associative connections with the R elements, thus eliminating interference from previously learned associations (see Table 4.1). Lair et al. (1969) found their experimental list to be acquired much more slowly than their control list by both middle-aged and elderly subjects. However, the disparity in learning rates was far more pronounced for their elderly subjects. This study implies that there are extreme transfer conditions in which elderly adults do seem to be more interference prone than younger adults.

In a later study with the A-B, A-Br paradigm, Kliegl and Lindenberger (1988) had the A-B list, as well as the A-Br list, learned in the laboratory. Their young and elderly subjects received successive paired-associate lists in which the same S and R words were repeatedly re-paired across lists. In two separate studies, they found their elderly subjects were much more likely than their young subjects to emit on test trials words that had been paired with S elements on preceding lists, rather than words paired with S elements on the present list. Again, with this extreme negative-transfer condition, elderly adults do appear to be more interference prone than young adults.

TABLE 4.1

Examples of the Kinds of Pairings Used in the Study of Age Differences in Transfer for the A-B, A-Br Condition

	List 1 (learned preexperimentally)		List 2 (learned in the laboratory)			
	All subjects		Experimental subjects		Control subjects	
Pair	S element	R element	S element	R element	S element	R element
A_1-B_1	Table	Chair	Table	Queen	Tennis	Queen
A_2-B_2	Fast	Slow	Fast	Chair	Flag	Chair
$A_n B_n$	King	Queen	King	Slow	Kind	Slow

An unusual negative-transfer condition was employed in a study by Winocur and Moscovitch (1983) with young adult subjects and both community-dwelling elderly subjects and elderly subjects living in an institutional setting (senior citizens' homes). Experimental subjects received two lists which the investigators identified as conforming to the A-B, A-C interference condition. However, the pairs in the first list consisted of semantically related words, such as *army-soldier*, and the second list consisted of the same stimulus elements paired with a new response, but one also semantically related to the stimulus and to the response element of the first list, as well (e.g., *army-battle*). Control subjects received only the second, or A-C, list. The three age groups were basically equivalent in performance on the A-C list in the control condition, which isn't surprising given the high degree of associative relatedness between S-R pairs. However, the two elderly groups performed at a significantly lower level on the A-C list in the experimental condition, with the age-related deficit being especially pronounced for the institutionalized elderly subjects. On the surface, these results imply greater interference proneness for elderly than for young adult subjects. However, the results are difficult to interpret from the perspective of a traditional transfer analysis. The use of related items within pairs and across lists creates a unique transfer condition with undoubtedly a number of processes other than interference per se. Moreover, the absence of an A-B, C-D control for nonspecific transfer complicates interpretation further. Interestingly, however, Winocur and Moscovitch (1983) discovered that the greater deficit for the institutionalized than for the community-dwelling elderly subjects disappeared in another experiment when the two lists in the experimental condition were practiced under environmental conditions that were highly distinctive for the separate lists. Apparently, the shift in context was especially useful for the institutionalized subjects as a means of discriminating the current list from the prior list, thereby reducing the amount of interference from the prior list. Community-dwelling elderly adults seemingly were able to make this kind of discrimination without support from an environmental shift.

There is another negative-transfer condition that should be of interest in aging research. It is one in which experimental subjects receive an A-B, C-B list sequence (whereas control subjects continue to receive an A-B, C-D list sequence). A C-B list carries over the R elements from the first list but replaces the prior S elements with new elements. For example, *apple-table* may serve as a first-list pair, whereas *anchor-table* serves as the second-list counterpart. Although some positive specific transfer is expected from the fact that the response-learning stage completed on the first list eliminates the need for further response learning in the second list, the fact is that overall negative specific transfer is often found in the C-B condition when young adults serve as subjects (e.g., Kausler & Kanoti, 1963). Its presence is explained by interference generated from competing R-S, or backward, associations during practice on C-B pairs (see Kausler, 1974, pp.

228–237, for elaboration). Note that a backward association within the first list, such as *table* → *apple*, does form the equivalent of an A-B, A-C interference relationship with the backward association of its second-list counterpart, such as *table* → *anchor*. What should make this transfer condition intriguing to geronto-logical psychologists is our earlier observation that elderly subjects generally man-ifest less R-S associative learning than do young adult subjects during practice on a paired-associate task. Given this diminished amount of R-S learning, elderly subjects should experience less backward interference than young adult subjects during practice on C-B pairs, and they should, therefore, show less specific nega-tive transfer than the young subjects.

This possibility has yet to be tested adequately in the laboratory. There have, however, been several studies (Boyarsky & Eisdorfer, 1972; Traxler & Britton, 1970) that have included the A-B, C-B condition in tests of age differences in retroactive inhibition. Interference theory maintains that there is a close rela-tionship between the amount of retroactive inhibition for the first list and the amount of negative transfer for the second list during practice on lists bearing any kind of interference relationship with each other. Conditions that alter the amount of negative transfer should also alter the amount of retroactive inhibi-tion. In this case, age is the critical condition. Because elderly subjects are ex-pected to show less negative transfer than young adult subjects for the A-B list preceding the C-B list, they are also expected to show less retroactive inhibi-tion for the A-B list preceding the C-B list. Unfortunately, methodological prob-lems inherent in the aforementioned studies make it impossible to evaluate age differences in amount of retroactive inhibition found with an A-B, C-B list se-quence (see Arenberg & Robertson-Tchabo, 1977, for further discussion of these problems).

Finally, what little is known about age differences in specific positive transfer comes from the previously mentioned study by Freund and Witte (1976). In-cluded in their study were experimental groups receiving A-B, A-B' list se-quences. The groups differed with respect to the degree of relatedness, high versus low, between B and B' response elements. We will consider only the condition employing a high degree of relatedness (defined in terms of word-association norms). The results obtained for this condition at each age level are plotted in Figure 3.6 along with the results obtained for the A-C and C-D groups. The scores are again the number of correct responses for each of four trials (again, maximum values = 12 and 6 for young and elderly subjects, respectively). Note that positive transfer was clearly present for the young subjects early in practice on A-B pairs (see top, Figure 3.6). The amount of positive transfer diminished with continuing practice, as indicated by the eventual convergence with perfor-mance on C-D pairs. The decrement in positive transfer surely resulted from an early ceiling effect found for A-B' pairs. A very different picture emerged for performance on A-B' pairs by elderly subjects (see bottom, Figure 3.6). Here, the amount of specific positive transfer was not distorted by a ceiling effect. Only slight positive transfer relative to C-D pairs appeared early in List 2 practice, and it eventually disappeared by the end of practice. Mediation on a transfer list seems to be as age sensitive as it is on an initial learning list.

Just as specific negative transfer extends to conditions other than the standard A-B, A-C condition, specific positive transfer extends to conditions other than the standard A-B, A-B' condition. For example, one such extension involves successively learned associations having identical R elements and related S elements (i.e., an A-B, A'-B condition; e.g., *table-pencil, chair-pencil*. Positive transfer is the general rule for young adult subjects receiving this sequence (see Kausler, 1974, pp. 235–236). Generalizing from what little is known about age differences in positive transfer with A-B' pairs is, of course, risky, but, in the absence of any research on age differences in other positive-transfer conditions, there is no alternative. Comparable age-related deficits are likely to be found in these other conditions, probably because of an age-related deficit in the proficiency of a mediating process. In the A-B, A'-B condition there is a further source of specific positive transfer through the transfer of response learning from the first to the second list (as in the A-B, C-B transfer condition). To what extent this positive transfer serves to mitigate the negative transfer expected for elderly subjects from a mediational deficit is unknown. Gaining knowledge of the extent of these age-related deficits should be an important objective of future experimental aging research. Much of everyday learning at all age levels does involve positive transfer from past learning. Once it is established that there are age-related deficits in such transfer, ways of compensating for these deficits may then be pursued. There is good reason to be optimistic that compensatory procedures will be discovered. In real-life positive transfer situations, elderly adults should have an important advantage over young adults, namely, a greater store of accumulated knowledge. Surely, ways could be found to utilize this knowledge as a means of compensation for whatever deficits exist in specific transfer mechanisms (e.g., mediation).

Comments

Many studies have been reviewed in this chapter and in Chapter 3. Collectively, they have contributed a great deal to our knowledge and understanding of adult age differences in verbal learning and transfer. We discovered that age-related deficits do exist on most kinds of learning tasks and that the age-sensitive processes accounting for many of these deficits have been identified. We also discovered that age differences in many transfer phenomena are slight and often nonexistent.

At the same time, we discovered that there remain significant gaps in our knowledge about age difference for various verbal learning and transfer phenomena. In fact, for some phenomena, such as stimulus selection in learning and transfer in the A-B, C-B and A-B, A'-B conditions, there really have not been studies directed at demonstrating the presence or absence of adult age differences. Whether or not these gaps will be filled in the near future is uncertain. They exist in areas that are viewed traditionally as belonging to associationism. Research linked to associationism in general has been viewed in recent years as belonging to experimental psychology's less than fruitful past, a past in which learning, rather than memory, was emphasized. Psychology has not reached a stage of development as a science in which any one conceptual model is clearly the correct one. Experimental aging research that has had its origins in associative concepts and principles has enriched our understanding of the effects of aging on learning and transfer (and on long-term retention as well, as we will discover in Chapter 10). Many of these effects do have important implications for adaptability to the world outside of the laboratory. Serious students of human aging should be as familiar with the contributions made in these areas as they are with the contributions made in more recent research on memory. Hopefully, some of these serious students will someday fill in the missing pieces needed for a full description and understanding of adult age differences and changes in verbal learning and transfer. There is some reason for being optimistic that they will do so. As Willingham, Nissen, and Bullemer (1989) observed, the current interest in procedural learning has directed the attention of cognitive psychologists to learning. Procedural learning need not be restricted to perceptual/motor-skill acquisition. Surely, the concept of "procedures" applies to verbal learning as well (e.g., learning-to-learn).

CHAPTER•5

Sensory Memory and Short-Term/ Primary Memory

Introduction

What did you have for lunch a week ago? Assuming your diet is somewhat more varied than a daily hamburger, a reasonable guess is that you do not remember what you did have to eat. In fact, if you grace various food establishments with your presence, you probably have difficulty remembering where you ate that day. Of course, if you happened to have dropped your tray in a cafeteria on that occasion, you may find the entire episode, including the contents of the tray, to be distinctive enough to be readily accessible for recall. This is far from being an isolated incident. What about the attempt at humor one of your professors made in class the other day? You may remember the gist of the humor, but not the finer details. Even a rigorous search of your memory system will probably fail to retrieve those missing details. How much do you remember of the last commercial you watched on television? Of the last sporting event you attended?

Memory of the kind illustrated above is obviously imperfect, and its imperfection is manifested throughout the life span. (In one of my favorite comic strips, a little girl informed her mother that her forgettery was better than her memory.) The ubiquitousness of memory failure in adulthood may be seen in the results obtained in an interesting study by Cavanaugh, Grady, and Perlmutter (1983). Their subjects, who ranged in age from 20 to 76 yr, maintained a memory diary for a period of time. In it, they kept a daily record of their failures to remember such things as an item they had intended to purchase at the supermarket. There was a pronounced age difference in the concern expressed by subjects about their memory failures. The older members of this sample reported themselves to be more upset with their failures than did the younger members. This shouldn't be surprising—many elderly adults list problems about memory to be one of their greatest concerns about growing old (e.g., Lowenthal et al., 1967). The number of actual memory failures recorded by the older subjects was actually only moderately greater than the number recorded by the younger subjects. The difference may well have underestimated the magnitude of daily memory problems confronting many elderly adults. If subjects in their 80s had been included in this study, the age difference would probably have been much greater. Moreover, we have to question the extent to which diary keeping really captures the full scope of memory problems. Most important, there may well be an age difference in the number of times a memory failure is itself forgotten before it can be recorded in a diary. Nor can the self-reports of elderly people be accepted as being fully reliable indices of their own memory capabilities. The correlation between severity of memory complaints and performance on laboratory memory tasks is often found to be essentially zero (see Chapter 4, p. 113, and Chapter 12, pp. 416, 423).

Not all memories are as trivial as remembering what one ate for lunch on a given day or remembering a professor's joke. Many memories greatly affect our everyday activities. Memory of a weather forecast determines the degree of preparation for a heavy snowstorm. Memory of whether or not you turned off the stove before leaving home could be instrumental in determining the presence or absence of a disaster. Memory of a stranger's face may make you either an excellent eyewitness or a poor eyewitness to a crime. Our list could go on and on—memory proficiency clearly plays an important role in determining how well we perform in the everyday world. There is an obvious need to evaluate the extent of age-related changes in the proficiency of memory and to determine the reasons for those changes. Conceivably, training procedures could then be found to reduce whatever deficits do occur in late adulthood. If such procedures fail to materialize, then there is need for an alternative strategy. Specifically, elderly people could be encouraged to employ memory surrogates as much as possible. Many of these surrogates are already widely used by people of all ages who do not quite trust their memory systems. They include copious note taking at meetings to assure important details are not forgotten, carrying an appointment book to record the time and place of all future commitments, listing all expenditures in a daily log, and so on. Objective records of these kinds compensate considerably for at least some shortcomings of the human memory system. Surely their value as memory surrogates will be expanded greatly by the eventual widespread use of home computers.

Our example of memory problems and failures are representative of what is called *episodic memory*. It deals with autobiographical information: "The essence of episodic memory is that it recaptures the temporal and spatial context of a person's past experience" (Lachman, Lachman, & Butterfield, 1979, p. 215). In other words, it retains information about personally experienced episodes or events in one's life—contents, and the time and place of their occurrences (i.e., contextual information). In a laboratory situation, one such episode might be *king*'s presence as a to-be-remembered item in a lengthy study list. *King*, of course, is not learned in the laboratory—it was acquired years before and stored forever in another component of the total memory system, namely *generic* or *semantic* memory (Tulving, 1972). Generic memory is a permanent long-term store where information is retained without reference to context, that is, the where or when it was acquired (see Chapter 12). What is now acquired, or rather remembered, is the occurrence of *king* in a particular temporal-spatial context (i.e., as part of a list practiced on a given day in a given laboratory). This occurrence is appropriately encoded and transmitted to a long-term episodic store. Conversely, to forget *king*'s episodic representation in no way means that *king*'s permanent representation has been forgotten or lost forever from your vocabulary. Nor does it necessarily mean that *king*'s memory trace has been "lost" from the episodic store. Conceivably, the trace may be available, but it may be, at least at the moment, inaccessible for retrieval (i.e., getting information out of the store).

The laboratory researcher's interest in list-inclusion episodes rests in the assumption that these episodes simulate those of real life—such episodes as remembering what items you are to purchase at the supermarket. These are the kinds of episodic events elderly people usually have in mind when they refer to their memory problems. Although the validity of this assumption can be questioned on ecological grounds, it can scarcely be denied that age-related deficits are found for list-inclusion episodes, just as they are for the everyday events elderly people claim to have trouble remembering. Laboratory studies may overestimate the magnitude of age-related deficits in episodic memory, but they may, nevertheless, serve effectively to identify the reasons why deficits of any magnitude occur in everyday episodic memory experiences. Normally aging individuals who show signs of modest to moderate memory problems were once classified as having "Benign Senescent Forgetfulness" (Kral, 1962). The currently preferred classification is that of "Age-Associated Memory Impairment" (AAMI) (Crook et al., 1986).

Unfortunately, what is known about age differences in learning has little relevance for age differences in episodic memory. Although one could argue (e.g., Smith, 1980) that the encoding of episodic information is actually learning, there is good reason, as we tried to convey in Chapter 1 (p. 4), for maintaining a distinction between learning and episodic memory. Traditional learning theories, namely, those derived from associationism, have contributed little, if anything, to our understanding of memories for personally experienced events. By contrast, information processing psychology has made episodic memory a focal point of its analysis of human behavior (see Solso, 1979, 1988 for extensive reviews of information processing psychology). Accordingly, our review of age differences or changes in episodic-memory proficiency will focus on research instigated by information processing models and analyses of the human memory system (see Craik, 1977; Craik & Jennings, 1992; Hultsch & Dixon, 1989; Kausler, 1985, 1989b; Light, 1991, 1992; Perlmutter et al., 1987; Poon, 1985; Walsh, 1975; for additional reviews). Our main objective in the present chapter is with two very transitory forms of episodic memory, namely, sensory memory and primary, or short-term, memory. Initially, however, we will begin with an overview of the human memory system. In Chapter 6 we will turn to the specific models of more permanent, or secondary, episodic memories that have served to guide aging research. These models differ largely in the way they deal with the processes and stores involved in the transmission of memory traces to a long-term store (LTS). Several additional chapters will be devoted to various secondary memory phenomena (e.g., organization, generation effect) and to various kinds of episodic memories (e.g., words, actions) that may be encoded and stored for later retrieval, and to long-term forgetting. Our coverage of age differences in memory will conclude in Chapter 12 with a discussion of generic memory and what psychologists call metamemory.

Overview of the Human Memory System

Shown in Figure 5.1 is a general model of the total-memory system that will guide our conceptualization of memory phenomena and age differences in those phenomena. There are indeed alternative models (e.g., Cowan, 1988), but the one illustrated in Figure 5.1 is, in our opinion, the model that provides the best fit to research on age differences in memory. Specific models of episodic memory per se, such as dual-store and levels-of-processing models, vary in terms of additions and/or deletions in the general model that serve to account for variations in the durability (or permanence) and retrievability of episodic-memory traces (see Chapter 6). Any model of episodic memory is directed at conceptualizing the flow of episodic information through the stages of *encoding, storage,* and *re-*

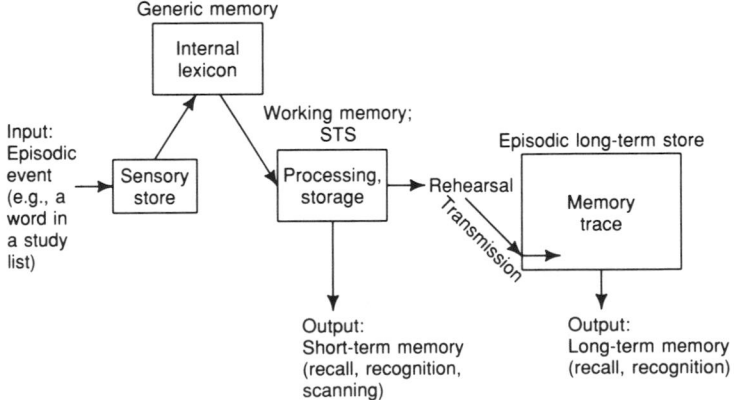

FIGURE 5.1   General model of the human memory system.

trieval. However, models differ in the emphasis they give to these stages. For example, in its original form, the levels-of-processing model focused almost exclusively on encoding and storage, with little attention being given to retrieval processes.

Both operative and storage structures are postulated to be involved in the flow of information within the system. Operative structures provide the space for the encoding of information to form an episodic-memory trace, the rehearsing of that information, and the transmitting of the resulting trace to a permanent episodic LTS. Our assumption is that this processing space resides in the limited capacity (and, presumably, a diminishing capacity from early to late adulthood) working-memory structures or its equivalent (e.g., the short-term-store (STS) in a dual-store model; to be described later). Four storage structures serve as repositories of information at different stages of representation of to-be-remembered information. The initial store is a place where input to the system (e.g., a word in a study list) resides briefly in sensory form while being subjected to the processes of pattern recognition. Here information is matched with information in a component of the permanent generic memory, the *internal lexicon* (a mental dictionary; see Chapter 12, pp. 388–391) and transmitted to working memory, where it resides in a limited capacity (and, presumably, diminishing capacity from early to late adulthood) STS. While in working memory, information may either be recalled directly (as for the short-term memory) or encoded/rehearsed and transmitted as a memory trace to the episodic LTS. If retained in the LTS, the information contained in the memory trace may eventually be retrieved and outputted in the form of recall or recognition. The phenomena of sensory memory and short-term, post-sensory memory are components of any specific model of episodic memory.

Adult Age Differences in Sensory Memory

Episodic-memory traces begin with information that reaches a sensory register. It is there that the information in sensory form is transformed into a psychological representation and is transmitted to other components of the memory system where encoding processes transfer the information further into a memory trace. The initial transformation of that information from sensory form requires time, and it is abetted by the brief storage of that information in the sensory register. That is, sensory memory occurs, with its capacity and duration being contingent on the specific sensory register involved in the transformation.

Iconic Memory

Does information held in a sensory receptor terminate as soon as the originating stimulus terminates? With visual stimuli, there is good reason to believe that it does not. Consider an array of letters flashed briefly (say, for 50 ms) by means of a tachistoscope. A subject's task is to identify, or name, as many of the letters as possible. The amount of information that can be seen in a glance is known as the *span of apprehension*. For young adults, the span has been known for many years to be four or five letters (Woodworth, 1938). There is some evidence (Schonfield & Wenger, 1975) indicating a modest decline in late adulthood. However, it has also been known for many years that subjects typically report to the experimenter that they actually see more than four or five letters—the problem is that the image of what they have seen seems to have faded away by the time they have named four or five letters. Most important, they report that images of the letters persist briefly after the visual stimulus ceases. Subjectively, they feel they are naming the letters seen in these persisting images, and they continue to do so until the images disappear. Thus, it appears that the visual system retains information briefly, with the information being in the form of an image, or icon, of a just-terminated stimulus. Not surprisingly, this form of retention of sensory information has been labeled *iconic memory* (Neisser, 1967).

Iconic memory plays an important adaptive role in information processing. It prolongs the time information is available for perceptual analysis and transformation to a psychological representation (e.g., a letter of the alphanet). That is, the processes of pattern recognition are not necessarily restricted to operating on information that is presently reaching the receptors of the retina; they may continue to operate on the memory of that information. The time extension permitted by iconic memory probably enhances the operations of selective attention as well. As observed by Solso:

> By preserving the complete sensory impression for a brief period we can scan the immediate events, picking out those stimuli which are most salient, and fitting them into the tangled matrix of human memory. When all works properly, no more or no less information is coded, transformed, or stored than is necessary for humans to carry on a normal existence (1979, p. 48).

Three questions come to mind immediately concerning iconic memory. The first concerns its locus. Is it really a peripheral phenomenon produced by continuing activity of retinal receptors (i.e., rods and cones)? Or is it a central phenomenon that reflects the encoding of information into some postsensory, or nonphysical, format? Here we find considerable division of opinion among basic researchers who have been investigating the nature of iconic memory. On the one hand, there is evidence to indicate that iconic memory stems from persisting activity of both rods (Sakitt, 1975) and cones (Adelson, 1978). On the other hand, there is also evidence to indicate postsensory factors are at least partially responsible for the existence of iconic memory (Holding, 1975; Merikle, 1980; Sakitt & Appleman, 1978). The second question concerns the duration of iconic memory. Here we cannot trust the subjective reports of subjects. What is needed are methods that permit rigorously controlled assessments of an icon's duration. Fortunately, two such methods have appeared in the past 25 yr. The third question, the one that concerns us most directly, follows naturally from the second: Are there adult age differences in the capacity and/or duration of iconic memory? To the extent that iconic memory is determined by the same, or highly similar, mechanisms that determine visual-stimulus persistence, we should expect duration to be longer for elderly adults than for young adults. A number of experimental aging studies have supported the notion that neural traces of visual stimuli persist longer for elderly adults than for young adults (see p. 36, and also Kausler, 1991, for further review of research on stimulus persistence).

The first method was introduced in a famous study by Sperling (1960). The method is basically an expanded version of the method used to measure the span of apprehension for letters. We noted earlier that this method consists of exposing an array of letters briefly and having subjects name as many of the letters as possible. Sperling continued to use this procedure, requiring his subjects on some trials to give what he called a whole report. Specifically, an array of 12 letters was exposed for 50 ms. As illustrated in part A of Figure 5.2, the array was arranged in 3 rows of 4 letters each. Immediately after the termination of the array's exposure, subjects on whole report trials began naming as many of the 12 letters as they could. In agreement with many early studies, Sperling found that they could name, on the average, about 4.5 letters (i.e., the span of apprehension). Stated somewhat differently, they could recall about 40% of what they had seen. Sperling's innovative touch consisted of the inclusion of another condition, one in which subjects gave a partial report rather than a whole report. In a partial report, only the letters in a single row had to be named. His subjects did not know in advance on any partial-report trial which one of the three rows was the one to be named. That knowledge came only *after* the physical display itself had been terminated, and it came in the form of a tone that signaled which of the three rows was the target for that trial (the rows varied randomly in being signaled over trials). A high-frequency tone signaled "name the top row," a medium-frequency tone signaled "name the middle row," and a low-frequency tone signaled "name the bottom row." One other highly innovative feature was added to the partial-report condition. Sperling varied the interval separating termination of the visual display and the signal cuing which row to name. This interval was set at 0 ms on some trials (i.e., the signal sounded as the display went off), and 150, 300, 500, or 1000 ms on other trials. The nature of this procedure is summarized in part B of Figure 5.2.

Sperling's (1960) results with the partial report condition are shown in Figure 5.3. Performance is expressed in terms of the percentage of row letters correctly named (i.e., out of the 4 letters in a row). Note that about 80% of the letters in a signaled row could be identified after a 0-ms delay. His subjects, of course, did not know on any given trial which row would be signaled for

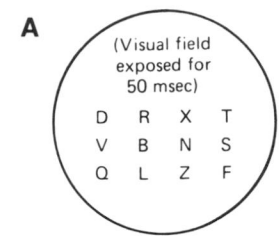

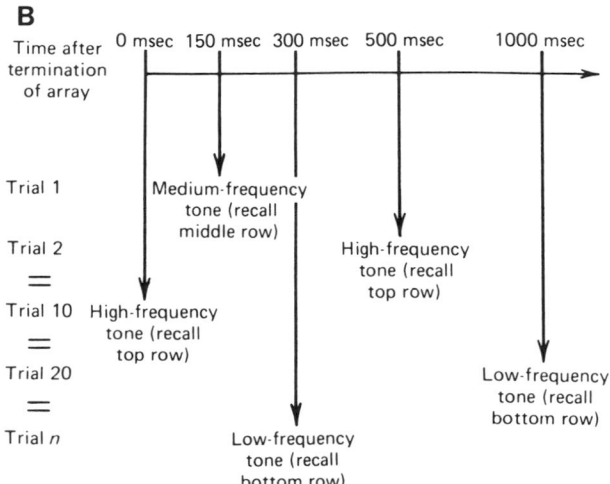

FIGURE 5.2 A: Typical array of letters exposed briefly for a Sperling task in which subjects give either a whole report (all letters) or a partial report (a single row). B: Example of the procedure followed in the partial report condition of a Sperling task.

identification. Thus, if 80% of the designated row could be identified, then the implication is that 80% of each of the other two rows could also have been identified. A reasonable estimate, therefore, is that the actual capacity of the iconic memory store is about 9.6 letters (i.e., 80% of 12) rather than 4.5 letters as estimated by the whole report procedure. The reason why the capacity of the store appears to be less in the whole report condition is that information stored in the form of icons fades as the subject begins to name the letters. By the time 4 or 5 letters have been transferred to a postsensory short-term store where they are held for reporting, the icons have disappeared completely, thereby prohibiting any further recall of what may have been seen. Now consider what happens with the partial report procedure when the signal is delayed 100 or more ms. During the delay, iconic information is fading rapidly, making fewer and fewer letters available for identification. By 500 ms, the percentage was down to 50% (see

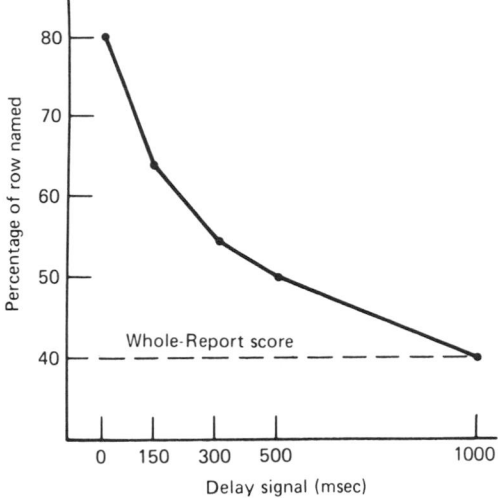

FIGURE 5.3 Percentage of the letters reported in a row (partial report) as a function of the delay between termination of the visual display and onset of the signal cuing which row to report. (Adapted from data in Sperling, 1960).

Figure 5.3), and by 1000 ms it had reached the 40% level found with the whole report procedure. A reasonable argument is that as long as partial-report recall exceeds full-report recall (in terms of percentage of letters recalled), some iconic memory remains. Once partial-report recall is reduced to the level of whole-report recall, only information that had been transmitted to the postsensory, STS before recall was signaled is available for recall. Thus, a comparison of partial- and full-report scores provides an estimate of the duration of iconic memory. Sperling's results (Figure 5.3) indicate that the duration for young adults is at least 500ms but less than 1 s.

Sperling's (1960) ingenious method offers a potentially valuable means of examining adult age differences in the capacity of the iconic store as well as the duration of iconic memory. Unfortunately, however, its use with elderly subjects encounters a number of obstacles (see Walsh and Prasse, 1980, for a detailed discussion). Indicative of these obstacles is the fact that 8 out of the 10 elderly subjects entering into a study by Walsh and Thompson (as reported in Walsh, 1975) were unable to perform under a partial-report condition. Their difficulty may have been one of attention rather than the absence of iconic memory per se. A partial report demands the rapid focusing of attention on a segment of the information held in the iconic store. With increasing age, the rapid shifting of attention becomes increasingly more difficult to accomplish. Another kind of problem encountered by elderly subjects was demonstrated in a study by

Salthouse (1976). His elderly subjects were characterized by an inefficient strategy in adapting to partial-report conditions. Specifically, they tended to focus their attention on only the top row of letters in the array. This is fine as long as recall of the top row is signaled. However, it makes the letters in another row virtually impossible to recall when that row is signaled. By contrast, his young adult subjects displayed a far more flexible strategy. Yet another problem stems from the time it takes to perceive and interpret the auditory cue signaling which row to report (Crowder, 1976). This duration is likely to be longer for elderly than for young subjects, thus allowing more time for the decay of elderly subjects' icons before a "read-out" of the icons ever begins.

Despite these methodological problems, there have been two more recent fairly successful attempts to compare young and elderly subjects in their whole-versus-partial-report performances (Coyne, Burger, Berry, & Botwinick, 1987; Gilmore, Allan, & Royer, 1986). In their study, Coyne et al. (1987) exposed arrays of 8 letters (2 rows of 4 letters each) for 50 ms. On whole-report trials, the young subjects reported about 62% of the letters, the elderly subjects about 44%. Only one partial-report condition was employed, one in which the row cue followed immediately after the offset of the array (i.e., a 0-ms delay). For the signaled row, young subjects reported correctly about 78% of the letters, the elderly subjects about 49%. Thus, a partial-report advantage was observed for both young and elderly subjects, but the advantage was much greater for the young subjects. On the surface, this outcome could be interpreted as indicating a diminished capacity of iconic memory in late adulthood. However, as noted by Coyne et al. (1987), young adults read out iconic information, and transfer it to short-term memory for verbal reporting, at a faster rate than do elderly adults (Cerella, Poon, & Fozard, 1982). The slower encoding of iconic information by elderly subjects implies greater opportunity for the fading of that information before it can be reported verbally. When a measure of encoding time (time needed to avoid backward masking of stimuli) served as a covariate, Coyne et al. (1987) discovered that the magnitude of the effect of age variation diminished considerably for both whole- and partial-report scores. Consequently, there appeared to be only a modest age-related deficit in the capacity of iconic memory. Since Coyne et al. (1987) did not employ varying delays between array offset and the partial-report cue, their study permits no age comparison for the duration of iconic memory.

The encoding time problem was seemingly eliminated in Gilmore et al.'s (1986) study by exposing the array of letters for a longer duration for their elderly subjects (200 ms) than for their young adult subjects (30 ms) and by sounding partial-report cues simultaneously with the presentation of the array. Under these conditions, no age difference was found for either whole-report or partial-report scores, with both age groups showing substantially larger scores for partial reports. In another experiment, they varied the delay for the partial report through 150 ms, with both age groups continuing to show a partial-report advantage through 150 ms. Unfortunately, still longer delays were not employed, making it impossible to determine the presence or absence of an age difference in the duration of iconic memory (i.e., the delay at which partial-report scores, in terms of percentages of letters recalled, equal whole-report scores.

The second method, one introduced by Eriksen and Collins (1967), is one in which successive identical stimuli (e.g., flashes of light) are presented with a varying interstimulus interval (ISI). It is a method used to investigate age differences in visual stimulus persistence. The measure of stimulus persistence is the critical ISI at which a subject reports seeing two successive stimuli rather than one continuous stimulus. For briefer intervals, the persisting trace of the first stimulus creates the illusion that the physical stimulus is still present. The critical interval was found with flashing lights to be about 90 ms for 70-yr-old subjects and only about 65 ms for 20-yr-old subjects—an age difference in agreement with the postulated greater persistence in late adulthood than in early adulthood (Amberson, Atkeson, Pollack, & Malatesta, 1979). A reasonable argument may be made that the duration of stimulus persistence is related, or even equivalent, to the duration of iconic memory. If true, then there is little reason to believe that its duration is less for elderly adults than for young adults—and it may even be longer for elderly adults (but, regardless of age, much briefer than it is as estimated by the partial-report procedure). The evidence regarding age differences in capacity and duration is ambiguous to say the least. Our best conclusion is that any changes with aging in either the capacity or the duration of iconic memory are likely to be slight, if they exist at all.

Echoic Memory

There is an auditory equivalent of iconic memory, namely *echoic memory* (Neisser, 1967). It has been widely investigated with young adult subjects. As with iconic memory, it refers to the persistence of an image of a physical stimulus. In this case, the image appears to preserve the sound features of an originating auditory stimulus. Solso has given us a clear description of the importance of echoic memory, or the "preperceptual auditory store" in his terms, to information processing:

> Preperceptual auditory store (PAS) is similar to preperceptual visual store (PVS; i.e., iconic memory) in the sense that the raw sensory information is held in it with true fidelity (in order that the pertinent features can be extracted and further analyzed) for a very short time. As in PVS, which allows us an additional time to view fleeting stimuli, PAS allows us additional time to hear an auditory message. If we consider the complex process of understanding common speech, the utility of PAS becomes obvious. Auditory impulses that make up speech are spread over time. Information contained in any small fraction of speech, music, or other sound is

meaningless unless placed within the context of other sounds. PAS, by briefly preserving auditory information, provides us with immediate contextual cues for comprehension of auditory information (1979, p. 45).

Five methods have served to assess directly the duration of echoic memory. Each, in principle, has the potential for extension to experimental aging research for the purpose of evaluating age differences in duration. However, implementing these methods is not easy to accomplish with elderly subjects (see Crowder, 1980, for a detailed account). One obvious problem is the fact that many elderly people experience hearing problems at the direct sensory level. That reason alone probably accounts for the fact that there has been relatively little aging research dealing directly with echoic memory.

The first method is the auditory analogue of Sperling's (1960) partial-report versus whole-report procedure (e.g., Darwin, Turvey, & Crowder, 1972; Moray, Bates, & Barnett, 1965). Three auditory messages (e.g., strings of digits) are presented simultaneously from three different spatial locations. In the whole-report condition, the subject attempts to recall as many digits as possible from all three locations immediately after hearing them. In the partial-report condition, a visual cue signals which one of the three locations is to be reported. Once more, the time between termination of the messages and the onset of the signal is a critical independent variable. A superior partial-report score relative to a whole-report score is viewed as indicating the continuing presence of echoic memory. With young adults, this superiority continues for perhaps at least a full second. Thus, echoic memory is believed to have a somewhat longer duration than iconic memory. Use of this method with elderly subjects is confronted by the same problems encountered in partial-report research on iconic memory. Consequently, it has been of little use in experimental aging research.

The second method (Effron, 1970) requires subjects to identify the offset of an auditory stimulus, with the difference between the true offset time and the perceived offset time providing an estimate of the duration of echoic memory. The third method (Plomp, 1964) is the equivalent of the "gap" method employed in research on visual stimulus persistence. That is, the ISI needed to perceive a silent gap between successive sound stimuli is determined. Research with both the second and third methods indicates that for young adults the duration of echoic memory is probably 200 ms or less. However, the duration is longer for children than for young adults (e.g., Wightman, Allen, Dolan, Kistler, & Jamieson, 1989), and the principle of an adult age difference in stimulus persistence implies that it should also be longer for elderly adults than for young adults. A variation of this method has been employed in two aging studies (Newman & Spitzer, 1983; Raz, Millman, & Moberg, 1989) yielding some suggestive evidence that this may be the case.

The fourth method, the suffix method, is a novel one. Subjects are given a number of serial recall lists, each of which is presented aurally. In serial recall, a string of items, such as digits, is presented for a single study trial, and subjects are asked to recall the items in the exact order presented. In effect, the task is much like that of a memory-span task, except for the fact that the number of items exceeds the number ordinarily spanned without error (i.e., the series is of supraspan length). To test the duration of echoic memory, a simple addition is made to half of the lists a subject receives (Crowder & Morton, 1969). The addition is that of a suffix in the form of an additional element heard at the end of the list. The suffix may be either another digit or letter that is not part of any of the lists or a completely unrelated element, such as the sound "uh." Whatever its nature, the suffix itself is not to be recalled. No suffix is added to the remaining lists (i.e., control lists). The presence of a suffix has a startling effect on recall of the to-be-remembered items. Specifically, the probability of recalling the last few items in the list is markedly below the level manifested for those same positions in the control lists. For other positions in the lists, the decrement produced by the suffix is much less pronounced and may even be nonexistent. The suffix effect was originally viewed as occurring because the tacked on sound at the end of a list blots out the echoic memory of the last few items in the list. Most likely, "blotted out" is the complete auditory information for the last list item and partial information for the immediate items preceding it. This persisting auditory information is available for control lists at the time of recall to aid in the retrieval of the last few items, but it is wiped out in the experimental lists by the masking provided by the auditory suffix.

This interpretation of the suffix effect, however, has been challenged by recent evidence indicating that the suffix need not be auditory in nature to produce the standard suffix effect (i.e., depressed recall of end items). For example, the effect is obtained when the suffix is mouthed by the experimenter and subjects lip-read its content—and even when all of the items are presented visually and subjects mouth them silently (e.g., Greene, 1986; Greene & Crowder, 1984, 1986). That is, a suffix effect is obtained when there is no direct auditory input during list presentation! However, the concept of echoic memory as a precategorical acoustical store (i.e., a store for information in physical form before it has been "categorized" or named) may be preserved if its conceptualization is broadened to include stored information about the mouth and vocal gestures needed to enunciate list items as well as direct auditory feature information (Greene & Crowder, 1984). In other words, echoic memory may contain not only sounds, but also mental, sound-related codes that are relevant to speech. In fact, echoic memory may be conceptualized as consisting of two separate phases or stages, one of brief duration (several hundred ms) and the other of much longer duration (perhaps as long as 20 s) (see Cowan, 1984). Presumably, information in the first stage consists of sound per se, whereas information in the second stage consists of mental codes. It is the duration of the first phase that is measured by the offset and gap methods described earlier. The suffix method seemingly offers a means of measuring the duration of the second stage.

There have been two interesting studies with the suffix method (Parkinson & Perey, 1980; Manning & Greenhut-Wertz, 1990) that provide some information about the proficiency of echoic memory in late adulthood. In Parkinson and Perey's (1980) study, young adult and elderly subjects who were matched for digit-span-performance scores were given a number of serial-recall lists, each composed of seven digits. In their suffix condition, "uh" followed the last digit after an interval of half a second (no "uh," of course, occurred in the control condition). The results obtained for their young subjects are shown in part A of Figure 5.4, and the results obtained for their elderly subjects are shown in part B. Note that their elderly subjects exhibited a suffix effect that did not differ greatly from that of their young subjects. Apparently, echoic memory does continue into late adulthood, and it has a duration of at least half a second. Unfortunately, however, this study does not permit an evaluation of age differences in duration of echoic memory. To accomplish this objective, additional conditions are needed in which the length of the interval separating the last list item and the suffix is varied systematically. The results obtained by Manning and Greenhut-Wertz (1990) were much like those obtained by Parkinson and Perey (1980). Their subjects received eight serial lists, with each list composed of the same six consonants. Each list had to be recalled in the order the items were presented (a different order for each list). The suffix for their experimental condition consisted of the aurally presented letter "Y." Recall for the next-to-last item and the last item, summated over the eight lists, averaged 7.06 and 7.75, respectively, for the young subjects in the control condition and 5.69 and 6.38, respectively, for the young subjects in the experimental (i.e., suffix) condition. At each of these two serial positions, the difference in recall was statistically significant, indicating the presence of a suffix effect at each position. Comparable averages for the elderly subjects were 6.44 and 7.25 in the control condition and 4.62 and 5.75 in the experimental condition. At each of the two positions, the difference in recall was again statistically significant, indicating a suffix effect for the elderly subjects as well as for the young subjects. In both of these studies, the magnitude of the suffix effect was at least as pronounced for the elderly subjects as it was for the young subjects.

Echoic memory is also presumed to enter into an episodic-memory phenomenon of considerable importance. The phenomenon is known as the *modality effect*. Assessment of the magnitude of this effect is the fifth method employed to measure the duration of echoic memory. Like the suffix method, it appears to measure the second, long-duration phase of echoic memory (Cowan, 1984). The modality effect refers to the difference in recall, whether serial or free, between list items

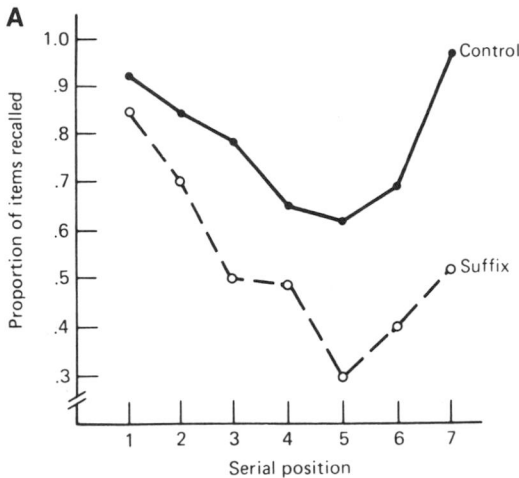

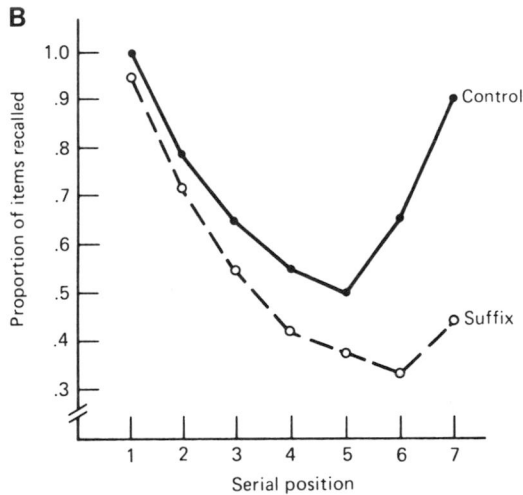

FIGURE 5.4 Magnitude of the suffix effect (depressed recall of end items relative to a control condition receiving no redundant suffix at the end of the list) for young adult (A) and elderly (B) subjects. (Adapted from Parkinson & Perey, 1980, Figure 2.)

presented aurally and list items presented visually (and at the same exposure rate for each modality). The nature of the effect may be seen in Figure 5.5. The results are those obtained by Madigan (1971) with young adult subjects and a serial-recall task. Note that recall of items near the end of the list was much higher

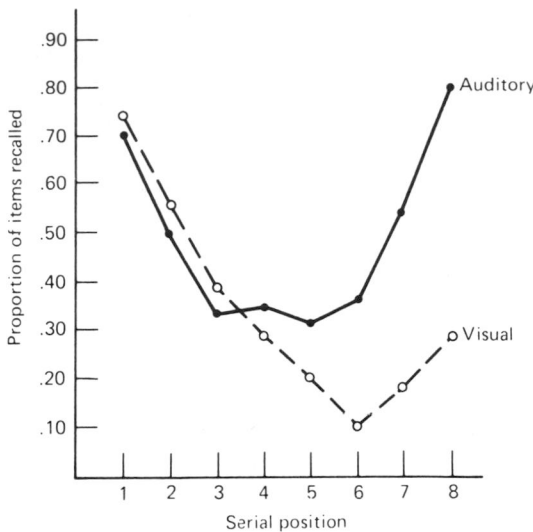

FIGURE 5.5 Superior recall for end items when presented auditorily than for end items when presented visually (the modality effect). (Reprinted from Madigan, 1971, Figure 1. Copyright 1971 by the American Psychological Association.)

when those items were presented aurally than when they were presented visually. It is this superiority for auditory presentation that defines the modality effect. By contrast, there was little difference attributable to modality of presentation for items occurring earlier in the lists. Why a modality effect for end items? According to O. C. Watkins and Watkins:

> The modality effect might have been predicted from the very fact of echoic memory as a psychological phenomenon. With auditory presentation, echoic information conforming to the final few list items should persist after list presentation and so facilitate their recall. Of course, a corresponding sensory store, referred to as iconic memory (again after Neisser, 1967) is usually assumed for visual presentations. But iconic information is, by most estimates, too transitory to be of any practical consequence in a typical immediate recall procedure (Sperling, 1960). Recency recall should therefore show positive effects of echoic memory but not of iconic memory. In this way, the concept of sensory storage provides a ready explanation of the modality effect (1980, p. 252).

The appearance of a modality effect for elderly subjects, therefore, offers an alternative to a suffix effect for demonstrating the continuation of echoic memory during late adulthood. Such a demonstration was given by Arenberg (1976). Both young and elderly subjects received a series of free-recall lists (i.e., subjects were free to recall the words in any order), each containing 16 words with either auditory or visual presentation. The results are shown in the part A (young subjects) and part B (elderly subjects) of Figure 5.6. At both age levels there was a modest, but consistent, modality effect spread over the last four items (i.e., the last four items in the input sequence for each free-recall list). The effect seems to be as pronounced for the elderly subjects as for the young subjects. (On the other hand, the probability of recalling items at *all* input positions, disregarding the modality of presentation, was clearly higher for young subjects than for elderly subjects—a comparable age-related deficit in serial recall occurred in the studies on the suffix effect cited earlier). A modality effect for the serial recall of consonants was also found for elderly subjects in the study by Manning and Greenhut-Wertz (1990) cited earlier. Included in their study was a condition in which the eight lists of six consonants each were presented visually rather than aurally. The elderly subjects averaged 5.31 and 6.19 consonants in the next-to-last and last serial positions. When these means are compared with the higher means in the auditory control condition for the suffix effect (6.44 and 7.25; see p. 144), they indicate a significant modality effect at each of these two serial positions. As in Madigan's (1971) study, the young subjects in Manning and Greenhut-Wertz's (1990) study clearly displayed a modality effect.

Other studies (Arenberg, 1968a; McGhie, Chapman, & Lawson, 1965; Talland, 1968; Taub, 1972, 1973) of relevance here have also reported an advantage of aurally presented items over visually presented items that was as pronounced for elderly subjects as for young adult subjects. Each of these studies involved short-term memory in which recall of items at the end of a series may be augmented by their continuing presence in echoic memory by both young and elderly adults. However, it should be noted that Botwinick and Storandt (1974) found a slight superiority on a short-term memory task, regardless of age, for visual presentation of items relative to auditory presentation. We will discover later that for secondary memory it is not unusual to find visual presentation of material to be superior to auditory presentation regardless of the age of subjects (see Chapter 8, pp. 282–283). Interestingly, both Arenberg (1976) and Robertson (1973) reported a slight advantage for visual presentation over auditory presentation, regardless of the age of the subjects, in the early serial positions of their lists. Memory for items in these positions is presumably from secondary memory (see Chapter 6, pp. 176–177). By contrast, Manning and Greenhut-Wertz (1990) found the opposite. That is, even in the early list positions there was an auditory advantage, again regardless of age. However, the lists in their study were much shorter (only six items) than in the earlier studies. It is possible that even the initial items in their lists had more residue remaining in the echoic store, but not in the iconic store at the time serial recall began, a residue that would abet recall only for the items presented aurally.

As with iconic memory, there seems to be no reason to believe that there are major age changes in echoic emory, at least for elderly adults without serious hearing dysfunctioning. However, the full limits of echoic memory and the mo-

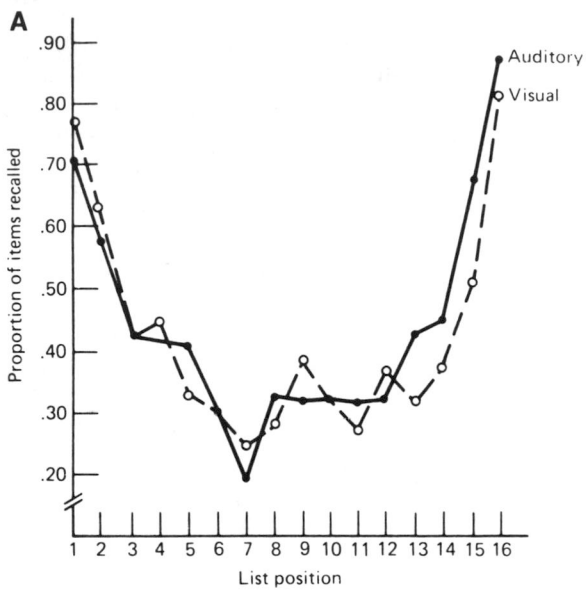

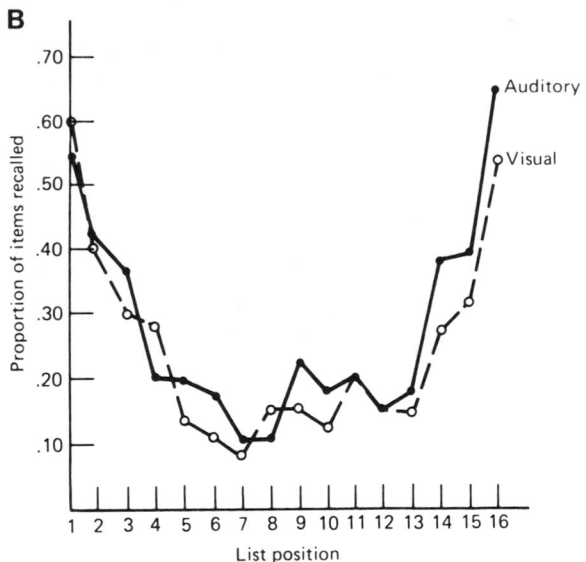

FIGURE 5.6 Magnitude of the modality effect found for young adults (A) and elderly adults (B). (Adapted from Arenberg, 1976, Figure 1.)

dality effect have yet to be tested with elderly adults. As reviewed thus far, the evidence for a modality effect, regardless of age, comes from studies in which "unmixed" lists are employed. That is, all items within a given list are presented in the same modality, whether it be auditory or visual. Remember that with such lists the advantage of auditory presentation is apparent only for end items of the lists. A recent study by Greene (1989a), with young adult subjects only, demonstrated that the auditory advantage applies to *all* list positions when the lists are "mixed" (i.e., half of the items in a given list are presented aurally, the other half visually). It is very unlikely that the auditory advantage found for early position items could be attributable to the retention of direct physical features of sound. Instead, Greene (1989a) reasoned that echoic memory contains additional information (besides the gestural information described earlier), such as the gender of the voice reading the items, that provides effective retrieval cues for auditorily presented items that are absent for visually presented items. When lists are unmixed, these retrieval cues suffer from cue overload (O. C. Watkins & Watkins, 1975). Thus, with unmixed lists, the auditory advantage is restricted to end items where physical information remains in echoic memory to enhance their recall. Hopefully, future aging studies will enable us to determine if elderly adults are as capable as young adults in the use of such supplementary information as effective retrieval cues.

Other Senses

The equivalent of iconic or echoic memory for each of the other senses has received relatively little attention. Of these other senses, the strongest case for the existence of a sensory store appears to be for the sense of touch (e.g., Gilson & Baddeley, 1969). To date, however, there have apparently been no studies dealing with age differences in memory for touch or any of the other remaining senses.

Adult Age Differences in Short-Term/Primary Memory

Postsensory episodic memories clearly differ in their durability and their accessibility. But, what accounts for this variability? According to William James (1890), in his classic book *Principles of Psychology*, the reason is the existence of two kinds of memory, *primary* and *secondary*. To James, primary memory is immediate memory, that is, memory of events that are in current consciousness. Secondary memory consists of memories that are no longer in immediate consciousness, but they are stored permanently and may become accessible to consciousness (i.e., return to primary memory) with effort.

After 75 years of dormancy, the distinction between the two kinds of memory was resurrected by Waugh and Norman (1965) in the form of the memory model shown in Figure 5.7. Their model expanded considerably on James's conceptualization of primary and secondary memory by postulating the existence of separate, but interacting, memory stores for the two forms, an STS for primary memory and a LTS for secondary memory.

There were other important elaborations as well, elaborations that specified more precisely the attributes and operations of the STS postulated to mediate primary memory. The STS was viewed as having a limited capacity for the amount of information it could hold at any one time. Of particular interest to us is the possibility that this capacity may diminish with normal aging. Included in their model was a specification of the paths by which information may enter the STS for storage. Note in Figure 5.7 that there are two such paths. One path, labeled "stimulus" in the model, is by way of new information that entered sensory memory and was encoded from information residing in generic memory (see Figure 5.1). The other path is from the LTS where previously stored (and now latent) information is accessed and returned to consciousness by entry into the STS. Finally, the model specified several operations that take place on information in the STS. First, information may be directly outputted from the store (see Figure 5.1) in the form of recall or recognition. Second, the information may be rehearsed in some way and transmitted to the LTS as a more permanent memory. Finally, the information in the STS may be "forgotten" if it is neither outputted immediately nor rehearsed sufficiently for transmission to the LTS. In effect, the information is displaced, and therefore lost, by new information reaching the STS. Waugh and Norman's model was, in turn, extended further in a model introduced a few years later by Atkinson and Shiffrin (1968). The presently popular working-memory model is also an extended version of Waugh and Nor-

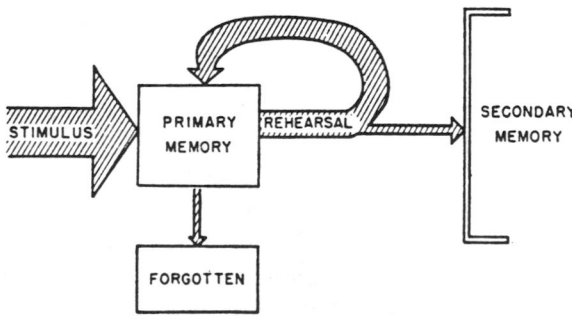

FIGURE 5.7   Waugh and Norman's two-store model of episodic memory. (Reprinted from Waugh & Norman, 1965, Figure 2. Copyright 1965 by the American Psychological Association.)

man's conceptualization of the STS. Both of these extensions, and their roles in aging research, will be covered in Chapter 6.

The processes and structures identified with the STS are nicely illustrated by the familiar experience of looking up a telephone number for dialing purposes. You often discover that several digits are forgotten (i.e., displaced from the STS) before you complete dialing. To avoid such forgetting, you may find yourself repeating the digits as you bridge the gap between reading them and dialing them. That is, you maintain the information by rehearsing it. Finally, an output occurs in the form of actually dialing the remembered sequence. For numbers that are called rarely, there is no need to rehearse them to the point that they become stored in the LTS—it would only be unnecessary cognitive effort that would add to the clutter of information stored there. Of course, it is a different matter for the telephone number of a relative or a close friend. Here the frequent dialing makes it worth the effort to rehearse the number sufficiently to assure its placement in the LTS from where it may be retrieved on demand. When it is retrieved on demand, it again enters the STS from which it is outputted.

In the remainder of this chapter, we will deal with research on adult age differences in various phenomena associated with primary memory and the STS. We will begin with the capacity of the STS.

Primary Memory: STS Capacity and Memory Span

Age differences in primary memory proficiency may result from an age-related change in the capacity of the STS. In principle, the amount of information that can be held temporarily may be less for elderly adults than for young adults. Such shrinkage would account nicely for the modest, but usually found, age deficits on memory-span tasks. On the surface, a span task would seem to measure the capacity of the STS, and age differences on such a task would seem to reflect an age difference in that capacity. A number of variations of a span task have been employed in aging research. They include forward and backward digit span, letter span, and word span. (Other variants associated with measuring working memory capacity will be discussed in Chapter 6, pp. 214–216. Still another variant associated with spatial memory will be discussed in Chapter 9, p. 316–317).

On a forward digit-span test, subjects are given a number of trials with series of digits that have to be recalled in the order given. The number of digits in the series increases over trials until the longest series that can be recalled without error is given. The length of that series defines a subject's forward digit span. A number of studies have reported a slight, but statistically significant, age-related deficit in digit span whether measured in a laboratory setting (e.g., Albert, Heller, & Milberg, 1988; Botwinick & Storandt, 1974a; Caird, 1966; Dirken, 1972; Friedman, 1974; Gilbert, 1941; Gilbert & Levee, 1971; Goldfarb, 1941; Hayslip & Kennelly, 1982; Heron & Chown, 1967; Hooper, Hooper, & Colbert, 1984;

Inglis & Ankus, 1965; Parkinson, 1982; Potvin et al., 1973; Robertson-Tchabo & Arenberg, 1976; Salthouse & Babcock, 1991; Taub, 1973; Wiegersma & Meertse, 1990) or a psychometric testing setting (e.g., Berkowitz, 1953; Wechsler, 1944, 1958, 1981, 1987). A number of other studies in a laboratory setting have also found a slight age difference, but one that did not attain statistical significance (e.g., Craik, 1968a; Drachman & Leavitt, 1972; Kriauciunas, 1968), and one study (Wingfield, Stine, Lahar, & Aberdeen, 1988) in which young and elderly subjects averaged equivalent scores (means of about seven digits spanned for each age group). In general, young adults average about 6.5 to 7 digits recalled correctly, elderly adults about 6.0 to 6.5, an age-related deficit, or "loss", of less than 10%.

The forward digit span, however, is not a fixed entity, but rather one that varies somewhat as a function of performance conditions and subject variables. Span length tends to increase as the rate of presenting the digits in a series decreases, but equally so for young and elderly subjects (Taub, 1966). Thus, the magnitude of the age-related deficit is relatively unchanged with variation in rate. Span length has usually been found to be greater when the digits are presented aurally rather than visually (Craik, 1968a; Talland, 1968; Taub, 1972, 1975); the opposite outcome, however, was reported by Botwinick and Storandt (1974a), but, again, equally so for young and elderly subjects. Nor do age-related deficits in span scores decrease with practice on a digit-span task (Taub, 1973; Taub & Long, 1972), even though both young and elderly subjects show modest gains in scores as practice progresses. Meaningfulness of the digits was varied in a study by Heron and Craik (1964). They found no age difference in span scores when the digits were read in Finnish, but they found an age-related deficit when the digits were read in English (the subjects' native language). Interestingly, the modest age difference in digit recall seems to be exaggerated even more when subjects perform under the everyday conditions of dialing the numbers on a telephone, rather than reporting them verbally (Crook, Ferris, McCarthy, & Rae, 1980), and the age difference is increased still more when dialing is delayed for several seconds by a busy signal (West & Crook, 1990). Digit-span proficiency of elderly adults has also been linked to the individual difference variables of intelligence level and health status. A digit-span test has long been a subtest on the various Wechsler intelligence tests (e.g., the Wechsler Adult Intelligence Scale-Revised [WAIS-R]; Wechsler, 1981). Span scores do correlate fairly highly with full-scale scores on the WAIS-R (Kaufman, 1990), a clear indication that they are reflecting individual differences in overall intelligence. Perlmutter and Nyquist (1990) found that self-report health status correlated positively and significantly with digit-span scores. In a longitudinal study covering 11 yr, Sands and Meredith (1992) discovered negative changes in blood pressure and hypertension over that period to be significantly related to declines in digit-span scores. It is tempting to conclude that poor health for elderly adults results in a decline in the capacity of the STS. On the other hand, improved health seems to have little effect on digit-span performance. Blumenthal et al. (1991) had their elderly subjects participate in a vigorous exercise program for many weeks. The result was a significant improvement in their physical health as measured by aerobic capacity—but little, if any, improvement in digit-span scores.

On a backward-digit-span task, the procedure is much like that for the forward-span task, with one important exception. Here subjects are required to recall the digits in the reverse order they were given. In general, backward-span scores average about one digit less than forward-span scores, although the age-related deficit is usually found to be greater than that found for the forward span, whether measured in a laboratory setting (e.g., Botwinick & Storandt, 1974a) or a psychometric testing setting (e.g., Berkowitz, 1953). A likely reason for the greater impairment for backward span than for forward span was given by Craik:

> It seems plausible that if subjects must reorganize the contents of their primary memory system, old subjects would be at a greater disadvantage; as well as maintaining the material, subjects must demonstrate mental flexibility and agility in order to rearrange the items (1977, p. 393).

In other words, one's performance on a backward-span task involves processes other than simply passively recalling the contents of a STS, processes likely to be highly age sensitive.

Letter-span and word-span testing procedures are also much like those for a forward-digit-span test, except that the items in the series of increasing length are either letters or words instead of digits. For letters presented serially and aurally, Botwinick and Storandt (1974a) reported mean span lengths of 6.7, 6.2, 6.5, 6.5, 5.5, and 5.4 for subjects in their 20s, 30s, 40s, 50s, 60s, and 70s, respectively. Thus, there was little decline from early to late adulthood until their subjects were in their 60s. A highly unique procedure for testing age differences in letter span was used by Salthouse et al. (1988a). Seven target letters were exposed simultaneously for 3 s on a computer screen (they were placed within an array of 25 letters, with the target letters made visually distinctive). Means for the number of letters recalled, averaged over four trials, for college-student young adults, noncollege-student young adults, middle-aged adults (40–59 years of age), and elderly subjects (60–79 years of age) in Salthouse et al.'s (1988a) second study are shown in Figure 5.8 (roughly comparable means were found in their first study. It may be seen that an age-related deficit was apparent by middle age, and it became greater by late adulthood. Expressed as a loss score, the deficit was about 16% for the elderly subjects relative to the college young adults and about 12% relative to the noncollege young adults.

In an early study of word span, Talland (1965a) reported no significant age difference in span length. A problem in this study, however, was the use of a free-recall procedure rather than the usual serial-recall procedure typical of span

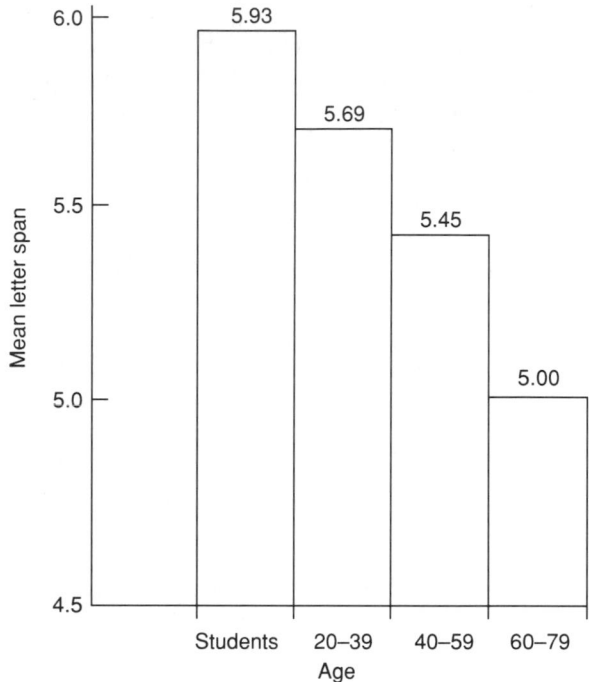

FIGURE 5.8 Mean letters recalled after a brief exposure. (Adapted from Salthouse, Kausler, & Saults, 1988a, Table 1.)

research. More recent studies (Kausler & Puckett, 1979; Salthouse & Babcock, 1991; Wingfield et al., 1988), however, have revealed an age-related deficit in word-span scores. In Kausler and Puckett's (1979) study, span length of young adult and elderly adult subjects was determined separately for lists composed of high-frequency and low-frequency words (as defined by frequency of occurrence in various publications). Expressed relatively, the age-related deficit was significantly greater for high-frequency words (22.9%) than for low-frequency words (17.5%). Salthouse and Babcock's (1991) subjects were assessed for digit-span length as well as word-span length. The correlation between age and span length was found to be greater for word span ($-.42$ in one study and $-.32$ in a second study) than for digit span ($-.34$ in the first study and $-.18$ in the second study). Wingfield et al. (1988) found span length to be about one word less for their elderly subjects (mean = 5 words) than for their young adult subjects (mean = 6 words; see also Chapter 6, pp. 216–217), an age difference roughly comparable to that found for digit-span scores in most studies.

Age-related deficits in word span have been linked to declines with normal aging in working memory by Kynette, Kemper, Norman, and Cheung (1990). Specifically, their analysis of working memory focused on the articulatory loop component of Baddeley and Hitch's (1974) model of working memory (see Chapter 6, p. 212). The articulatory loop is essentially an STS for holding information via articulatory processes. Baddeley, Thomson, and Buchanan (1975) discovered that word-span length is determined by the rate at which words can be repeated and held within the limited storage capacity of the articulatory loop. Consequently, word-span length is smaller for words that take a longer time to pronounce than for words that take a shorter time to pronounce (e.g., Schweikert & Boruff, 1986). It is also known that articulation rate declines with normal aging (e.g., Liss, Weismer, & Rusenbek, 1990). Thus, even with one-syllable words, elderly subjects are expected to have a slower repetition rate and therefore a shorter word-span length than young adults. This was confirmed by Kynette et al. (1990). Their young adult subjects averaged a repetition rate of 1.47 words per second and a word-span length of 4.6 words. Comparable values for their elderly subjects were 0.93 and 3.5.

Collectively, these many aging studies on memory span suggest that there is a modest decline in STS capacity from early to late adulthood. Memory theorists (e.g., Craik, 1977; M. J. Watkins, 1977), however, believe that performance on memory-span tasks is not determined exclusively by the capacity of the STS. Age differences in span scores may well be the consequence of age-sensitive secondary memory processes rather than diminished STS capacity in late adulthood. Greater rehearsal of items residing in the STS by young than by elderly subjects is one possible reason. The result would be more information transmitted as memory traces to the LTS, and subsequently retrieved from the LTS during recall on a span task, by young adults than by elderly subjects. The net effect would be an increase in the age-related deficit in recall above that attributable to an age-related decline in STS capacity. This is seemingly the reason why the age difference in word span is greater for high-frequency words than for low-frequency words (Kausler & Puckett, 1979). High-frequency words are likely to receive more rehearsal, and especially so by young adults, than low-frequency words.

Repetition of a series of items is also likely to increase the extent to which secondary memory contributes to the recall of that series. That is, the amount of rehearsal each item in the series receives should increase with each repetition, thus enhancing transmission to the LTS and later recall from the LTS. This was demonstrated by Hebb (1961) with a procedure in which young adult subjects received a number of digit series for immediate serial recall. Some of the series were repetitions of earlier series, thereby providing opportunity for extended rehearsal of that single series. A natural prediction is that such repetition should lead to greater increments in recall for young adults than for elderly adults, given the greater benefit of rehearsal expected for young adults. However, the evidence in support of this prediction is somewhat contradictory (Caird, 1964, 1966; Heron & Craik, 1964).

As the length of a series of items increases from span length to supraspan length, the involvement of secondary memory should also increase and, seemingly, so should the magnitude of age-related deficits in recall of the series. This was the case in a study by Friedman (1966) in which letter series varied in length from 4 to 12 items. A somewhat similar outcome was found by Taub (1968) with letter series, although the magnitude of the age-related deficit for supraspan series was not as pronounced as in Friedman's (1966) study. Surprisingly, Craik (1968a) failed to find a statistically significant Age X List Length interaction effect for lists of digits that varied in length from 4 (subspan length) to 9 (supraspan length). However, in a later study (Craik, 1968b) did find the expected interaction for word series. For some series, the words were names of English counties, and, for other series, they were either names of animals or unrelated words. The extent of the Age × List Length interaction was far more pronounced for unrelated words and animal names than for English counties (and also for digit series). Note that the word pool from which series items were drawn was smaller for English counties than for either animals or, of course, unrelated words. Craik's explanation of the word-pool effect is that "younger subjects are less penalized by the inadequate retrieval information inherent in large word pools" (1977, pp. 395–396). (Digits, of course, come from an especially small "word" pool.) The availability of retrieval information is another kind of secondary memory process. Variation in the meaningfulness of the letters in a supraspan series should result in variation in the number of letters recalled. This is, indeed, the case. In a study by Kinsbourne (1973) meaningfulness was varied for eight-letter series by varying the approximation of the series to meaningful English words. Recall of the letters increased substantially the closer the series approximated a word—and equally so for young and elderly subjects. This is a somewhat unexpected outcome in that, on the one hand, an age-sensitive organizational process indigenous to secondary memory was likely to be increasingly involved the closer a series approximated a word, thus favoring recall for young adults (see Chapter 8, p. 277–278). On the other hand, a frequent position in aging research is that age-related deficits in recall scores should be less for meaningful material than for meaningless material. If this is the case, then the age-related deficit in Kinsbourne's (1973) study should have decreased as the letters more closely approximated a word.

A vastly different means of involving nonprimary memory processes is through the chunking of elements that are components of a series of to-be-remembered items (e.g., digits on a digit-span task) (Miller, 1956). Chunking is an encoding process somewhat similar, at least in some cases, to subjective organization in free recall (to be discussed in Chapter 7). Through it, successive items in a series are related to one another. For example, a digit series of 3 8 1 4 9 2 5 could be organized into four rather than seven chunks, once "1492" is identified as a famous historical year. The advantage of chunking is that several items rather than only one may then occupy the space of a single storage unit in the STS. The requisite process, presumably part of the secondary memory system, and in this example the retrieval of information from generic memory, is again more likely to be present for young subjects than for elderly subjects.

Convincing evidence for an age difference in chunking comes from a study by Taub (1974). Young, middle-aged, and elderly subjects were given 12 letters to recall in serial order. In a low chunking condition, the letters provided little opportunity for chunking (e.g., *PBSKOJUHRMGA* as a series). In a high chunking condition, successive groups of four letters each formed a meaningful word (e.g., *JUMPHOGSBARK*). All subjects participated in both conditions, and they had no advance information describing the presence of words in the high chunking condition. Age differences favoring young adults were far greater in the high chunking condition than in the low chunking condition, in agreement with our preceding analysis. Chunking in this case, as in our "1492" example, made use of information (i.e., words) stored in generic memory. Chunking may be induced in another way without involving generic memory. This is by the use of spatial boundaries separating "chunks" of a meaningless series presented visually (e.g., *RGT WKLV* for a letter series) or by a pause after each "chunk" presented aurally. This is akin to the way telephone numbers are chunked for easier remembering (e.g., 499 1598). Chunking spatially in this way has been found to facilitate the recall of otherwise meaningless series of items by young adults (e.g., Severin & Rigby, 1963). In a series of studies by Allen (Allen, 1990, 1991; Allen & Coyne, 1988a, 1988b, 1989; Allen & Crozier, 1992), age differences have been examined for the way letter series are organized into chunks in the absence of experimenter-identified spatial boundaries. For example, the series *TKCFZW* could be organized into *TKC FZW* or *TK CFZW* chunks. At stake is where subjects set their own "chunking boundaries" for mastering letter series (N. F. Johnson, 1978). Allen's research has revealed that there are no significant age differences in functional chunk capacity. However, it has also revealed that on a recognition memory test of the series-letter content, elderly subjects make more transposition errors on a recognition memory test (i.e., assigning a letter to the wrong chunk) than do young adult subjects.

Primary Memory: STS Capacity and the Recency Effect

The evaluation of age differences in STS capacity clearly requires a method that eliminates contributions of secondary memory processes to the recall of to-be-remembered items. One method suggested by the postulated nature of the STS (e.g., Glanzer & Cunitz, 1966) involves the assessment of what is called the *recency effect* in the free recall of word lists. On a free-recall list subjects are presented a lengthy series of items (usually words), and they are "free" to recall them in whatever order they wish. The recency effect emerges when subjects are given a number of successive free-recall lists, each for a single study trial, followed by a recall test trial. When the probability of recalling list items for all of the lists combined is plotted across the ordinal position of those items during study trials, the resulting function takes the form shown in Figure 5.9. The last few items in study trials have an unusually high probability of recall relative to the probability of recalling midlist items, a disparity that defines the recency effect. Variation in the magnitude of the recency effect may be either in the magnitude of the heightened probability or in the number of items from the end of the list over which the heightened probability spreads. The effect may be presumed to result from the direct recall of item information held in the STS. Items at and near the end of the list are still in the store when item presentation ceases, and they are, therefore, in residence when recall of items begins. That is, there are no additional items to displace them from storage, making them available for direct recall from the STS. By contrast, earlier items in a list are followed by a number of additional items, and they must, therefore, be booted out of the store to make room for new incoming items. These items must be recalled from the LTS, if they are to be recalled at all. The first few items in a list have a greater probability of being transmitted to the LTS than do midlist items. Consequently, there is also a *primacy effect*, defined in terms of the heightened probability of recalling early list items relative to midlist items (see Figure 5.9). We will turn to the importance of the primacy effect in experimental aging research in Chapter 6.

Primacy and recency effects in free recall clearly resemble the serial position effects that characterize serial-anticipation learning (see Chapter 3, p. 99). For each task, performance is superior for the items at the two ends of a list than for items in the middle of the same list. The resemblance ends there, however. Quite different processes are postulated to underlie the superficially similar phenomena.

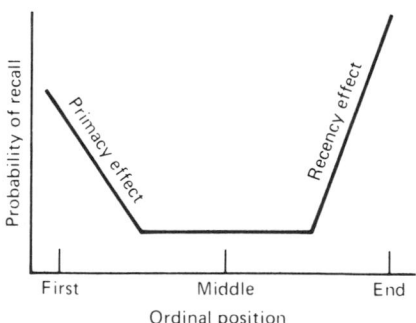

F I G U R E 5.9 The nature of primacy and recency effects in the recall of items from multiple free-recall lists.

In serial anticipation learning, subjects must acquire information pertaining to each item's position in the total list as well as acquire information regarding what specific words serve as list items. It is the former process that presumably accounts for serial-position effects. That is, order, or position, information is learned earlier for the items at the two ends of the list than for items in the middle of the list. The availability of the items themselves is not presumed to vary across serial positions (Jensen, 1962a). In free recall, separate components of the total memory system are responsible for the heightened performances at the two ends of the list—the STS for one and the LTS for the other. (Alternatively, different levels of processing are postulated for terminal items than for beginning or midlist items—an alternative analysis of free recall that will be discussed more thoroughly in Chapter 6).

The nature of the recency effect for elderly subjects is of great interest. If its attributes match those found for the recency effect manifested by young subjects, then the argument may be made that the capacity of the STS is basically unaltered by age. The results here are conflicting, however. Craik (1968b), in a careful analysis of age differences in the recency effects obtained with various kinds of words, concluded that the capacity of the STS is about the same for elderly adults as it is for young adults. Raymond (1971) came to the same conclusion. However, only elderly subjects participated in her free-recall study. Raymond compared the attributes of this effect (i.e., its height and its extension from the end of the list toward the middle of the list) with those reported in a number of studies with young adult subjects (e.g., Glanzer & Cunitz, 1966) and found few, if any, differences. Craik (1971) also found little effect attributable to age variation when a recognition test substituted for a recall test.

On the other hand, the recency effects for young and elderly subjects apparent in the study by Arenberg (1976) cited earlier do show an important difference. For his young subjects (part A of Figure 5.6) the proportions of last and next-to-last items recalled averaged (combined over modalities) about .85 and .57, respectively. For his elderly subjects (part B of Figure 5.6) the comparable proportions were about .60 and .37. These disparities could be viewed as indicating a diminished storage capacity of the STS in late adulthood. Parkinson, Lindholm, and Inman (1982), Salthouse (1980), and R. E. Wright (1982) have also reported results from free-recall studies that revealed a pronounced age-related deficit in the probability of recalling recency items. The study by Parkinson et al. (1982) is especially informative. They employed several procedures (e.g., Tulving & Colotla, 1970) designed to measure the extent of the recency effect in recall protocols. The age-related "loss" in the magnitude of the recency effect was as much as 20% (relative to young adults). This age differential is much greater than that found on digit-span tasks (less than 10% loss). Moreover, the age-related deficit for recency items was as great as the age-related deficit found for earlier items in the list, items presumably retrieved from the LTS. Similar outcomes, that is, equivalent age-related deficits for primary and secondary memory components of free recall, were reported by Foos, Sabol, Corral, and Mobley (1987) and Rissenberg and Glanzer (1987). The implication is that primary memory is as age sensitive as is secondary memory.

A similar age-related deficit was found by Parkinson (1980) with a running-memory-span task instead of a free-recall task. His young and elderly subjects received strings of digits that varied in length from trial to trial. Following the presentation of the last digit on a given trial, subjects tried to recall the last five items in the string, starting with the terminal item. No age difference was found for the very last item. However, beginning with the next-to-last item and extending through all of the remaining items, young subjects clearly recalled a higher proportion of items than elderly subjects. This deficit also implies a diminished storage capacity in late adulthood.

The results of these studies, however, conflict somewhat with the results obtained by Delbecq-Derouesne and Beauvois (1989). Their task involved a modification of the usual free-recall procedure. Their subjects, who ranged in age from 20 to 86 yr, were required to recall the final words in each list before they could recall the other words in the lists. They argued, reasonably, that this forced early recall of words in recency positions offers a more reliable assessment of direct recall from the STS than does the assessment based on truly free recall. Words were counted as being recalled from primary memory if no more than seven words (during study or during recall) intervened between their presentation and their recall. All other words that were recalled were scored as being recalled from secondary memory. There was a very slight age-related deficit in primary memory scores, with the ratio of recall scores for the young adults (20–25 yr) to the recall scores for the elderly adults (65–86 yr) being .93. By contrast, there was a pronounced age-related deficit in secondary memory scores, with the elderly adult–young adult ratio being a strikingly low .36. This outcome certainly differs from those studies noted above that found the age-related deficit in primary memory scores to be nearly equivalent to that in secondary memory scores.

In general, the evidence from various sources suggests that there may be a moderate decline in the capacity of the STS by late adulthood. Our conclusion must be tempered, however, by our awareness that not all memory theorists hold to the concept of a limited capacity STS. Again, we will discover in Chapter 6 that these other theorists have an alternative way of explaining such phenomena as the recency effect in free recall.

Primary Memory: Flexibility of Representation

Information held in the STS consists ordinarily of sound representations of inputs into our sensory registers. For example, if the letter V is a visually presented list item, it is the sound *ve* that is likely to enter the STS. Support for this position comes from studies (e.g., Conrad, 1964) in which strings of letters make up the items for a recall test. With retention intervals of several seconds, it is not unusual to discover errors of recall involving letters that are phonemically similar to to-be-remembered items. For example, V may be recalled as B (see also Chapter 6, p. 181). On the other hand, it is unusual to discover errors involving letters that are orthographically similar but phonemically dissimilar to to-be-remembered items (e.g., recalling Y instead of V). At the same time, there does seem to be considerable flexibility in the kind of representations that may be stored in the STS. For young adults, visual representations of sensory inputs are capable of residing in the STS for at least several seconds. One way of demonstrating visual short-term memory is through the use of the Posner chronometric method (Posner, Boies, Eichelman, & Taylor, 1969). Subjects receive pairs of letters having the same name. In one condition, the letters are of the same case (e.g., AA); in another condition, they are different in case (e.g., Aa). In either condition, the correct decision is the same. To test for the presence of visual representations in the STS, the investigator also varies the time separating the exposures of the two letters in a pair. When that time is no more than 2 s, decision time is faster for Aa-type pairs than for Aa-type pairs (Posner et al., 1969). A visual image of A, the first letter exposed, seems to be retained over this 2-s interval, thus making it possible to match the second A with that stored information. Such a match is not possible when the second letter is a. Here the decision of sameness can be made only on the basis of a common name for the two letters. When the retention interval is longer than several seconds, there is no longer visual information available in the STS, information that would permit direct matching. Consequently, the decision can be made only on the basis of the common name, just as it is in the Aa condition, and there is no longer an advantage to be gained for AA pairs. A retention interval of 2 s, of course, implies the underlying process cannot be that of iconic memory (it persists for less than 1 s) and must, therefore, be a postsensory, or STS, process.

The overall difficulty that elderly people have with imaginal activity implies that they may also have difficulty in constructing visual representations for STS storage. There have apparently been no aging studies, however, that have employed either the above method or one of several alternative methods (e.g., Kroll, Parks, Parkinson, Bieber, & Johnson, 1970). Consequently, we do not know if the flexibility for storage offered by visual representations diminishes in late adulthood. However, there have been a number of aging studies (e.g., Adamowicz, 1976, 1978; Adamowicz, & Hudson, 1978; Arenberg, 1977, 1978, 1982; Davies, 1967; Farrimond, 1967; Kendall, 1962; Mergler, Dusek, & Hoyer, 1977; Riege, Kelly, & Klane, 1981; Robertson-Tchabo & Arenberg, 1989; Trembly & O'Connor, 1966) in which short-term retention (i.e., retention over seconds) has been tested with such visual stimuli as mosaic patterns and geometric designs. These studies have found pronounced age-related deficits in short-term memory as measured by both recognition of the visual stimuli and reproduction of those stimuli, but with the deficits being less for recognition than for reproduction. Interpretation of these deficits is difficult, however. They could be the consequence of poorer visual representations in the STS for elderly subjects than for young subjects, but they could also be the consequence of poorer translation of visual stimuli into verbal representations by elderly subjects than by young subjects. Verbal translations could be transmitted to the LTS for later retrieval of relevant stimulus information. Whatever the case, long-term memory for designs has also been found to be susceptible to greater age-related deficits than long-term memory for words, even when the materials have been equated for difficulty with younger subjects (Tubi & Calev, 1989). Visual representation in the STS is an important problem area, one that merits further investigation of age differences with the kind of chronometric methodology described earlier.

Nor does the flexibility of representations in the STS and here. There is ample evidence to indicate that deaf individuals who are skilled in sign language store kinesthetic representations of the movements required to produce signs for verbal information (e.g., Shand, 1982). But what about semantic representations in the form of meanings of list items? Isn't the name of A stored long enough to permit its matching with a on the Posner task? As we noted earlier, the name is likely to have been stored in the LTS, and it is this long-term information that mediates the match. This raises the important distinction between short-term memory (and forgetting), in general, and memory (and forgetting) mediated directly by the STS. Short-term memory is an empirical phenomenon identified by the retention of information over a brief interval (usually a matter of seconds). Most important, short-term memory may actively involve the storage in, and the subsequent retrieval from, the LTS as well as, or instead of, retrieval from the STS. We will discover shortly that there is short-term retention of semantic information. If there is indeed a STS, it seems unlikely to hold semantic information for direct recall, suggesting that short-term memory for such information is actually a secondary memory phenomenon.

Primary Memory: Rate of Loss of Information

Age differences in primary memory proficiency may result from an age change in the rate with which information is lost, or forgotten, from the STS. Short-term memory forgetting, that is, forgetting over intervals of seconds instead of minutes, hours, or days, is widely studied in basic memory research through the use of a procedure introduced around the same time by Brown (1958) and Peterson and Peterson (1959) and, therefore, commonly referred to as the Brown-Peterson procedure. The strategy is a simple but potent one. Subjects are given a single nonsense syllable to hold in memory over a retention interval that varies across trials from 0 to 18 s. To prevent rehearsal of that syllable during the retention interval (and, therefore, to prevent its constant reentry into the STS— and its entry into the LTS as well), subjects are required to count backwards by threes, starting with a three-digit number that is given immediately after the syllable is presented. Each subject receives many trials, with each trial involving the retention of a different nonsense syllable. On some trials the retention interval is set at 0 s (i.e., subjects recall the syllable immediately after its presentation), on some trials at 3 s (filled with counting backwards), and still other trials at longer intervals, up through 18 s. Performance may then be measured in terms of the proportion of subjects recalling syllables at each of the retention intervals.

The results obtained by the Petersons (1959) with young adult subjects are plotted in part A of Figure 5.10. Note the very rapid forgetting of information presumably held in the STS at the onset of the retention interval. Memory psychologists have proposed various explanations for the rapid rate of forgetting found with the Brown-Peterson task. It should be noted initially that the typical forgetting curve found with this task is commonly presumed to reflect both recall from the STS and recall from the LTS. The rapidly dropping segment of the curve results from the loss of information held in the STS, a loss that is fairly complete by 12 s. The asymptotic segment, at about 12 s and beyond, results from the limited amount of information sufficiently encoded to have been transmitted to the LTS. To some (e.g., Brown, 1958) the rapid loss from the STS results from the spontaneous decay of information residing there; to others it results from either the displacement of letters from the store by the numbers recited in counting backwards (e.g., Reitman, 1971) or the kind of interference postulated by interference theorists to account for proactive inhibition (Keppel & Underwood, 1962; see Chapter 10, p. 359).

These theoretical issues remain largely unresolved. Support for an age difference in rate of decay came from an early study by Fraser (1958). An aurally presented series of letters was exposed at either a fast rate or a slow rate, with recall occurring immediately after the last letter. An age-related deficit in recall was found for the slow rate, but not for the fast rate. A slow rate, of course, permits more time for decay to occur than does a fast rate, thus providing a recall disadvantage for elderly subjects, if, indeed, they do have a faster rate of decay than do younger adults. Further support for an age difference in rate of decay was obtained by Schonfield and Donaldson (1966). The first and second halves of digit series were presented at different rates of exposure. For some series, the sequence was "slow" for the first half and "fast" for the second half. For the other series, the order was reversed. A recall advantage for digits in the slow-fast condition over the fast-slow condition was found for the elderly subjects but not for the young subjects, an age difference the investigators attributed to faster decay of information by elderly adults than by young adults. In the slow-fast condition,

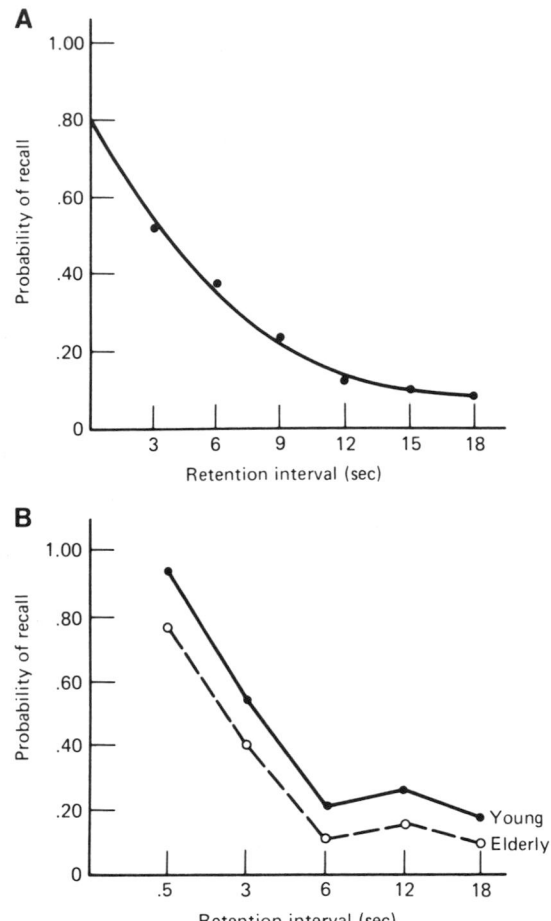

FIGURE 5.10 A: Rate of forgetting in short-term memory as found by the Petersons for young adult subjects. (Adapted from Peterson & Peterson, 1959, Figure 3.) B: Age differences in rate of short-term memory forgetting. (Adapted from Schonfield, 1969a, Table 3.)

digits are in the store for a shorter time, on the average, than in the fast-slow condition, making this a particular advantage for individuals with a faster rate of decay (presumably this includes elderly adults).

Other evidence, however, has not been as supportive of an age difference in rate of decay. Kinsbourne (1973) reported results that conflicted directly with those of Fraser (1958). That is, the age-related deficit was greater for a fast rate of exposure than for a slow rate. With visually presented items, Taub (1966) found the magnitude of the age-related deficit in recall to be no greater for a slow rate of exposure than for a fast rate. The results from these two studies are difficult to reconcile with the hypothesis that, if information in the STS does decay spontaneously, then it decays at a faster rate for elderly adults than for young adults (Craik, 1977). Most investigators in experimental aging research seem to rely more heavily on the principle that loss of information from the STS takes place either by displacement from the store by new information or by interference produced by new information. In fact, explanations of the rapid loss of information over a few seconds need not even involve the postulation of a STS, as is the case for the interference explanation. Here interference is produced proactively for a given item by previously presented items (Keppel & Underwood, 1962). Our interest, however, is not in the reasons for the rapid forgetting of information over a few seconds when rehearsal of that information is prevented, but rather in the possibility of adult age differences in the rate of loss. Our focus is on those studies that have examined age difference in short-term memory as defined empirically. Specifically, does the rate of forgetting over short retention intervals increase from early to late adulthood?

There have been several studies comparing young and elderly subjects on the basic Brown-Peterson task. Early studies were conducted by Schonfield (1969a), Talland (1967), Kriauciunas (1968), and Binks and Sutcliffe (1972). The results obtained by Schonfield (1969a) are shown in the part B of Figure 5.10 (comparable results were obtained in the other early studies). Note that the rate of forgetting was essentially the same for the two age groups. Recall simply began at a higher level (i.e., as found at the 0.5-s retention interval) for the young subjects, probably because they encoded the linguistic elements more proficiently than did the elderly subjects. The age difference remained about the same, however, at each successive retention interval, suggesting that the rate of losing information was about the same for each age group (although the age difference immediately after item study presents a problem in accepting this interpretation; see Chapter 10, pp. 356–357). If elderly subjects forget at a faster rate than young subjects, we would expect the magnitude of the age difference in amount recalled, favoring young adults, to increase as the retention interval increased. An absence of an age difference in rate of short-term forgetting was also found by Keevil-Rogers and Schnore (1969) with digits as the to-be-remembered items and color naming as the interpolated rehearsal-preventing activity and by Craik (1971) with a recognition test rather than a recall test.

These results, however, were later challenged by Inman and Parkinson (1983). They identified potential problems in the earlier studies that may have made the absence of an age difference in the rate of forgetting an artifact. For example, elderly subjects may count backwards more slowly than young adults, thus yielding less interference from the distractor task. Alternatively, elderly subjects may expend less of their resources on the distractor task than do young subjects, thus allowing them greater opportunity to conduct uncontrolled covert rehearsal of the to-be-remembered items. The net effect would be to "slow down" the rate of forgetting those rehearsed items. The number of letters in each to-be-recalled item was either 3, 4, or 5. The interpolated task of interest to us required subjects to add two single-digit numbers together and then determine if the sum was odd or even. The digit pairs were presented at a rapid rate (one pair per second), making the task seemingly difficult enough to prevent covert rehearsal of the letters. Finally, the retention interval was varied by requiring only one pair of digits to be added before signaling for letter recall on some trials (i.e., a 2-s retention interval), and either 3, 5, or 7 pairs on other trials (retention intervals of 6, 10, and 14 s). Our emphasis will be on the three-letter condition. Here there was no age difference in the probability of recall after only one interpolated digit pair, with both age groups having a recall probability of 1.0. However, after seven interpolated pairs, there was a striking age difference, with young subjects averaging a recall probability of about .90, elderly subjects about .70. Thus, the rate of forgetting was considerably faster for elderly than for young subjects. Even faster forgetting by the elderly subjects also occurred with longer to-be-remembered items. In addition, Inman and Parkinson (1983) also measured each subjects letter memory span, and found that span scores correlated moderately highly with recall scores on the Brown-Peterson task for both young and elderly subjects.

The results obtained by Inman and Parkinson (1983) are strongly suggestive of faster short-term forgetting for elderly than for young adults. However, the story doesn't end here. In still later studies by Parkinson, Inman, and Dannenbaum (1985), Puckett and Stockburger (1988), Puckett and Lawson (1989), and Dobbs and Rule (1990), no age difference in rate of forgetting was found. These studies had several important methodological innovations. Parkinson et al. (1985) exposed their to-be-remembered items for a longer period for their elderly than for young subjects, thereby assuring age group comparability in the encoding of information prior to the retention interval and eliminating the problem noted earlier in connection with Schonfield's (1969a) study. Dobbs and Rule (1990) employed digits as to-be-remembered items and a self-paced antonym-naming task as the distractor activity during the retention interval. Puckett and Stockburger (1988) and Puckett and Lawson (1989) employed word series as their to-be-remembered items, with the length of each subject's series being set at that subject's previously determined word-span length. Thus, on the average, the series were slightly longer for their young subjects than for their elderly subjects. Most important, Puckett and Stockburger also employed a method introduced by Reitman (1974) to identify subjects who surreptitiously engaged in rehearsal of the to-be-remembered words while performing on the interpolated distractor task. For young and elderly subjects clearly identified as being nonrehearsers, there was no difference in rate of forgetting. If there is an age difference in rate of short-term forgetting, it seems to be modest to the point where it may be found in some studies and not in others, contingent on the performance conditions extant in those studies.

Other evidence indicating the probable absence of any pronounced age difference in the rate of short-term forgetting comes from studies employing a variation of the Brown-Peterson procedure that was introduced by D. Wickens (e.g., Wickens, Born, & Allen, 1963). With this modified procedure, triplets of words serve as the to-be-remembered items. After each triplet is presented, subjects perform on a rehearsal-preventing activity during a specified retention interval (e.g., 18 s) and then attempt to recall the three words. In a control condition, the triplets have the same form of relatedness on each of four consecutive trials. For example, each triplet may consist of the names of three different animals (e.g., fox, lion, bear on the first trial; zebra, monkey, seal on the second trial; and so on). With young adult subjects, recall of the words declines progressively over the four trials. That is, proactive inhibition (interference on current material from previously acquired material) increases steadily from trial to trial. In an experimental condition, the only change is in the nature of the triplet presented on the critical fourth trial. Instead of animal names, words from a different taxonomic category (e.g., vegetables) now make up the triplet (e.g., lettuce, corn, turnip). With young adult subjects, proactive inhibition again increases over the first three trials. However, there is typically a *release-from-proactive-inhibition* effect on the critical fourth trial. That is, recall of the words is dramatically higher than recall of the words given on the same trial for subjects in the control condition.

The release phenomenon does not necessarily mean that information may be encoded semantically in the STS. The phenomenon could well be one of secondary memory. Our concern, however, is only with age differences in the extent of release as a short-term memory empirical phenomenon. Several studies (Elias & Hirasuna, 1976; Lorsbach, 1990; Mistler-Lachman, 1977; Moscovitch & Winocur, 1983; Puglisi, 1980; Schonfield, Davidson, & Jones, 1983) have examined age differences in the release phenomenon. The results have been virtually identical in these studies. Plotted in Figure 5.11 are the results obtained by Elias and Hirasuna (1976). Note that proactive inhibition increased (i.e., the amount of recall decreased) at about the same rate for young and elderly subjects in the control condition. Moreover, the extent of the release from proactive inhibition was about the same for the two age groups. That is, the greater recall in the experimental condition relative to the control condition on Trial 4 was about the same for elderly subjects as for young subjects. Once more, we have reason to believe that short-term forgetting is not markedly affected by age over the adult life span. The only age difference favoring young adults was in the overall level of recall that was apparent on the first trial and continued over the remaining trials (see Figure 5.11). This superiority is most likely attributable to the more

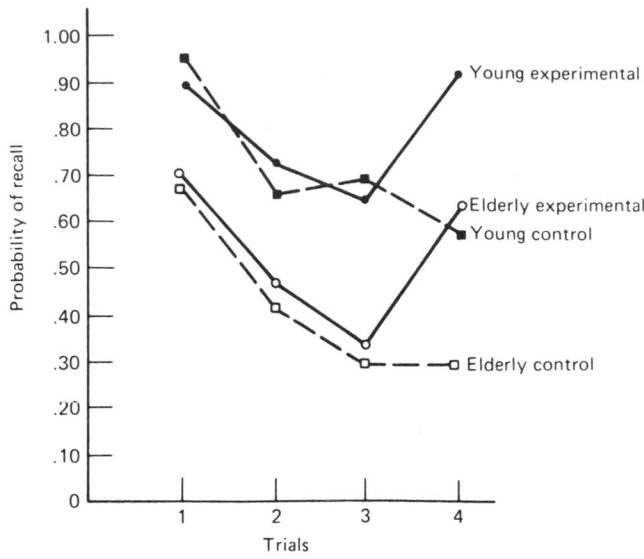

FIGURE 5.11 Magnitude of release from proactive inhibition (experimental minus control) for young and elderly subjects. (Reprinted from Elias & Hirasuna, 1976, Figure 1. Copyright 1976 by the American Psychological Association.)

proficient encoding of the triplets for transmission as memory traces to the LTS by young subjects at the time the items are presented (a superiority that again presents a problem for concluding equal rates of forgetting over Trials 1–3 for young and elderly subjects). A normal release effect, however, seems to be found only for normally aging individuals. Moscovitch and Winocur (1983) discovered no release for institutionalized elderly individuals under standard conditions. However, release was found when the letters of the final triplet were printed in a color that differed from the color of the letters for the prior triplets. Similarly, Goggin (1975) found a normal release effect for individuals who scored above 50 on the Wechsler Memory Scale, but not for individuals who scored below 50.

Primary Memory: Search of Content

The nature of short-term memory scanning has been one of the most thoroughly studied topics in basic memory research over the past 25 yr. What is meant by scanning may be illustrated by a simple example. Suppose you hear a television sportscaster say, "Today's winners in the National League were the Dodgers, Padres, Reds, Cardinals, Pirates, and Cubs." Then someone in the next room asks you, "Did the Braves win today?" Your "no" answer cannot be given until you have searched, or scanned, the contents of your STS and discovered the absence of a Braves' representation.

Interest in scanning began with several striking discoveries by Sternberg (1966, 1969b). The task introduced by Sternberg (subsequently labeled the Sternberg task) was itself highly original. His young adult subjects received a memory set of items (usually digits but sometimes letters or words) on each of many trials. The size of the set varied from trial to trial. On some trials, a single digit was presented for study and registration in the STS. On other trials, the set was expanded to 2, 3, 4, 5, or 6 digits displayed successively (with an exposure rate slightly greater than 1 s per digit). Following exposure of the last digit in a memory set, his subjects received a test stimulus (or probe). On half of the trials for each set size, the test stimulus was a digit that had been part of the just-presented memory set (a positive probe; e.g., 7 1 3 as a memory set and 1 as the positive probe); on the other half, the test stimulus was not part of the prior memory set (a negative probe; e.g., 2 as the probe for the 7 1 3 memory set). On each trial, a subject's task was to respond yes or no to the probe—pushing one button for yes, a different button for no—to indicate whether or not the probe was a member of the memory set. The dependent variable was the reaction time in pressing the appropriate button (errors are unusual—subjects rarely press the wrong button). Sternberg's striking discoveries may be seen in part A of Figure 5.12, where mean reaction time is plotted as a function of the set size (i.e., number of digits in the set). The first discovery is that it really made no difference whether the probe was positive or negative—mean reaction time was about the same for each. The second is that reaction time increased linearly as the size of the set increased. Because positive and negative probes did not differ in reaction times, they were combined for purposes of plotting the best fitting line (A, Figure 5.12) to represent the relationship between reaction time and variation in set size. Not apparent in Figure 5.12 is another one of Sternberg's discoveries. For positive probes, he found reaction time to be independent of a probe's position in the preceding memory set. Thus, if the memory set consisted of 7 1 3, the reaction time was about the same for 7 as the probe as it was for either 1 or 3 as the probe.

Collectively, these results revealed to Sternberg the fundamental nature of a search through the content of the STS. Specifically, the search appears to be both *serial* and *exhaustive*. It is serial in the sense that the items in the store are searched consecutively at a constant rate to determine the presence of the probe stimulus. The rate of progression through the series is roughly the same in going from the first to the second representation as it is from the second to third representation, and so on. The net effect is the linear increment in total reaction time as the number of items in a set increases. The search is exhaustive in the sense that it continues even after the probe stimulus itself has been matched with a representation of an item in the store. Thus, for our 7 1 3 set, a subject continues to

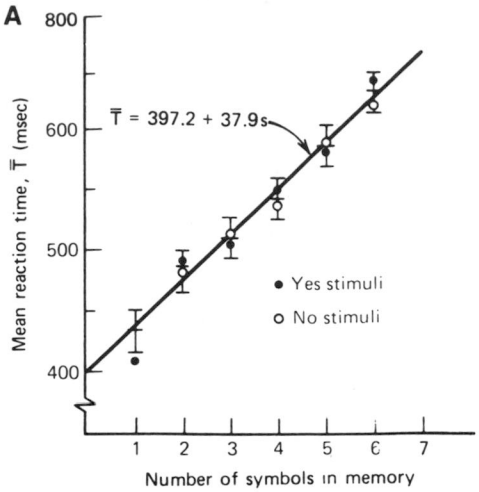

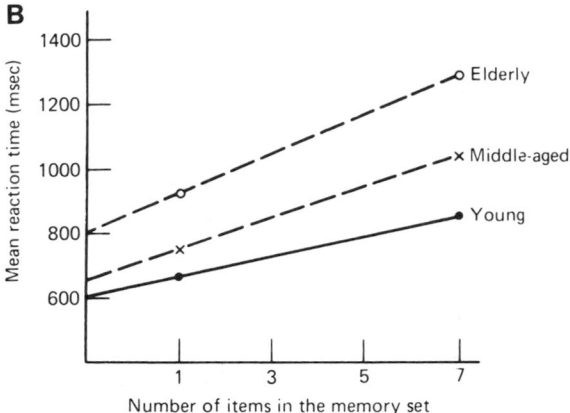

FIGURE 5.12   A: Sternberg's results for reaction time to a test stimulus as a function of the number of items searched in the short-term store. (Reprinted from Sternberg, 1966, Figure 1. Copyright 1966 by the AAAS.) B: Age differences in reaction time on the Sternberg task. (Reprinted from Anders, Fozard, & Lillyquist, 1972, Figure 1. Copyright 1972 by the American Psychological Association.)

examine representations of 1 and 3 in the store even when 7 is the probe stimulus, and a match occurs immediately. It is the equality of reaction times for positive and negative probes at each set size that convinces us that the search must be exhaustive. If it were self-terminating (i.e., ending as soon as the representation of a positive probe is located in the store), then mean reaction time would be expected to increase more steeply as set size increases for negative probes than for positive probes. Sternberg (1969b) has argued quite effectively that an exhaustive search leads to more proficient memory operations than does a self-terminating search.

Quantitatively, two measures were introduced by Sternberg (1966) to summarize the attributes of a search. Both are very useful in evaluating age differences in the proficiency of the underlying processes. The first is the slope of the best fitting line shown in part A of Figure 5.12. From that slope, the rate of scanning information in the STS may be estimated for the average member of a group of subjects. The slope indicates that the average young adult scans at the rate of about 25 digits per s—obviously a high-speed operation. The second measure is the point at which the straight line intersects the ordinate. From part A of Figure 5.12, it may be seen that this intercept is about 400 ms. A widely held belief is that this value estimates the average time it takes a young adult to encode the probe stimulus in preparation for its trip through the STS to seek out its equivalent in that store.

Does the nature of a memory search change over the adult life span? Studies by Anders, Fozard, and Lillyquist (1972) and Eriksen, Hamlin, and Daye (1973) suggest strongly that the qualitative attributes of a memory search are unaltered by age. Thus, for elderly adults, reaction time continues to be about the same for positive and negative probes, it continues to increase linearly as memory set size increases, and it is independent of the serial position occupied by a positive probe in the memory set. In other words, the search remains both serial and exhaustive. On the other hand, there appear to be important changes with aging in the quantitative attributes of a memory search (although these changes have not always been found; Bacon, Wilson & Kaszniak, 1982; Kirsner, 1972). These changes may be seen in part B of Figure 5.12 for the elderly subjects in the study of Anders et al. (1972) (comparable results were obtained in the study of Eriksen et al., 1973). The changes are obvious when slope and intercept values found for elderly subjects are compared with the values obtained in the same study for young (and middle-aged) subjects. The slopes indicate that elderly subjects scan items at a much slower rate, about 14 items per s, than young subjects, about 26 items per s (in close agreement with Sternberg's, 1966, earlier finding). Middle-aged subjects also appear to scan at a much slower rate than young subjects, averaging about 16 items per s. Intercept values indicate that elderly subjects encode a probe stimulus more slowly than do young subjects, averaging about 800 ms, relative to the 600 or so ms taken by young subjects (an estimate somewhat greater than that of Sternberg, 1966). By contrast, encoding time for middle-aged subjects seems to be about the same as that of young subjects. The overall pattern fits the concept of a general slowing down of mental activities in late adulthood, a slowing down that affects the scanning of the STS and the encoding of a probe stimulus, as well as many other activities (see Chapter 6, pp. 208–212).

The slower rate of searching the STS by elderly adults than by young adults has been challenged, however. Kirsner (1972) suggested, reasonably, that the decision times measured with the Sternberg task include the times to perform other operations in addition to searching the STS. For example, they include the time to perform the yes-no decision response. These times are likely to be slightly greater for elderly adults than for young adults. To provide a correction for these "surplus" times, Kirsner (1972) included trials in which subjects simply had to read the probe word, rather than decide whether or not it had been in the prior memory set. With this time as a correction factor, the age-related deficit in scanning rate all but disappeared. It seems likely that the age difference in search rate per se is somewhat exaggerated in the studies by Anders et al. (1972) and Eriksen et al. (1973).

Thus far our discussion has concerned only searching under a condition in which the content of the memory set varies from trial to trial (i.e., a varied set procedure). This condition corresponds closely to the varied mapping condition employed in visual-search research (see Kausler, 1991). However, the Sternberg task may also be structured so that it corresponds to the consistent mapping condition employed in visual search research. One apparent way to accomplish this objective is to use a fixed memory set (Sternberg, 1969b). That is, the same items, whether digits, letters, or any other kind of item, constitute the to-be-remembered set on each trial. With a fixed set procedure, representations of the repeated items should be stored in the LTS, and secondary memory processes should become involved in the yes—no decisions (Atkinson & Juola, 1973; Waugh & Anders, 1973). In consistent mapping for visual search, the search process eventually becomes automatic to some degree. A similar outcome is expected for a memory-search task (Schneider & Shiffrin, 1977). Automaticity in this case should be manifested by a zero-slope line fitting the reaction-time set size function. That is, reaction time for a yes-no decision should be as fast for a set of, say, five items as it is for a set of, say, two items.

Age differences under fixed set conditions have been examined by Anders and Fozard (1973), Madden and Nebes (1980), and Menich and Baron (1990). Faster decision times for young adults continued to be manifested in these studies. Madden and Nebes (1980) also found a trend toward automaticity for both young and elderly subjects with extended practice on the fixed set items. That is, slope values decreased systematically over many trials, but, even for young adults, they did not reach zero. On the other hand, a zero-slope function relating reaction time to memory set size was found for both young and elderly subjects in a unique study by Puglisi (1986). Strictly speaking, a varied set procedure was employed. However, the to-be-searched items in a set were always from the same category. Interestingly, the items were all statues, instead of words or digits, with the statues for half of the trials coming from one category (statues of children), the statues for the other half of the trials coming from a different category (Christmas statues).

Age differences in searching the LTS have also been investigated by Coyne, Allen, and Wickens (1986) with a different procedure, one introduced originally by Wickens, Moody, and Dow (1981). The procedure calls for combining the varied set procedure with the Brown-Peterson procedure. Varied sets of either two or four items (words) were presented for study, and then followed by 12 s of performance on a distracting task. A positive or a negative probe was then presented at the end of the 12-s retention interval for a yes-no decision. Information contained in the STS is presumably "wiped out" during the retention interval, thereby permitting decisions only on the basis of item information that had been transmitted to and stored in the LTS. Also included in Coyne et al.'s (1986) study were trials without the interpolated distractor activity. That is, they were trials on a standard varied set task involving search of the STS. Mean reaction times for positive probes are shown in Figure 5.13 for both primary memory searches (i.e., without the distracting activity) and secondary memory searches (i.e., with distracting activity). Note that serial scanning seems to be as characteristic for a secondary memory search as for a primary memory search, regardless of age. Note further the far greater slowing down on reaction time with aging in the secondary memory condition than in the primary memory condition. The reason for this pronounced age effect in the secondary memory search condition could result from the greater difficulty older adults have, relative to young adults, either in transmitting information to the LTS or in retrieving what information has been transmitted.

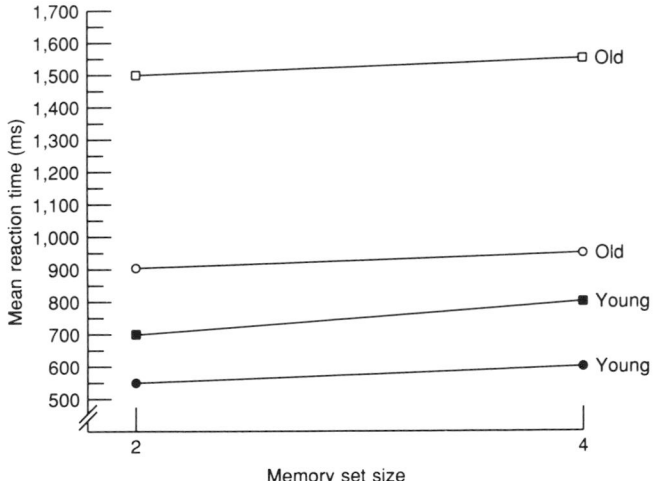

FIGURE 5.13. Reaction times to positive probes as a function of memory set size for primary memory (circles) and secondary memory (squares) searches. (Adapted from data in Coyne, Allen, & Wickens, 1986.)

To complete our coverage of age differences in searching memory sets, we need to discuss yet another variation of the Sternberg task, one in which the memory sets are components of permanent or generic memory. Consider, for example, this question: Is Montreal in the Eastern Division of baseball's National League? The generic memory store of a baseball fan includes the information that Chicago, Florida, Montreal, New York, Philadelphia, Pittsburgh, and St. Louis have teams in the National League's Eastern Division (but this will change when baseball shifts to three divisions in each league). Thus, the memory set size held in permanent memory is seven. Conceivably, a positive probe, such as Montreal, is answered affirmatively following a high-speed search of information in the generic memory set. A laboratory counterpart of this task was used in an interesting study by Thomas, Waugh, and Fozard (1978). One fixed set of items used in their study consisted of the letters $A\ B\ C\ D\ E\ F$, letters organized sequentially in both the letter set given their subjects and in the generic memories of those subjects. Age differences in reaction times to both positive (e.g., C) and negative (e.g., X) probes were far less pronounced than they were to a fixed set of letters that violated the kind of organization extant in generic memory (e.g., $P\ G\ K\ T\ R\ I$ as a fixed set of scrambled letters). This outcome is consistent with other evidence indicating the relative absence of age changes in generic memory phenomena (see Chapter 12).

CHAPTER 6

Models of Long-Term Episodic Memory

Introduction

In Chapter 5 our focus was on short-term, or primary, episodic memory. In the present chapter, and in several following chapters, our focus changes to long-term, or secondary, memory. Our concern in this chapter is with models of memory and how they explain adult age differences in long-term memory in general. In Chapters 7, 8, and 9 we will extend our coverage to adult age difference in various specific long-term episodic memory phenomena. These are phenomena that have usually been investigated somewhat independently of any general model of memory.

Dual-Store Models

Nature of Dual-Store Models

A dual-store model is one in which separate short-term (STS) and long-term stores (LTS) are postulated to exist (Atkinson & Shiffrin, 1968; Waugh & Norman, 1965). The basic nature of such a model is shown in Figure 6.1. Major components of a dual-store model are the limited capacity STS and the primary memory phenomena it mediates. Adult age differences in these phenomena were reviewed in Chapter 5. Our present interest is in the rehearsal transmission component of the model (see Figure 6.1). It is age differences in this transmission process that seemingly account for many age-related deficits in secondary episodic memory. Our analysis to this point suggests that primary memory deficits are relatively moderate in late adulthood. The implication, therefore, is that secondary memory processes are responsible for most age-related deficits found in episodic memory.

A phenomenon commonly viewed as being one of secondary memory and, therefore, an appropriate one for examining age differences in secondary memory

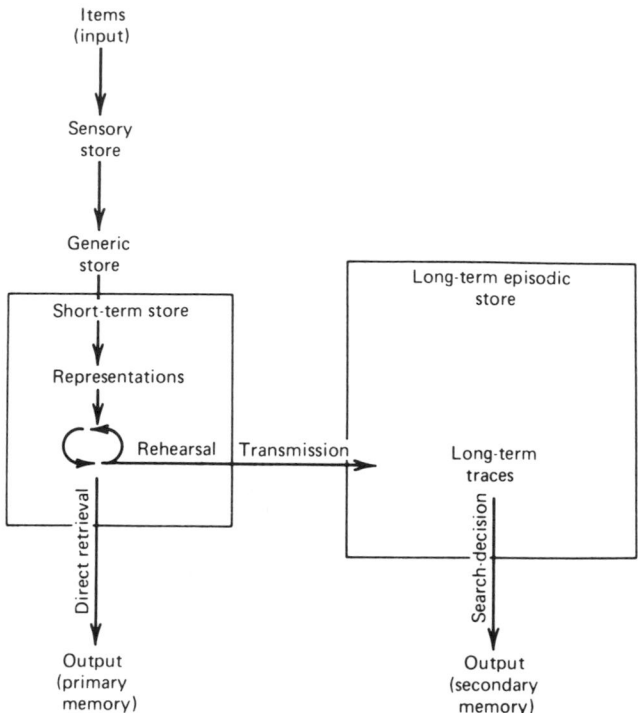

FIGURE 6.1 A dual-store model of episodic memory containing separate, but inter-acting, short-term (primary memory) and long-term (secondary memory) components.

proficiency is that of the primacy effect in free recall (see p. 158 and Figure 5.9). The primacy effect is characterized by a heightened probability of recall for the early items in a free recall list and a declining probability of recall from the first item to midlist items. Some idea of the magnitude of the age difference in the primacy effect may be gathered by comparing the probabilities of recalling the first few list items for the young and elderly subjects in the study by Arenberg (1976) described earlier (see Figure 5.6). For his young subjects, the proportions of first and second items recalled averaged (combined over modalities) about .75 and .60, respectively. For his elderly subjects, the comparable proportions were about .58 and .40. Age disparities this large have also been found in several other studies (e.g., Craik, 1968b; Parkinson et al., 1982; Salthouse, 1980).

Explanation of Age Differences in Secondary Memory

To understand the reason for these age-related deficits, we must first consider the explanation of the primacy effect given by proponents of dual-store models.

They view the primacy effect as simply reflecting a gradient in the amount of rehearsal items receive while they are residing in the STS. The argument is that the probability of transmission, or transfer, of information from the STS to the LTS in the form of a memory trace increases linearly as the amount of rehearsal increases. As that probability increases, so does the probability of recalling information from the LTS. The early items in a list are assumed to be rehearsed more than later items, with the amount of rehearsal decreasing progressively from the first item on. Indirect support for this position comes from studies (e.g., Glanzer & Cunitz, 1966) in which rate of presenting free-recall items is varied. A slow rate results in heightened probability of recall for all items of the list other than those near the end (although even these items may be affected; see Bernbach, 1975), relative to a fast rate of presentation. A slow rate provides more rehearsal time and, therefore, more rehearsal responses throughout the list. The result is increased transmission of item information to the LTS, except for items near the end of the list where recall is mediated largely, if not entirely, by the STS. More direct support comes from studies (e.g., Rundus & Atkinson, 1970) in which subjects are required to rehearse overtly, or out loud, during a study trial. By tape recording each subject's overt-rehearsal activity, it becomes possible to count the actual number of rehearsal responses each item in the list receives. The results obtained by Rundus and Atkinson (1970) with this procedure are plotted in part A of Figure 6.2. Shown in this figure are both the mean number of rehearsal responses each item received and the probability that that item was recalled. Note that the number of rehearsal responses each item received decreased from the first input position in a list through the sixth input position—and so did the probability of recalling the items at those positions. Beyond this gradient of decreasing recall (the primacy effect), the number of rehearsal responses leveled off at a modest level—and so did the probability of recall, at least until the recency segment of recall emerged at the 18th input position (with direct recall from the STS presumably taking over).

Increasing the number of rehearsal responses seemingly increases the probability of transmission to, and retrieval from, the LTS. There are several possible reasons for the direct covariation between number of rehearsal responses and proficiency of recall (see Crowder, 1976, for a detailed discussion). One possibility is that the number of rehearsal responses determines the strength of an item's representation as a single memory trace in the LTS. Another is that each rehearsal response transmits a different copy of that representation in the store (i.e., multiple traces rather than a single trace varying in strength). The ease of recalling an item from the store may be assumed to increase directly as either its strength increases or its number of copies increases. In either case, there is a ready explanation for the age deficit in secondary memory proficiency as such proficiency is evaluated by probabilities of recalling nonrecency items for free recall. Elderly subjects are likely to emit fewer rehearsal responses than young subjects

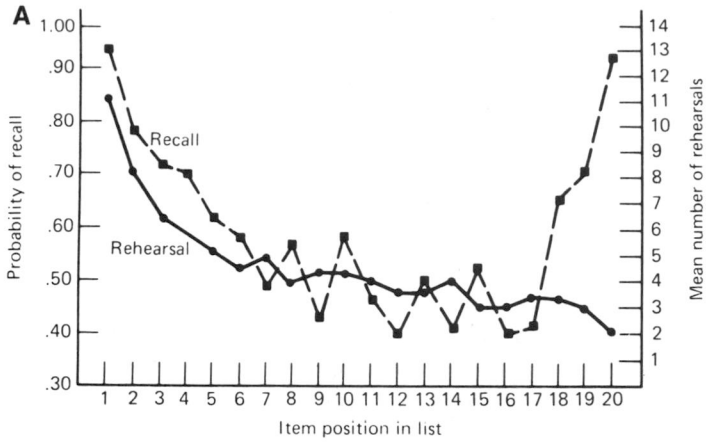

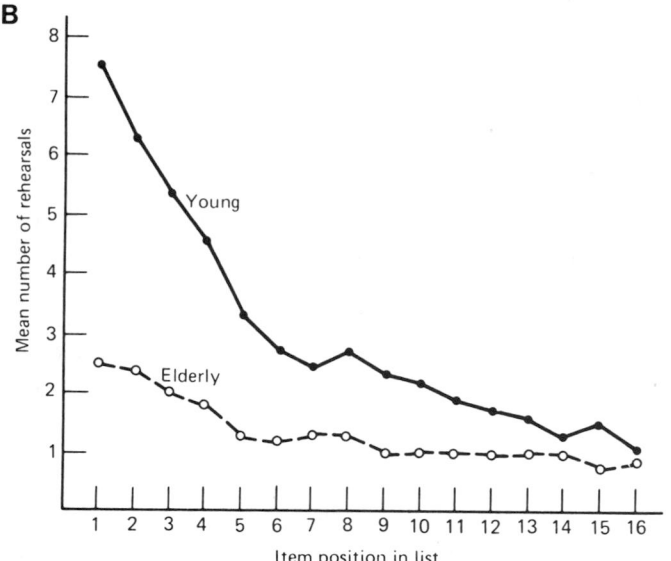

FIGURE 6.2   A: Results obtained by Rundus and Atkinson for both the probability of recalling items as a function of their input positions and the number of rehearsals per item as a function of input position. (Adapted from Rundus & Atkinson, 1970, Figure 1.) B: Age differences in number of rehearsal responses. (Adapted from Sanders, Murphy, Schmitt, & Walsh, 1980, Figure 2.)

at each nonrecency position in a study list. The overall decrement in number of rehearsal responses should be revealed when elderly subjects as well as young subjects are required to rehearse overtly and their responses are tape recorded.

The expected age differential in number of rehearsal responses was indeed found by Sanders, Murphy, Schmitt, and Walsh (1980). Their results may be seen in part B of Figure 6.2. Note that elderly subjects averaged fewer responses at each position in the list, with the age differential being especially pronounced at the nonrecency positions.

Explanation of the age deficit in secondary memory in terms of an age deficit in the number of rehearsal responses fits nicely the conception of a general slowing down of mental activities, including those activities relevant to memory phenomena (Salthouse, 1980; Waugh & Barr, 1980: see p. 208 for elaboration). In effect, age deficits in memory are reduced to quantitative changes, much like those involved in changes in the rate of rehearsal responses presumed by associationists to underlie much of the age-related deficit in paired-associate learning. We discovered earlier, however, that quantitative changes in rehearsal activity are less likely than qualitative changes in that activity to be responsible for age differences in associative learning. A similar possibility exists in the encoding of information for transmission to long-term episodic memory (Kausler, 1978). That is, the critical factor underlying age deficits in secondary memory may be the kind of processes in which young and elderly subjects engage. This position is the one advocated by proponents of a levels-of-processing approach to age differences in secondary memory, and it will be discussed in detail in the next section. Initially, however, we should report some evidence supporting this interpretation, evidence that comes from studies employing the externalized rehearsal procedure of Rundus and Atkinson (1970). Specifically, our interest rests in the question: How does recall under the overt-rehearsal condition compare with recall under the standard covert-rehearsal condition (i.e., silent rehearsal of the kind usually employed in free-recall research)?

This comparison was made by Kellas, McCauley, and McFarland (1975) with young adult subjects. Recall without overt rehearsal was clearly superior to recall with overt rehearsal. Similar contrasts were made for both young and elderly subjects by Sanders et al. (1980). Their results are shown in Figure 6.3. In agreement with the results obtained earlier by Kellas et al. (1975), recall proficiency for young subjects deteriorated when overt rehearsal was demanded (see Figure 6.3). Note that recall with covert rehearsal exceeded recall with overt rehearsal at every position in the list except the last. By contrast, no systematic difference favoring covert rehearsal was found for elderly subjects. The implication is that overt rehearsal by young adults forces the rote repetition of items, thereby prohibiting the more efficacious kind of elaborative rehearsal engaged in by young adults when they are left on their own (as in the covert condition). Sanders et al. (1980) did find evidence of such elaborations in the response protocols of their young adult subjects. On the other hand, elderly adults are unlikely to engage in elaborative rehearsal even when rehearsal is covert. This too was evident from the response protocols collected by Sanders et al. (1980).

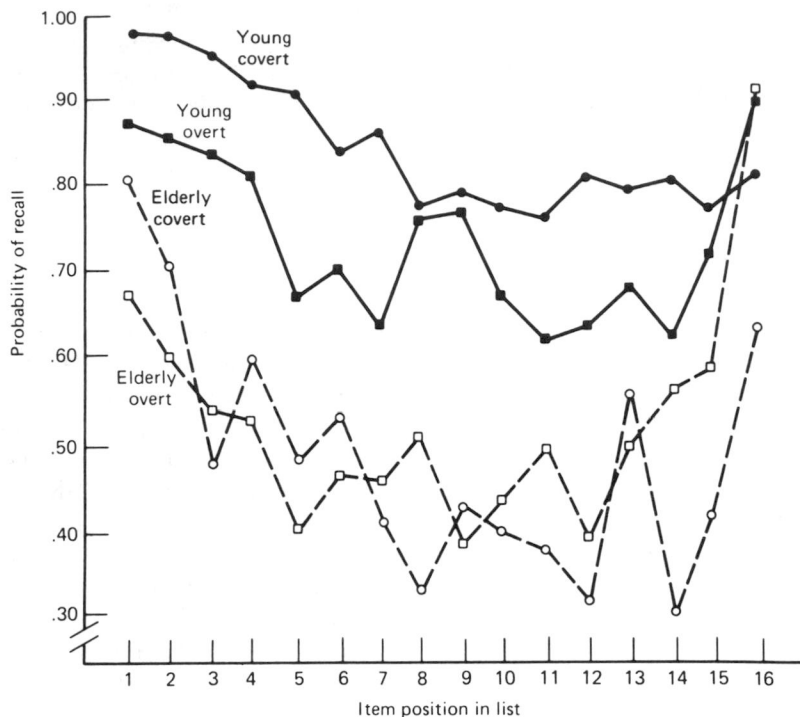

FIGURE 6.3 Age differences in recall as a function of the type of rehearsal activity (overt or covert). (Adapted from Sanders, Murphy, Schmitt, & Walsh, 1980, Figure 1.)

Consequently, the restriction placed on rehearsal by making it overt makes little difference to elderly subjects. However, there is also evidence indicating that the failure of elderly people to use elaborative rehearsal is largely a production deficiency that can be overcome with appropriate training (Schmitt, Murphy, & Sanders, 1981; see Chapter 12, p. 430).

There is also the possibility that the critical difference in rehearsal responses between young adults and elderly adults lies not in age difference in the number of rote responses but rather in the distribution of those responses. With young adult subjects only, and with overt rehearsal, Modigliani and Hedges (1987) discovered that rote rehearsal responses of an item that are distributed over a study trial (i.e., they occur when the rehearsed item itself is not physically present) result in a heightened probability of recall relative to rehearsal responses that are entirely massed (i.e., they occur only when the item is physically present). Rehearsal of an item when it is physically absent forces the retrieval of that item's memory trace from the long-term episodic store and enhances later retrievability of that item on the recall test (see Chapter 7, p. 268). Conceivably, distributed rehearsal is less likely to occur for elderly adults than for younger adults.

The major focus of dual-store models is on getting new information into the LTS, with little attention directed at retrieving information from that store. However, Atkinson and Shiffrin's (1968) version of a dual-store model does include the concept of a self-addressable memory bank in the LTS. Information is presumed to be stored in locations that are identified by their contents, contents that may later be addressed during recall. Unfortunately, this concept has had little, if any, influence on aging memory research.

Dual-store models served their purpose well in stimulating research on age differences in episodic-memory proficiency. Especially important was their impact on short-term memory research. The model's influence diminished considerably, however, in the 1970s with the advent of the levels-of-processing model. Largely affected was the concept of a separate short-term memory system that mediated many of the phenomena of short-term memory. Nevertheless, history does have a way of repeating itself. In this case, repetition occurred in the form of the currently popular working-memory model. A short-term store is a basic component of working memory, thus revitalizing the concept of the STS—but, most important, it is not the only component. Working memory is commonly viewed as composed of a limited-capacity processing component as well as a limited-capacity storage structure.

Levels-of-Processing Model

Nature of the Levels-of-Processing Model

The levels-of-processing model was introduced by Craik and Lockhart in 1972, and it became immediately popular in stimulating considerable memory research, both basic and gerontological. The starting point for the model is its rejection of a separate STS. That is, the model assumes there is only one episodic-memory store. What is transmitted to that store is contingent on the depth of perceptual processing, or analysis, conducted on to-be-remembered episodic events, such as *king* as an item on a free-recall list. Depth of processing falls on a shallow-to-deep continuum. *Shallow processing* means that only king's sensory features (i.e., its phonemic and orthographic components) stored in the internal lexicon of generic memory (see Chapter 12, pp. 389–390) are analyzed and encoded as the memory trace transmitted to the episodic store. A sensory-based memory trace is assumed to be fragile and susceptible to rapid forgetting. *Deep processing* means that *king* is analyzed and encoded in terms of its meaning, or semantic features, that are stored in the lexicon. A semantic-based memory trace is assumed to be robust and temporally durable. The relevance of the model to age differences in episodic memory becomes immediately apparent simply by postulating that elderly adults engage spontaneously in less deep processing of episodic events than do young adults. If true, the episodic-memory traces of elderly adults are expected to be less durable than the traces of younger adults.

There is another component of the levels-of-processing model that has considerable relevance for explanations of age deficits in episodic memory. This component stresses the existence of two different kinds of rehearsal activity that follow the initial processing of to-be-remembered events (e.g., words in a free-recall list). The first is called *maintenance rehearsal*. In effect, it amounts to the rote repetition of a word's auditory representation. Such rehearsal is seen as perpetuating a word in consciousness (i.e., it is attended to), but, at the same time, as having relatively little effect on increasing the eventual retrievability of that word's long-term trace. Maintenance rehearsal serves mainly to keep a word available for immediate recall without increasing greatly its availability for delayed recall. Thus, a used-only-once telephone number receives maintenance rehearsal while awaiting its dialing—without leaving a more permanent memory trace. The functional equivalence of maintenance rehearsal to both rote rehearsal, as that concept is employed by associationists, and to rehearsal, as viewed from the perspective of dual-store models, is obvious. However, the postulated absence of a direct relationship between the amount of rehearsal and delayed recall proficiency runs contrary to one of associationism's (and a dual-store model's) basic tenets, namely, that repetition per se leads to gains in associative strength (or memory-trace strength). There is evidence with young adults (e.g., Glenberg & Adams, 1978) to indicate that the retrievability of a memory trace does increase somewhat as the amount of maintenance rehearsal increases (see Greene, 1987, for further review). Nevertheless, the gain is not nearly as pronounced as would be expected from the perspective of either associationism or dual-store models. At any rate, age changes in the amount of maintenance rehearsal are unlikely to account for many of the age-related deficits reported in the literature.

By contrast, the other kind of rehearsal, *elaboration*, is of considerable interest to experimental aging researchers. Elaboration is essentially a still deeper form of semantic analysis whereby the semantic features of a to-be-remembered word "trigger associations, images, or stories on the basis of the subject's past experience with the word" (Craik & Lockhart, 1972, p. 675). In effect, elaboration is a further analysis of information that has already been analyzed deeply in the sense of identifying semantic features, as illustrated in Figure 6.4. As the degree of elaboration increases, the durability of the resulting memory trace is expected to increase (see Figure 6.4). Thus, elaboration is akin to what stage analysts call mediated rehearsal, only it is viewed as being regulated by a subject's own control processes rather than by the transfer of a generalized habit. Given the well-known

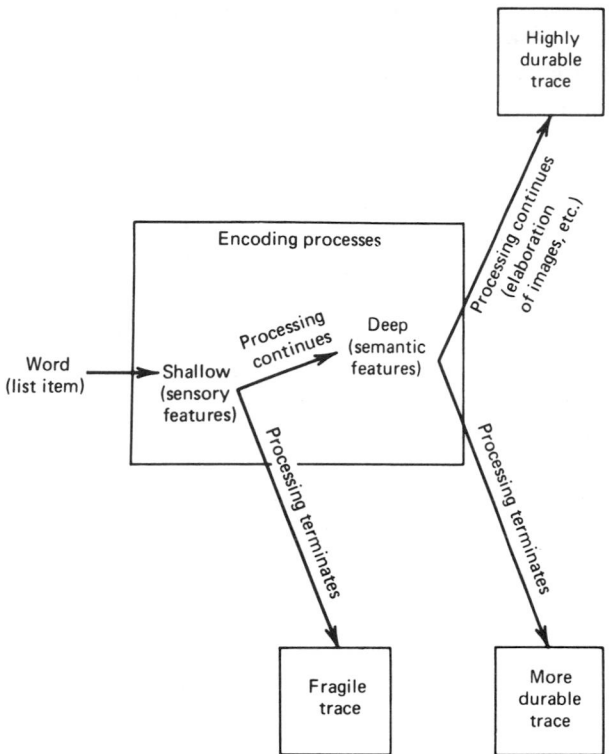

FIGURE 6.4 A levels-of-processing conceptualization of variations in the encoding of memory traces. Processing may be seen to vary along a shallow-to-deep (sensory-features-to-semantic-features) dimension. In addition, deep features may be further processed by elaboration. Durability of a memory trace is assumed to vary in accordance with the kind of processing entering into the formation of that trace.

existence of age differences in the use of imaginal and verbal mnemonics, the implication is that age changes in the extent of elaborative rehearsal may account for much of the age deficit in episodic memory.

Orienting Tasks and Variation in Depth of Processing

For some years, researchers (e.g., Saltzman, 1953) have known that incidental memory of item content need not be below the level of intentional memory of that same content. The critical factor is not the presence or absence of intent to commit to memory, but, rather, the nature of the processing of information at the time it is being perceived. A widely cited study by Hyde and Jenkins (1969) provided a convincing demonstration of how processing activities influence the memorability of items. Three groups of young adult subjects, each performing under an *incidental memory* condition (i.e., the subjects were not informed in advance that they would eventually be tested for memory of item content), differed with respect to the orienting task they performed during exposure to each item (a word) of a 24-item list. An orienting task is an activity a subject performs to assure attention is directed at each list item. The first orienting task required subjects to evaluate each item in terms of the pleasant or unpleasant feeling that item aroused. The second task required a decision for each item as to whether or not it contained the letter *E*, and the third task required an estimate of the number of letters contained in each item. In addition, there was another group of subjects performing under a control *intentional memory* condition, that is, with intent to commit the list items to memory (and without an orienting task to perform). The mean number of items recalled in each condition is shown in Figure 6.5. Note that recall was as high with the first orienting task (pleasant/ unpleasant decisions) as it was with intentional memory. On the other hand, recall with the other two orienting tasks was well below the level found with intentional memory.

Why should incidental memory following pleasant/unpleasant evaluations be equivalent to intentional memory? According to the levels-of-processing model, a decision about a word's emotional connotation requires an examination of that word's meaning as it is stored in the internal lexicon of generic memory. To make

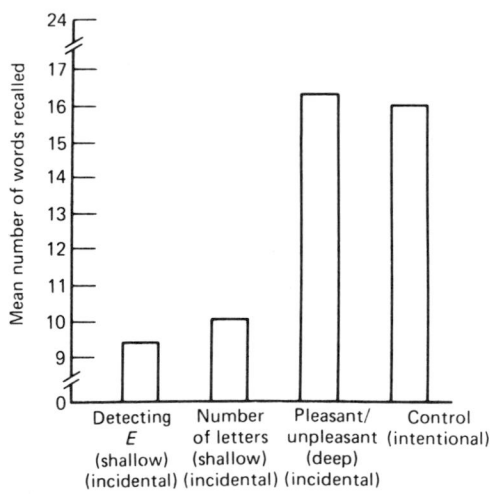

FIGURE 6.5   Results obtained by Hyde and Jenkins for the recall of items as a function of the depth of processing they received. (Adapted from Hyde & Jenkins, 1969, Table 1.)

this examination, subjects must first encode the item per se deeply, that is, in terms of its meaning. This is the kind of encoding operation postulated by the levels-of-processing model to lead to a relatively permanent memory trace, quite independently of any intent to memorize that item. Consequently, a trace of that operation is likely to be available for recall after the orienting task is completed. Most important, this is the same kind of deep processing engaged in by young adults when they study a list of words with the intent to recall those words. Thus, there should be little difference between incidental and intentional memory when the orienting task guiding incidental memory forces the deep processing of incoming items. The processing demand is very different, however, for the other two orienting tasks employed by Hyde and Jenkins (1969). Only shallow processing is needed to determine either the presence or absence of a specific letter or the number of letters in a word. The result in each case is a more fragile memory trace and, therefore, lower recall than expected with either intentional memory or incidental memory following deep processing.

The Hyde and Jenkins procedure has considerable relevance for testing alternative hypotheses about age deficits in episodic-memory phenomena. The alternatives closely approximate the mediational deficit versus production deficit hypothesis encountered earlier in our analysis of age differences in learning (see also Salthouse, 1991). On the one hand, elderly adults may be viewed as being less proficient than young adults in memory because the former have suffered a true decrement in the ability to engage in deep processing. On the other hand, elderly adults may simply be less likely than young adults to initiate deep processing spontaneously. In either case, recall of items under an intentional memory condition is expected to favor young adults. The critical condition is for incidental memory with an orienting task that forces deep processing. If the age difference in recall disappears, then it is obvious that the deficit present under intentional memory is only a production deficit. That is, once deep processing is prodded by an appropriate orienting task, episodic memory would appear to be as proficient for elderly adults as it is for young adults. Consequently, the age deficit apparent in intentional memory would appear to be due simply to the failure of elderly people to engage spontaneously in deep processing.

These alternative hypotheses were tested initially in an important study by Eysenck (1974) that followed closely the procedural guidelines set by Hyde and Jenkins (1969). There were four incidental memory groups, two receiving shallow-processing orienting tasks, and two receiving deep-processing orienting tasks. One shallow task required subjects to count the number of letters in each item (word), whereas the other required them to name a rhyming word for each item. One deep task required subjects to form an image of each item and then rate the vividness of each image, whereas the other required them to name a modifying adjective for each item. In addition, an intentional-memory condition was included for both young and elderly subjects. The results found for total number of items recalled from the 27-item list are shown in Figure 6.6. Shallow processing clearly led to inferior performance relative to both intentional memory and incidental memory by means of deep processing at both age levels. Moreover, recall following shallow processing did not differ between the two age levels. Thus, there appears to be no change with aging in the ability to conduct shallow processing. Most important, the deep processing tasks did not eliminate the age deficit found with intentional memory (see Figure 6.5), although the magnitude of the age deficit was reduced somewhat in the deep incidental conditions, relative to the intentional-memory condition.

Eysenck's (1974) results would seem to indicate that elderly adults have a true deficit in semantic processing, and not merely a production deficit. The age-related deficit, if present, is presumably the consequence of the diminished cognitive resources of the elderly adult (Craik & Byrd, 1982; Craik & Rabinowitz, 1984). Semantic processing is cognitively effortful, and it places a strain on these diminished resources. There are problems in accepting this conclusion, however. In the first place, there have been a number of studies since Eysenck's (1974) that have examined age differences with various shallow and deep orienting tasks. In most of these studies the basic outcome of his study (i.e., age-related deficits with

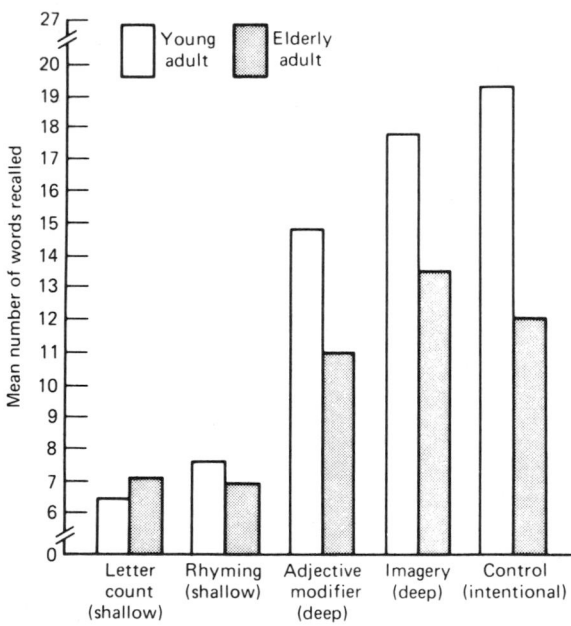

FIGURE 6.6   Age differences in recall of items as a function of depth of processing. (Adapted from Eysenck, 1974, Table 1.)

deep orienting tasks that are greater than age-related deficits with shallow orienting tasks) has been replicated (e.g., Duchek, 1984; Erber, 1979; Erber, Herman, & Botwinick, 1980; Lauer, 1976; Light & Singh, 1987; Mason, 1979; Perlmutter, 1979a; Rankin & Collins, 1986; E. Simon, 1979; A. D. Smith, 1979a; S. White, as reported in Craik, 1977). That is, there is a significant interaction between age and type of processing via variation in an orienting task. A similar outcome has been found when other procedures are used to manipulate levels of processing (e.g., Buschke, 1988; Dorfman, Glanzer, & Kaufman, 1988; Macht & Buschke, 1983, 1984). However, there have been exceptions in which elderly adults closely approached the performance level of young adults under deep orienting task conditions (Barrett & Wright, 1981; Craik & Simon, 1980; L. K. Johnson, 1973; Mitchell & Perlmutter, 1986; Moscovitch, 1982; Rankin & Hyland, 1983; Shaw & Craik, 1989; Zelinski, Walsh, & Thompson, 1978) and other exceptions in which the age-related deficit in recall is relatively unaffected by a variation in processing level (e.g., Bäckman & Mäntylä, 1988; Bäckman, Mäntylä, & Erngrund, 1984; Buschke & Macht, 1983; Guttentag, 1988). Moreover, age differences following a deep orienting task are often much less pronounced when memory for the words is tested by recognition rather than by recall (e.g., Erber et al., 1980; Perlmutter, 1979a; S. White as cited in Craik, 1977). Our best conclusion is one shared with Verhaeghen et al. (1993), namely that "the nature of the orienting task does not reliably affect age differences in recall (p. 161)."

One fact does emerge from these conflicting results. Elderly subjects do encode semantically when forced to do so—they simply have difficulty actively recalling the encoded information. This retrieval problem is largely overcome by the use of a recognition memory test or a cued recall test. There remains the question of semantic encoding by elderly adults when they are "on their own," that is, no orienting task is used to prod semantic encoding. The results obtained by Eysenck (1974; and others) in his intentional memory condition imply that they are less likely to do so than are young adults, thus resulting in poorer intentional memory of study list words (see Figure 6.5). However, there is the possibility that the age deficit in intentional memory stems from the difficulty elderly subjects have in retrieving memory traces, even when they are composed of semantic information, and not from any difficulty in initial encoding.

Noncued Recall versus Cued Recall: Encoding or Retrieval as the Locus of Age Differences in Episodic Memory

A commonly used procedure in memory research to distinguish between age-sensitive encoding and retrieval processes is to provide subjects with a retrieval cue, or aid, for each study list item at the time that memory proficiency is being assessed (Tulving & Pearlstone, 1966). Recall proficiency may then be compared with these cues (*cued recall*) and without these cues (*noncued recall*; i.e., free recall). In noncued recall, failure to recall may result from either (or both) (1) inadequate encoding during a study trial, with no durable registration of traces in the episodic store or (2) inadequate searching during a test trial of those traces that were encoded and registered in the store. In cued recall, retrieval cues presumably gain access to stored information. Consequently, recall failure in this condition may be the result of an encoding deficit. However, if the age deficit apparent in noncued recall is eliminated in cued recall, then encoding per se appears to be age insensitive.

One form of retrieval cue consists of synonyms for previously studied items. For example, with *late* as a study list item, *tardy* may be the retrieval given as an aid to recall the prior item. In a study involving incidental memory and a deep orienting task, E. Simon (1979) found that these cues enhanced the recall scores of young adults relative to a noncued recall condition, but they did not enhance the scores of elderly adults. The implication is that her elderly subjects did not encode the to-be-remembered words semantically, thus making semantic retrieval cues useless as an aid to recall. However, E. Simon's (1979) results are rather an exception. Others (Craik & Masani, 1969; Erber, 1984; Rankin & Hinrichs, 1983; Rankin & Hyland, 1983; A. D. Smith, 1977; West & Boatwright, 1983; West & Cohen, 1985) have found that semantic cues do enhance the recall scores of elderly adults and that such cues may even serve to eliminate the age difference in recall (e.g., Erber, 1984). (Other kinds of cues, for example, initial letters of the study list items, have also been found to enhance recall scores for elderly adults; Drachman & Leavitt, 1972). Representative of the results from these studies are those obtained by A. D. Smith (1977). His subjects received a 20-item list for a single study trial. For each item, the retrieval cue consisted of the taxonomic category subsuming that item (e.g., *a bird* as the cue for *robin*). Recall with such cues was then compared with noncued or free recall. Retrieval cues aided the recall of older subjects more than they aided the recall of young subjects. That is, the age-related deficit in recall was less with cued recall than with noncued recall. Thus, it seems highly likely that elderly subjects do spontaneously encode semantic information. Nevertheless, a pronounced age difference favoring young subjects persisted in cued recall as well as noncued recall, thus implying the presence of an age-sensitive encoding process other than semantic encoding. In addition, A. D. Smith's (1977) study implies that the retrieval process is also age sensitive. The implication follows from the fact that the age deficit in recall was less pronounced with cued recall (retrieval demand made easier) than with noncued recall.

There is ample evidence from other sources to indicate that elderly adults do indeed encode words semantically. One line of evidence comes from those studies reviewed earlier that have demonstrated release from proactive inhibition by elderly subjects (Chapter 5, p. 167). Release occurs when items from one taxo-nomic category are followed by items from another taxonomic category. It would not be possible unless semantic information (i.e., category membership) is en-coded by elderly subjects at the time the relevant items are studied.

A second line of evidence comes from experimental aging studies employing the *false recognition procedure* (Coyne, Herman, & Botwinick, 1980; Dick, Kean, & Sands, 1989; Rankin & Kausler, 1979; A. D. Smith, 1975a). This is a modifi-cation of a recognition test in which two classes of new test items (or distractors) are employed by the investigator. One class consists of words that are unrelated to prior study list words (as in a standard recognition memory test). The other class consists of words that are related through synonymity to prior study list words (e.g., *late* as a study list item, *tardy* as a test list item). Of interest is the difference in false alarm rates between these two classes of new items. A higher false alarm rate for synonyms than for unrelated words, a *false recognition* effect, reveals that subjects have been misled by the commonality in meaning between a study list item and a test list item that is semantically related to that study list item. Coyne et al. (1980), Rankin and Kausler (1979), and A. D. Smith (1975a) all found a clear false recognition effect for their elderly subjects. This effect would be possible only if elderly subjects do encode both study list items and test list items semantically.

A third kind of evidence comes from the application to aging research of a procedure introduced by Shulman (1970). Subjects are presented a study list of words and are then tested with a probe stimulus that is either identical to one of those words (e.g., *late* as both a study list item and a probe item) or a synonym of a study list item (e.g., *late* as a study list item, *tardy* the probe item). Lorsbach and Simpson (1984) discovered no age effect in the identification of probes that were synonyms of study list items, again implying that elderly adults encode semantically as well as young adults do.

Finally, Mitchell and Perlmutter (1986) and Shaw (1991) demonstrated that the *flanker effect* (Shaffer & LaBerge, 1979) is as pronounced for elderly subjects as it is for young subjects. A series of words is presented, with subjects required to name for each word the taxonomic category to which it belongs (e.g., *maple*, "tree"). Some of the words have exposed above and below them a word from the same category (e.g., *cedar*), while others have either a nonword *fzvb* or a word from a different taxonomic category (e.g., *lion*). Decision times were found to be significantly faster when the surrounding words were from the same category than from either of the other conditions for both young and elderly subjects. That is, the same category words produced a facilitation of word recognition. What hap-pens when the nontarget words are from a different category will be discussed later (p. 222). Again, the implication is that elderly adults are just as sensitive to semantic information as are young adults.

Elaboration as the Locus of Age Differences in Episodic Memory

A more likely reason for age deficits in episodic memory than the failure of elderly adults to encode at the semantic level is the greater difficulty elderly adults probably have than young adults in conducting elaborative rehearsal. Elaboration does seem to require effortful processing that would be adversely affected by the diminished cognitive resources of older adults.

The great advantage elaboration has for young adults was effectively demonstrated by Craik and Tulving (1975). The to-be-remembered words were presented within sentence frames, with the subjects' task being to decide whether or not a word would fit meaningfully within the sentence (half of the words did, half did not). The sentences varied in complexity from simple, for example, "He dropped the _____," to complex, for example, "The old man hobbled across the room and picked up the valuable _____ from the mahogany table." Consider *watch* as the word presented along with each sentence frame. For both frames, "yes" should be the appropriate response in that a meaningful sentence exists in each case with *watch* as the inserted word. However, Craik and Tulving (1975) expected the probability of *watch* being recalled later to be much greater for subjects receiving the complex sentence than for subjects receiving the simple sentence. In their words, "Although the second sentence is no more predictive of the word, it should yield a more elaborate encoding and thus superior memory performance" (1975, p. 283). That is, the memory trace containing information about the word should be more elaborate in the sense of containing additional information in the complex sentence condition than in the simple sentence condition. Their subjects received initially a free, or noncued, recall test, followed by a cued recall test in which the sentence frames were reinstated and subjects recalled the word belonging in the blank space. As may be seen in Figure 6.7, their results clearly confirmed their prediction—recall increased greatly on both kinds of tests as the degree of elaboration increased. (The "No" word recall is for those words that did not fit the sentence frames—e.g., *jungle* for the previous sentences.)

An age-related deficit in such elaboration is apparent from the results obtained by E. Simon (1979) in a study that partially replicated and extended that of Craik and Tulving (1975). Following a series of sentence frame/word items, her young, middle-aged, and elderly subjects were given either a free-recall test for the words or a cued-recall test in which the sentence frame served as the cue. When cued with the sentence frame, the young subjects recalled substantially more words (about 80%) than they did in free recall (about 50%). By contrast, both the middle-aged subjects and the elderly subjects recalled essentially no more words when cued than noncued (about 30% and 25% for the two age groups in each condition). Apparently, Simon's (1979) older subjects did not take advantage of

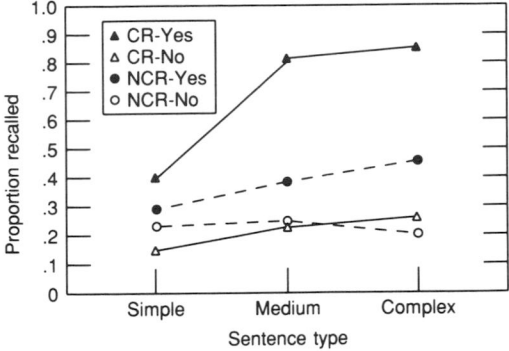

FIGURE 6.7 Proportion of words recalled as a function of sentence complexity (Experiment 7). CR, cued recall, NCR, noncued recall. (Reprinted from Craik & Tulving, 1975, Figure 6. Copyright 1975 by the American Psychological Association.)

the information provided by a sentence context to enrich the encoding of the word accompanying that context. Consequently, the level of encoding was no greater than it would have been without the presence of the sentence frame. In support of this position, Rankin and Collins (1985, 1986) found that their elderly subjects generated less elaborate sentences than did their young subjects when they were asked to provide the equivalent of their own sentence frames for list words. They also found that the generation of elaborators either had no benefit for subsequent memorability at either age level (Rankin & Collins, 1985), or the benefit was greater for young adult than for elderly subjects (Rankin & Collins, 1986). On the other hand, Hashtroudi, Parker, Luis, and Reisen (1989) were successful in having their elderly subjects generate elaborators that were as precise as those generated by their young adult subjects. The net effect was a greatly reduced age-related deficit in the recall of target words in the sentences, relative to a condition in which the elaborators were provided rather than generated. In addition, Erber, Galt, and Botwinick (1985) found that elderly adults did not benefit in memorability for words when they were presented in the context of a story, relative to memorability of the same words when they were components of a standard study list. A story context surely offers the opportunity for increased elaboration of to-be-remembered words, again relative to elaboration of the same words when presented in isolation.

A study by Cherry, Park, Frieske, and Rowley (1993) nicely demonstrates that elderly adults are able to make effective use of elaboration to enhance memorability when the environment provides sufficient support for their use. Consider the sentence, "The grimacing man held the cheese while the mousetrap sprang on his finger." Note that the modifying phrase explains adequately why the man is grimacing. Their subjects received a cued-recall test for such adjectives as *grimacing* with the remainder of the sentences as the cues. Cherry et al. (1993) found negligible age differences in recall of the adjectives under these elaborative conditions. On the other hand, they found a pronounced age-related deficit in recall when the phrases at the ends of the sentences failed to explain why the adjectives were appropriate in the context of the sentences (e.g., "while he prepared to slice it" instead of "while the mousetrap sprang on his finger").

Age differences in elaboration have also been investigated for picture memory by Puglisi and Park (1987). The pictures were line drawings of common objects that were presented with varying degrees of contour completeness. Their reasoning was that incomplete pictures should require greater amounts of perceptual analysis (which they identified with elaboration) than should complete pictures, and, in agreement with the elaboration principle, should result in greater memorability for the incomplete pictures. Their results confirmed their prediction, at least for moderately incomplete pictures. Most important, both young and elderly subjects remembered more incomplete than complete pictures, leading to their conclusion "that older persons are capable of engaging in active, elaborative processing of pictorial stimuli when those stimuli are presented in such a way as to encourage cognitive elaboration" (Puglisi & Park, 1987, p. 161). The implication is that age-related deficits in elaboration are largely production deficits that may be overcome by appropriate prodding. There are problems in accepting this conclusion, however. The age difference in recall scores favoring young adults in their study was as least as large for incomplete pictures as for complete pictures. If the failure of elderly adults to apply elaboration to the same degree as young adults is the consequence of only a production deficit, then the age difference in recall scores should disappear when that deficit is overcome. This, of course, was not the case in their study. Moreover, elaboration of the kind entering into picture memory may not be equivalent to elaboration as it enters into word memory. It may be argued that the perceptual analysis of incomplete pictures requires greater cognitive effort than does the perceptual analysis of complete pictures—and that it is the differential effort involved that affects subsequent memorability. However, with verbal materials, efforts to vary the degree of cognitive effort deployed by young adults have yielded conflicting results regarding the effect of that variation on item memorability. Tyler, Hertel, McCallum, and Ellis (1979) did find a positive effect when subjects unscrambled anagrams and were later tested for memory of the solution words. Anagrams that presumably required a high degree of cognitive effort to solve (e.g., *croodt, doctor*) yielded solution words that were better remembered than anagrams that required a low degree of effort (e.g., *dortoc, doctor*). However, this positive effect of effort has proved to be difficult to replicate (Zacks, Hasher, Sanft, & Rose, 1983).

Cognitive Resources and Cognitive Support

Why are elderly adults less capable of encoding and retrieving information than are younger adults? Craik (1983, 1985, 1986; Craik & Byrd, 1982) has argued, quite justifiably, that the reason must lie in the diminished capacity of some general cognitive resource. His recent research has, in fact, centered on working memory as the likely specific resource (see pp. 216–217). Because of the diminished resource, elderly people are less proficient than younger people in conducting elaboration as a means of encoding new information and in conducting active searches of the episodic LTS in order to recall previously stored information. He has also argued, again quite justifiably, that the performance decrements of elderly adults may be reduced by providing support to them either through internal stimulation or through external stimulation. Similar arguments have been raised by Bäckman (Bäckman, 1985a, 1986, 1989; Bäckman, Mäntylä, & Herlitz, 1990). Internal stimulation may be given by prodding elderly adults to engage in deep processing of new information they need to acquire. This is, of course, what mnemonic training programs are largely about. Internal stimulation may also be given by presenting to-be-remembered material in more than one sensory modality (e.g., visual and aural; Bäckman, 1986). External stimulation may be given in the form of cues for recall of information (i.e., a cued-recall test) or by giving a recognition test instead of a recall test. Both internal and external stimulation undoubtedly enhance the episodic long-term memory proficiency of elderly adults. We have already discovered that deep processing by elderly subjects leads to better memory scores than shallow processing, as does the substitution of a recognition test for a recall test. However, young adults also benefit greatly from such stimulations, so much so that the extent of age differences in memory performances are either unchanged or may even become greater. From the results of recall of several lists, Verhaeghen and Marcoen (1993) concluded that age-related deficits in recall are quantitative in nature and not due to qualitative age differences in encoding processes. In the next chapter we will discover other forms of internal and external stimulation that enhance memory performances, regardless of age. Of course, it is elderly adults, rather than young adults, who ordinarily express the need for memory enhancement and who may be performing at a seriously low level without such stimulation.

Trace Distinctiveness as the Locus of Adult Age Differences in Episodic Memory

Several of the basic principles of the levels model have been severely criticized by basic memory researchers since the model's inception (e.g., Baddeley, 1978; Morris, Bransford, & Franks, 1977; T. O. Nelson, 1977). Foremost among the principles under attack is that of the fragility of memory traces composed of sensory attributes. A number of studies have indicated that sensory-based memory traces can be robust and, therefore, can be available for retrieval long after a study phase is completed. Such durability is, of course, contrary to the basic tenets of the levels-of-processing model. Much of the current thinking deals with structural differences produced by shallow and deep processing rather than temporal, or durability, differences (e.g., Hunt & Elliott, 1980). Briefly, sensory-based traces are usually less distinctive than are semantic-based traces. Phonemically encoded traces are bound to share many attributes with each other, given the limited number of phonemes there are in a spoken language. By contrast, semantically encoded traces are far less restricted in their content, given the many meanings that are communicated by words. A reasonable hypothesis is that the more distinctive a memory trace is, the more accessible it is in the LTS for retrieval. Thus, semantically encoded traces should have an advantage in retrievability over sensorily encoded traces.

Another reasonable hypothesis, one that is especially applicable to age differences in episodic memory, is that the same words may be encoded semantically in varying degrees of distinctiveness, resulting in varying degrees of accessibility contingent on the degree of distinctiveness. Most important, elderly adults may encode words semantically in a way that leads to less distinctive traces than is the case for young adults. This possibility was proposed originally by Rabinowitz and Ackerman (1982):

> It is hypothesized that old people encode material in a rather general, prototypic manner on the basis of similarities with past experiences. Only general, or global features of the event are encoded at the expense of specific features of the immediate context which are likely to differentiate the event from other similar events. In contrast, the encodings of younger people are likely to be more specific and will include those aspects of the immediate experimental context that are likely to differentiate each event from other similar events" (pp. 146–147).

The concept of differentiation as used by Rabinowitz and Ackerman (1982) seems to refer to the discriminability of memory traces based on how distinctively they were encoded. Consider a word list that contains both *lion* and *horse* as items. A general encoding of "animal" for both items, likely to be characteristic of elderly adults, would yield traces that would be difficult to differentiate. A specific encoding of "wild animal" for *lion* and "domesticated animal" for *horse*, likely to be characteristic of young adults, would yield traces that are more distinctive and readily differentiated. In a test of the distinctiveness/differentiation hypothesis, Rabinowitz and Ackerman 1982; (see also Rabinowitz, Craik, & Ackerman, 1982) had their young and elderly subjects generate a semantic associate to each word in a lengthy study list. After this task had been completed, they were given an unexpected cued recall test for the words in the study list. Half of the items were cued by the associates the subjects themselves had generated (e.g., *tiger* as the cue for recalling *lion*); the other half of the items were cued by their category names (e.g., *animal* for recalling *lion*). (It should be noted that, when instructed to do so, elderly adults seem to be as capable as young adults of generating distinctive modifiers of words; Rankin & Firnhaber, 1986.) Shown in Figure 6.8 are the proportion of words recalled by each age group for each type of cue. Note the presence of an interesting interaction between age and cue type. The elderly adults recalled about as many words with category cues as they did with associate cues. By contrast, the young subjects recalled substantially more words with associate cues than with category cues. Rabinowitz and Ackerman (1982) concluded that:

> These results suggest that older people are just as likely to encode general aspects of the presented material as are young people but are less likely to encode specific features of the presented context, even when this context is one that they themselves have generated. Our conclusion is that the memory traces of the older people contain relatively more general than specific information as compared with those of the younger people (pp. 148–149).

Other evidence implying an age difference in encoding distinctiveness comes from studies by Hess and Higgins (1983) and Hess (1984) in which homographs

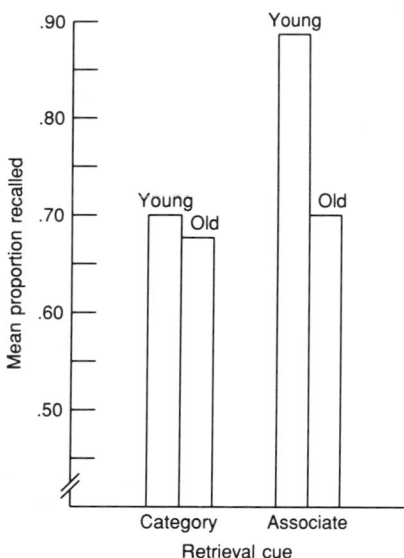

FIGURE 6.8 Proportion of words recalled to two kinds of retrieval cues. (Adapted from Rabinowitz & Ackerman, 1982, Table 1.)

served as items. They were surrounded by words that influenced their encoding in terms of one of their alternate meanings (e.g., a triad consisting of *river bank shore*, with *bank*, the to-be-remembered item, encoded semantically with respect to a body of water rather than with respect to a repository for money). On a recognition memory test, elderly subjects had substantially more false alarms than young subjects to new words that were surrounded by prior old words that preserved the general meaning of the prior study list triad (e.g., *river beach shore*, with *beach* the new word tested for inclusion in the prior study list). This outcome is the expected one if elderly subjects were basing their decisions on more general information encoded from the triads. Perhaps an even more convincing demonstration of an age difference in encoding distinctiveness would be simply to give young and elderly subjects a standard free-recall study list containing such categorizable words as *lion*. Cued recall would follow in which the cues are either general, such as "animal" or specific such as "wild animal." Our understanding of the suspected age difference in encoding distinctiveness leads us to expect the specific cue to be far more beneficial for young subjects than for elderly subjects. If this expectancy were to be confirmed, perhaps then we will be able to accept distinctiveness as a more viable explanation of age differences in episodic memory than the other possibilities derived from the levels-of-processing model.

Primary Memory and the Recency Effect Reconsidered

One of the hallmarks of the levels-of-processing approach to episodic memory phenomena is its elimination of the distinction between primary and secondary memory. Phenomena attributable to the primary (short-term) memory system by dual-store theorists must be explained solely by means of processes consonant with the concepts of the levels-of-processing model. Illustrative of these phenomena is the recency effect so clearly manifested in free recall by both young and elderly subjects. To dual-store theorists, the recency effect is the product of the direct recall of item information from the STS, and an age deficit in the effect results from a diminished capacity of this store in late adulthood. How satisfactory is this account? Not very, according to Craik and Lockhart (1972) in their highly influential introduction of the levels-of-processing model.

The reason for concern begins with a consideration of the procedure typically used in studies dealing with the recency effect (e.g., Glanzer & Cunitz, 1966; Raymond, 1971). The procedure calls for giving subjects many free-recall lists, often as many as 14 or 15, each with a single study-test trial. The probability of recalling items in end positions of these lists are then determined by pooling together all of the lists and finding the average probability at each list position. What happens when each list is analyzed separately? In principle, each list, including the first one received, should yield a recency effect of the approximate magnitude found when all of the lists are pooled together. From the perspective of a dual-store model, nothing changes over the successive lists. For each list, the recency effect reflects direct recall from the limited capacity STS. Because that capacity does not change from list to list, the magnitude of the recency effect should not change either.

The invariance of the recency effect over lists is not the case, however, as demonstrated initially by Keppel and Mallory (1969). They analyzed separately each of the six successive free-recall lists their young adult subjects received, determining for each list the probability of recalling the last few items in that list. Their results for the last and next-to-last item are graphed in Figure 6.9. Note that the probability of recall was far from being constant over lists. It was moderate for the last item of the first list, but it increased dramatically for the last item of the second list (and remained high for the last item of each remaining list). In addition, probability of recall for the next-to-last item increased regularly from the first through the sixth list. Comparable results with young adults have also been reported by other investigators (e.g., Maskarinec & Brown, 1974).

To account for these changes in the magnitude of the recency effect, proponents of the levels-of-processing model argue that subjects change the nature of their rehearsal strategy during the course of receiving successive free-recall lists (e.g., M. Watkins & Watkins, 1974). For the first few lists, subjects attempt to rehearse each item elaboratively, including end items. However, with later lists, they switch to maintenance rehearsal for end items while continuing to use elaborative rehearsal for earlier list items. Maintenance rehearsal yields shallow processing and, therefore, results in fragile memory traces of a sensory content format. To make these fragile traces available for immediate recall, the switch in rehearsal is accompanied by a switch in retrieval, or outputting, strategy (Maskarinec & Brown, 1974). For the first few lists, early items tend to be retrieved and recalled before end items. For later lists, end items assume a higher priority in the order with which items are recalled. That is, the end items are recalled immedi-

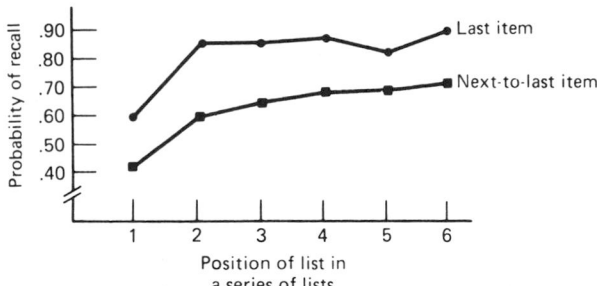

FIGURE 6.9 Probability of recalling end items of a free-recall list as a function of position in a series of lists. (Reprinted from Keppel & Mallory, 1969, Figure 2. Copyright 1969 by the American Psychological Association.)

ately after the study trial terminates and, therefore, while their fragile traces are still available for recall. The outcome is the eventual emergence of a pronounced recency effect.

A study by Wright (1982) revealed that this switch in strategy is as characteristic of elderly subjects as it is young subjects. Her young and elderly subjects received 10 consecutive free-recall lists. The order of recalling items by subjects of both age levels is illustrated in part A of Figure 6.10. Positive scores (maximum value = +1) indicate recall of items early in an output sequence; negative scores (maximum value = −1) indicate recall of items late in an output sequence. For convenience, mean order scores are plotted for the first two lists averaged together, the fifth and sixth lists averaged together, and the last two lists averaged together. Both age groups clearly reversed their outputting strategy as they pro-

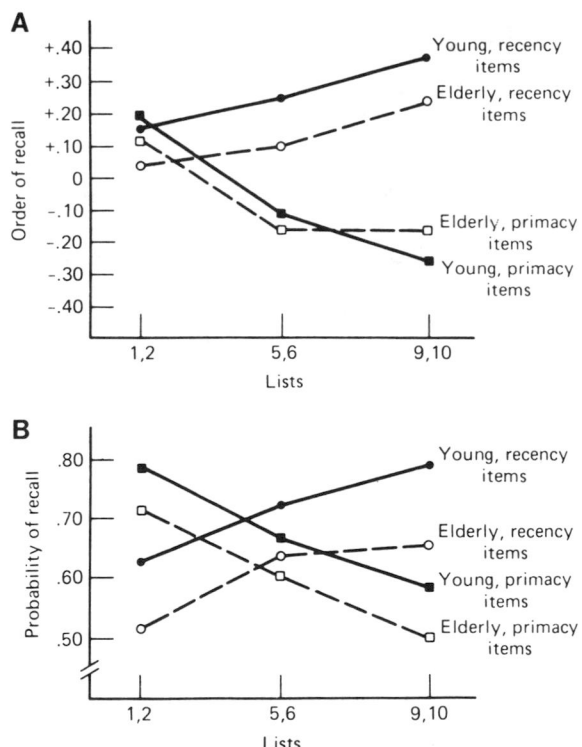

FIGURE 6.10   A: Age differences in the order of recalling primacy and recency items as a function of position in a series of lists. B: Age differences in probability of recalling primacy and recency items as a function of position in a series of lists. (Adapted from data in Wright, 1982.)

gressed from the initial lists to the final lists. For the initial lists, primacy items were recalled early in the output sequence, that is, prior to recency items. For the final lists, recency items were recalled early in the sequence, whereas primacy items were among the last ones to be outputted. Most important, the interaction between age and lists fell far short of statistical significance. Thus, no age difference was apparent in the overall shift in the order of outputting items. The consequence of this change in output strategy is illustrated in part B of Figure 6.10. For both age groups, the magnitude of the recency effect increased progressively from initial to final lists. This outcome is in complete agreement with the results obtained by Keppel and Mallory (1969), which are graphed in Figure 6.9. At the same time, it may be seen in Figure 6.10 that the magnitude of the primacy effect decreased from initial to final lists. This outcome is also in agreement with the results obtained by Keppel and Mallory (1969). Holding back on the outputting of primacy items until recency items have been recalled means that the primacy items are subjected to increasing amounts of output interference (see Chapter 7, p. 267) across lists, thus accounting for the decreasing probabilities of recalling these early lists from the initial to the final lists.

The results obtained by Wright (1982) suggest strongly that the age deficit in the magnitude of the overall recency effect found when lists are pooled together (see p. 158) are attributable to some factor other than different outputting strategies by young and elderly subjects. Most likely the deficit is simply the product of more maintenance rehearsal responses of end items by young subjects than by elderly subjects. There is evidence in basic memory research to indicate that increments in the number of rote rehearsal responses do yield moderately more durable memory traces and, therefore, higher probabilities of recall (e.g., T. O. Nelson, 1977).

It should be noted that the total number of words recalled tends to decrease over successive lists for both young adult and elderly subjects. While some investigators have found the rate of decrease to be greater for elderly subjects than for young adult subjects (e.g., Hartley & Walsh, 1980), others have found the rate to be equivalent for young and elderly subjects (e.g., Craik, 1968b). Thus, prior lists produce a form of negative nonspecific transfer in contrast to the positive nonspecific transfer found for paired-associate lists (see Chapter 4, pp. 120–123). The decrement in recall is largely the consequence of the decrement in the primacy effect over successive lists for both young and elderly subjects (see Figure 6.10B).

Comments

Of concern is the ecological validity of levels-of-processing research for understanding the everyday memory problems characteristic of late adulthood. The levels model itself is intended to apply to a wide range of human memory phenomena. Yet tests of the model have been nearly exclusively limited to memory phenomena indigenous to the multiple-item free-recall task. (Of course, tests of dual-store models have also focused largely on free-recall phenomena). How representative of real-world episodic-memory experiences, especially those of older people, are the episodes generated by encounters with free-recall lists? Most likely, not very. The closest real world counterpart to a free-recall list would seem to be a shopping list you carry in your head to the supermarket (age-related deficits have been found when a shopping list provides the material for a laboratory free-recall task; e.g., McCarthy, Ferris, Clark, & Crook, 1981). Even then, such lists may not exceed six or seven items. Of course, it may be argued, and it often is by some experts, that the processes studied in free recall are highly general ones. The task itself simply provides a convenient means of capturing these processes and studying them carefully under tightly controlled conditions. Further questions may be raised about the ecological validity of the controlled laboratory procedure employed in aging research on free-recall memory. In the laboratory, subjects are faced with paced presentations of the individual items, and they have no opportunity to use extrinsic mnemonic aids if they so desire. These conditions are highly unlikely to be encountered in the everyday world. In fairness to laboratory research, however, it should be noted that age differences in recall scores do not disappear (and, in fact, may actually be increased) when subjects set their own study pace for each word, and they are allowed to take notes during the study phase (Rabinowitz, 1989a; see also p. 430).

Many other laboratory memory tasks indoubtedly have an air of artificiality about them. These tasks, as well as the free-recall task, are intended primarily to permit identification and manipulation of psychological processes under controlled conditions. It is at the process level that correspondence between everyday memory tasks and their laboratory simulations is critical—and not at the level of overlap in specific content (Bruce, 1989; Kausler, 1989a; Mook, 1989). To accomplish this objective, a researcher may find it necessary to use materials in a task that have seemingly little ecological relevance (Banaji & Crowder, 1989; Bronfenbrenner, 1977).

Despite these reasonable arguments, many contemporary experimental aging researchers have turned away from free-recall research to research with other tasks that they believe have greater ecological relevance, such as memory for discourse, memory for the noncontent attributes of episodic events (e.g., temporal, i.e., when they occurred), and memory for self-performed activities. Research on these topics is usually conducted quite independently of the levels-of-processing model. Research on age differences for these kinds of tasks will be reviewed in later chapters.

Moreover, even with traditional word list tasks, the levels-of-processing approach has been largely replaced in current research by alternative approaches. One approach is to seek explanation (as does Craik himself) of why elderly adults have processing or encoding deficits in the first place. The by now familiar assumption is that they experience a decrement in some limited capacity general resource. Limited resource models are presently much in vogue. Research on age differences in episodic memory as guided by these models will be reviewed in the next section. Another approach has been to emphasize the breadth of encoding rather than the depth of encoding. Here the emphasis is on the encoding of contextual information that is congruent with content information, and the utilization of this contextual information in the retrieval of content information. Research stemming from this approach will be reviewed in the following chapter. Finally, there has been a movement away from broad conceptual models to more specific models that are directed at explanation of a limited episodic phenomenon or phenomena (e.g., organizational effects, generation effects). Research on age differences in several of these phenomena will also be reviewed in the following chapter.

General Resources

Overview

There is a remaining kind of model that has become a central feature of contemporary explanations of age-related deficits in cognitive performances. This feature was aptly described by Salthouse, Kausler, and Saults (1988b):

> An important theoretical perspective on cognitive aging is what may be called *resource theory*. This theory is seldom explicitly stated, but many researchers seem to subscribe to the belief that age differences in certain cognitive tasks are not due to impairments in task-specific components or strategies, but instead are at least partially attributable to an age-related reduction in the quantity of some type of general-purpose processing resources considered necessary for efficient functioning in a broad assortment of cognitive tasks. There is much controversy concerning the specific cognitive tasks presumed to be resource-dependent or effortful and those presumed to be resource-independent or automatic, and little consensus exists regarding the exact nature of the hypothesized processing resource. Some version of a resource theory nevertheless seems to be accepted by large numbers of researchers because references to resource-like concepts such as working-memory space, attentional energy, and processing time pervade the contemporary research literature in cognitive aging (p. 158).

The position taken by many cognitive aging researchers is that there is indeed some general resource within the information processing system that is adversely affected by aging. The hunt to identify that single resource has served as cognitive aging's pursuit of the Holy Grail. If a single resource accounts for age-related deficits on a wide range of cognitive tasks, then there is little reason to continue efforts to identify specific age-sensitive processes. However, even if there is a general resource whose degeneration with normal aging is responsible for many age-related deficits on cognitive tasks, there remains the possibility that there are those tasks that are exceptions to the resource-diminished principle. We will discover in Chapter 9 that a major exception has been postulated to exist for those tasks that are processed automatically in the sense that the processes mediating performance on them bypass the limitations of a general resource (see p. 306).

The nature of a strong general-resource model is shown as Model 1 (Salthouse et al., 1988b) in Figure 6.11. Note that age is postulated to affect a general resource whose proficiency, in turn, determines performance level. A weaker version of a general-resource model is shown as Model 3 in Figure 6.11. Note that age affects a general resource, but it may also affect performance directly on some tasks by altering the specific processes indigenous to those tasks. Finally, Model 2 in Figure 6.11 depicts the situation in which age affects each task separately by altering only the specific processes mediating performances on those tasks. Ac-

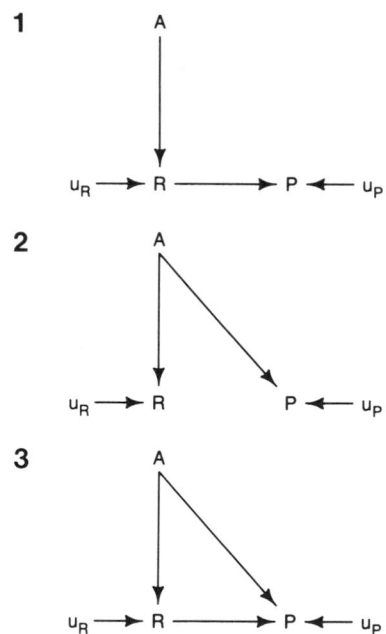

FIGURE 6.11 Illustration of three alternative models of the interrelations among age (A), processing resources (R), and cognitive performance (P). The μ_R and μ_P terms represent unmeasured sources of variance in processing resources and cognitive performance. (Reprinted from Salthouse, Kausler, & Saults, 1988b, Figure 1. Copyright 1988 by the American Psychological Association.)

cording to Model 2, a general resource would have no relevance for predicting performances on specific cognitive tasks.

An age-related reduction in some general cognitive resource has implications for age-related deficits not only on truly cognitive tasks but also on tasks that, on the surface, would seem to be unaffected by that reduction. For example, control of one's posture while standing is likely to be affected adversely by diminished cognitive resources (Teasdale, Bard, LaRue, & Fleury, 1993). There is ample evidence to indicate that normal aging is accompanied by an increase in postural swaying (e.g., Era & Heikkinen, 1985). Maintenance of an upright position is often needed while a person is engaged in some other activity, such as carrying on a conversation. Thus, control of a stable posture must compete with the cognitive processes needed for conversation, a competition placing a strain on the diminished resources of elderly adults. Some evidence for the role played by diminished resources in the difficulty many elderly adults have in maintaining a stable posture was provided by Teasdale et al. (1993).

Processing Rate and Working-Memory Models

The two most popular versions of a general-resource model are those that stress either a spatial analogy, known as working memory, or a time analogy. The spatial analogy argues in terms of a limited-capacity mechanism in which that capacity diminishes from early to late adulthood. Capacity refers either to the space available for storing information briefly or to the space for processing task-relevant information—or both. The storage component functions much like that of the STS component of dual-store models. Like the STS, the primary representation of information held in working memory has been found to be phonological in young adults (D. M. Jones & Macken, 1993; Salamé & Baddeley, 1989). The spatial analogy has been especially a favorite one among memory researchers. The alternative ways in which this resource may be adversely affected by aging are illustrated in Figure 6.12. Note that aging may be postulated to result in a diminished storage capacity or a diminished processing capacity—or both.

The time analogy stresses the rate at which information is processed, with that rate presumed to be slower for elderly adults than for younger adults. That is, there is a general "slowing down" in processing rate from early to late adulthood. The "slowing down" principle had its historical roots in early arguments that there is a slowing of neural transmission with aging, presumably attributable to an increase in neural noise with aging (Birren, 1964, 1965; Birren, Riegel, & Morrison, 1962; Crossman & Szafran, 1956; Gregory, 1957; Welford, 1958). The principle became more precisely formulated in the 1980s due largely to the theorizing of Cerella (e.g., Cerella, 1985; Cerella, Poon, & Williams, 1980) and Salthouse (e.g., 1982, 1985a, 1985b, 1988a, 1988b). There has been some limited evidence in support of an adult age difference in the amount of neural noise

(P. A. Allen, Namazi, Patterson, Crozier, & Groth, 1992; but see also Salthouse and Lichty, 1985). Several alternative explanations for the slowing down of processing with normal aging have been proposed. One is that there is a uniform slowing of transmission of neural impulses across synapses (Birren, 1974). There is also evidence to indicate that elderly adults with slower EEG activity in the left temporal lobe have poorer memory than elderly adults with faster EEG activity (Rice, Buchsbaum, Hardy, & Burgwald, 1991). A more mathematical explanation has been offered by Myerson, Hale, Wagstaff, Poon, & Smith, 1990) in which they reason that there is an age differential in the loss of information during each neural transmission.

The core of the principle is the slowing down/complexity hypothesis in which each process on a given task slows proportionately to the same degree, relative to the time young adults require to complete the same process. Suppose, for example, we conduct an aging study in which there are three variations of a task that increase in complexity as the number of processes needed for performance increases. For Task 1, only Process A is involved; for Task 2, both Process A and Process B are involved, and for Task 3, Process A, B, and C are involved. Suppose further that each process requires an average of 100 ms for a young adult to execute, and the processes in each variant of the task are executed serially (i.e., the Process B begins after process A is completed, and Process C after Process B is completed). The total performance time for young adult subjects should there-

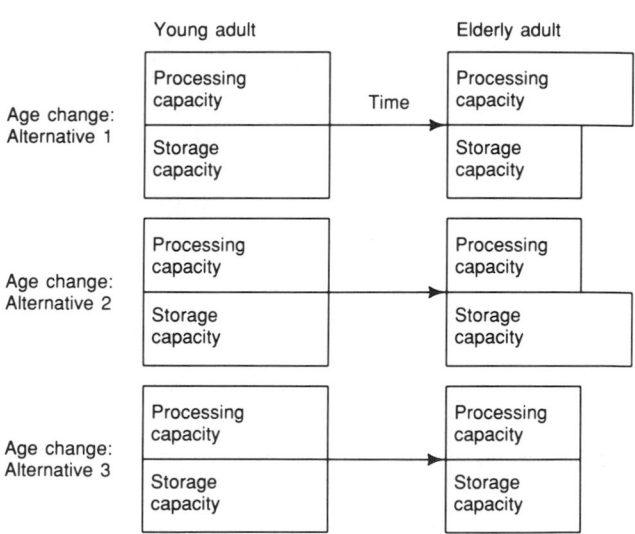

FIGURE 6.12 Alternative conceptualizations of an age-related decrement in working memory's capacity. (Reprinted from Kausler, 1989b, Figure 2.6. Copyright 1989 by Springer Publishing Company, Inc., New York.)

fore average 100, 200, and 300 ms for Tasks 1, 2, and 3, respectively. We are likely to discover that the average time for a group of elderly subjects is 150 ms for Task 1, 300 ms for Task 2, and 450 ms for Task 3. If we then plot the mean time scores for young and elderly subjects as a function of task completity, we would discover the Age × Task interaction shown in part A of Figure 6.13. The implication of the interaction is that we have introduced a specific age-sensitive process as we increased task complexity (see Kausler, 1991, for the interpretation of interactions involving age as a variable).

However, as illustrated in part B of Figure 6.13, there is an alternative way of plotting the outcome of our hypothetical study. The mean scores for the elderly subjects are plotted as a function of the mean scores earned by the young adult subjects (now known as a Brinley-plot, after the gerontologist who introduced

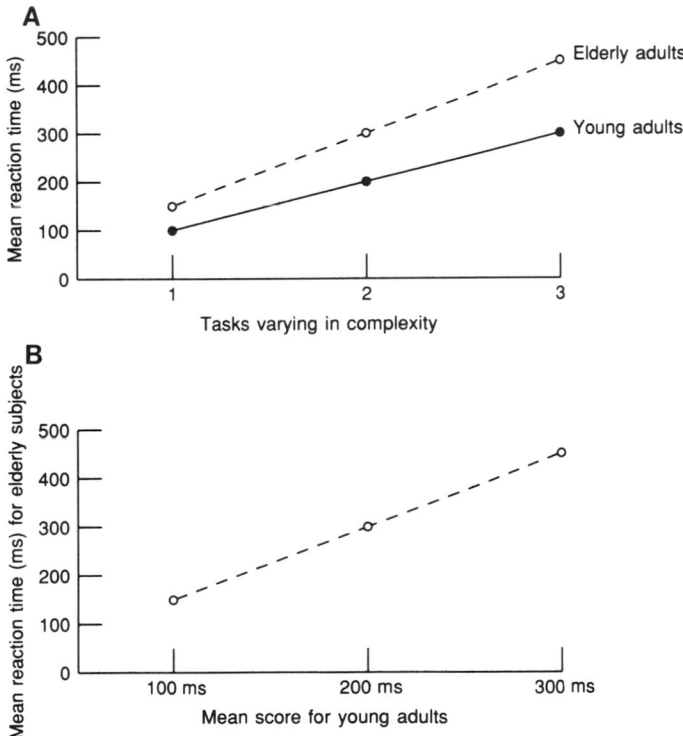

FIGURE 6.13 A: A conventional analysis of age differences in performance as a function of task complexity, revealing a significant interaction effect. B: A restructuring of the results shown in A, showing mean reaction-time scores for elderly subjects as a function of mean scores by young subjects on the same tasks.

the procedure; Brinley, 1965). The result is a linear relationship with a slope indicating that mean scores for the elderly subjects increase at a rate of 1.5 times the mean scores of the young subjects. A similar linear relationship is also often found in a meta-analysis in which the mean reaction times for elderly subjects from many studies are plotted as a function of the mean reaction times for young adult subjects included in the same studies (e.g., Cerella et al., 1980). Across these studies, the complexity of the tasks being performed varied considerably, but they usually involve variations in reaction time tasks. Increasing task complexity simply adds processes to performance, but each process added would appear to be equally age sensitive in the sense that each one takes about 1.5 times longer for elderly adults to execute than it takes young adults, in accordance with a general slowing-down principle. Our present interest in the processing rate or slowing-down principle is in its implications for episodic long-term memory, implications that we will address shortly. The principle also has implications for adult age differences in generic or semantic memory (see Chapter 12, p. 399).

The slowing-down principle, as observed by Salthouse (1980), leaves little reason to continue the hunt for specific age-sensitive processes:

> In fact, if we accept the implication that the central nervous system is functioning at a slower rate in older adults, mental operation time may be the principal mechanism behind age differences in nearly all aspects of cognitive functioning. It certainly seems more reasonable and parsimonious to suggest that the elderly are doing the same things as the young but merely at a lower rate, than to suggest that for some unknown reason they have shifted to a strategy utilizing less imagery, less organization, or less depth of encoding (p. 61).

But what qualifies as being "nearly all?" There are studies revealing no adult age difference in the speed of various behaviors. For example, Waugh, 1980) found no adult age differences in the rate of reading words, Nebes and Andrews-Kulis (1976) in the rate of forming sentences, Nebes (1978) in vocal reaction time (in contrast to the highly age-sensitive reaction time measured by a manual response), and Amrhein and Theios (1993) in the increase in latency to draw a picture of a given word relative to drawing a picture when given a picture. Allen, Madden, Weber, and Groth (1993) also failed to support a general slowing-down principle for the time needed to identify words on a lexical decision task (see Chapter 12, pp. 399). At a physiological level, both Bashore, Osman, and Heffley (1989) and Strayer, Wickens, and Braune (1987) failed to find a slowing with aging in the latency of the cortical evoked potential. Moreover, Salthouse et al. (1988b), in a further analysis of their multiple-task study (Salthouse et al., 1988a; see p. 70), failed to find convincing support for a strong general resource model, either the working-memory model or the processing-rate model (see Salthouse, 1988a, 1988b, 1991) for discussions of other problems confronting any general-resource model). Various other logical and theoretical criticisms of the processing-rate model per se have also been raised (Fisk & Rogers, 1991; A. Hartley, 1992). Nevertheless, many studies in the past 12 or so years have yielded at least partial support for the processing-rate model.

Inhibition Model

The latest model that may be considered, to some degree, a general-resource model is one that stresses an age-related decline in inhibitory mechanisms (Hasher & Zacks, 1988). Actually, the model expands on the concept of working memory. The assumption is that there is an age-related breakdown in the inhibitory processes that control the contents of working memory. Inhibition may be for either irrelevant external stimuli, namely material that is irrelevant with respect to to-be-remembered material, or irrelevant internal stimuli, namely thoughts that are tangential to the ongoing memory task. In either case, the failure of elderly adults to inhibit these stimuli means that working memory is loaded to some degree with irrelevant information, thus placing a further strain on the diminished capacity of their working memory for processing task-relevant information. The inhibitory mechanism qualifies as a general resource in that it applies to a wide variety of memory tasks and to other kinds of tasks as well (e.g., attentional). The concept of an age-related decrement in inhibitory processes is itself not a new one. It had been widely employed earlier to explain age-related declines in the proficiency of selective attention (e.g., Rabbitt, 1965; see Kausler, 1991, for review) and even in the proficiency of a particular memory task (Kausler & Kleim, 1978; see pp. 220–221). (See also Stoltzfus, Hasher, Zacks, Ulivi, and Goldstein, 1993, for recent support of an age-related deficit in inhibition on a selective attention task, and Hasher, Stoltzfus, Zacks, & Rypma, 1991, for support on other kinds of tasks.)

Network Theory

As general-resource models added momentum to research on adult age differences during the 1980s, a number of basic cognitive researchers and theorists were becoming increasingly disenchanted with the approach to human cognition taken by these models. The approach is embedded within the view of the human organism as a computerlike information processor. Much of the disenchantment stemmed from concern about the computer as a conceptual model for cognitive processes. W. F. Hill (1990) has nicely summarized one of the bases for discontent:

> Neurons operate a great deal less quickly than transistors, and it seemed increasingly unlikely that humans could think as effectively as they do (perhaps we should say 'even as effectively as they do') if they operated in the same step-by-step way as computers. However, the neurons in the brain are organized in complex ways, with

each connecting with many others, so that it would be possible for the brain to increase its proficiency considerably by having different sets of neurons working on a problem at the same time in various complex ways. Moreover, as psychologists and physiologists studied those animal nervous systems that were simple enough to analyze in detail, they found evidence that they operated more like a network than like the single processing unit of a computer. Maybe the difference between a computer's hardware and a person's or animal's 'wetware' really does make a difference! (p. 175).

This concern has led to new models that stress *parallel distributed processing* within neural networks in which neurons are interconnected by many synapses (thus, the term *connectionism* is also applied to this approach) (e.g., McClelland & Rumelhart, 1985). Research within network theory is still in its infancy, even with young adult subjects. Most important, the approach has had virtually no impact on research to date in cognitive aging (but see Salthouse, 1988c, for an analysis of adult age differences in form perception from the perspective of what may be considered a network model and Cerella, 1990, for an analysis of adult age differences in response latencies from the same perspective). Consequently, we will not attempt to explore the network model further.

Processing Rate and Adult Age Differences in Episodic Long-Term Memory

Why should a slower processing rate produce adverse consequences for the episodic memories of elderly adults? Several intriguing explanations have been offered by Salthouse, one of which is as follows:

> We postulated that the memory process that would most likely be affected by age-related speed loss was rate of rehearsal. A speculative model indicating the manner in which rate of rehearsal might affect memory performance is illustrated in Figure 6.14. Assumptions implicit in the processes portrayed in Figure 6.14 are (1) that rehearsal is continuous with both fast and slow rehearsal; (2) that item strength increases a fixed amount with each rehearsal and decays at a constant rate between rehearsals regardless of rehearsal speed; and (3) that the strength of an item trace accumulates if residual strength remains from the preceding rehearsal.
>
> As can be seen in the two parts of the figure, these assumptions lead to items rehearsed at a fast rate having a greater trace strength over the same period of time as items rehearsed at a slow pace (1980, p. 56).

What makes this hypothesis intriguing is that it shifts the reason for the age-related deficit in memory away from an age differences in the number of rehearsal responses per se to an age difference in the time separating successive rehearsal responses. The slowing down of rehearsal rate in late adulthood means a longer separation between consecutive responses. Consequently, more decay of the trace built by prior responses should occur for elderly subjects than for young subjects (see Figure 6.14). The core of this hypothesis, of course, is the concept of spon-

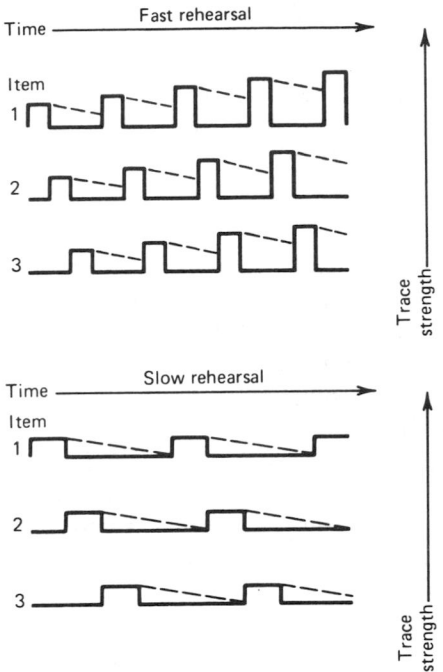

FIGURE 6.14 Postulated effects of rate of rehearsal on strength of memory traces. (Adapted from Salthouse, 1980, Figure 2.2.)

taneous decay of a memory trace over time, a concept that many memory psychologists find difficult to accept (see Kausler, 1974). The rehearsal rate or trace decay hypothesis fits well into a dual-store model's conceptualization of why there are age differences in secondary memory performances. As we discovered earlier (pp. 178), elderly adults do rehearse words in a free-recall list at a slower rate than do young adults. However, it is less clear how the hypothesis fits into the levels-of-processing model where qualitative, rather than quantitative, aspects of encoding/rehearsal are emphasized. Of course, it may be argued that elaboration of item information occurs more slowly as people age. With a limited time available for each word in a study list, elderly adults should manifest fewer complete elaborations of those words than young adults, thereby transmitting less durable memory traces to the episodic store.

How useful age changes in processing rate are as an explanation of age changes in episodic memory proficiency depends on our ability to assess age differences in processing rate independently of the age differences on the tasks to which the concept is applied. Without such independent assessment, the reservation Baddeley (1981) expressed about the concept of working memory applies equally well to the concept of processing rate:

> Given almost any poorly understood performance decrement, it is possible to attribute it to the inadequate performance of . . . (working memory). Hence, if the concept is to be useful, it is important that an attempt is made to ensure that it is not simply used as a label for one's ignorance of the underlying cause of a given decrement (p. 18).

Stated somewhat differently, without independent assessment of processing rate, and evidence that these assessments covary with performance on some memory task, we are in danger of circular reasoning. That is, why did the elderly subjects perform more poorly than young subjects on this memory task? Because they have a slower processing rate. How do we know they do? Because they performed more poorly on the memory task!

In his own research, Salthouse (e.g., 1982, 1985a, 1985b, 1988a, 1992b) has employed a variety of speeded tests to serve as an overall measure of processing rate. Scores on these different tests show moderately high positive intertest correlations for both young and elderly subjects (Salthouse, 1988a), suggesting that they are measuring a common factor (presumably processing rate). The favorite choice of a measure has been the digit-symbol test. Elderly adults do perform at a much slower rate on this test than do young adults. With this measure of individual differences in processing rate, the processing rate model has met with moderate success. For example, in one of his studies (Salthouse, 1985a) the correlation between age and scores on a free-recall task was about $-.75$. This correlation was reduced considerably (to about $-.45$) when individual differences on the digit-symbol test were controlled or partialed out. Thus, controlling for the slower processing rate of elderly subjects, as operationalized by scores on the digit-symbol test, greatly attenuated the magnitude of the age deficit in free-recall scores, a finding replicated in two later studies (Salthouse, 1993; Salthouse, in press). Unfortunately, a similar analysis of scores on a paired-associate learning task (Salthouse, 1985a) was less supportive of the processing-rate model. This is surprising because paired-associate learning is a task where rehearsal rate is expected to be especially important in determining performance proficiency. However, in later studies (Salthouse, 1992b, 1993, in press), several speed tests were employed, tests of both motor and perceptual-cognitive speed. This time statistical control by a composite speed score was found to attenuate greatly age-related deficits in the accuracy of paired-associate learning scores. A similar attenuation of age-related deficits has also been found for the serial recall of digits and letters (Salthouse & Coon, 1993).

On the surface, there are several kinds of evidence provided by other researchers that appear contradictory to the processing-rate model. For example, Macht and Buschke (1984) reported an analysis showing that on a free-recall test trial elderly subjects recall items at the same rate as do young subjects. They concluded that "certain kinds of complex mental processes do not show age-related slowing" (p. 442). However, in a thorough critique of this study, Salthouse (1985a) pointed out that several conditions present in it severely limited its power to test the processing-rate model.

As another example, Craik and Rabinowitz (1985) varied presentation time per study item, much the way it has been varied in the past with the paired-associate learning task (see Chapter 3, p. 86). This time, however, the task was a single trial free-recall task under conditions of either intentional memory without an accompanying deep orienting task or intentional memory with the orienting task. The words in the list were presented for either 1.5, 3, or 6 s. On the basis of the processing-rate model, Craik and Rabinowitz (1985) predicted an interaction between age and presentation time. They expected to find the recall disadvantage for elderly subjects to decrease as presentation time increased. That is, increased study time was expected to compensate for the slower processing rate of the elderly subjects. Mean recall scores under all conditions are shown in Figure 6.15. Note that the elderly subjects did not differentially benefit from the longer presentation time in either task condition (a result obtained earlier by A. Smith, 1976). In fact, there was a trend toward increasing age differences in recall scores as presentation time increased. They argued that "although there is no doubt whatsoever about the reality of mental slowing with increasing age or about the importance of this phenomenon for many age-related differences in cognitive performances (Salthouse, 1982; Waugh & Barr, 1980), these changes in 'mental

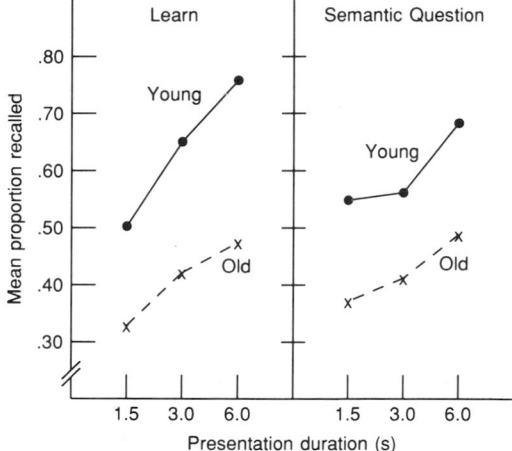

FIGURE 6.15 Mean proportion of words recalled as a function of encoding condition, age, and rate of presentation. (Adapted from Craik & Rabinowitz, 1985, Figure 1.)

tempo' cannot account for all such age-related decrements" (p. 314). Also viewed as being challenging to the processing-rate model are the results obtained by Allen (1991) with a variation of the Sternberg memory scanning model. How seriously these results challenge the validity of the processing-rate model may be questioned. Consider the results obtained by Craik and Rabinowitz (1985). There are means other than rehearsal rate by which the slower processing rate of elderly adults may be detrimental to their ability to remember the words in a free-recall list (e.g., see Salthouse, 1982, pp. 194–197). At any rate, the processing-rate model has been gaining momentum in recent years, and it has been serving increasingly as an explanatory mechanism for the presence of age differences for various memory tasks other than free recall, such as memory for auditorily pre-sented sentences (Stine, Wingfield, & Poon, 1986). Most important, as we will soon see, it has become integrated with the working memory model as a means of enhancing our understanding of adult age differences in memory phenomena of various kinds.

Working Memory and Adult Age Differences in Episodic Long-Term Memory

The working-memory model seems to be the most popular choice of propo-nents of diminished resources with aging as the basic source of age-related deficits in episodic memory. The fundamental concept of a limited-capacity center that combines storage and processing operations has been a familiar one in gerontol-ogy for over thirty years. However, its early use was restricted to an informal explanation of age-related deficits on problem solving and reasoning tasks (Tal-land, 1965b; Welford, 1958; Wright, 1981).

Interest in working memory's role in other cognitive phenomena, including those of episodic memory, was greatly stimulated by Baddeley and Hitch's (1974) seminal model of the components and operations of working memory. They viewed working memory as being composed of an executive control system and an articulatory loop that held information in STS via articulatory rehearsal (see Chapter 5, p. 155). The former is comparable to the limited-capacity processing component of working memory and the latter to the limited-capacity storage component of the working-memory model introduced earlier (p. 203). As we discovered then, application of the working-memory model to the diminished resources that accompany aging has three alternatives, one postulating dimin-ished storage capacity only, another diminished processing capacity only, and the third both diminished storage capacity and diminished processing capacity. There has been another theoretical development in the conceptualization of working memory that has had special relevance to age differences in episodic-memory phenomena. Hasher and Zacks (1979) postulated that the encoding of some kinds of episodic information (e.g., the frequency with which events occur) by-passes working memory and therefore takes place *automatically*. Since the diminished capacity of working memory is an irrelevant factor in determining age differences in the proficiency of encoding these events, there should be an absence of age differences in the resulting memory traces (see Figure 6.16). By contrast, the encoding of other events (e.g., the contents of words in a free-recall list) is cognitively *effortful*, and takes place through the operations of working memory. Given the diminished capacity of working memory for elderly adults, there should be age-related deficits in the resulting memory traces (see Figure 6.16). Research on age differences in presumably automatic forms of memory will be reviewed in Chapter 9.

Indirect evidence in support of a diminished capacity of working memory in late adulthood would be provided by evidence showing that elderly subjects are affected to a greater degree than younger subjects by the division of attention between a memory process and some secondary nonmemory process. That is, elderly adults should have less capacity than young adults for performing either an encoding process or a retrieval process while performing simultaneously on another task. With either encoding or retrieval, elderly adults' memory scores under divided attention should decline more, relative to scores on the memory task when it is performed alone, than the scores of young adults under identical conditions. Park, Smith, Dudley, and Lafronza (1989), however, received only partial support for this prediction. The expected age differential in decline in memory scores under divided attention was found when the secondary task was

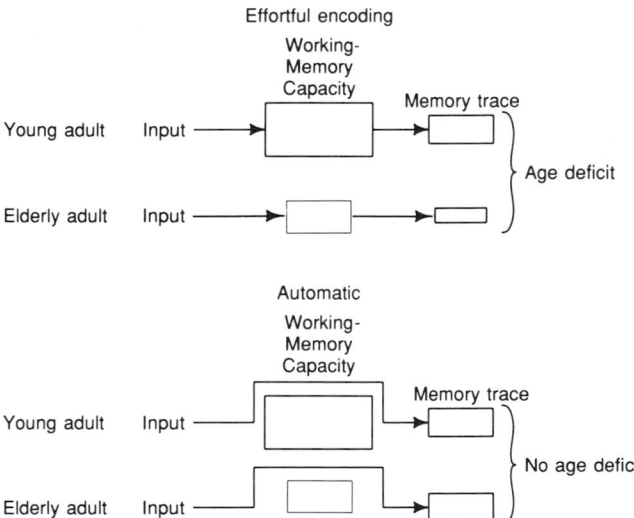

FIGURE 6.16   Postulated aging effects for effortful and automatic encoding of episodic events.

performed during encoding of a free-recall list—but not when it was performed during recall of the words in the list. This is surprising, given the common belief in the highly cognitively effortful nature of recall.

The problem especially haunting application of the working-memory model to age differences in effortful episodic memory is the same problem confronting application of the processing-rate model, namely the availability of a valid means of assessing individual differences in working-memory capacity. A valid test is one that would yield scores that both reflect the expected diminished capacity of working memory in late adulthood and correlate significantly with episodic memory scores on tasks believed to be affected adversely by that diminished capacity. In addition, different kinds of working-memory tests should yield scores that correlate highly with each other, if working memory is indeed being assessed by each of the tests. A standard forward digit-span test is apparently of little use. At best, it assesses only the capacity for passively storing information, and it fails to address the capacity for actively processing information. Moreover, age differences on this test are relatively modest (see p. 151). A standard backward digit-span test is more promising. To-be-remembered digits not only have to be held in store while new members of the series are presented, they also have to be processed in a manner that permits their recall in reverse order. This test has, in fact, been used as a measure of working-memory capacity with some degree of success by some experimental aging researchers (e.g., Salthouse, 1988c).

Not surprisingly, new tests of working-memory capacity have appeared since the publication of Baddeley and Hitch's (1974) model. For example, Dobbs and Rule (1990) introduced one in which a series of digits is presented, and subjects have to recall at various points in the series the digit just heard, the digit presented one digit before the digit just heard, or the digit presented two digits before the one just heard. The test does seem to involve both a passive storage component and an active processing component. Moreover, age difference on Dobbs and Rule's (1990) working-memory test are far more pronounced than are age differences on either a forward or a backward digit-span test. However, to date there is no evidence to indicate how successful the test is in its correlations with scores on episodic-memory tasks. A text-span test was introduced by Norman, Kemper, Kynette, Cheung, and Anagnopoulos (1991). Subjects listen to a prose passage that is interrupted occasionally by pauses. At each pause, they are asked to recall the words immediately preceding the pause. The young adult subjects recalled more words than the elderly subjects (i.e., they had a larger text-span score). Text-span scores were found to correlate significantly with both forward and backward digit-span scores.

An intriguing recent test is the computational-span test introduced by Salthouse and employed in a number of his studies (e.g., Babcock & Salthouse, 1990; Salthouse & Babcock, 1991; Salthouse, Babcock, & Shaw, 1991; Salthouse & Mitchell, 1989; Salthouse, Mitchell, Skovronek, & Babcock, 1989). Subjects are given a series of simple equations to solve, for example, $4 + 1 = ?$, $5 - 2 = ?$, $8 + 4 = ?$, and $4 - 3 = ?$. Their task is to solve each equation while simultaneously holding in memory each of the second digits in the equations so that they can be recalled in order after the last equation has been solved. The test is especially designed to evaluate age differences in processing capacity. This is accomplished by varying the complexity of the equations containing the to-be-remembered digits. Although the evidence provided by Babcock and Salthouse (1990) suggests that the test may be only moderately successful in achieving this objective, later evidence (Salthouse & Babcock, 1991) has been more promising (to be discussed shortly). Age-related deficits in computational-span scores have been found to account, in part, for age-related deficits in memory for scenes (Frieske & Park; see also Chapter 7, pp. 258–259).

Other tasks that are presumed to assess adult age differences in working memory include a spatial-line-span task (Babcock & Salthouse, 1990) and a task in which subjects have to produce the digits 1 through 9 in a random order (Wiegersma & Meertse, 1990). Pronounced age differences, favoring young adults, have been found for both tasks. The spatial-line task has been further demonstrated to correlate moderately highly ($r = .40$) with computational-span scores (Babcock & Salthouse, 1990), and computational-span scores with listening-span scores (see below; $r = .68$; Salthouse & Babcock, 1991), as they should if these tests are all assessing individual differences in working-memory capacity.

Perhaps the most popular test in aging research is one introduced by Daneman and Carpenter (1980). Subjects are required either to read or to listen to a series of sentences with the intent to recall the last word in each sentence. A subject's score is the longest number of sentences spanned without making an error (i.e., either a reading-span or a listening-span score). The test does seem to require both passive storage of words and active processing of words, thus making it highly relevant to the working memory concept. Moreover, with young adult subjects Daneman and Carpenter (1980) found that their span scores correlated fairly substantially with scores on a reading comprehension task, a task that does place demands on working memory. Application of the span test in aging research, however, has had mixed success. For example, J. Hartley (1986) found mean reading-span scores to be identical for her young and elderly subjects (each group averaged 2.88 sentences spanned without error). A test to be used to measure age differences in working-memory capacity can scarcely be useful if its scores reveal no age-related deficit in capacity. On the other hand, L. L. Light and Anderson (1985) did find a significantly greater mean reading-span score for their young subjects (mean = 3.44 sentences) than for their elderly subjects (mean = 3.02 sentences), thus fulfilling the first prerequisite of a valid test of working-memory capacity. However, they failed to find significant correlations between scores on the span test and scores on their episodic-memory task (memory for paragraphs), thus failing to fulfill the second prerequisite. Pratt, Boyes,

Robins, and Manchester (1989) also found their elderly subjects to score significantly lower (mean = 2.32) than either young adult subjects (18 to 25 yr; mean = 2.70) or somewhat older subjects (26 to 55 yr; mean = 2.73). This time a significant relationship was found, both within and between age groups, between sentence-span scores and memory-task scores (retelling a story). Despite the negative evidence provided by L. L. Light and Anderson (1985), there is now ample evidence to indicate that age-related declines in memory for discourse materials (see also Chapter 8, p. 305) are caused by age-related declines in working-memory capacity (Cohen, 1988; Kemper, 1988).

A modification of the basic sentence-span test has yielded a measure of working-memory capacity that is much more promising in terms of the task's potential validity (Gick, Craik, & Morris, 1988; Morris, Gick, & Craik, 1988; Stine & Wingfield, 1987a; Wingfield, Stine, Lahar, & Aberdeen, 1988). The modification calls for an addition to the basic task in which subjects have to make a verification decision (i.e., true/false) about each sentence's content as well as holding the last word of each sentence in memory for eventual recall. Thus, for some of the sentences, the correct response is true, for others it is false (e.g., "A river is usually larger than a *stream*" or "An ocean is not larger than a *stream*, with *stream* the to-be-remembered word; Gick et al., 1988). The verification component forces the active processing of incoming information from a new sentence, while maintaining in memory the last words of each prior sentence. The net effect is to capture more fully the full scope of working memory's dual operations than is possible with the simple sentence-span task. Pronounced age differences are found with this revised test, as may be seen in part A of Figure 6.17 for the results obtained by Wingfield et al. (1988). Also shown in this figure are the age differences found for the same subjects on a forward digit-span test and a simple word-span test. Note that the age-related deficit in the number of items spanned is far greater for the "loaded" word-span test (i.e., the modified Daneman and Carpenter, 1980, test) than for either of the other potential measures of working-memory capacity.

Our confidence in the modified sentence-span test should be strengthened even more by Stine and Wingfield's (1987a) discovery that individual differences in their modified listening-span test scores accounted for a sizable segment of the variance in scores of young and elderly subjects on their episodic-memory task (recalling short prose passages). Thus, important validating evidence of the second kind (i.e., correlation between working-memory test scores and episodic-memory test scores) was obtained.

Unresolved by such evidence is the question of where the major decline in working memory with aging occurs, that is, in its processing component or in its storage component. Welford (1958) proposed some years ago that age-related deficits in performance should increase as the complexity of a task increases. When applied to working memory (Craik & Rabinowitz, 1984), an interaction between age and task complexity implies that it is largely the processing compo-

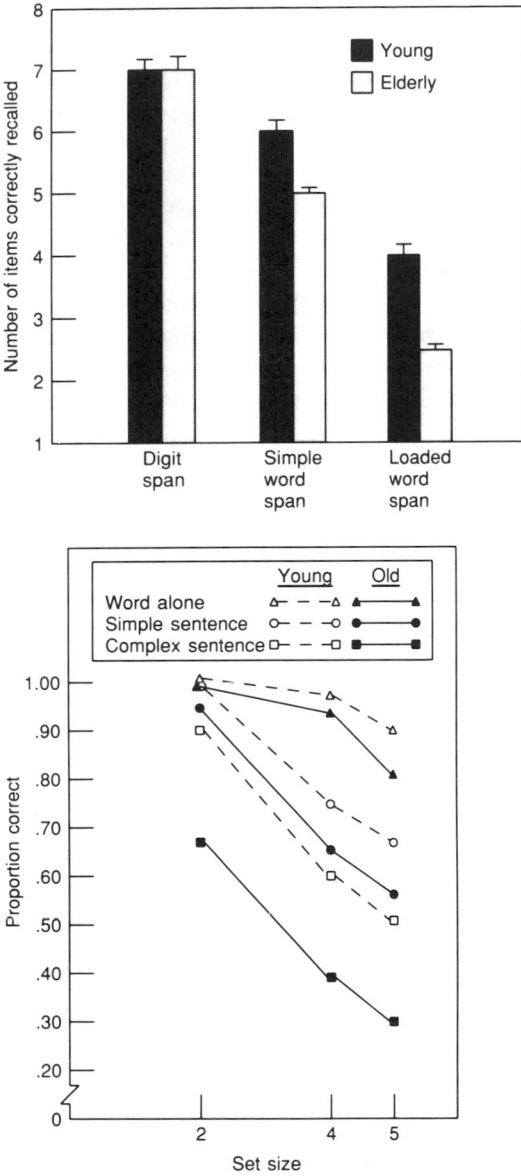

FIGURE 6.17 A: Mean number of words correctly recalled with three span measures. (Reproduced from Wingfield, Stine, Lahar, & Aberdeen, 1988, Figure 1; © Beech Hill Publishing Company.) B: Proportions of words recalled as a function of set size and experimental condition. (Adapted from Gick, Craik, & Morris, 1988, Figure 1.)

nent that is affected adversely by aging. By contrast, the presence of main effects for age and task complexity, but the absence of an interaction between the two, implies that it is the storage component of working memory that is largely affected by aging. To test this hypothesis, Gick et al. (1988) and Morris et al. (1988) introduced several other variations in the nature of a reading-span test. Most important was the variation in sentence complexity. Simple sentences were viewed as ones conveying positive statements (e.g., "Cats usually like to hunt *mice*"), complex sentences as ones conveying negative statements (e.g., "Bookcases are not usually found by the *sea*"). As in Wingfield et al.'s (1988) study, they also included the equivalent of a word-span test by having a condition in which subjects simply received series of words, with each word presented alone. Shown in part B of Figure 6.17 are the proportions of words recalled as the number to be recalled increased from two to five. Note the modest age difference for words presented alone (in agreement with Wingfield et al., 1988), combined with the much greater age-related deficit for terminal words in sentences (again, in agreement with Wingfield et al., 1988). Moreover, there was a significant interaction between age and sentence complexity. The magnitude of the age-related deficit was much greater for complex sentences than for simple sentences. Gick et al. (1988) concluded that ". . . older people have greater difficulty with the ongoing processing aspects of working-memory tasks, and thus they are less able to add additional words to the rehearsal loop, especially when complex sentences are presented (p. 360)."

The implications for the aging of working memory are clear. The capacity of working memory diminishes differentially, with the active processing component diminishing considerably more than the passive storage component. Other investigators have also reported a significant Age × Task Complexity interaction that seemingly reflects the greater performance decrement for elderly adults than for young adults as the processing demands on working memory increase (Salthouse, Mitchell, Skovronek, & Babcock, 1989; Salthouse & Skovronek, 1992). However, it should be noted that Babcock and Salthouse (1990) failed to find the expected interaction.

Perhaps the most important step in decomposing working memory into age-sensitive storage and age-sensitive processing components was made by Salthouse and Babcock (1991). Their view of the processing component was in terms of *processing efficiency* rather than processing capacity. In their second study, over two hundred adults ranging in age from to 18 to 82 yr performed on a number of tests. Two of these tests were of working memory (computation-span and modified listening-span tests). Each subject was assigned a single working-memory score based on a composite of scores on the two tests. In addition, each subject completed two simple span tests (digit-span and word-span) to provide assessments of working memory's storage capacity, several tests designed to measure processing speed (e.g., letter comparison and pattern comparison), and several tests to measure processing proficiency (a simple addition test and a sentence comprehension test). Hierarchical regression analyses revealed that age-associated variance in working-memory test scores was greatly reduced when individual differences in simple speed scores were controlled. Salthouse and Babcock (1991) summarized the outcome of their study by means of the path analysis shown in Figure 6.18. As noted by Salthouse and Babcock, "The most interesting aspect of Figure 6.18 is that all the age-related effects on processing efficiency, storage capacity, and working memory are indirect, rather than direct. In other words, all the significant relations between age and measures of these constructs appear to be mediated through age-related reductions in simple speed" (1991, p. 773). Their analysis would seemingly add greatly to the validity of the processing-rate model. Working memory itself seems to vary in proficiency as a function of one's processing rate. The slower rate of processing of elderly adults would therefore account for their age-related deficits in both storage and processing proficiency. It should be noted, however, that this conclusion is challenged somewhat by the results obtained by Hultsch, Hertzog, Small, McDonald-Miszczak, and Dixon (1992). They measured longitudinal decline over three years in scores on two tests of working memory for a large sample of elderly adults. They found that the extent

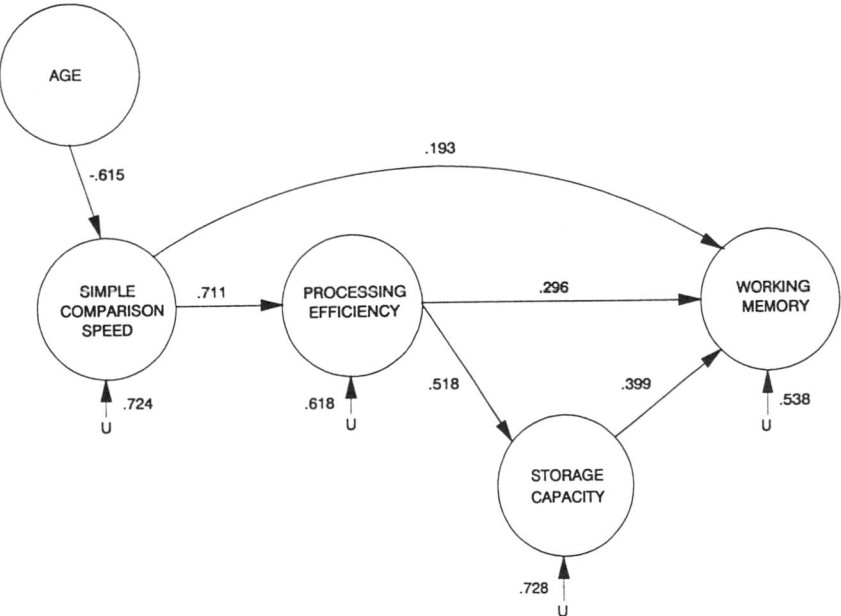

FIGURE 6.18 Path analysis relating processing efficiency, storage capacity, and working memory. (Reprinted from Salthouse & Babcock, 1991, Figure 6. Copyright 1991 by the American Psychological Association.)

of the decline was not greatly attentuated by statistically adjusting for the accompanying decline in processing rate as measured by several tests.

Other conceptualizations of the fate of working memory with aging continue to appear, and they are likely to continue to do so in the future. For example, Foos (1989a) presented evidence to show that the adverse effect of aging on storage capacity may have been underestimated in other studies. He employed tasks for which the stored information (e.g., linear ordering of information contained in sentences) was more complex than the words or digits usually required for storage. Similar evidence for storage capacity being the primary locus of age-related declines in working-memory capacity was presented by Foos and Wright (1992) with a procedure in which subjects had to allocate their resources either to the storage of new information (names of persons) or to the processing of new information (solving addition problems)—or both.

Inhibition and Adult Age Differences in Episodic Long-Term Memory

An age difference in memory performance, favoring young adults, attributed to an age-related decline in an inhibitory process was reported by Kausler and Kleim (1978). In their study, the irrelevant information that needed inhibition occurred from external stimulation on a multiple-item recognition memory task (or verbal discrimination, as it is often called; Kausler, Pavur, & Yadrick, 1975). The procedure for this task calls for exposing two or more items at the same time during a study trial. In each exposure, one of the items is arbitrarily designated "correct" by the investigator, whereas the other item(s) is designated "incorrect." The distinction between correct and incorrect items is made by simply underlining the correct item of each combination of items. On a subsequent test trial, subjects attempt to identify which items had been previously designated correct when confronted by the item combinations in the absence of the distinctive markings.

In effect, correct items may be viewed as conveying relevant information, whereas incorrect items convey irrelevant information. The most effective strategy for mastering such a task is to focus attention on only correct items and inhibit attention directed at incorrect items. An impaired inhibitory process would therefore place elderly subjects at a disadvantage relative to younger subjects (Kausler, Kleim, & Overcast, 1975). Moreover, the extent of the age-related deficit should increase as the number of incorrect items combined with each correct item increases. Kausler and Kleim's (1978) young and elderly subjects received study lists in which correct items were combined with either one or three incorrect items. Their results, expressed in terms of mean number of errors in mastering the lists, are plotted in Figure 6.19. Note that an age difference favoring young subjects was clearly present in both conditions. Most important, as predicted by the inhibition model, the magnitude of the age difference in-

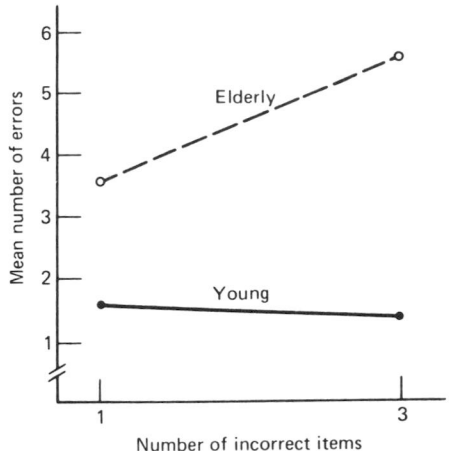

FIGURE 6.19 Age differences in multiple-item recognition memory as a function of number of incorrect items paired with each correct item. (Adapted from Kausler & Kleim, 1978, Table 1.)

creased as the number of incorrect items increased (comparable results have been reported when elderly subjects are required to give frequency judgments of correct and incorrect words that varied in terms of the numbers of items in which they appeared; Kausler and Hakami, 1982). What may appear to be a puzzling outcome in Kausler and Kleim's (1978) study is the fact that the young subjects, if anything, increased in proficiency as the number of incorrect items increased. This seemingly paradoxical outcome has been found with young subjects by other investigators (e.g., Radtke, McHewitt, & Jacoby, 1970). Actually, this outcome is readily explained by the major theory of multiple-item recognition memory (Ekstrand, Wallace, & Underwood, 1966). The theory itself does not concern us here. What does concern us is the fact that we have uncovered a situation in which the susceptibility of elderly people to an impairment in inhibiting irrelevant external stimuli reduces considerably their proficiency in performing on the task at hand.

Interestingly, there appears to be the absence of an age difference in inhibiting attention to irrelevant item information when task conditions approximate those of a nonsearch visual attention paradigm (i.e., one in which identification of a target stimulus amid irrelevant nontarget stimuli does not require searching an array of stimuli; see Kausler, 1991, for a discussion of this paradigm). This was demonstrated in a free-recall study by Pavur, Comeaux, and Zeringue (1984). Words were presented in the form of a simulated shopping list. Some items on the list were preceded by the word "get," whereas other items were preceded by the words "don't get." The results indicated that both young and elderly subjects were equally capable of inhibiting attention to the "don't get" items. No search of items was necessary to determine which ones were relevant to the fictitious shopping trip. That is, advance cues served to identify which items needed to be processed and which ones did not.

The flanker effect (see p. 189) provides another situation for testing an adult age difference in the efficacy of inhibitory processes. We discovered earlier that both young and elderly subjects show a facilitation effect in naming the category of a word when other words above and below that word are from the same category. Our present concern is with what happens when the contextual words are from a different category. Here attention to the external irrelevant stimuli needs to be inhibited in order to name the target word rapidly. An age difference in this inhibitory process implies that elderly subjects will direct more attention to these irrelevant stimuli than will young subjects. The net effect is that elderly subjects should show a longer latency in naming the category of the target word than young subjects, relative to naming the category when the context consists of nonwords. Unfortunately, the results here are conflicting. A significantly greater inhibition effect for elderly subjects than for young subjects was found by Shaw (1991) but not by Mitchell and Perlmutter (1986).

Direct evidence for an age difference in the ability to inhibit internal irrelevant stimuli was provided by Hartman and Hasher (1991). In the first part of their study, young and elderly subjects were given sentence frames with the last word missing, for example, "She ladled the soup into her _____." They were asked to predict the last word for each sentence. There is a high probability at each age level that the predicted word will be *bowl*. On some sentences the predicted word did indeed appear. However, for critical sentences the predicted word did not subsequently appear. Instead an unlikely word, such as *lap* for our example, appeared. In the second part of the study, the subjects were given an indirect test of memory involving the words from the first part of the study (an indirect test is one of implicit memory; see Chapter 11 p. 372). Sentence frames with the last word missing were again given, with subjects filling in the last word. Examples of these sentences are "Scotty licked the bottom of the   " and "The kitten slept peacefully on her owner's   ." Half of their subjects had received the prior "soup" sentence in the first part of the study; the other half had not (a control condition). The proportions of subjects completing the sentences in the control condition with "bowl" and "lap" were .499 and .470 for the young and elderly subjects, respectively. For each age group, the difference between this proportion and the proportion of sentences completed by subjects receiving prior sentences like the "soup" sentence defines a *priming effect* (see Chapter 11, p. 371, and Chapter 12, p. 396, for other forms of priming effects). The young subjects had a priming effect of .123 for the "kitten" sentence and .011 for the "bowl" sentence. Thus, a significant priming effect was evident when the prior sentence word was the correct word (i.e., the word physically presented;

e.g., *lap*) but not when the prior sentence word was not physically presented (e.g., *bowl*). By contrast, the elderly subjects had equivalent priming effects of .060 for both kinds of sentences in the indirect memory test. The age difference is presumably attributable to the greater difficulty of elderly subjects than young subjects in inhibiting thoughts about "bowl" during the initial first part of the study.

Indirect evidence for an age difference in the inhibitory process for irrelevant internal stimuli comes from studies in which subjects receive successive word lists for study and test. Of interest is an age difference in occurrences of words from a previous list when being tested on a new list. These errors are called intrusion errors. An age-related impairment in the inhibition of irrelevant thoughts (i.e., of words once relevant to a prior list but irrelevant to a present list) implies that there should be more intrusions for elderly subjects than for young subjects. In agreement with the inhibition model, slightly more intrusion errors for elderly than for young subjects have been reported in several studies (e.g., Drachman & Leavitt, 1972; Fuld, Katzman, Davies, & Terry, 1982; Hartley & Walsh, 1980a; Stine & Wingfield, 1987a; Taub, 1966). Of further interest are studies of negative transfer in which subjects also need to inhibit thoughts of responses from a prior list while practicing on a current list. In fact, the concept of interference proneness bears a close relatedness to the concept of inhibition. We discovered earlier (Chapter 4, pp. 125–126) that the evidence indicating greater interference proneness (or, in other words, less efficient inhibition) for elderly adults than for young adults is limited to the A-B, A-Br-negative transfer paradigm.

The inhibition model does show promise for stimulating research on various long-term episodic memory phenomena. We will discover in Chapter 8 that it has been applied to adult age differences in discourse memory as well as to the forms of memory discussed in this section. However, it should be noted that there is one bit of evidence that conflicts directly with the tenets of the inhibition model. Giambra (1989) discovered that intrusions by task-irrelevant thoughts while performing on a simple vigilance task actually occurred more frequently in young subjects than in elderly subjects. This is certainly not to be expected if it is elderly adults who have difficulty in inhibiting task-irrelevant thoughts. On the other hand, Arbuckle and Gold (1993) did find significant correlations for their elderly subjects between scores on several tests believed to measure deficits in inhibiting task-irrelevant thoughts (e.g., Wisconsin Card-Sorting Test) and degree of verbosity expressed during an interview. Verbosity is defined as excessive "talkativeness," and it may be caused in part by failure to inhibit task irrelevant thoughts during conversations.

Generality of Resource Decrements

There is a need for a parsimonious explanation of the reductions of nearly 40% in the efficiency of processes involved in reasoning, spatial, and memory abilities between the twenties and the sixties. The proposal that age-related reductions in some type of general-purpose processing resources for at least some of these effects is still plausible, and therefore serves a useful integrative function (Salthouse, 1988a, pp. 235–236).

The estimate of nearly a 40% reduction in memory ability may be unduly large, but there is no doubt that laboratory studies do reveal a pronounced age-related deficit in episodic-memory proficiency. Much of the deficit surely could be attributed to reductions in "some type of general-processing resources." However, is a reduction in processing resources necessarily a consequence of "normal" human aging? Conceivably, other factors that often accompany normal aging are often the cause for diminished resources, and not aging qua aging. Questions about such factors are usually raised about age-related declines in intelligence test scores (e.g., Arbuckle, Gold, & Andres, 1986; Baltes, 1987; Schaie, 1983a,b; see Kausler, 1991, for elaboration), but they may also be raised about episodic-memory performances. Jenkins (1974, 1979) has made the telling point that memory performances are determined by patterns of interactions between acquisition variables, test variables, material variables, and subject variables. Especially important are subject variables, other than age per se. The general concern expressed by such considerations is commonly called contextualism. As applied to memory, a clear statement of contextualism was made by Arbuckle, Gold, Andres, Schwartzman, and Chaikelson:

> Adoption of a contextualist position implies that, to gain a fuller understanding of the aging process as it relates to memory, it is necessary to take into consideration the individual characteristics and life experiences that provide the nonnormative context that the learner brings into the experimental situation (1992, p. 25).

Physical health is certainly one such contextual variable. Physical ailments, such as cardiovascular diseases, are more prevalent in late adulthood than in early adulthood, ailments that could have negative effects on amounts of cognitive resources. Of course, an age differential in health status shouldn't be a factor in many aging studies that have revealed substantial performance decrements on episodic-memory tasks for elderly subjects. Almost without exception, only elderly subjects who report their health to be good or excellent are employed in these studies. Nevertheless, it is conceivable that a number of elderly subjects either are unaware of their health problem or they have overstated their health status. Perhaps these subjects are the only ones who contribute to the observed episodic-memory deficits. We do know that elderly subjects who report their health to be poor perform worse on a serial learning task than do other subjects who report their health to be good or superior (Milligan, Powell, Harley, & Furchtgott, 1984). As we observed earlier, this is also true for several other learning and memory tasks (e.g., Perlmutter & Nyquist, 1990; see p. 152). However, we also observed earlier (p. 71) that variation in self-reported health status had little relationship with performance on a paired-associate learning task (Salthouse et al., 1990), surely a task that places considerable demand on cognitive resources. There is some evidence that elderly subjects with cardiovascular problems tend to score below the level of elderly subjects without these problems (or, at least, they don't report them to the investigator) on a free-recall task, but only when the words are relatively unfamiliar ones (Barrett & Watkins, 1986). The implication is that the negative effects of poor health are experienced only when the memory task is difficult enough to tax the diminished resources accompanying the poor health. However, as noted by Barrett and Watkins (1986), "Because no attempt was made to separate the actual disease process from the use of drugs to control the process, it may be that this recall effect is due to the disease process, a drug effect, or some combination of both (p. 223)." The health issue is a critical one, but it remains largely unsettled. Nevertheless, it does seem reasonable to expect deteriorating health in late adulthood to affect cognitive resources adversely.

Physical exercise is a means of combating the possible declining physical health experienced by many elderly adults. Of particular interest to us is the further possibility that physical exercise may reverse memory problems experienced by some elderly adults. The evidence to date, however, is not very promising. Blumenthal and Madden (1988), Madden, Blumenthal, Allen, and Emery (1989), and Blumenthal et al. (1991) discovered no significant difference in scores on several memory tasks, tasks on which scores are seemingly affected by working memory's capacity, between participants and nonparticipants in an intensive and extensive aerobic-exercise program. This was the case for both middle-aged men (30–58 yr; Blumenthal & Madden, 1988) and elderly men and women (60–83 yr; Madden et al., 1989; Blumenthal et al., 1991), despite the fact that aerobic capacity did increase for subjects in each age group participating in the exercise program. However, a somewhat different outcome was reported by Hill, Storandt, and Malley (1993). Their elderly subjects in the exercise group received 12 mon of intensive aerobic training; comparable subjects in their control group did not participate in the training program. Their memory test was the Logical Memory subtest of the Wechsler Memory Scale (Wechsler, 1945). The test consists of memory for short paragraphs, and it is scored in terms of the number of ideas recalled from the paragraphs (see Chapter 8, p. 281). On the pretest the exercise group and control group averaged 11.51 and 11.57 ideas recalled, respectively. On the posttest (i.e., after 12 mo), mean scores were 11.08 and 9.41, respectively. The two groups differed on the posttest but not on the pretest. However, the group difference on the posttest was due to the decline in scores for the control group rather than a gain in scores for the exercise group. It could be argued that intensive exercise does not enhance memory proficiency— but it does serve to retard decline. A problem with this interpretation, as observed by the investigators, is that the magnitude of the decline manifested by the control subjects over only one year was unusually large and unexpected. A replication of this study is clearly needed.

What about elderly adults who have been regular exercisers for many years? How do they compare with more sedentary elderly adults who have been nonexercisers? The answer is, quite favorably. Clarkson-Smith and Hartley (1989) found the exercisers to score considerably higher on several reasoning tests, tests that surely involve working memory to a high degree, than the nonexercisers. Of course, unknown is the cognitive status of current exercisers and nonexercisers when they were young adults. Conceivably, the current exercisers were more intelligent young adults than the current nonexercisers when they too were young adults. Nevertheless, if vigorous exercise does promote increased cognitive proficiency in older adults, it may need to begin early in adulthood and to continue throughout the remainder of life.

Another potential contextual factor is the diminished mental activity level of many elderly adults. Young adults, and especially the college students who serve as the young subjects in most aging memory studies, are generally viewed as being more mentally active than elderly adults. Conceivably, it is only those elderly subjects who are living relatively inactive mental lives who are responsible for performance decrements on episodic-memory tasks. Some evidence in support of this position comes from a study by Craik, Byrd, and Swanson (1987). They found that elderly residents of a retirement community that provided them with a physically and mentally active and enriched environment scored considerably higher on several memory tasks than did other elderly subjects living more passively. Moreover, the active elderly subjects scored as high on these tasks as did their young subjects (college students). In addition, self-ratings of mental and social activity have been found to be a significant predictor of free-recall scores for elderly subjects (Arbuckle et al. 1986) and of the extent of longitudinal decline by elderly subjects over 5 yr for scores on a memory for designs test (Shichita, Hatano, Ohashi, Shibata, & Matuzaki, 1986). Other positive evidence for the benefits of mental activity on memory comes from a study by Clarkson-Smith and Hartley (1990). Elderly adults who played bridge regularly were compared with other elderly adults who were not bridge players on several tests the investigators believed to measure working-memory capacity. Surely, bridge is a game that does demand a high level of mental activity. On all three tests the bridge players scored higher than the nonplayers. The investigators were aware, of course, of the possibility that people who play bridge already had more cognitive resources at the time they learned the game than nonplayers did at the same age. Finally, Hultsch, Hammer, and Small (1993) found a significant positive correlation between the degree to which older adults live an active lifestyle and scores on several memory tests, including one of working-memory capacity. An active lifestyle for elderly adults, in turn, may often depend on the amount of social support they have, a factor found by Arbuckle et al. (1992) to correlate positively with scores on several different memory tests.

Less supportive evidence for the positive effects of mental activity comes from studies comparing elderly subjects who are currently college students (and therefore experiencing many memory demands) with elderly subjects who have been removed for years from an academic setting. Zivian and Darjes (1983) did find that middle-aged college students performed as well on a free-recall task as young college students, with both groups scoring well above the level of middle-aged subjects who were not college students. However, elderly college students were not included in this study. Nor were they included in a study by Ratner, Schell, Crimins, Mittelman, and Baldinelli (1987) in which the age deficit in discourse memory was found to be greater when elderly subjects were compared with college students than when they were compared with noncollege student young adults. Could we expect to find age deficits in episodic-memory scores to be eliminated, or at least to be markedly attenuated, when elderly adults who are presently college students serve as subjects? Probably not, judging from the results of two studies in fulfilling this condition (Hartley, 1986; Parks, Mitchell, & Perlmutter, 1986). Other negative evidence was provided in the study by Salthouse et al. (1988a). Correlations between frequency of participating in vigorous mental activities (e.g., playing chess or bridge) with scores on the several memory tasks included in their study were found to be essentially zero. Even older chess experts who show remarkable memory for placement of chess pieces perform no better than older nonexperts for memory tasks that do not involve chess (Charness, 1981a, 1981b). Despite these conflicting findings, research on individual differences in mental activity should have a high priority for future researchers who are concerned about how general the decrement in processing resources may be in the total elderly population.

Not to be ignored is the possibility of certain personality characteristics affecting the cognitive resources of elderly adults to a greater degree than the resources of younger adults. A leading candidate is the presence of severe depression, a mental condition assumed to affect adversely scores on various memory tests (e.g., Hasher & Zacks, 1979). It is not uncommon to see statistics reporting the incidence of depression to be higher in late adulthood than in early adulthood (e.g., Gurland, 1976; Leon, Gillum, Gillum, & Gouze, 1979; Zemore & Eames, 1979). However, the higher incidence of depression in elderly people may be attributable to their frequent listing of somatic, or physical, symptoms of depression, such as insomnia and fatigue, that are indigenous to normal aging and are not necessarily related to depression, at least in elderly adults (e.g., Gatz & Hurwicz, 1990). It seems unlikely that the estimates of the decline in resources with normal aging have been markedly exaggerated by a higher incidence of depression in elderly subjects than in young subjects. Moreover, there is substantial evidence to indicate that depressed elderly adults actually perform no differently than nondepressed elderly adults (Kahn, Zarit, Hilbert, & Niederehe, 1975; Niederehe & Camp, 1985; Rohling & Scogin, 1993; West, Crook, & Barron, 1992). For example, West et al. (1992) found age to be a far better predictor of performances on a variety of tasks designed to simulate everyday-memory tasks (e.g., memory for telephone numbers, memory for names) than scores on a test of depression.

Finally, degree of neuroticism was found by Arbuckle et al. (1992) to be correlated with memory test scores in their sample of elderly adults. However, it is known that neuroticism is a personality trait that is rather stable over the adult life span (e.g., Costa et al., 1986), and it is therefore no more likely to affect memory performances for older adults than it is younger adults. Earlier we noted that individual differences in anxiety seem to be similar for elderly adults and young adults (see p. 10). Our best conclusion is that personality characteristics of elderly people are an unlikely contributing factor to their lower performances on memory tests, in general, and working memory tests, in particular.

Long-Term Episodic Memory:
Effortful Phenomena

Introduction

Memory for words in a free-recall list is an example of rehearsal-dependent memory. That is, memory performance is contingent on how proficiently to-be-remembered information is rehearsed. Such memory is ordinarily intentional, although, as we discovered in Chapter 6 (p. 185), incidental memory may be as proficient as intentional memory when an orienting task forces the use of the same kinds of encoding processes engaged in during intentional memory. Rehearsal-dependent memory requires cognitive effort, and it is therefore often called "effortful" memory. Being effortful, it calls upon the organism's limited cognitive resources, and it is therefore likely to be affected adversely by whatever decrement occurs in those resources with aging. A number of encoding and retrieval phenomena will be examined in this chapter and in Chapter 8. Many of them involve the kinds of list memory tasks described in Chapter 6. These phenomena will be covered in the present chapter. Others involve memory for discourse, such as the content of sentences, paragraphs, and longer passages. They will be covered in Chapter 8.

Adult Age Differences in Organizational Processes

In Chapter 6 we considered only episodic-memory traces of discrete items that are independent of one another. Memory traces need not involve just single items, however. A memory trace for one item may be related to the memory trace of another item or to the traces of several other items. That is, two or more discrete items may be organized into a complex memory trace that preserves some inherent relatedness among those items (Mandler, 1967, 1979). Not surprisingly, existence of organizational processes has attracted considerable attention in experimental aging research. Organizational processes are presumed to enhance

229

memorability, and they are therefore often stressed in various mnemonic training programs (see Chapter 4, p. 115). Research on organizational processes has been conducted without specific reference to either the dual store model or the levels of processing model (e.g., Hultsch, 1971a, 1971b). However, age-related deficits in organization may certainly be explained in terms of a diminished resources model. In this section we will review the contributions that have been made to our understanding of age differences in several kinds of organization.

Categorical Organization

Consider a free-recall list containing the 20 items shown in Table 7.1. The items are grouped in five sets, each containing four items. Within a set, the items are all instances of the same taxonomic category. The five categories represented in the list are also identified in Table 7.1. The items/instances are scattered randomly through the list during a study trial, whereas the category names themselves are omitted from the list. Following the study trial, subjects are free to

TABLE 7.1

Examples of the Kind of Material Used to Test the Presence of Categorical Organization

Category	Items/instances	Order of items in study trial
A bird	Robin	Chair
	Sparrow	Robin
	Cardinal	Apple
	Canary	Sofa
A fruit	Apple	Canary
	Plum	Horse
	Pear	Copper
	Banana	Lamp
An article of furniture	Chair	Lion
	Sofa	Sparrow
	Desk	Banana
	Lamp	Gold
A metal	Iron	Plum
	Tin	Dog
	Gold	Desk
	Copper	Iron
A four-footed animal	Dog	Bear
	Horse	Tin
	Lion	Cardinal
	Bear	Pear

recall the names in any order they wish. Beginning with a famous study by Bousfield (1953), many studies (see Kausler, 1974, for a review) have observed an intriguing phenomenon in the output sequences of young adult subjects for this kind of list. The phenomenon is that of *categorical clustering*—items from the same taxonomic category tend to be recalled consecutively at a level well above chance expectancy despite their separation during the study trial.

The implication of these studies is that information stored in episodic memory emulates the structure of its storage in the lexicon of generic memory. That structure, at least to many memory theorists, is hierarchical, with superordinates subsuming subordinates (see Chapter 12, pp. 390, 404). Episodic memory traces may be similarly organized (Tulving & Pearlstone, 1966). Given multiple instances of the same category, subjects construct episodic structures in which the category name is the superordinate, or higher order unit, with the list instances forming subordinate units. The resulting memory traces extant at the time retrieval processes become operative are hypothesized to be much like those shown in Figure 7.1. According to Tulving (1968), retrieval of organized memory traces is a two-stage process. The first stage consists of gaining access to the higher order units (i.e., category names). Once a higher order unit is retrieved, the subordinate units (i.e., items/instances) stored with it are then searched and recalled. The net effect is the successive recall of related items (i.e., clustering), as illustrated in Figure 7.1. Categorical organization does appear to enhance recall, at least for

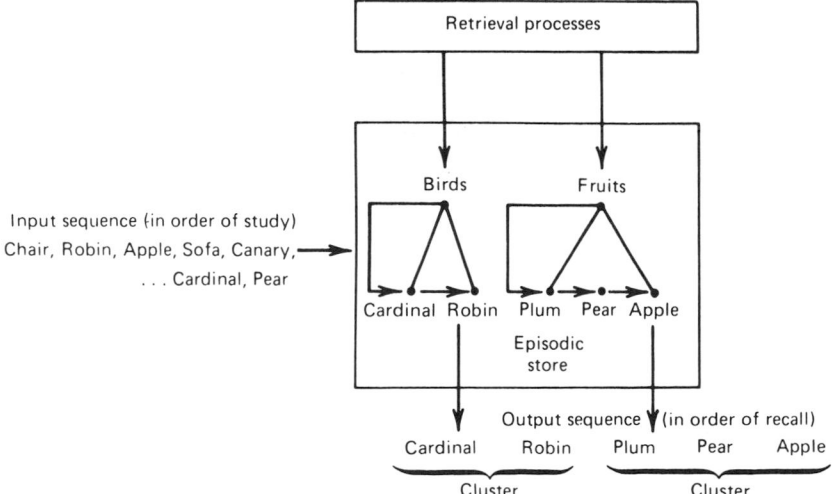

FIGURE 7.1 Schematic representation of organization for a list of items that are instances of various taxonomic categories.

young adult subjects. That is, recall scores tend to be higher for a list of categorically related items than for a list of unrelated items (e.g., Puff, 1970).

Performance proficiency on a categorized list is multiply determined. It is
contingent on the ability to encode information in a structured format that
includes information both for each individual item and for the relatedness among
items from the same taxonomic category (as illustrated in Figure 7.1). It is also
contingent on the ability to retrieve the higher order units from each structure
(i.e., category names) and the ability to retrieve the specific item traces stored
with each higher order unit. Any one of these processes may be age sensitive.
Tests of the age sensitivity of these various processes involve comparisons between age groups on a categorizable list under both noncued- and cued-recall
conditions. The contrast in recall scores between the two conditions offers a
mean of distinguishing, hopefully, age-sensitive encoding-storage processes from
age-sensitive retrieval processes.

Before reviewing the relevant studies that have used this procedure, we should
point out the existence of a potentially confounding methodological factor. The
problem rests in the comparability of categorical instances for adults of different
ages. For example, is *canary* a less (or more) familiar instance of the category *bird*
for elderly adults than for young adults? If so, then age differences in performance
on a categorized list could be due to this differential familiarity rather than to age
differences in either encoding or retrieval processes. Fortunately, the problem is
not a serious one. This may be seen in the responses given when young and
elderly subjects are asked to name instances of various categories (e.g., name
several birds). The responses of elderly subjects (Howard, 1980) are much like
those of young adults (Battig & Montague, 1969).

In the first study to evaluate age differences in performance on a categorical
list, Laurence (1967) compared noncued recall (i.e., free recall) with cued recall
in which the category names were available during the test trial that followed a
single study trial. Young adults were clearly superior to elderly adults on the
noncued-recall test. However, the age difference all but disappeared on the cued-
recall test. The resulting interaction effect between age and type of test suggests
that the encoding of categorical information is age insensitive, whereas gaining
later access to the higher order units is age sensitive. Category names as retrieval
cues presumably lead to stored information that is otherwise inaccessible through
a direct search of the store. Ceci and Tabor (1981) also discovered the age-related
deficit on a noncued-recall test to disappear with a cued-recall test. However, an
age-related deficit on the cued-recall test may have been masked by a ceiling
effect.

A different outcome was obtained in a more thorough study by Hultsch
(1975). His study list contained 40 items, 4 instances from each of 10 taxonomic
categories. The proportion of words recalled from this list by three age groups
under both noncued- and cued-recall conditions are plotted in part A of Fig-

ure 7.2. It can be seen that, contrary to Laurence's (1967) results, recall by young subjects exceeded that of older adults with cued recall as well as with noncued recall. Conceivably, the older subjects in this study encoded and, therefore, stored less categorical information than the young subjects. As a result, retrieval cues failed to eliminate age differences in recall scores. However, the improbability of this account of the age-related deficit manifested in cued recall was revealed by two additional analyses conducted by Hultsch.

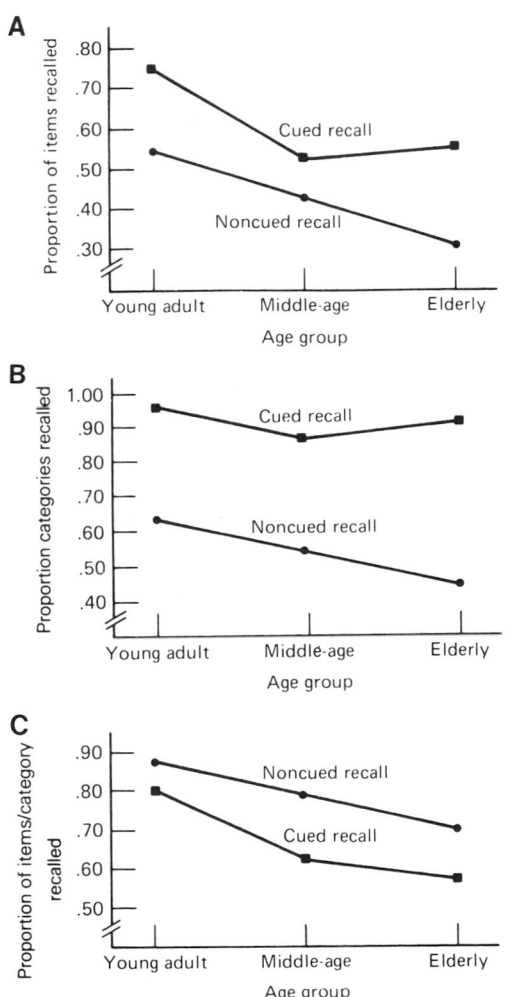

FIGURE 7.2 Age differences in total items recalled (A), category names recalled (B), and instances per category recalled (C). (Adapted from Hultsch, 1975, Tables 1, 2, 3.)

The first analysis compared his age groups on the proportion of the 10 categories retrieved during recall. A category was considered to be retrieved in both the noncued- and the cued-recall condition if at least one item/instance of that category was recalled. Thus, if *robin* was recalled by a subject, then it was assumed that the subject had gained access to a successfully encoded and stored higher order unit, namely that of *a bird*. The proportions of such higher order units retrieved by the three age groups are plotted in part B of Figure 7.2. An interaction is apparent—age differences were found for noncued recall but *not* for cued recall. The overall age-related deficit in encoding and storage does not seem to have its locus in the encoding and storage of the higher order units. If it were, then cued recall should be as ineffective as noncued recall for older subjects. Again, if information has not been encoded and stored successfully, then no amount of retrieval aid can recover it. However, older subjects do appear to have greater difficulty than young subjects in locating these higher order units in storage, a difficulty that is eliminated when category names per se serve as retrieval cues.

The second analysis examined the proportion of items/instances recalled from each category. If a subject recalled two names of birds that had been in the study list, then the subject's score for that category would be .50 (i.e., two out of four instances). Mean scores for this measure (averaged over all 10 categories) are plotted in part C of Figure 7.2. It may be seen that age differences, favoring young subjects, existed for both noncued- and cued-recall conditions. Zivian and Darjes (1983) and Witte, Freund, and Brown-Whistler (1993) also reported significantly more items per category recalled by young than by elderly subjects in a noncued-recall condition. One interpretation of this outcome is that the encoding of specific instances declines in proficiency with increasing age, in contrast to the encoding of higher order information which, as noted earlier, appears to be age insensitive. Conceivably, only so much item information can be subsumed under any given higher order unit (the cue overload principle noted in Chapter 6, p. 149), with the limit being less for older than for younger individuals. There is an alternative interpretation, however, one suggested by the fact that more instances per category were retrieved at all age levels with noncued recall than with cued recall (see part B of Figure 7.2). Basic memory researchers (e.g., Rundus, 1973) have identified a form of output interference that occurs when category names serve as retrieval cues. The nature of this interference will not concern us, however, in that it does not seem to be any greater for elderly subjects than for young adult subjects (Hultsch & Craig, 1976).

A more likely possibility, however, is that elderly subjects simply encode less item-specific information than do young adults. An organizational approach to episodic memory emphasizes the discovery and utilization of relationships among words. In the case of categorical organization, the relationship is among words from the same taxonomic category. The utilization of that relationship should result in related words being stored together under the same superordinate unit. Little emphasis is given to the processing of the individual words within a list, that is, the kind of emphasis stressed by the levels-of-processing approach. Einstein and Hunt (1980; Hunt & Einstein, 1981) have reasoned that optimal memory should occur when the two approaches are integrated together, that is, when subjects are forced simultaneously both to engage in deep processing of individual words (item-specific processing; e.g., via an orienting task) and to discover interword relationships of the kind represented by common categorical membership. Their results with young adult subjects provide firm support for this integration hypothesis. Moreover, there is evidence that elderly adults also benefit from conditions promoting the integration of item and interitem processing (Bäckman & Larsson, 1992; Guttentag, 1988; Luszcz, Roberts, & Mattiske, 1990). Conditions that facilitate the integration of specific item information with relatedness information should reduce the strain on the diminished capacity of elderly adults' working memory, resulting in a decrease in the age-related deficit in recall of words from a categorizable list. Some evidence in support of this position was provided by Bäckman and Larsson (1992). The items in a taxonomically categorizable list consisted of either words or objects represented by those words (e.g., either the words *sofa* and *chair* or toy objects of these instances of furniture). The investigators reasoned that objects would be richer in encodable features than would words themselves, resulting in deeper item-specific processing for the former than for the latter and therefore enhancing item-specific processing for the former, especially for elderly subjects, and reducing the age-related deficit in item recall. On a cued recall test with category names as the cues, the age-related deficit in total item recall was less for the objects list than for the word list, in agreement with their reasoning. Relational processing by elderly subjects as well as by young adult subjects also benefited greatly from the use of objects rather than words as items. The relational advantage of objects over words was revealed by significantly higher clustering scores for the objects than for the words. Most important, the correlation between clustering scores and total items recalled was statistically significant for elderly subjects with objects as items but not with words as items.

Whether or not there are age differences in the amount of clustering observed in noncued recall is debatable. Several early studies (Bäckman & Nilsson, 1984; Eysenck, 1974; Gordon, 1975; Howard, McAndrews, & Lasaga, 1981); Rankin, Karol, & Tuten, 1984) found no age difference in clustering, while several other studies (Denney, 1974; Horn, Donaldson, & Engstrom, 1981; Mueller, Rankin, & Carlomusto, 1979; Sanders et al. (1980) reported greater clustering by younger subjects than by elderly subjects. These early studies, however, used rather gross measures of clustering that failed to take into account the age difference in the total number of items recalled. To assess the amount of clustering during recall, corrected for the number of items recalled, Zivian and Darjes (1983) used the adjusted ratio of clustering score (ARC) developed by Roenker, Thompson, and Brown (1971). ARC scores range in numerical value from 0 (chance) to 1.00 (maximum possible clustering), and they adjust for group differences in total number of items recalled. The mean score was .30 for their young adult subjects and .16 for their elderly subjects, values somewhat lower than those reported later by Bäckman and Larsson (1992), also with ARC scores. Zivian and Darjes (1983) found a moderate positive correlation ($r = .33$) between amount of clustering and number of words recalled. Witte et al. (1993) found the correlation between clustering scores and items recalled to be even larger for both their young and their elderly subjects. Clustering as a form of organization does seem to enhance the number of words recalled from a categorizable list—the greater the amount of clustering, the greater the number of words recalled, regardless of age level. The implication is that a contributing factor to the age-related deficit in total item recall is an age-related deficit in clustering during recall. However, neither Bäckman and Larsson (1992), Fisher and McDowd (1993), Rankin, Karol, and Tuten (1984), nor Witte et al. (1993) found an age difference in clustering with scores adjusted for the length of the list and for age differences in the total number of words recalled. Nevertheless, the young adult subjects in these studies clearly recalled more items than did the elderly subjects. Our best conclusion is that the age-related deficit in clustering is slight, if it exists at all. Age-sensitive processes other than relational processing seemingly account for most of the age-related deficit in item recall from a categorizable list of words. One of these processes, of course, is the aforementioned processing of specific item information.

However, the results obtained by Witte et al. (1993) suggest that the absence of an age difference in clustering scores may be an artifact attributable to the use of only one study-test trial in most studies comparing young and elderly subjects in taxonomic organization. Their subjects received 5 study-test trials on a list composed of 40 words, 5 taxonomic instances from each of 8 categories. For half of the categories, the instances were high in their associative relatedness (e.g., *table* and *chair* as instances of *furniture*); for the other half, they were low in associative relatedness (e.g., *canary* and *ostrich* as instances of *birds*). Shown in part A of Figure 7.3 are the total recall scores for each of the five trials. It may be seen that the young subjects showed a greater practice effect over the trials than the elderly subjects and that at each age level more words with high associative relatedness were recalled than words with low associative relatedness. Of particular importance are the increments in ratio of clustering (RR) scores plotted over trials in part B of Figure 7.3. As noted above, there was no significant main effect for age. However, it is apparent from Figure 7.3 that the Age × Trials interaction was significant. On the first trial, their elderly subjects actually clustered more items than did their young subjects. Beyond that trial, slightly more clustering occurred for their young subjects than for their elderly subjects. Witte et al. (1993) analyzed further their recall data in terms of another form of organization

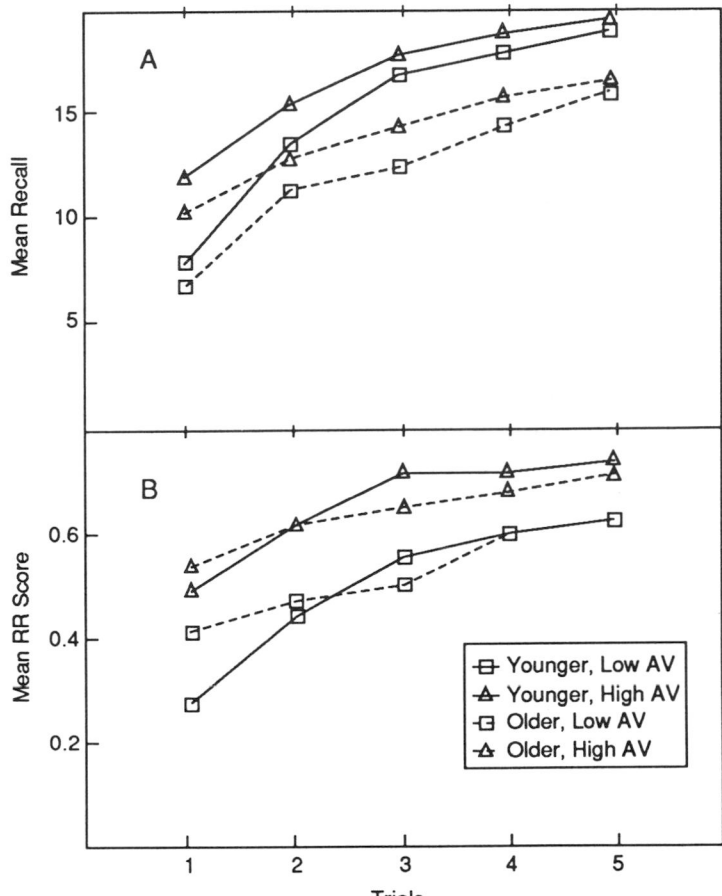

FIGURE 7.3 Practice effects for the recall of words with high- and low-associative relatedness. AV, Association value; RR, clustering score. (Adapted from Witte, Freund, & Brown-Whistler, 1993, Figure 1.)

during recall, namely seriation (i.e., recalling the words in the order they were presented on a study trial). Their young subjects relied heavily on seriation for the first test trial, thus limiting their use of categorical clustering, while their elderly subjects manifested little use of seriation. As observed by Witte et al., "The finding that younger, but not older, adults exhibit a seriation strategy would make it unlikely that studies using only one recall trial would find age differences in category clustering" (1993, p. 25). In agreement with the existence of an age difference in the use of seriation are the results of earlier studies reporting the magnitude of an age-related deficit in item recall to be larger when recall is scored with respect to order in the study list than when it is scored without regard to order (Friedman, 1966, 1974; Kinsbourne, 1973).

Recall of words in a taxonomically categorizable list should be enhanced when subjects are forced to do deep processing of the individual items (e.g., rating each word in list for degree of pleasantness). The net effect should be a combination of deep individual item processing and relational processing among items as prodded by their preexperimental relatedness. There is ample evidence to indicate that enhanced recall does occur for young adults (e.g., Einstein & Hunt, 1980). However, the evidence for elderly adults is more ambiguous. Luszcz et al. (1990) failed to find the expected increase in recall for elderly subjects when deep individual item processing was performed on items in a categorizable list relative to recall of items in a list composed of unrelated words (surprisingly, they also failed to find it for their young subjects). By contrast, Fisher and McDowd (1993) reported a striking increment in recall for their elderly subjects as well as their young adult subjects. Nevertheless, their elderly subjects continued to recall far fewer words than their young subjects even with the most favorable combination of encoding conditions.

Other Forms of Intrinsic Organization

Relationships among items may involve attributes other than common categorical membership. Semantic relationships, for example, may be based on information other than common categorical memberships. Consider the words *table, desk, bed, waiter, teacher, nurse, restaurant, school,* and *hospital* as words in a free-recall list. As presented here, they are grouped according to taxonomic categories (*furniture, occupations, buildings*). However, they may also be grouped according to conforming to scripted events that "go together" in the everyday world ("eating out"—*table, waiter, restaurant;* "in the classroom"—*desk, teacher, school,;* "being sick"—*bed, nurse, hospital*). Interestingly, Arbuckle, Gold, and Andres (1986) discovered that when elderly adults were asked to sort these nine words into whatever groups they thought most appropriate, nearly all of them sorted on the basis of scripted events. Unfortunately, young adult subjects were not included in their study, making it impossible to determine if there is an age difference in preference for type of organization. What is known is that a schematic organization, such as that of scripted events, results in higher levels of item recall for young adults than does taxonomic organization (Rabinowitz & Mandler, 1983). However, the results obtained by Hess, Flannagan, and Tate (1993) suggest that a similar advantage of schematic organization over taxonomic organization may not apply to elderly adults. Their subjects received 36 short phrases. In one condition, the phrases were organized taxonomically. For example, in one set of six phrases, each phrase was in reference to an article of furniture (e.g., *get into bed, work at a desk*). In another condition, the phrases were organized in the form of a scripted event. For example, in one set of six phrases, each phrase was in reference to going out to eat (e.g., *drive to a restaurant, order from the waiter*). The proportions of phrases recalled by the young subjects were .37 in the taxonomic condition and .49 in the scripted condition, thus replicating earlier results for young adults. By contrast, the elderly subjects recalled only .30 of the phrases in *each* condition, thus indicating no advantage of scripted organization over taxonomic organization.

Lists may also be organized in terms of preexisting *schema*, or knowledge systems, such as knowledge about the behaviors associated with particular personality traits (e.g., friendliness, shyness). Hess and Tate (1991) gave their subjects sets of nine behavioral descriptions for each of eight dominant traits. Of the behaviors for each trait, six were likely to be performed by persons possessing that trait and three were unlikely to be performed. On a subsequent recall test, their young adult subjects recalled significantly fewer of the likely behaviors (62%) than the unlikely behaviors (74%). By contrast, their elderly subjects recalled only slightly less of the likely behaviors (44%) than the unlikely behaviors (48%).

Phonological commonality among words is another possible basis for organization. Research with young adult subjects has revealed that rhyming words (e.g., *chair* and *share*) tend to cluster together during recall trials, even though the words are widely separated during study trials (see Kausler, 1974). Organizational processes seem to account for the emergence of this form of clustering. Mueller et al. (1979) demonstrated that elderly subjects display both less total item recall and less clustering for rhyming words than do young subjects. Moreover, the age-related deficit in number of items recalled occurred for both noncued and cued recall conditions, which is in general agreement with Hultsch's (1975) results obtained with categorically related items. Both young adult and elderly adult subjects have also been found to cluster homophone pairs of words (e.g., *surplus* and *surplice*) contained in a list (Laurence & Trotter, 1971).

Another form of clustering commonly found for young adult subjects occurs when pairs of synonyms (e.g., *ocean* and *sea*) serve as items of a free-recall list (see Kausler, 1974). As with rhyming words, synonyms tend to be recalled together, even though they were widely separated in the study list. Denney (1974) compared middle-aged and elderly subjects in their performance on such a list. Her middle-aged subjects emulated the performance of young adult subjects by showing a statistically significant amount of synonym clustering. Moreover, there was a substantial positive correlation between the amount of clustering and the total number of items recalled. By contrast, her elderly subjects failed to show a significant amount of clustering, nor were their clustering scores significantly correlated with their recall scores. Not surprisingly, the middle-aged subjects recalled significantly more words than the elderly subjects. The implication is that of an age-related deficit in the proficiency of relational encoding processes when syno-nymity forms the basis of the relationships extant within a list. The diminished capacity of working memory with normal aging seems to reduce the proficiency of recall by elderly adults regardless of the nature of the relatedness of items within an organizable list.

Subjective Organization

Organization of list items is by no means limited to items that are preexperi-mentally related to one another. Even items that are seemingly unrelated, at least to the investigator who selected them as components of a study list, can become unitized. Young adults often find a connecting link between so-called unrelated words. The connecting link may then serve as a higher order unit for subsuming the traces of the discrete items. For example, consider *late* and *robin* as items in a study list. A clever subject might find a link between them by reversing an old proverb (i.e., the *late robin* never gets the worm). The modified proverb would become the higher order unit for accommodating both list items. During the test trial, a search of the episodic store would presumably retrieve the higher order unit first, followed by retrieval of the traces of the specific items nested under that unit. Consequently, *late* and *robin* would be recalled consecutively, even though the items may have been widely separated in the study list.

We have described what is called *subjective organization* by basic memory re-searchers (Tulving, 1962, 1964). Its existence is established by the fact that the probability of recalling items like *late* and *robin* consecutively increases as the number of study-test trials on the same list increases. Most important, increments in the amount of subjective organization with practice are expected to increase the number of items recalled from the list. Thus, subjective organization is viewed as being a potent process underlying increments in total recall scores with contin-uing practice on a list of so-called unrelated items (Tulving, 1962, 1964).

There have been a few aging studies employing the multiple study-test trial procedure (with list items in a different random order on each study trial) that have permitted an analysis of age differences in subjective organization. In the earliest study, Laurence (1966) found lower total item recall scores by her elderly subjects than by her young adult subjects, even though the two age groups did not differ in amount of subjective organization. This finding contradicts the prin-ciple that it is increments in subjective organization that make possible incre-ments in total item recall. It also contradicts the expected age difference, favoring young adults, in the extent of subjective organization emerging with multiple study-test trials. However, there was a methodological problem in Laurence's (1966) study. The scoring system used to measure subjective organization was one that did not take into account subjective units that incorporated more than two items. With many study-test trials on a given list, subjects have the opportunity to unitize three or more items. For example, the item *meal* could eventually be linked to *late* and *robin* in the reverse early bird proverb functioning as a higher order unit. However, it should be noted that Jackson and Schneider (1982) also failed to find an age difference in amount of subjective organization.

Other investigators (Hultsch, 1974; Rankin et al., 1984; A. D. Smith, 1979b, 1980; Witte, Freund, & Sebby, 1990) have found both an age-related deficit in amount of subjective organization and in total item recall. Hultsch (1974) made use of a more sophisticated scoring system, one taking into account longer sequences of linked items than that of Laurence (1966). Witte et al. (1990) used various formulas for measuring amount of subjective organization, and they found an age-related deficit regardless of the specific formula used. Rankin et al. (1984) discovered that both elderly and younger subjects increased the amount of subjective organization as the number of test trials increased, but the gain in amount was greater for younger subjects. Witte et al. (1990) identified an important difference between the studies finding no age differences in amount of subjective organization and those that did, namely a pronounced difference in the number of items included in the study list. That is, much shorter lists were used in the null effect studies than in the other studies. As noted by Witte et al. (1990), with relatively few items in a list, list acquisition is easy for young subjects, and there is little reason for them to make use of subjective organization. Witte et al. (1990) also found moderately high positive correlations between the amount of subjective organization and the number of words recalled for both their young adult and elderly subjects. These correlations are in agreement with the principle that subjective organization enhances individual item recall, a principle that seemingly applies to adult subjects of all ages.

Age differences in subjective organization have also been investigated through the use of a method introduced by Mandler (e.g., Mandler & Pearlstone, 1966). Subjects are given a stack of cards, each card containing a word that is unrelated to the words on the other cards. The subject's task is to sort the cards and words into two or more piles. Each pile represents an artificial category shared in some way by words sorted into that pile. Thus, subjects must find connections of some kind among the words assigned to the same category. This forced categorization leads to organizational structures that enhance the later (and unexpected recall) of the individual words, relative to control subjects who either simply study the individual words without sorting them or sort them into piles designated by people other than themselves (and, therefore, into categories that are not relevant to their own subjective organization). This procedure was applied initially in an aging study by Hultsch (1971b) and later repeated in a study by Worden and Meggison (1984). Hultsch (1971b) found an age deficit in number of words recalled with both the relevant-sorting task and the control task. However, relevant sorting improved recall scores for elderly subjects as well as for young subjects and, in fact, more so for the elderly subjects. Consequently, the age deficit in recall was less pronounced in the sorting condition than in the control condition.

In Worden and Meggison's (1984) study, different groups of both young and elderly subjects were required to sort the 48 cards/words (high-frequency words for half of the subjects, low-frequency for the other half) into either 2, 4, 6, or 8 artificial categories. As may be seen in Figure 7.4, the outcome was puzzling. Recall scores for the young subjects were markedly affected by the number of categories, with recall being greater for either 6 or 8 categories than for either 2 or 4 categories. This is to be expected on the basis of the cue overload principle— that is, the fewer the number of categories, the greater the "load" assumed by each individual category. What is puzzling is the absence of any effect for variation in number of categories on recall scores for the elderly subjects. Moreover, although the Age × Number of Categories interaction was statistically significant, the main effect for age on recall scores was not. Worden and Meggison (1984) concluded that "This is remarkable and certainly does not suggest a picture of the elderly individual as having a poor memory because of a decline in the use of active means of organization in recall. Rather it shows that old adults can bring resources to the memory situation that are highly effective, even if mysterious, compared to what we know about young adults" (1984, p. 324). Of course, their results do indicate less sensitivity to organization as an aid for memory by their elderly subjects than by their young subjects. What is mysterious is the absence of a cue overload effect for this unique group of elderly subjects when each of just a few categories has to subsume a large number of subordinates.

A similar absence of a cue overload effect for elderly subjects was found in a later study by Basden, Basden, and Bartlett (1993). This time the subjects had no

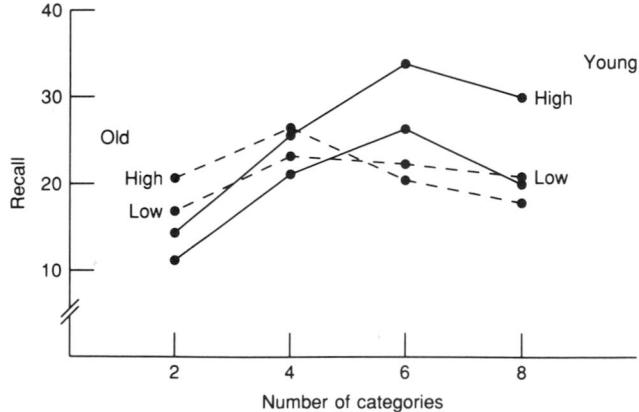

FIGURE 7.4 Number of words recalled as a function of age, number of categories, and word frequency. (Adapted from Worden & Meggison, 1984, Figure 1.)

restrictions on the number of categories into which the words could be sorted. For 100 unrelated words, the number of categories was approximately equal for their young subjects (mean = 25.05 categories) and elderly subjects (mean = 23.25 categories). Unlike the results obtained by Worden and Meggison (1984), the number of words recalled on a free-recall test was much greater for the young (mean = 62.30) than for the elderly subjects (mean = 41.95). As in Worden and Meggison's (1984) study, the number of words recalled was linearly related to the number of categories in the prior sort for the young subjects but not for the elderly subjects, thus again indicating the absence of a cue overload effect for the elderly subjects.

Of further interest is the presence of an age difference in recall when subjects are given general instructions regarding the advantage for item recall of organizing a list of words in some way. Presumably, some form of subjective organization is likely to be prodded by such instructions. In a study by Hultsch (1969), a potential way of organizing the list was created by having each word begin with a different letter of the alphabet. Relative to a control condition in which no prior stress on organization was given, Hultsch (1969) discovered that simply informing older subjects (45–54 yr) about the advantage of organization resulted in superior recall, relative to the control condition, but only for those subjects of high verbal ability. In fact, the high verbal older subjects recalled about the same number of words as did high verbal young subjects (16–19 yr). However, older subjects of low verbal ability recalled far fewer words in either condition than either high or low verbal young subjects. The difference in recall between high and low verbal ability elderly subjects is an important one. The difference is likely to be an indication that they differ in overall cognitive ability, including working memory's capacity. Subjective organization, like categorical organization, surely involves both item-specific and relational processing, and it is therefore likely to be affected adversely by decrements in working memory's capacity.

Multitrial Free Recall

Most studies on adult age differences in free recall have been ones in which subjects receive only one study-test trial for each list included in those studies. However, there have been some studies in which subjects are given more than one study-test trial on a given list. Of interest is the age difference in the proportion of words recalled over trials. Increments in this proportion reveals increasing learning of the item content of that list with practice (blurring further the distinction between "learning" and "memory" (see Chapter 1, pp. 3–4). These studies reveal a standard learning curve for both young adults and elderly, usually a negatively accelerated one. In question, however, is a possible age difference in the rate of learning. Some studies have found larger increments from the first to the last trial for young subjects than for elderly subjects. This is the case in the study by Witte et al. (1993). The learning curves for their young and elderly subjects may be seen in part A of Figure 7.3. Note the negatively accelerated curves for both age groups, but note also the increasing age difference in amount recalled as practice continued. Comparable results (i.e., differential learning rates) have been found with lists of unrelated words (Macht & Buschke, 1983; Mueller et al., 1979; Query & Megran, 1983; Rankin & Firnhaber, 1986; Worden & Sherman-Brown, 1983) and lists of names (Crook & West, 1990). On the other hand, there have been studies reporting equal increments over trials for young and elderly subjects (Furchtgott & Busemeyer, 1979; Hultsch, 1974; Keitz & Gounard, 1976; Rankin et al., 1984) and even one study reporting unequal increments in some conditions and equal increments in other conditions (Witte et al., 1990). One thing is clear—elderly adults are highly unlikely to show greater increments in recall with practice than young adults. Whether or not they show smaller increments seems to be determined by as yet undetermined subject and/ or task variables.

Generation Effect

Among the many task variations known to affect episodic memory perfor- mances of young adults is one producing the *generation effect*. The generation effect refers to the superior recall of words subjects generate themselves, relative to the recall of words they only passively read. For example, consider *coat* as an item in a study list. In the passive reading condition, subjects simply read the word as it is presented. In the generating condition, they are asked to produce a synonym of a cue word that begins with a designated letter (e.g., *jacket*—c; only the generated word, *coat*, is to be recalled later). Superior recall for generated words was demonstrated initially by Slamecka and Graf (1978), and it has since been found in many other studies with young adult subjects (e.g., McFarland, Frey, & Rhodes, 1980). The reason for the positive effect of self-generation is unclear. However, there are two general classes of explanation, each with some support. The first stresses processes at the level of the lexicon (e.g., McElroy & Slamecka, 1982). Lexical features of a word are presumed to be activated by generation that are not activated by ordinary reading. These added features serve subsequently as effective retrieval cues for accessing the generated word. The second class of explanation stresses some derivative of the act of generation itself. For example, generation may enhance memorability because of the greater cog- nitive effort it requires, relative to passive reading (e.g., McFarland et al., 1980). We discovered in Chapter 6 (p. 192) that the amount of cognitive effort needed to process an episodic event has been viewed by some memory researchers as an alternative to depth of processing as a general memory principle (but not without conflicting evidence).

Whatever the mechanism accounting for the generation effect, it seems to be operating effectively in late adulthood. Johnson, Schmitt, and Pietrukowicz (1989), McFarland, Warren, and Crockard (1985), Mitchell, Hunt, and Schmitt (1986), and Rabinowitz (1989b) have all reported a significant generation effect (i.e., higher test scores following generation than following reading) with their elderly subjects. The results obtained by Mitchell et al. (1986) are shown in Figure 7.5. The procedure called for giving their subjects (subjects diagnosed as having senile dementia of the Alzheimer's type (SDAT) were included, along with young adult and normally aging elderly subjects), the subjects received 20 sentences, with the object being generated for 10 of the sentences (e.g., The horse jumped the _____), and simply read for the other 10 (e.g., The horse jumped the *fence*). A cued recall followed in which the subjects of the sentences served as cues. Note the robust generation effect for the normally aging elderly subjects, and the clear absence of the effect for the SDAT subjects (an absence also found by Dick and Kean, 1989). Note further that self-generation of items did not eliminate the age-related deficit in recall. Rabinowitz's (1989b) subjects were given a recognition test, rather than a cued-recall test, but the outcome was much the same as that found by Mitchell et al. If anything, the magnitude of the generation effect was greater for his elderly subjects than for his young subjects—but scores of the elderly subjects remained well below those of the young subjects. Johnson et al. (1989) also gave their subjects a recognition test, and found no age difference in the extent of the generation effect.

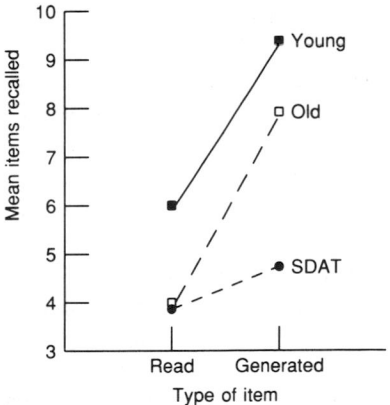

FIGURE 7.5 Mean number of read and generated words recalled by young and old adults and SDAT patients. (Adapted from Mitchell, Hunt, & Schmitt, 1986, Figure 1.)

Encoding Variability and the Lag Effect

As you might expect, the recallability of words in a free-recall list increases as they are repeated within a single study trial. For example, words repeated twice are recalled better than words presented only once (e.g., Waugh, 1963). Item repetition clearly benefits elderly subjects as well as young adult subjects (e.g., Cohen, Sandler, & Schroeder, 1987; Rabinowitz, 1989b). Explaining why item repetition enhances recall isn't as easy as it may seem. Some theorists have postulated simply that repetition increases the "strength" of a memory trace, and therefore its accessibility for recall (e.g., D. A. Norman & Wickelgren, 1965). However, evidence supporting the strength principle is not very convincing (e.g., Wells, 1974). Many basic memory researchers have preferred instead an alternative explanation. Repetition of an item means that it is exposed in two different positions in the list, and therefore the item has been preceded by a different set of other items on the second occasion than on the first occasion. The set of items preceding each occasion of the repeated item may be regarded as part of the external context for that item. Contextual information may, in turn, influence the encoding of the repeated item. Thus, a different set of sensory or semantic features may be encoded on the second occasion than on the first, a principle known as *encoding variability*. Qualitatively different memory traces should therefore be transmitted to the episodic store on each occasion, thereby enhancing eventual retrievability of the item (i.e., two chances at retrieval are better than one). The change in context, however, is likely to be minimal when the second occasion follows closely after the first, and it should become increasingly greater as the number of intervening different items increases (i.e., the lag separating the first and second presentations of the repeated item). The consequence should be progressively increasing recall for repeated items as the lag increases, a *lag effect* frequently demonstrated in basic memory research (e.g., Melton, 1970; see *top*, Figure 7.6).

Alternatively, contextual information may become associated with an item's content. Since context changes are likely to be greater for widely separated repetitions of items than for massed repetitions, more context-item associations are expected to be formed for the former than for the latter, again yielding a retrieval advantage for items having repetitions that are widely spaced (Glenberg, 1979; Greene, 1989b).

There is another factor to consider, however, in evaluating the effects of lag on subsequent recall. In studies such as that of Melton (1970; A, Figure 7.6), recall of repeated items occurs after an entire lengthy study list has been presented. Thus the retention interval between the second presentation and recall averages out to be fairly long. Increasing recall with increasing lag has been found to be true only when the retention interval is long (i.e., a number of seconds). With short retention intervals (i.e., a few seconds), recall of repeated items either

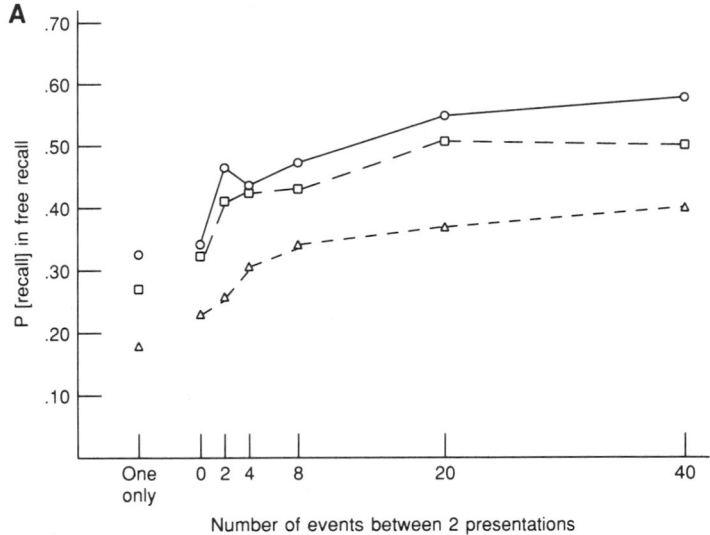

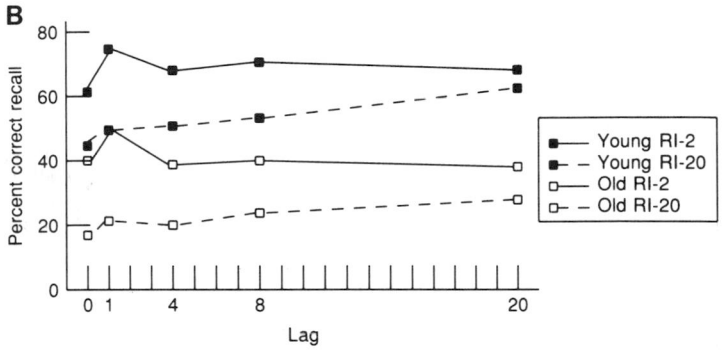

FIGURE 7.6 A: Probability of recall of words that occur once or twice, with varying number of words between presentations, when presented visually at rates of 1.3, 2.3, and 4.3 per word (young adults only). (Adapted from Melton, 1970, Figure 1.) B: Mean percentage correct recall for twice-presented pairs as a function of age, retention interval (RI), and lag. (Reprinted from Balota, Duchek, & Paullin, 1989, Figure 1. Copyright 1989 by the American Psychological Association.)

remains constant or may actually decline as the lag increases (e.g., Glenberg, 1976). The probable reason for the interaction between the interpresentation interval and the retention interval is a complicated one that will not concern us in detail (see Balota, Duchek, & Paullin, 1989, for a thorough description). Briefly, the critical factor is the degree of overlap between the context at the time of encoding and the context at the time of retrieval. The degree of overlap is contingent on both the interpresentation lag and the time between a pair's second presentation and the test for that pair.

Tests of this interaction hypothesis require substituting paired words for single words as the items in a lengthy study list, such that the first word of each pair may serve as the cue for the recall of the second word at any designated retention interval. With this cued-recall procedure, Balota et al. (1989) tested the generalizability of the predicted interaction to elderly subjects. The retention interval was set at either two intervening pairs (short interval) or 20 intervening pairs (long interval), and the interitem lag was set at 0 (i.e., consecutive presentations of the same pair), 1, 4, 8, or 20 items. As may be seen in part B of Figure 7.6, the predicted interaction was as apparent for their elderly subjects as for their young subjects, although over all levels recall was considerably greater for the young subjects. Balota et al. (1989) also fitted their data to a stimulus fluctuation mathematical model developed by Estes (1955, 1959). From the application of this model they concluded that elderly adults encode less contextual information than do young adults (a point we will cover in greater detail in a later section) and that contextual information changes more slowly over time than it does for young adults.

A very different approach to an age difference in encoding variability was taken by Mäntylä and Bäckman (1990). They gave their young adult and elderly subjects a list of words with instructions to generate for each word several properties (e.g., *apple*—a fruit, usually red). This procedure was repeated several weeks later for half of the original words. The elderly subjects were found to show less "intrasubject overlap" than their young subjects. That is, fewer properties from the first generation were repeated on the second generation for elderly than for young subjects, an indication of greater encoding variability of words by the former. For the other half of the words from the first test, subjects were given a cued recall test in which the properties each subject listed on the first test served as that subject's retrieval cues. The young subjects recalled about 15% more words than the elderly subjects. However, the age effect was eliminated when the age difference in intrasubject overlap was partialed out. This pattern of results may be interpreted in terms of the principle of encoding specificity (see p. 261). The recall testing situation confronting the young subjects was much more like what they encountered during the initial encoding of the target words (i.e., the words in the list) and the contextual information they themselves generated (i.e., the properties) than was the case for the elderly subjects (who were seemingly less likely to be associating those properties with the target words at the time of the recall test). Mäntylä and Bäckman (1990) pointed out further that their results do not imply an age-related change in the structure of the internal lexicon (which we will argue later remains stable with aging; see Chapter 12, pp. 388–395); they imply only an age-related change in the variability of processing information in the lexicon. However, it is conceivable that their young subjects simply had greater implicit memory (see Chapter 11, pp. 374–383) of the events from the first session than did their elderly subjects, and that this age disparity affected the age difference in explicit memory (cued recall).

Recognition Memory

Single-Item Recognition Memory

We have had frequent occasion to refer to recognition memory tests in earlier sections of this chapter and in Chapter 6, and many more references are yet to come (e.g., recognition memory tests for pictures and faces; pp. 255–259 and pp. 259–261). Our present purpose is to discuss more general characteristics of recognition memory tests and to identify why they are so often employed in aging research on episodic-memory phenomena. Our concern is with single-item recognition memory in which to-be-remembered items occur individually on a study trial, usually as members of a lengthy series of events. An alternative form of recognition memory, namely multiple-item recognition memory, was discussed in Chapter 6 (pp. 220–221) in the context of an inhibition model and will not be discussed further here.

There are various forms of single-item recognition memory tests. The most common one requires presenting subjects with a lengthy series of test items, some of which are "old" (i.e., they are items that were in the prior study list) and others are "new" (i.e., they were not in the study list). Subjects are asked to respond "old" or "new" to each item. Their hit rate is the proportion of old items to which they respond correctly "old," and their false alarm rate is the proportion of new items to which they respond incorrectly "old." New test items are usually unrelated to prior study list items, unless the false recognition effect is being investigated (see Chapter 6, p. 189). An alternative test form consists of presenting multiple-choice test items each containing an old study list item and one or more new items (distractors or foils) with subjects being asked to choose the "old" item.

Many studies have compared young and elderly subjects with one or the other of the above methods. Some studies have reported either no age difference in recognition test performance (Schonfield & Robertson, 1966; Craik & McDowd, 1987) or only slight age differences (e.g., Craik, 1971; Gordon & Clark, 1974a). However, most studies have reported at least a moderate decrement in recognition memory proficiency with increasing age (e.g., Fozard & Waugh, 1969). Representative of these studies is one by Erber (1974). She administered a multiple-choice test in which each old item was combined with four new items. Correct identifications of old items averaged 80.7% and 69.2% for young and

elderly subjects, respectively. Nevertheless, age differences are usually less pronounced for a recognition test than for a recall test (e.g., Erber, 1974).

Consistent age-related deficits have also been reported for yet another form of
a recognition memory test, namely a continuous recognition memory test. Here
subjects receive a lengthy list of items (usually words), some of which are repeated
at later points in the sequence. As each item is exposed, subjects decide if it is
old (i.e., repeated) or new (i.e., exposed for the first time). Representative of the
outcomes with this procedure are those obtained by Rankin and Kausler (1979).
Their young, middle-aged, and elderly subjects averaged respectively 93.9%,
80.8%, and 76.4% accuracy in identifying truly old items as old. Superior hit rate
scores for young adult subjects relative to elderly subjects was also found by Erber
(1978) and Wickelgren (1975). Signal detection analyses of hit rates and false
alarm rates (see McCormack, 1984, for a discussion of problems encountered in
such analyses) have been employed by still other investigators (Gordon & Clark,
1974b; Harkins, Chapman, & Eisdorfer, 1979; Le Breck & Baron, 1987) as a
means of evaluating age differences in recognition memory scores. Again, superior scores (expressed as d' values) by young adults have been found, indicating
their greater sensitivity to the presence of memory traces.

The use of signal detection methodology to evaluate the nature of adult age
differences on recognition memory tests is especially important. There is the
possibility that greater cautiousness by elderly subjects than by young subjects is
responsible for many of the lower accuracy scores found for elderly subjects. That
is, elderly subjects may be reluctant to respond old to a test item unless they are
absolutely certain of its oldness. A conservative response bias of this nature would
serve to lower considerably the number of old items identified as being old. There
would be another important consequence of this conservative bias as well, namely
a lower false alarm rate for elderly subjects than for more liberal young adult
subjects. That is, elderly subjects would be expected to respond old to new test
items less often than would young subjects. Surprisingly, this is not the case. If
anything, elderly subjects have been found in a number of studies (e.g., Harkins
et al., 1979; Rankin & Kausler, 1979) to have a higher false alarm rate than
young adult subjects and to have response bias scores that are at least no greater
than those of young adult subjects (e.g., Le Breck & Baron, 1987).

A recent development in basic memory research has been to separate recognition memory into memory through either recollection or familiarity (e.g., Gardiner, 1988). (This is an issue of considerable relevance to research on implicit
memory, and it will be discussed further in Chapter 11). Recollection means
remembering the prior occurrence of a word qua item in a study list by remembering having associated a word to that item or having imaged that item during
its presentation. Familiarity means "knowing" an item had occurred recently
without recollecting the context in which it occurred. The results obtained by
Parkin and Walter (1992) suggest strongly that it is largely recollection that is af-

fected adversely by aging and thus accounts for age-related deficits on recognition-memory tests. Both young-old (average age = 67.7 yr) and old-old (average age = 81.6 yr) subjects were included in their study, along with young adult subjects. Each subject received a 36-word study list, followed by a 72-word test list (36 old words and 36 new words). For each test word, subjects placed either an R (for recollection) or a K (for knowing without recollection) for each word recognized as being from the prior study list. Shown in Figure 7.7 are the proportions of prior study-list words identified as either R or K by each age group. The older subjects were clearly less able of recollecting whether or not a word had been in the study list than the young subjects. Why the age-related decline in recollection but not in familiarity? Parkin and Walter (1992) reasoned that recognition through recollection, but not through familiarity, is a frontal lobe function. Both physiological evidence (e.g., Gerard & Weisberg, 1986; Haug et al., 1983) and neuropsychological evidence (Albert & Kaplan, 1980; Haaland, Vranes, Goodwin, & Garry, 1987; Mittenberg, Seidenberg, O'Leary, & DiGuilo, 1989; Parkin & Walter, 1991) have revealed declining frontal lobe functioning with normal aging, a decline that would account for the diminished proficiency of elderly adults in recollection. Limited support for this position was obtained by Parkin and Walter (1992). R scores were found to correlate significantly with scores on a neuropsychological test of frontal lobe functioning for the old-old

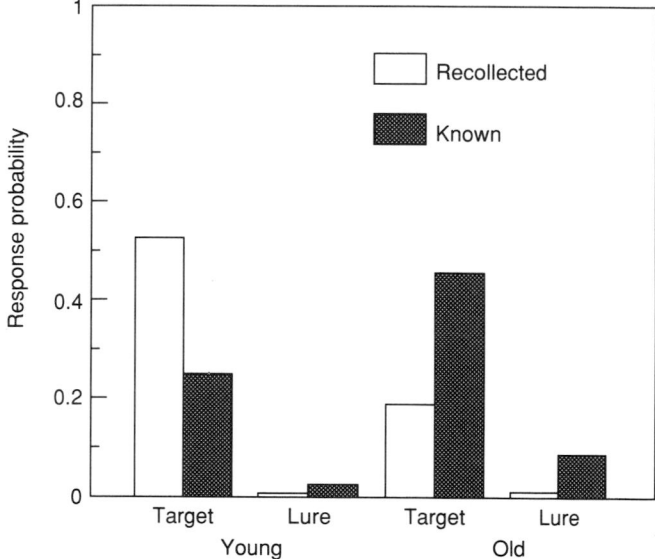

FIGURE 7.7 Proportions of study-list words identified as recollected (R) or known (K). (Reprinted from Parkin & Walter, 1992, Figure 1. Copyright 1992 by the American Psychological Association.)

subjects in their study but not for the young-old subjects. Thus the low R scores for the young-old subjects (see Figure 7.7) remains unexplained.

Our focus on recognition memory in this section has been on words as study-test items. Age differences as they apply to pictures and face as items will be discussed in a later section of this chapter and to actions and activities in Chapter 9. We should note that age-related deficits in recognition memory are also observed when still other kinds of items are employed (e.g., bird calls and tactual stimuli; Riege & Inman, 1981; theme songs from television shows; Maylor, 1991). Moreover, pronounced age-related deficits have been found even when common everyday objects have been tested for accuracy of recognition memory. For example, Foos (1989b) compared young and elderly adults in their ability to recognize from multiple alternatives the correct drawing of the top side of a penny. Thirty percent of the young subjects were able to identify the correct drawing— but none of the 30 elderly subjects were correct. This age-related deficit is surprising, given the fact that exposure to the ordinary Lincoln penny began when current elderly adults were much younger. That is, the "study list" is certainly not equivalent to one in which new material is presented for the first time to both young and elderly subjects. It is unlikely that the age-sensitive process is an initial acquisition process. A more likely explanation is pronounced forgetting among the elderly subjects produced by interference generated by encounters with other coins and other similar objects over many years.

Although recognition memory accuracy tends to be less proficient for elderly adults than for young adults, several ancillary recognition memory phenomena appear to be quite similar for young and elderly adults. One of these phenomena is the *word-frequency effect*. It refers to the higher accuracy of recognition scores for words that have a low frequency of occurrence in everyday materials than for words that have a high frequency (the reverse is true for recall of words). Numerous studies (e.g., Gorman, 1961; Schulman, 1967) have demonstrated the word-frequency effect for young adults, and a comparable effect has been demonstrated for normally aging adults (but not for abnormally aging adults; Wilson, Bacon, Kramer, Fox, & Kaszniak, 1983). Another phenomenon found to be quite comparable for young and elderly adults is the *consistency effect*. It refers to the better recognition of episodic events that are inconsistent with one's expectations (based on a pre-existing schema or knowledge of the events) than recognition of events that are consistent (Pezdek, Whetstone, Reynolds, Askari, & Dougherty, 1989). In an interesting demonstration of the generalizability of the consistency effect over age levels, Mäntylä and Bäckman (1992) had their young and elderly subjects walk into an office with the intent to remember the objects in that office, some of which were commonly found in an office, others rarely, if ever. On a subsequent old/new recognition memory test, the age difference was slight for unexpected objects (mean d' score = 3.7 for young adults and 3.5 for elderly adults) but moderately large for expected objects (mean d' score = 2.7 for young subjects and 2.2 for elderly subjects). Note that recognition memory at each age level was more accurate for the unexpected objects than for the expected objects, in agreement with the consistency effect. The consistency effect obviously has much in common with the word-frequency effect.

Recognition versus Recall

Although the encoding or storage of information is a probable factor in producing age differences in episodic-memory performances, it is unlikely to be the only factor. Performance on such tasks as free-recall depends on the proficiency of retrieving information from the episodic store as well as the proficiency of getting information into the store. In principle, it is conceivable that a retrieval deficit is the major factor responsible for age deficits in free-recall performance and could even be the *only* factor underlying performance deficits (see p. 187).

The nature of retrieval in episodic-memory performances becomes apparent when recall of to-be-remembered items is compared with recognition of those items. Recall demands an active, self-initiated search of the episodic store's contents (Atkinson & Shiffrin, 1968; Craik, 1986; Craik, Byrd, & Swanson, 1987). Once a trace is located, a decision must then be made as to whether or not the trace matches the content of a prior to-be-remembered item. Recognition presumably bypasses the necessity of searching the store. That is, the test item itself may be a to-be-remembered item, and only a decision based on the familiarity of that item need be made (Gardiner, 1988; Mandler, 1980). Recognition tests, therefore, offer a potential means of determining whether or not the age deficits manifested in recall are due to inefficient encoding processes or inefficient search processes. If age deficits disappear when a recognition test replaces a recall test, then it would seem that the search component of retrieval is the only age-sensitive process. However, if age deficits remain even on recognition tests, as they usually do, then it may be reasonable to conclude that less information is encoded and placed in storage by elderly adults than by young adults. Actually, less information needs to be encoded about to-be-remembered items to promote recognition than is needed to promote recall (McNulty & Caird, 1966). That is, partial information may be sufficient to allow recognition of an item but not its recall. When both recall and recognition tests are given to the same subjects, a common finding (e.g., Erber, 1974; White & Cunningham, 1982) is that the age deficit for recall is much greater than the age deficit for recognition. The implication is that both encoding and retrieval are age-sensitive processes. There are problems in this kind of analysis, however. There are reasons to believe that the separation of encoding and retrieval processes by means of recall/recognition comparisons is not as simple as it has been described here (Brainerd, 1985). For example, recognition itself may not always be completely free of the involvement of a search process component (Schonfield, 1967). Fortunately, other procedures for separating the contributions of encoding and retrieval processes to age differ-ences in effortful episodic memory have been introduced in recent years (Howe, 1988; Wilkinson & Koestler, 1983). Their use in aging research to date, however, has been rather limited.

Nevertheless, it does seem apparent that recall is more cognitively effortful than is recognition, and it therefore places a greater strain on the limited cogni-tive resources of elderly adults than does recognition. A major difference is the amount of environmental support offered by a recognition test in contrast to a recall test (Craik, 1986). That is, the study-list items themselves are reinstated on a recognition test, thus diminishing the need for a constraining self-initiated search of the memory store. Evidence in firm support of this position comes from studies in which subjects perform a secondary task while either recalling or rec-ognizing prior study-list items (Craik & McDowd, 1987; Macht & Buschke, 1983). For example, Craik and McDowd (1987) compared reaction times on a secondary task that was either performed alone or simultaneously with recall or recognition. Relative to the alone condition, reaction times for elderly subjects were markedly slower when recalling prior items, but they were unaffected when recognizing prior items. Only the recall task was sufficiently effortful to reduce the resources available for performing the secondary task. By contrast, their young adult subjects performed nearly as well on the secondary task when recalling prior study list items as when performing it alone.

Adult Age Differences in Picture and Face Memory

A picture is worth a thousand words—or so it seems in terms of memorability. Several studies have revealed the startling ability of young adults to recognize with great accuracy pictures of scenes (selected from magazines), even though hundreds and even thousands of pictures were presented for a single study trial. For example, Shepard (1967) found a hit rate of 96.7% when subjects were tested immediately after study with a subset of 612 pictures, and 99.7% when tested with a new subset 3 hr later! In the same study, Shepard (1967) also tested sub-jects for memory of words in a lengthy series (540 words). When tested immedi-ately after study with a subset of the words, the hit rate was quite high (88.4%), but, nevertheless, well below the hit rate for pictures. The advantage that pictures have over words in recognition is known as the *picture superiority effect*. This effect is consistent with an important theory of memory that postulates the exis-tence of separate, but interacting, picture memory and word memory systems (Paivio, 1969, 1971). Pictures are more likely than words to be encoded in both systems—two memory traces result in better retrieval than a single memory trace.

Dual coding theory also explains why concrete words have a recall advantage over abstract words for young adult subjects in a free-recall task (e.g. Paivio,

1967), and in a recognition–memory task (Gorman, 1961), an advantage known as the *concreteness effect*. Concrete words are more likely than abstract words to elicit images while being studied, and therefore more likely to benefit from a dual encoding. However, Rissenberg and Glanzer (1987) failed to demonstrate a similar benefit for their normally aging elderly subjects. Their young adults recalled 65% of the concrete words and only 54% of the abstract words in their study lists. By contrast, their elderly subjects recalled 43% and 40%, respectively, a difference that was not statistically significant. In a later study, Dirkx and Craik (1992) did find a concreteness effect for their elderly subjects, but the magnitude of the effect was significantly less than that found for their young adult subjects. In their meta-analysis of these studies, Verhaeghen et al. (1993) concluded that variation in concreteness does not affect the magnitude of age-related deficits in recall.

Conceivably, the picture memory system is highly age sensitive, making dual encoding of items far less likely than in earlier adulthood. We know that elderly adults have difficulty in generating images to words spontaneously, even when the words are highly concrete (see Chapter 3, pp. 95–96). Especially convincing evidence for the difficulty elderly adults have in producing images comes from the study by Dirkx and Craik (1992). Their subjects received lists of concrete words under several conditions that varied what they experienced after the exposure of each word on a screen. In a control condition the screen was absent of content. In a passive interference condition the screen contained two identical patterns of intersecting lines, with subjects simply viewing the patterns. In an active interference condition, the screen contained two line patterns that were identical for some prior words and different for other prior words, with the subjects being required to make a same or different judgment for each pair of patterns. The decline in the number of words recalled from the control and passive conditions relative to the active condition was much greater for the young subjects than for the elderly subjects. Having generated images of the prior words, young adults experience considerable interference in the recall of those words when they are forced to process further pictorial information during the interword intervals. By contrast, having produced fewer mental pictures of prior words, elderly adults experience little interference from interpolated visual processing.

Picture Memory

Perhaps a fairer test of the age sensitivity of a picture memory system is to compare young and elderly subjects when pictures themselves serve as study list items. Several investigators have tested for the presence of the picture superiority effect in elderly subjects with a recall test (Keitz & Gounard, 1976; Maisto & Queen, 1992; Rissenberg & Glanzer, 1986; Winograd, Smith, & Simon, 1982) (see A. D. Smith & Park, 1990, for further review). The procedure calls for presenting subjects with either a list containing line drawings of common objects or a list containing words that name the objects depicted in the other list. With either list, it is the names of the objects that have to be recalled. The magnitude of the picture superiority is usually found to be slightly greater for young adult subjects than for elderly subjects, and the magnitude of the age difference in recall scores is, if anything, slightly greater for pictures than for words as list items. The results obtained by Winograd et al. (1982) are shown in part A of Figure 7.8.

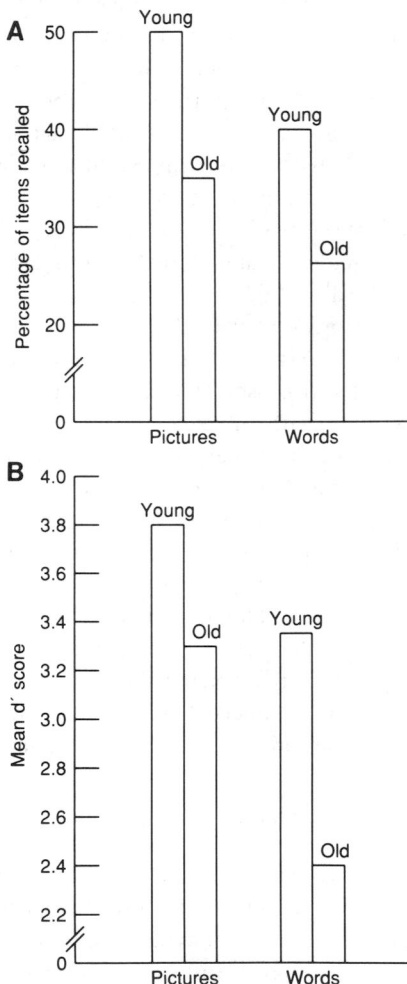

FIGURE 7.8   A: Age differences in recall of pictures and words. (Adapted from Winograd, Smith, & Simon, 1982, Table 3.) B: Age differences in recognition of pictures and words. (Adapted from Park, Puglisi, & Sovacool, 1983, Table 2.)

Maisto and Queen found further that the slight age difference increased substantially when pictures and words were presented simultaneously rather than pictures alone, an effect they assumed was attributable to the greater difficulty of elderly subjects, relative to young adult subjects, in dividing attention between a picture and the word naming that picture. The results have been somewhat less consistent when a recognition test replaces a recall test (Howell, 1972; Park & Puglisi, 1985; Park, Puglisi, & Sovacool, 1983). Sometimes a greater picture superiority has been found for elderly subjects than for young subjects, with the net effect being a less pronounced age-related deficit for pictures than for words (Park et al., 1983; see the bottom section of Figure 7.8). However, a greater effect for young adults, with a resulting greater age-related deficit for pictures, has also been reported (e.g., Park & Puglisi, 1985; Waugh & Barr, 1989).

Adult age differences in memory for pictures of common objects per se (i.e., without contrasting it with memory for words) has also been of interest. Trahan, Larrabee, and Levin (1986) tested age differences in picture recognition memory (line drawings of objects) with the continuous recognition procedure (see p. 250). Their subjects ranged in age from 10 to 89 yr. The older adults in their sample were far less proficient on this task than were the younger adults (e.g., mean d' = 3.10 and 2.25 for the age ranges of 18–29 yr and 66–77 yr, respectively). A cued-recall procedure was employed in a study by Park, Smith, Morrell, Puglisi, and Dudley (1990). In the control condition of their study, line drawings of to-be-remembered common objects (e.g., a spider) were presented along with an unrelated cue in juxtaposition with the target (e.g., a drawing of a cherry). On the recall test, the unrelated cues were reinstated, and the subjects attempted to recall the target items paired with them. Of 32 target items, the young adult subjects recalled an average of 16.18 and the elderly subjects an average of only 5.79. Park et al. (1990) also demonstrated that the memorability of target items could be enhanced by altering the relationship between the targets and the cues exposed along with them. In one condition, the two pictures in each pair were shown as interacting with each other (e.g., the spider eating the cherry). Here the young and elderly subjects averaged 14.53 and 9.66 targets recalled, respectively. In a third condition, each target was exposed in juxtaposition with a semantically related picture (e.g., an ant next to the spider). Now recall averaged 23.78 and 16.59 targets for the young and elderly subjects, respectively. Note that the increase in recall promoted by adding either an interacting or a semantic relationship between the target and its context (i.e., the cue picture) was greater for the elderly subjects than for the young subjects. Park et al. (1990) appropriately viewed this age differential as evidence for the advantage of providing environmental support to aid the memory of older people (see also Chapter 6, p. 192, for further support in a study by Puglisi and Park, 1987).

There is no reason to doubt that picture memory as it involves memory of pictures of simple and common objects diminishes from early to late adulthood.

One probable reason for this age-related deficit stems from the greater likelihood of young adults, relative to elderly adults, to name the depicted objects verbally to themselves as they are presented. Thus, from Paivio's (1969, 1971) perspective, they are more likely to have the benefit of a dual coding. In support of this position, Rissenberg and Glanzer (1986) discovered that their elderly subjects displayed the picture superiority effect only when they had to name overtly the objects in the pictures as they were presented, thus assuring dual coding. On the other hand, their young subjects displayed the picture superiority effect whether or not they were required to name the objects.

Unanswered by the above studies, however, is the extent of age differences when the to-be-remembered pictures are more complex and of such a nature that covert verbal naming with a single word is highly unlikely. In an early study by Farrimond (1968), subjects in their 20s through their 60s viewed under incidental memory conditions a series of scenes (e.g., a boy inflating a bicycle tire) on a silent film. Very little decline on a surprise recall test was found until subjects were in their 60s, with the age-related disparity then being a moderate 12% relative to young adult subjects. Till, Bartlett, and Doyle (1982) found only a slight age difference in recognition memory favoring young adult subjects when scenes from magazines served as study-list materials. In several experiments, Park, Puglisi, and Smith (1986) provided further evidence for negligible age differences in scores on a recognition memory test for complex pictures. The pictures were line drawings depicting complex scenes (e.g., an infant on the floor of a room with various objects in the area). Mean d' scores were, if anything, slightly higher for their elderly subjects (3.42) than for their young subjects (3.27). They also discovered that young and elderly subjects benefited equally from the embellishment of such pictures (i.e., increasing the amount of detailed information). This is especially interesting in that elderly adults apparently remember fewer details of pictures than do young adults (Pezdek, 1987), and they have greater difficulty than do young adults in discriminating between originally studied scenes and slightly altered test scenes (Frieske & Park, 1993; Till et al., 1982). As noted by Park et al. (1986), their results "present an unusually optimistic view of age-related memory changes with respect to complex, meaningful pictures (Park et al., 1986, p. 16)." A. D. Smith, Park, Cherry, and Berkovsky (1990) also found only slight age-related deficits in recognition memory for complex scenes of line drawings of objects in a relevant context (e.g., a chest and other old objects in an attic). However, the age-related deficit was much greater when drawings of abstract figures replaced the drawings of familiar objects. The pronounced age-related deficit for abstract figures is much like that found for the short-term memory of abstract designs (see Chapter 5, p. 161). Finally, Denney, Miller, Dew, and Levav (1991) reported only moderate age-related deficits for memory of scenes whether they were either the targeted to-be-remembered items or the background for words as the targeted items, and Frieske and Park (1993) found the age-related deficit in scene memory to be accounted for in part by an age-related deficit in working-memory capacity.

Scenes like those of old objects realistically stored in an attic conform to what may be considered a script. In this case, the script involves a series of objects that seem to go together rather than a series of actions that go together (see p. 238). Of interest is what happens to memory when some objects in a scene fail to follow a script (e.g., a kitchen scene containing unexpected objects, such as a roller skate and a lantern), while other objects do (e.g., a refrigerator and a stove). Hess and Slaughter (1990) found that recognition memory was more accurate for the nonscripted objects than for the scripted objects. This was true for both their young and elderly subjects. However, the difference was statistically significant only for their elderly subjects.

Face Memory

Age differences in memory for pictures of faces presented under laboratory conditions have been found to be rather pronounced (Crook & Larrabee, 1992; Ferris, Crook, Clark, McCarthy, & Rae, 1980; Flicker, Ferris, Crook, & Bartus, 1989; Mason, 1986; A. D. Smith & Winograd, 1978). Crook and Larrabee (1992) found the decline in face recognition memory to be apparent by the fifth decade of life, but to be especially pronounced in the seventh decade. The standard procedure is to present a series of pictures of faces (lifted, for example, from a college yearbook), and then test for memory with a list consisting of a mixture of old and new faces. The study by A. D. Smith and Winograd (1978) is especially informative. It demonstrated that the age-related deficit found for the deep processing of words as study-list items applies equally to the processing of pictures of faces. Deep processing during incidental memory was stimulated by having subjects decide for each study-list face if it appeared friendly, whereas shallow processing was stimulated by having subjects decide if each face had a big nose. Surprisingly, an age difference favoring young adults in the hit rate for recognizing old faces as old was found with shallow processing as well as with deep processing (an age difference with words as items is usually found with deep processing, but not with shallow processing). In addition, their elderly subjects had considerably higher false alarm rates for new test faces than their young subjects, regardless of the processing conditions. Other researchers have found little age difference in hit rates for correctly recognizing old faces but a large age difference in false alarm rates for incorrectly recognizing new faces as old (Bartlett & Fulton, 1991; Bartlett, Strater, & Fulton, 1991; Fulton & Bartlett, 1991)

Elderly adults have been found to be no more accurate in the recognition of old faces serving as target items than in the recognition of young faces (Bäckman, 1991; Fulton & Bartlett, 1991). How recognition accuracy varies for young adults with the age of the faces is uncertain. Bäckman (1991) found it to be greater for old faces, but Fulton and Bartlett (1991) found it to be greater with young faces. Elderly adults have also been found to be less accurate than young adults in recognizing changes in faces from study to test (e.g., changes in facial expression or perspective of viewing; J. C. Bartlett & Leslie, 1986; J. C. Bartlett, Leslie, Tubbs, & Fulton, 1989).

These results have important implications for a number of real-world phenomena (see Winograd & Simon, 1980; Yarmey, 1984; Yarmey & Kent, 1980, for elaboration). One of these implications pertains to possible age differences in the reliability of eyewitness testimony. Witnessing a criminal commit a crime often occurs under incidental memory conditions and often with shallow processing. The implication, of course, is that elderly witnesses may be less likely than young adult witnesses to identify the face of the criminal (i.e., a hit). Even more disturbing is the possibility that elderly witnesses may be more likely than young adult witnesses to identify falsely an innocent person as the criminal (i.e., a false alarm). Yarmey's studies (1984; Yarmey, Jones, & Rashid, 1984) have also indicated, with laboratory simulations of crimes, a markedly higher false alarm rate for elderly than for young subjects. The potential problem of the elderly witness is compounded by evidence indicating that the false alarm rate for elderly subjects is greater when the study-list faces are of young adults than when they are of elderly adults (Mason, 1986). Criminals, of course, are more likely to be young adults than elderly adults. Adult age differences in the accuracy of recall of details of a simulated crime viewed on videotape (e.g., objects present in the crime scene) have been investigated in several studies, but with conflicting results. There is evidence to indicate that elderly subjects are less complete than young adults in the details they remember from a simulated crime scene (List, 1986; Yarmey et al., 1984), but there is also evidence to indicate no age difference in the recall of main details (Adams-Price, 1992). Adams-Price (1992) did report a modest age-related deficit in the accuracy of recognizing the criminal from the previously viewed crime scene.

Of course, under both laboratory conditions and everyday eyewitness memory conditions, face recognition memory is tested for faces exposed usually only once and then quite briefly. In most everyday memory situations, we are not limited to single brief exposures to faces. Consider, for example, a professor meeting his or her class over the period of weeks making up a term or a semester. Surely, we would expect to find no age differences in recognition memory following such "overexposure." A study by Bahrick (1984a) seems to confirm this expectancy. Older professors (in their 60s) were just as proficient in recognizing faces of students in their relatively small introductory classes as were younger professors (in their 30s and 40s) several days after the end of the term. The sample sizes were small, however, and the subjects were undoubtedly from an elite population. Nevertheless, these results would probably generalize to other situations in which adults of all ages are exposed frequently to faces, such as those of the checkers in a supermarket where they shop regularly. Extensions of Bahrick's (1984a) study to everyday recognition memory of faces by subjects from the more general population are greatly needed.

Adult Age Differences in Retrieval

As we discovered earlier, retrieval processes are important contributors to age-related deficits in episodic-memory performances. The contribution is likely to be considerable unless retrieval information is made to be especially effective (Schonfield, 1965). Elderly adults may have memory traces present in the long-term store, but they may often have difficulty in gaining access to that information. This difficulty was nicely demonstrated in a study by Buschke (1974). His young and elderly subjects received one study trial on a 20-word free-recall list. The single study trial was followed by repeated test trials. For the young subjects, words that were recalled on one test trial were also likely to be recalled on the other test trials. That is, there was consistency in retrieval and therefore in recall. This was not the case for the elderly subjects. Words recalled on one test trial were often not recalled on other test trials. Recall of a word on a given test trial implies that a memory trace for that word exists in the LTS. Failure to recall the same word on a later trial indicates the inability to retrieve that trace at a particular time. Thus, Buschke's (1974) elderly subjects revealed many more retrieval failures than did his young subjects.

The retrieval of traces from the episodic LTS involves various processes, and it takes place in various ways. These processes and mechanisms may vary in their degree of age sensitivity. One such process is that of recognition of previously encoded information. We discovered earlier (p. 249) that moderate age differences exist on recognition memory tests. We also discovered at that time a basic problem in interpreting these age differences. They could be the result of either inefficient retrieval or inefficient encoding—or both. Obviously, retrieval of Item X cannot be successful if that item's informational content had never been encoded and transmitted to the LTS. In this section, we will review studies dealing with age differences in other aspects of retrieval.

Encoding Specificity

The encoding of information accompanying to-be-remembered items affects eventual retrieval of the to-be-remembered items in another important way. At stake is the influence of contextual information on the eventual retrieval of to-be-remembered episodic events, and the operations of a principle known as *encoding specificity*:

The encoding specificity principle of memory (Tulving & Thomson, 1973) states that memory is best when information available at encoding is also available at retrieval. In other words, cues that are present at encoding are the maximally effective ones for facilitating retrieval. This principle is important because it provides a general theoretical framework for understanding how context variables influence memory. According to the encoding specificity principle, how information can be retrieved depends upon how it was encoded (Tulving, 1979). To the extent that contextual information accompanying to-be-remembered items is encoded with those items, the contextual information should provide effective retrieval cues for accessing the to-be-remembered information (Puglisi, Park, Smith, & Dudley, 1988, p. P145).

In other words, "memory is best when encoding and retrieval conditions are compatible" (Park, Puglisi, Smith, & Dudley, 1987, p. 423).

The encoding specificity principle has particular relevance in the psychology of aging because of the belief that elderly adults are less proficient in encoding contextual information than are young adults (Burke & Light, 1981; Craik & Simon, 1980). In effect, the breadth of encoding, as extended to contextual information, may be more age sensitive than the depth of encoding to-be-remembered items. If true, elderly adults should clearly have a retrieval disadvantage, relative to young adults, as illustrated in Figure 7.9. This is an interesting hypothesis, but it does demand understanding as to what defines contextual information. Here is the definition offered by one prominent basic memory researcher:

The term context is most frequently taken to refer to the immediate physical surround of a target stimulus. Thus in a memory experiment the context may be

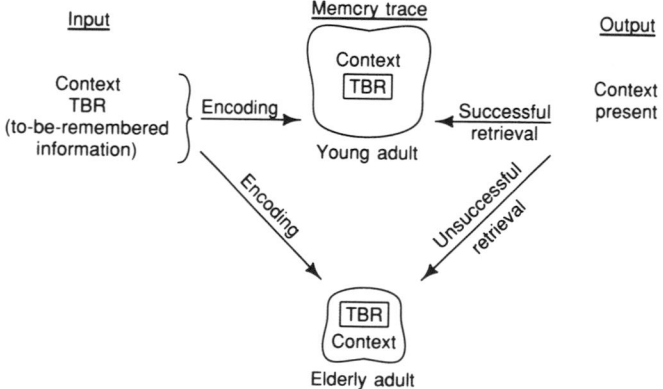

FIGURE 7.9 Schematic representation of age differences in the operations of encoding specificity.

defined as the word preceding, or the word paired with, a target word. . . . Or the context may refer to more global features of the environment in which the stimulus is presented, such as under water or on land (Godden and Baddeley, 1975) or, less exotically, in one room or another. The experimental manipulation of this form of context entails a change in the physical surround with the physical properties of the core stimulus remaining largely unchanged (Lockhart, 1988, p. 323).

The global physical context does seem to have an effect on memory for younger adults as was exotically demonstrated in the study by Godden and Baddeley (1975). Groups of divers studied a list of words for free recall either on land or under water. They then attempted to recall the words either in the same physical context (e.g., studied under water, retrieved under water) or in an altered context (e.g., studied under water, retrieved on land). Recall was strikingly higher in the same context condition than in the altered context condition. This is, of course, exactly what is predicted by the principle of encoding specificity. Less exotic are variations of the physical context by having subjects study a list of words for recall or recognition in a specific room and then test memory for those words either in the same room (physical context reinstated) or in a physically very different room (physical context altered). In general, research with young adults indicates some memory advantage when the test occurs in the same room as the study occurred (e.g., S. M. Smith, Glenberg, & Bjork, 1978), but this advantage has not always been found (Fernandez & Glenberg, 1985).

Words accompanying to-be-remembered words also have been demonstrated with young adults to operate in accordance with the encoding specificity principle. In fact, in the early studies (e.g., Thomson & Tulving, 1970) on encoding specificity, context for a given to-be-remembered word consisted of a weakly associated word. For example, *black* was a to-be-remembered word that was paired with *train* during the study trial. Subjects were informed that it was *black* that was to be remembered, and that *train* was there only to help them to remember *black*. After the study trial, subjects received a cue for each word to help them retrieve that word. Some subjects received the weakly related words from the study list (e.g., *train*), while others received words not in the study list, but rather ones strongly associated preexperimentally with the to-be-remembered words (e.g., *white*). Recall was considerably higher with the reinstated cues from the study list than with the strongly associated cues. Only the weakly related cues present at retrieval reinstate the context present at encoding, thus conforming to the conditions of encoding specificity.

A later study by Tulving and Thomson (1973) demonstrated a related phenomenon in which cued recall with words like *train* yielded higher scores than did recognition of the target words (e.g., *black*) when presented in the absence of any retrieval cues. The recognition test occurred after the study trial. The subjects were asked to give word associates to stimulus words that were certain to elicit prior target words as associates. For example, *white* was a stimulus word that

elicited *black* as one its associates. The subjects then examined each list of associates, and, for each, attempted to identify any associate that had been a prior
target item on the study list. The probability of recognizing *black* as a target was
actually less than the probability of recalling *black* to *train* as a retrieval cue. This
is indeed an intriguing finding in that recognition test scores are usually much
higher than cued-recall scores for the same targets. The memory trace of *black*
that is formed in the presence of *train* is apparently quite different than the
memory trace of *black* formed in the absence of contextual information. Access
to the contextually modified trace requires reinstatement of the original context.

Apparently, there have been no studies employing elderly divers in and out of
water and only one study on room shifts (it involved memory for activities, and
it will be discussed in Chapters 9 and 10). However, there have been several
aging studies in which words provided the contextual information. Little support
for the differential operation of encoding specificity in young and elderly adults
was found in a study by Puglisi, et al. (1988) that replicated the basic procedure
of Thomson and Tulving (1970). Weakly associated words were paired with target
words on a study trial, and were then either reinstated as retrieval cues or replaced
by words strongly related to target words on a cued-recall test trial. Their results
are plotted in part A of Figure 7.10. It may be seen that the probability of recall
was much greater for their elderly subjects as well as their young subjects in the
weak cue condition. A similar outcome was obtained by Park et al. (1987) with
pictures rather than words as target items. Their objective was to determine the
extent of age differences in recognition memory when encoding and retrieval
conditions were either compatible or noncompatible. The to-be-remembered
items were pictures of common objects that were accompanied during study by
another picture of an unrelated object. The subjects were then tested for recognition of the target pictures either in the presence or in the absence of the
unrelated pictures. As may be seen in part B of Figure 7.10, their results indicated
that recognition accuracy, expressed as d' scores, was much greater for all subjects
when the conditions extant during encoding were reinstated during testing. That
is, there was no interaction between age and study-retrieval conditions, an interaction that would be expected if elderly subjects encode less contextual information than do young subjects. Comparability of the encoding specificity principle
for young and elderly adults is indicated further by the demonstration that elderly
adults show the same "when recall is greater than recognition" phenomenon as
do young adults (Rabinowitz, 1984; Shaps & Nilsson, 1980).

On the other hand, evidence of age asymmetry in the operations of encoding
specificity comes from studies by Rabinowitz, Craik, and Ackerman (1982) and
Duchek (1984). Rabinowitz, Craik, and Ackerman (1982) found an encoding
specificity effect for their elderly subjects only when words strongly related to
target words were present at both encoding and retrieval. By contrast, their young
adult subjects displayed an encoding specificity effect both with strong-strong *and*

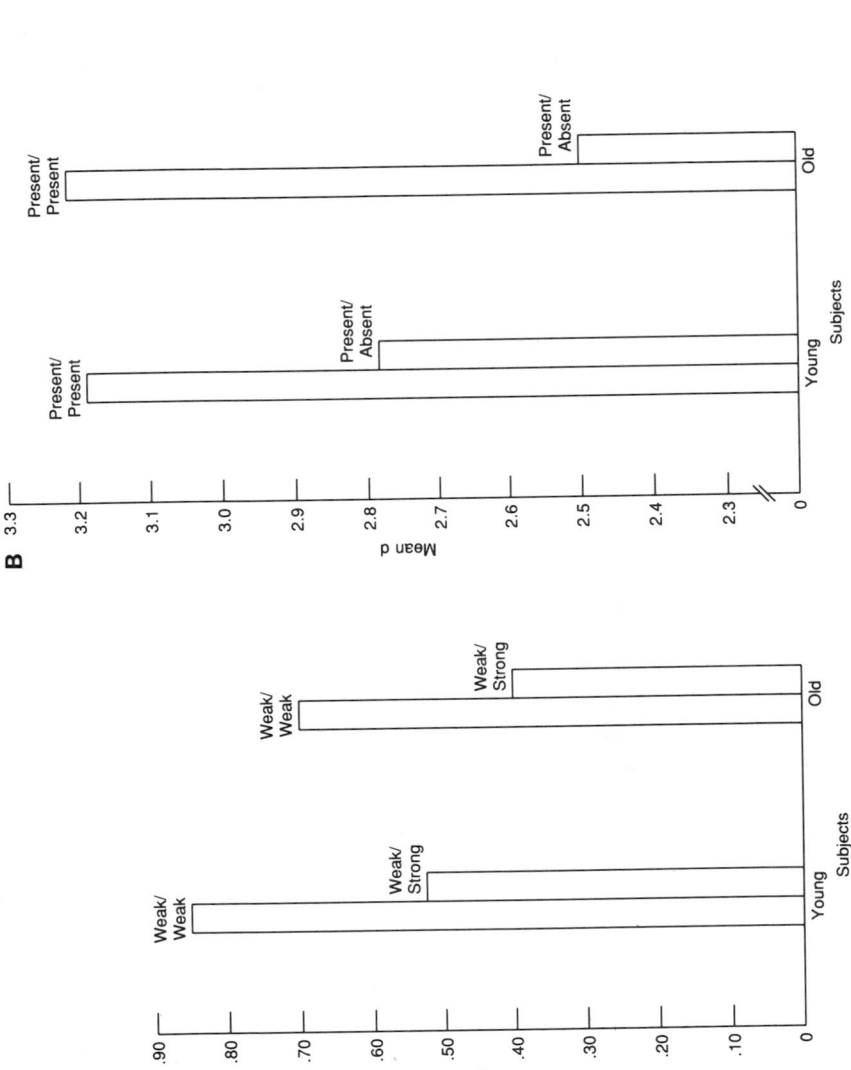

FIGURE 7.10 A: Cued recall probability with (weak/weak) and without (weak/strong) study list cues reinstated during retrieval. (Adapted from Puglisi, Park, Smith, & Dudley, 1988, Table 1). B: d' scores for recognition of pictures with (present/present) and without (present/absent) study-list cues. (Adapted from Park, Puglisi, Smith, & Dudley, 1987, Table 1.)

weak-weak conditions. They suggested that the limited processing capacity of elderly adults restricts severely their ability to integrate weakly related cues to target words. In agreement with this position, Puglisi et al. (1988) discovered in a second experiment that the encoding specificity effect found in their first experiment disappeared for elderly subjects, but not for young subjects, when the study of list items was shared with a secondary task (monitoring auditorily presented digits). The resources required to perform the secondary task were sufficient to limit the resources available for elderly subjects to integrate cue-target information.

Duchek's (1984) subjects received a semantic orienting task consisting of questions about a target word's category membership (e.g., "Is it a bird?" followed by *robin*). At retrieval they were given cue words that were either semantically related to the targets or semantically unrelated (rhyming words of the targets) to aid recall. In agreement with the principle of encoding specificity, both young and elderly subjects recalled more targets with semantic cues than with rhyming cues. However, the advantage of the semantic cues over the rhyming cues was considerably greater for the young subjects, leading Duchek to conclude that "it appears that older individuals do not simply show a deficit in semantic coding, but rather, show a deficit in their ability to use a semantic retrieval cue to reinstate the specific semantic context that was encoded earlier" (Duchek, 1984, p. 1179).

Asymmetry in encoding specificity for young and elderly adults obviously remains a largely unresolved issue. Whether or not elderly adults benefit in retrieval from the reinstatement of contextual information seems to depend on undetermined task conditions. In general, however, it appears that the ability to integrate contextual information with target information is not beyond the capacity of elderly adults. Our conclusion is reinforced by evidence provided by Park, Puglisi, and Sovacool (1984) in which a somewhat different meaning of context was employed. Their materials were cartoons, and context was defined as the presence of background detail. Pictures studied with background details present were recognized with much greater accuracy when the details were also present during the test trial than when they were absent—and equally so for elderly and young subjects—suggesting, in their words, "a strong encoding specificity effect for young and elderly people" (Park et al., 1984, p. 214).

Our focus thus far has been only on encoding specificity as it involves external contextual variation. However, context may be internal as well as external. The internal context refers to both one's physiological state and one's emotional, or mood, state. To-be-remembered information may be encoded differently when one is in a drug-altered state than when in a normal state. In accordance with the encoding specificity principle, young adults remember more information when they are tested in the same state (whether altered or normal) they were in at the time the to-be-remembered information was encoded (Eich, Weingartner, Stillman, & Gillin, 1975). In other words, memory tends to be *state dependent*. To some degree, young adults also tend to show *mood-dependent* memory. Again in accordance with the encoding specificity principle, memory performances tend to be better if they are tested in the same mood (e.g., happy or sad) they were in at the time the to-be-remembered material was presented than if they are tested while in a different mood (e.g., Bower, 1981). To what extent state dependency and mood dependency apply to elderly adults appears to be largely unknown.

Output Interference

Retrieval proficiency may also be affected by the occurrence of *output interference* during the recall of study list items. The outputting, or active recalling of some items from the episodic store, is expected to decrease the availability of other items that remain in the store and await recall (Tulving & Arbuckle, 1963). Some evidence of greater proneness to output interference by elderly adults than by young adults was reported by Taub and Walker (1970). In one of their conditions, subjects had to respond with a redundant item on each list prior to recalling the items that were specific to a given list. In effect, responding with this prefix item may be expected to generate output interference for the recall of the list-specific items. Performance of their elderly subjects suffered more from this added output requirement (relative to a control condition in which the redundant prefix was absent) than did their young subjects, which is in agreement with the hypothesis of an age difference in proneness to output interference.

More rigorous tests of this hypothesis by A. D. Smith (1974, 1975b), however, failed to provide support. In his 1975 study, the to-be-remembered items were eight paired associates that were presented for a single study trial. Tulving and Arbuckle (1963) had used the same materials and procedure in their earlier study with young adults. They argued that paired-associate learning may be viewed as an episodic-memory phenomenon. A trace of paired items may be transmitted to the LTS, just as a trace of a single item may be transmitted. In fact, one could argue that the stimulus item of a pair functions as a context that is integrated with the to-be-remembered item (the response element). Returning to A. D. Smith's study (1975b), after the single study trial was over, stimulus elements of the pairs were presented as retrieval cues for recalling their paired response elements. The order of these cues was systematically varied so that pairs that were first in the input sequence (i.e., during the study trial) were sometimes tested first in the output sequence, sometimes second, and so on, through the eighth output position. Similarly, pairs in the second input position were tested from the first through the eighth output position, and so on. A. D. Smith's results (1975b), showing recall probability as a function of position in the output sequence (as averaged over all eight input positions) are illustrated in Figure 7.11. Output interference was clearly present for young, middle-aged, and elderly subjects. That is, for all three age groups, there was a progressive decline in recall as the number

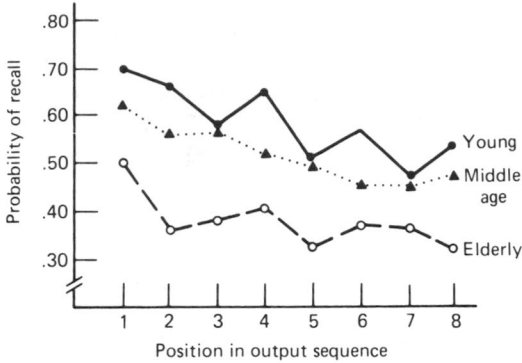

FIGURE 7.11   Age differences in output interference. (Adapted from Smith, 1975b, Figure 1.)

of prior items recalled (or outputted) increased. More important, however, there was no significant interaction between age and output position. Thus, output interference was no greater for elderly subjects than for younger subjects. It seems likely that the age differential in output interference reported by Taub and Walker (1970) was actually due to the confusion created by having to preface each recall sequence with the prefix item. That is, the adverse effect of this confusion was probably greater for their elderly subjects than for their young subjects.

Effects of Prior Retrieval on Later Retrieval

A number of basic memory studies have demonstrated that prior retrieval of study list items enhances later recall of those items (e.g., Allen, Mahler, & Estes, 1969; Darley & Murdock, 1971; Hogan & Kintsch, 1971). However, it has also been found that an initial recall test has little effect on a final recognition test (Darley & Murdock, 1971), suggesting that the effects of prior recall are on the accessibility, rather than on the availability of study list items. As observed by Bjork, "A critical aspect of the maintenance of knowledge is maintaining access to that knowledge in memory. The key to maintaining such access is to use that information: The act of retrieving an item from memory facilitates subsequent retrieval access to that item" (Bjork, 1988, p. 396). In other words, recalling an episodic event shortly after it has occurred should serve to make that same event more accessible for retrieval at a later time. This is an important principle that should be known to those psychologists who offer training on how to improve your memory. Despite the principle's importance, it has received relatively atten- tion by experimental aging researchers, and little is known about its generaliza- bility to older adults. There have been, however, several studies employing elderly subjects with results promising enough to indicate the need for further research. Only the study by Rabinowitz and Craik (1986) will concern us here. It involved effortful memory processes and words as items. The other studies involved automatic memory processes, and activities or actions as "items." We will report on the outcome of these studies in Chapter 9.

Rabinowitz and Craik (1986) made use of a modified Brown-Peterson short-term memory procedure. On each trial subjects received two sets of three words each, with each set being instances of a different taxonomic category. After a retention interval filled with counting backwards, they were cued to recall the three words from only one of the two categories encountered on the study trial. On any given study trial, subjects never knew until after the retention interval was over which of the two categories would be cued. Consequently, all six words required processing and encoding, even though only three would be recalled on the short-term test. This procedure continued for a number of study trials. At the end of the study trials, the subjects were asked to recall *all* of the words from the study trials. As may be seen in Figure 7.12, both the young and the elderly subjects recalled a substantially larger proportion of words that they had previously attempted to recall than words that had never experienced attempted recall. Rabinowitz and Craik concluded that "retrieval practice may be an effective mnemonic technique for elderly adults—techniques of self-testing under conditions that optimize the likelihood of initial retrieval could easily be taught in group settings" (1986, p. 374). Note in Figure 7.12 that the items "practiced" by elderly subjects approached the recall level of young subjects for "nonpracticed" items. It is not unusual for elderly adults with retrieval practice to approximate the performance level of young adults who haven't received practice (see p. 332 and p. 341).

Cued Recall and Indirect Retrieval

Cues related to to-be-remembered episodic events serve to enhance recall of those events for both young adults and elderly adults, even when the cues were not present during study trials. We discovered this to be true for categorical names as cues for recalling previously encountered instances of those categories (see p. 232). Such cues seemingly aid recall by gaining direct access to hierarchically ordered memory traces. Cues may also aid recall indirectly when implicit associates of those cues overlap with implicit associates of their related target items that were activated during a study trial (McEvoy & Holley, 1990; McEvoy, Nelson, Holley, & Stelnicki, 1992; D. L. Nelson, Schrieber, & McEvoy, 1992). When direct recall of a target item does not occur, the overlapping implicit associate elicited by the cue may prompt recall by its linkage to the target item. McEvoy and her associates reasoned that the smaller the set of associates to a target item, the greater the likelihood of finding the linking associate to the target's

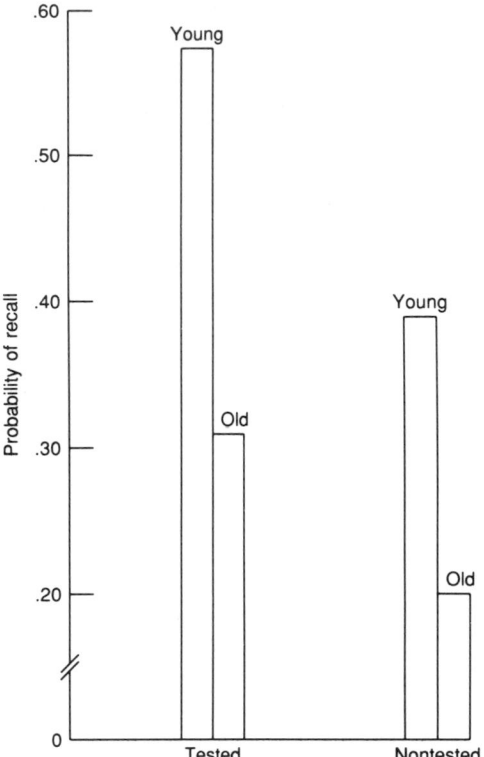

FIGURE 7.12 Probability of long-term recall of previously tested (short-term) and nontested items. (Adapted from Rabinowitz & Craik, 1986, Table 1.)

representation in the LTS. Thus, indirect recall should be greater for targets having a small set size than for targets having a large set size. McEvoy and Holley (1990) did find a set size effect for both their young and their elderly subjects. Probability of recall by the young subjects was .76 and .52 for small and large set sizes, respectively. Comparable values for their elderly subjects were .57 and .42. Note that the set size effect was much greater for the young than for the elderly subjects. The age difference seemingly reflects the poorer utilization of indirect retrieval routes by elderly subjects than by young subjects.

Fan Effect

We discovered earlier (p. 234 and p. 242) that hierarchically organized memory traces can accommodate a limited number of subordinate units (a cue overload principle), with the limit being less in late adulthood than in earlier adulthood. Even when that limit is not exceeded, the speed of retrieving a sub-ordinate unit decreases as the number of such units increases. The decrease in speed of retrieval with increasing units is known as the *fan effect* (Anderson, 1974). The effect presumably results from the interference caused by the compe-tition among the facts sharing the same superordinate. Demonstration of the fan effect in the laboratory requires initially that subjects learn a series of facts (sub-ordinates) about each of several concepts (superordinates). For example, subjects may learn that a doctor (as a concept) took a car on a test drive, cut an apple pie into six pieces, and so on (as facts stored hierarchically with the concept). They are then given a recognition test in which the previous facts are intermingled with foils similar to previous facts. For young adults, the reaction time of respond-ing on the test trial increases as the number of stored facts increases, say, from one to three (e.g., Anderson, 1974). Both G. Cohen (1990) and Gerard, Zacks, Hasher, and Radvansky (1991) found the magnitude of the fan effect to be greater for elderly subjects than for young subjects. For example, in Gerard et al.'s (1991) study, the mean reaction time for their young subjects increased by 387 ms from one to three facts, whereas it increased by 710 ms for their elderly subjects. The greater fan effect for elderly subjects seemingly indicates that they have more difficulty than young adults in inhibiting the interference from competing facts at the time of retrieval in agreement with inhibition theory (see Chapter 6, pp. 220–223).

Adult Age Differences in Prospective Memory

All of the components of episodic memory discussed thus far are variations of retrospective memory (Meacham & Leiman, 1975). That is, memory consists of a trace of some prior episodic event (or remembrance of things past). There is another variation of episodic memory, however, one labeled *prospective memory* by Meacham and Leiman (1975). Here is one psychologist's description of pro-spective memory:

> It consists of remembering to perform planned actions at an appropriate time in the future. Thus, we instruct ourselves in the morning to take home a specific book upon leaving the office in the evening, or take our medicine after eating breakfast. The planned action will be executed only to the extent that its episodic trace is retrieved at the appropriate time for execution. It is this component of episodic memory that is commonly associated with the ancient gimmick of tying a string on one's finger to serve as a 'reminder' (i.e., a retrieval cue) to perform a planned action.
>
> The imperfections of prospective memory are evident from the fact that, more often than we care to admit, we do leave behind the book in question and we do forget to take the prescribed medicine on schedule. Even highly practiced planned activities are not free of failures to perform on schedule. For example, Lee Trevino,

an experienced professional golfer, 'forgot' to sign his card following a round of the PGA Golf Tournament, thereby disqualifying him from further participation in that year's tournament. The imperfections of prospective memory are what people usually have in mind when they refer to themselves as being 'absent minded'. Problems associated with prospective memory are certain to be among those listed by elderly people—and yet we know little about how aging does affect prospective memory. In fact, little is known about prospective memory in general" (Kausler, 1985, pp. 118–119).

The early studies comparing young and elderly subjects in proficiency of prospective memory followed a rather standard nonlaboratory procedure (see Sinnott, 1989; West, 1986, for further review). Young and elderly subjects are given a task to perform in their own environs, one in which a designated action is to be performed at a number of different times. Usually the action consists of calling a given telephone number at specific times over several weeks (Maylor, 1990a; Moscovitch, 1982; Poon & Schaffer, 1982; Sinnott, 1984; West, 1984) or mailing postcards to the experimenter at designated times (Patton & Meit, 1993). These studies generally found that elderly subjects remember to make more of the scheduled calls or to mail more of the postcards than do young adult subjects (e.g., 90.3% of the scheduled calls were made by Poon and Schaffer's (1982) elderly subjects, only 80.3% by their young subjects).

On the surface, the implication is that of a reverse age-related deficit! However, not all researchers have found the rate of making telephone calls at scheduled times over a lengthy period of time to be as high as that reported by Poon and Schaffer (1982). In a control group of elderly subjects employed by Sczomak (1989), the rate was only 50.4%. His subjects made the calls under the guise of believing they were participating in a sleep study and that they were to report each day on the nature of their sleep during the previous night. Interestingly, Sczomak (1989) found the rate to be much higher (over 70%) for other elderly subjects who were cued in various ways to remind them to make the calls (e.g., a reminder sticker placed prominently in their homes). The age level of older adults also seems important. In a skillfully executed study, Park, Morrell, Frieske, and Kincaid (1992) monitored compliance of young-old (age 70 and younger) and old-old (age 71 and older) to their schedules of taking medications. The young-old showed a higher rate of compliance (94%; a rate that was as high with no intervention by the researchers as it was with such interventions as providing a medication organizer) than did the old-old subjects (84%). External aids, however, have been found to increase medical compliance by very old adults (Cockburn & Collin, 1988; see Park, 1992, for further review). One such aid consists of verbal and postcard reminders (Leirer, Morrow, Pariante, & Doksum, 1989). Especially effective aids are containers that have medicines organized with respect to days of the week and times of the day in which the medicines are to be taken (Park, Morrell, Frieske, Blackburn, & Birchmore, 1991; Park, Morrell, Frieske, &

Kincaid, 1992). In addition, some researchers (e.g., West, 1988; Cockburn & Smith, 1988, 1991; Dobbs & Rule, 1987; West, 1988) found elderly adults to be more likely than young adults to forget to perform some future action over an extended period of time.

The problem with comparing young and elderly subjects in proficiency of prospective memory by means of such tasks as making telephone calls at designated times at home is well recognized by the investigators themselves. Factors other than an age difference in prospective memory per se may be responsible for the outcomes. Particularly important is the probably greater motivation for conforming to the task demands experienced by elderly subjects than by young subjects. Interview data from Poon and Schaffer's (1982) study indicated that their young subjects remembered when it was time to call—their preoccupation with other, more important activities, simply prevented them from calling. Similarly, Patton and Meit's (1993) elderly subjects rated their postcard mailing task to be more important to them than did their young subjects, indicating greater motivation for the elderly subjects to perform the actual mailings. However, Sinnott (1986) did find the absence of an age difference in remembering to do certain requested things in a field setting. Her subjects were participants in the Baltimore Longitudinal Study, and their planned activities were part of what was scheduled for them on one of their annual visits to the testing center. Other more naturalistic studies of this kind would certainly be welcomed.

Our confidence in the age insensitivity of prospective memory would be strengthened greatly if age comparability was also found on laboratory tasks that simulate the involvement of everyday prospective memory processes. Such simulation was provided in a study by Harris and Wilkins (1982) in which subjects were instructed to perform a specific action at some designated time while watching a movie. However, Harris and Wilkins did not examine age differences in their study. Adult age differences in a laboratory setting were examined in studies by Cockburn and Smith (1988, 1991), Dobbs and Rule (1987), Einstein and McDaniel (1990), and Maylor (1993), with elderly subjects being only slightly more likely to forget to perform some future action than younger subjects. In each of these studies, subjects participated in an experiment unrelated to prospective memory, and they were instructed to perform the designated action at some point during their participation. Cockburn and Smith's (1991) subjects were told to ask for a future appointment at a given signal (a kitchen timer sounding off), and Dobbs and Rule's (1987) subjects were told to ask for a red pen at some given time in the experiment. Einstein and McDaniel's (1990) subjects received 42 short-term memory trials with words as the to-be-remembered items. They were instructed both to recall the words on each trial and to monitor the words for the presence of a target word. Whenever the target word appeared, they were to press a designated key on a computer keyboard. The target word was present on three of the short-term memory trials. The age difference in the number of key presses at the appropriate times was not statistically significant, implying that prospective memory is indeed age insensitive rather than age sensitive as implied by the other laboratory studies. Maylor's (1993) middle-aged and elderly subjects viewed a series of 30 faces and responded to two of them on each of many trials. The two age groups did not differ in correct responses to the target faces on the first block of trials. However, only the middle-aged subjects increased their correct responses over further blocks of trials.

If prospective memory is indeed largely age insensitive, then it is a surprising exception to the general suspectibilty of long-term memory to age-related deficits. As noted by Einstein and McDaniel (1990), prospective memory seemingly requires a self-initiated retrieval process of the kind entering into free recall of a word list, a retrieval process commonly viewed as being highly age sensitive (see p. 253). Interestingly, Einstein and McDaniel (1990) also reported the absence of covariations between prospective memory test scores and scores on each of several retrospective memory tests (e.g., free recall of a word list) for both their young and their elderly subjects. Prospective memory may well be a unique component of episodic memory.

Whether or not prospective memory is age sensitive may depend on the type of prospective memory involved. Einstein and McDaniel (1991) and Einstein, Holland, McDaniel, and Guynn (1992) noted that there are actually two kinds of prospective memory, one that is event-based and the other that is time-based. For event-based memory, an external cue is present to serve as a reminder to perform an action (e.g., the timer in Cochran and Smith's, 1991, study and the appearance of a target word in Einstein and McDaniel's, 1990, study). For time-based memory, there is no external cue, and subjects must remember to perform an action at some given time or after some period of time has lapsed. Einstein and his associates have reasoned that time-based prospective memory, with its need for self-initiated processing, is likely to be more age sensitive than event-based prospective memory. In agreement with this position, Einstein and Mc-Daniel (1991) found a significant age-related deficit in performance under time-based conditions (pressing a computer key every 10 min) but not under event-based conditions (pressing the key to the presence of a target word).

The situation regarding event-based prospective memory is unclear, however. Both the presence and the absence of age differences have been found with event-based procedures (Cochran & Smith, 1991; Einstein & McDaniel, 1990, 1991; Mäntylä, in press a, b). What seems to be the critical factor determining the presence or absence of age-related deficits is the complexity of the external cues and the amount of self-initiating processing required before performing the appropriate action. With a procedure comparable to that of Einstein and McDaniel (1990), Einstein et al. (1992) found their elderly subjects to be less likely than their young subjects to perform the designated action when there were multiple target words as external cues rather than a single word as a cue. Presumably, the extent of self-initiated processing increases as the number of external cues increases, and the extent of the age-related deficit in performance of the designated action increases accordingly. Similarly, Mäntylä (in press a, b) found that the extent of the age-related deficit is contingent on the nature of the external cues. In these studies, the cues were instances of a specified category (e.g., *liquids*), with subjects performing an action at the occurrence of each instance. On some occasions, the instance was a typical one for that category, and on other occasions it was an atypical one (e.g., *milk* and *ink* as typical and atypical instances, respectively, of *liquids*). A significant age-related deficit in prospective memory performance was found when the external cues were atypical instances but not when they were typical instances. The extent of self-initiated processing is presumably greater for atypical cues than for typical cues and therefore so is the age-related deficit in prospective memory.

Long-Term Episodic Memory: Discourse

Introduction

Memory psychologists do not devote all of their time and effort in research involving discrete items in a list. For many years, memory of discourse was a topic of modest interest (e.g., F. C. Bartlett, 1932). This interest has intensified greatly in the last twenty or so years (e.g., J. R. Anderson & Bower, 1973; Kintsch, 1974). Accompanying the increase in basic research has been an increase directed at age differences in memory for discourse, that is, memory for meaningful series of words at the levels of individual sentences, paragraphs, and stories/essays. Much of this interest has been guided by the belief that discourse memory is more ecologically relevant to memory in the everyday world than is memory for discrete items; therefore it should more adequately reflect the extent of age-related deficits in episodic memory that occur outside of the laboratory.

Some gerontological psychologists (e.g., Hulicka, 1967a, 1967b; Kay, 1955) have argued that age differences favoring young adults should be less pronounced for the meaningful material characteristic of, say, sentences than for the meaningless material characteristic of, say, free-recall lists. The argument is a familiar one—elderly adults are presumed to be less motivated when confronted by meaningless material than when confronted by meaningful material. Consequently, adverse performance factors are less pronounced for elderly subjects with meaningful material than with meaningless material. Other gerontological psychologists (e.g., Craik & Masani, 1967), however, have argued that, if anything, age-related deficits should be greater for meaningful material than for meaningless material. They believe that the differential rests in age-sensitive organizational processes that enter into memory of meaningful material but not into memory of meaningless material. In defense of their position, Craik and Masani (1967) cited evidence reported by Heron and Craik (1964). In that study, no age deficit in digit span was found when the digits were read in Finnish, but an age-related deficit was found when the digits were read in English (the subjects' native language). The contrast between Finnish and English digits was regarded by Craik and Masani (1967) as being simply one form of the more general contrast between meaningless and meaningful material. They, therefore, expected the effect of this kind of contrast on age differences to apply to other kinds of material that may vary in meaningfulness, including word strings. We have encountered evidence from other studies that seem to support their position. For example, age differences, favoring young adults, are more pronounced for a word-span task when the words are high in meaningfulness than when they are low in meaningfulness (Chapter 5, p. 154), and for a letter string memory task when chunking via meaningful words is possible than when it is not (Chapter 5, pp. 156–157).

Adult Age Differences in Sentence Memory

Syntactic and Semantic Constraints

One way of testing these opposing views of the interaction between age and the degree of meaningfulness is to compare young and elderly subjects in their memories for material that ranges from being a random string to being a completely meaningful sentence. Do age differences favoring young adults increase or decrease as the meaningfulness of the strings increases? A useful set of materials for such tests was constructed by Miller and Selfridge (1950). They prepared strings of words that varied in their order of approximation to meaningful English text. A zero-order string consists of randomly selected and randomly ordered words. Successively higher order approximations increase progressively in their conformity to English syntax and in their likelihood of conveying a meaningful content. This may be seen in Table 8.1 where 20-word strings of zero-, first-, third-, and fifth-order approximations are listed along with another string that constitutes meaningful English text (i.e., it is a syntactically and semantically legitimate sentence). Material of this nature (only the strings were 30 words in length rather than 20) were read to young adult and elderly subjects by Craik and Masani (1967). Mean recall scores (number of words recalled) for each group improved greatly as the strings increased progressively in their approximations to text. However, the magnitude of the age difference favoring young adults also increased progressively. The result is a divergent relationship. That is, the magnitude of the age-related deficit increased as overall performance scores increased. The implication is that different age-sensitive processes become involved in the transition from meaningless to meaningful material. Zero-order strings are equivalent to a word list composed of unrelated items. Consequently, the organizational processes governing the encoding of the material are those that govern subjective organization. Increasing the approximation to textual material means that both syntax and semantic content become increasingly involved. The

TABLE 8.1

Word Strings of Varying Approximations to English text[a]

Zero order
betwixt trumpeter pebbly complication vigorous tipple careen obscure attractive consequence expedition pane unpunished prominence chest sweetly basin awoke photographer ungrateful
First order
tea realizing most so the together home and for were wanted to concert I posted he her it the walked
Third order
family was large dark animal came roaring down the middle of my friends love books passionately every kiss is fine
Fifth order
road in the country was insane especially in dreary rooms where they have some books to buy for studying Greek
Text
more attention has been paid to diet but mostly in relation to disease and to the growth of young children

[a] Adapted from G. A. Miller and Selfridge, 1950, by permission of University of Illinois Press.

constraints offered by normal syntax provide an effective organization for ordering words correctly and should, therefore, lead to a major reduction in the number of errors made in recalling the string. For example, the sequence *has been paid* in the textual string listed in Table 8.1 follows that of normal text. To recall it as *been has paid* would clearly violate the rules of syntax. Similarly, the constraints offered by semantic content provide an effective organization for ordering words correctly. If the content of the textual string in Table 4.1 is encoded correctly, it would make no sense, for example, to reverse the positions of *diet* and *disease* in recalling the sentence—the meaning would be altered drastically.

The divergent relationship found by Craik and Masani (1967) suggests that syntactic–semantic organizational processes suffer a greater decrement in proficiency from early to late adulthood than do subjective organizational processes of the kind described earlier (Chapter 7, pp. 240–243). However, the Age × Approximation interaction was not replicated in a later study by Craik and Masani (1969), nor was the interaction found in a later study by Kinsbourne (1973) in which letter strings varied in their approximation to English words (see Chapter 5, p. 156). As observed by Craik, "Given these contradictory results, the most reasonable conclusion at present appears to be that while older groups generally do less well than a young group at recalling long strings of words or letters, both groups can make equally good use of the linguistic rules inherent in higher orders of approximation to English" (1977, p. 403).

Normal Sentence Recall

An age deficit in the recall of normal sentence content was also found in early studies by Gordon (1975) and Whitbourne and Slevin (1978). The study by Whitbourne and Slevin (1978) is especially informative. Two kinds of sentences were constructed. In one kind, the subject and object of each sentence were concrete nouns of high-imagery value, whereas in the other kind, they were abstract nouns of low-imagery value. A number of studies with young adult subjects (e.g., Begg & Paivio, 1969) have found far superior recall of content for sentences containing high imagery words than for sentences containing low imagery words. Presumably, imaginal representations of a sentence's content enhance recall of that content. Such representations, of course, are more likely to occur with high-imagery words than with low-imagery words. As illustrated in Figure 8.1, Whitbourne and Slevin's (1978) results indicated that elderly subjects benefit as much from high-imagery words as do young subjects. Consequently, the age difference in recall scores favoring young adults was no greater for sentences containing low imagery words than for sentences containing high-imagery words. The additive nature of the relationship between age and imagery variation suggests that the use of imagery to encode sentence content changes little over the course of the adult life span. This outcome is somewhat surprising in that elderly adults do not seem to show the same advantage for concrete words (i.e., high imagery) over abstract words (i.e., low-imagery words) that young adults do on a free recall task (see Chapter 7, p. 255).

Another interesting finding was reported by Botwinick and Storandt (1974a). Their subjects received foolish, or anomalous, sentences, that is, word strings that

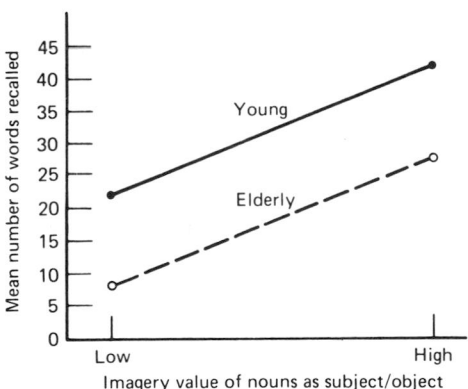

FIGURE 8.1 Age differences in words recalled from sentences of low- and high-imagery value. (Adapted from Whitbourne & Slevin, 1978, Table 1.)

were syntactically sound but semantically meaningless. For example, one of their sentences was, "The Declaration of Independence sang overnight while the cereal jumped by the river." If the age-related decrement in recall of sentence content is due only to an age-related deficit in the ability to use semantic constraints, then age differences in recall should disappear when those constraints are no longer relevant. That is, young subjects should be as disadvantaged as elderly subjects when confronted by foolish sentences. Our reasoning follows from the application of the deletion method (in this case, it is the process of semantic constraint that is deleted; see Kausler, 1991, for a description of the deletion method). However, Botwinick and Storandt (1974a) did not find the age deficit in recall to disappear. Nevertheless, the magnitude of the deficit was not as pronounced as the magnitude found with normal sentences. The implication is that semantic organization is an age-sensitive process.

However, more recent evidence presented by Wingfield, Poon, Lombardi, and Lowe (1985) and Stine and Wingfield (1987a) seems to challenge this conclusion. The young adult and elderly subjects in these two studies listened to a number of word strings that were exposed at varying rates. At a normal conversational rate (180 words per min), word strings that were both normal sentences and were read with a normal prosodic intonation were recalled about as well by their elderly subjects as by their young subjects. When read at a very fast rate (360 words per min), there was a substantial age-related deficit in sentence recall in Stine and Wingfield's (1987a) study but not in Wingfield et al.'s (1985) study. Moreover, when comparable sentences were read without normal prosodic intonation (i.e., in a monotone), the age-related deficit appeared with slower rates of reading than was the case for sentences with normal intonation. Tun, Wingfield, Stine, and Mecsas (1992) found a similar Age × Speech Rate interaction effect. Interestingly, they also found that the interaction was not exacerbated in a divided attention condition. Wingfield, Wayland, and Stine (1992) provided further evidence for age-related deficits in sentence recall being minimal when sentences were presented at a normal conversational rate and with a prosody that conforms to the syntactic structure of those sentences. These results indicate that elderly adults do make effective use of both semantic organization and prosodic organization in their comprehension and memory of auditorily presented word strings. Spilich and Voss (1982) demonstrated further that elderly adults, like young adults, make effective use of the contextual information provided by preceding sentences in aiding memory of target sentences. Here too there appears to be little age-related deficit in the use of semantic organization to aid individual sentence recall.

Given the conflicting findings on sentence memory, there is the obvious need for further research to determine the basis for the discrepant findings. Of interest would be a study comparing age groups on distorted sentences that are semantically valid but syntactically out of order, such as, "Neighbors sleeping noisy wake parties" (Marks & Miller, 1964). Comparisons of age-related deficits found with these kinds of sentences and with foolish sentences would offer a means of evaluating the relative contributions of syntactic and semantic organizational processes to age differences in memory for normal sentences.

Adult Age Differences in Paragraph Memory

Recall of Ideas

A paragraph relates consecutive sentences together into an integrated content. A number of the ideas of the kind illustrated in Table 8.2 are represented in a single paragraph. Memory proficiency for the content of this paragraph may be evaluated by determining how many of the 16 ideas embedded within it are recalled after reading it once. Whether or not the individual ideas are recalled in exactly the same words present in the paragraph is unimportant. What is important is recall of the basic ideas and not their specific phrasings. For example, recall of the last idea in the paragraph ("no casualities were reported") would be scored as being correct if it took the form, "there were no casualities."

Early studies on age differences in memory proficiency for paragraphs generally used fairly short paragraphs, and their concern was often only with reporting the magnitude of the age difference. That is, there was little attempt to vary such characteristics as the difficulty of the paragraph. Age differences in memory proficiency were simply evaluated by comparing mean idea recall scores for various age groups. This simple procedure was applied in a study by Wechsler (1945). He found a modest decline by age 50 in the number of ideas recalled from paragraphs of the kind illustrated in Table 7.3. A later study by Hulicka (1966) used the materials from Wechsler's study and extended the age variation to people in their 80s. The decline observed by Wechsler was found to continue steadily through late adulthood, with subjects in their 80s recalling about one-fourth fewer ideas

TABLE 8.2

Paragraph Used to Test Age Differences in Memory for Connected Discourse[a,b]

Thousands of persons/ have been evacuated/ from their homes/ in two/ Mexican states/ after more than forty-eight hours/ of rains/ that have caused/ disastrous floods./ Several lowland sections/ in three cities/ were reported under water./ One flooding river/ has covered/ almost a half-million acres./ No casualties were reported.

---

[a]From: Botwinick and Storandt, 1974a. (Courtesy of Charles C. Thomas, Publisher, Springfield, Illinois.)
[b]Slash marks denote separate ideas, each given a score of 1 if recalled.

than subjects in their 20s. A more precipitous decline was found by Botwinick and Storandt (1974a). The paragraph shown in Table 8.2 is one of two received by their subjects. The second paragraph contained 25 ideas, thus making 41 the maximum possible recall score for the two paragraphs combined. It can be seen from the mean recall scores, as plotted in Figure 8.2, that the performance proficiency of 70-year-old subjects was about half that of 20-year-old subjects. A number of other studies have also reported substantial age-related declines for the ideas contained within a paragraph (e.g., Kear-Calwell & Heller, 1978: Moenster, 1972; Schneider, Gritz, & Jarvik, 1975). Age deficits have also been found when a recognition test replaces a recall test (Gordon & Clark, 1974a,b; Taub, 1976).

Modality of Presentation

Most of the other early studies on age differences in paragraph memory centered on the issue of the modality of presentation for the to-be-remembered material. That is, is the magnitude of the age-related deficit affected by the visual-versus-auditory mode of presenting the content? Taub (1975) discovered that, regardless of age level, the mean number of ideas recalled was greater following visual presentation than following auditory presentation. However, the magnitude of the age-related deficit was about the same for each modality. Taub's (1975) procedure allowed subjects to review the paragraph while reading it. That is, as each new idea occurred, a subject could refer back to earlier segments of that paragraph. This review was not possible with auditory presentation. When review is prohibited with visual presentation, Taub (Taub & Kline, 1976) discovered

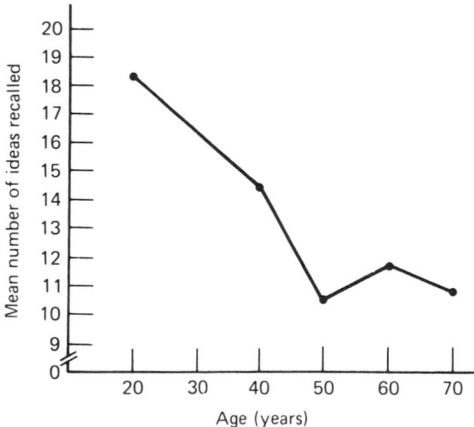

FIGURE 8.2 Age differences in ideas recalled from paragraphs. (Adapted from Botwinick & Storandt, 1974a, Figure 11.)

that recall of paragraph content is not affected by modality of presentation, again regardless of age level. In other studies, Taub (Taub, 1976; Taub & Kline, 1978) compared age differences in recall scores when subjects read silently versus reading aloud. This variation was found to have virtually no effect on memory scores for either young or elderly subjects. Consequently, the age difference favoring young subjects was about the same in each condition.

Attributes of the Text

More recent studies have broadened the focus as well as increasing the lengths of the passages (typically 80 or so words). That is, the focus is no longer on simply reporting age-related deficits. Instead, it has been on the extent to which these deficits are related to attributes of the text and attributes of the subjects themselves. In addition, the concept of a *proposition* (Kintsch, 1974; Kintsch & van Dijk, 1978) has largely replaced the concept of an idea. Propositions have the advantage of being scorable in terms of their importance to the content of any discourse (e.g., high, moderate, and low). Consequently, age differences may be examined separately for propositions at different levels. In terms of textual attributes, the magnitude of age-related deficits has been found to be essentially unaffected by either word length (Zelinski, Light, & Gilewski, 1984) or propositional density (i.e., the number of propositions contained in a fixed-length text; Stine, Wingfield, & Poon, 1986).

On the other hand, the magnitude of the age-related deficit in recall does seem to be affected by the level of propositions. Stine and Wingfield (1987b) gave their young and elderly subjects, classified as high and average verbal ability on the basis of vocabulary test scores, two passages, each containing about 80 words. Shown in Figure 8.3 are the percentages of high-, medium-, and low-level propositions recalled by high and average verbal ability subjects at each age level. Note that the age-related deficit overall was most pronounced for low-level propositions and least for high-level propositions. Note further that the age-related deficit was much greater for average verbal ability than for high verbal ability elderly subjects. Kemper (1987a) discovered that elderly subjects have particular difficulty in recalling propositions that are embedded within syntactically complex sentences. On the other hand, Wingfield and Stine (1986) reported that elderly subjects are as sensitive to syntactic boundaries within normal sentences as are young adult subjects.

Comprehension of Content

The implication of these studies is that there is an age-related deficit in memory of the content of paragraphs. The important question, however, is the locus of the deficit. The deficit may well be the result of an initial comprehension

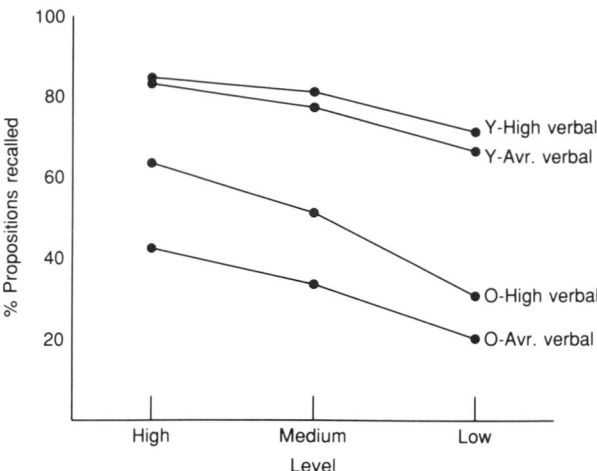

FIGURE 8.3 Percentage of propositions recalled as a function of age (Y, young subjects; O, older subjects), verbal ability, and level of importance. (Reproduced from Stine & Wingfield, 1987b, Figure 1; © Beech Hill Publishing Company.)

problem (see L. L. Light, 1988a; L. L. Light & Albertson, 1988; L. L. Light & Burke, 1988; Spilich, 1985; Stine, Wingfield, & Poon, 1989, for further review). What is comprehended is what is likely to be encoded for storage in memory. Consequently, an age-related deficit in comprehension is, in effect, equivalent to an age-related deficit in encoding. Memory, of course, can scarcely be accurate if encoding of content is inadequate. Alternatively, initial comprehension/encoding may be age insensitive, with the locus of age-related deficits in memory for content being in retrieval processes. The importance of age differences in comprehension as a contributing factor to age differences in paragraph memory was identified in early studies by Belmore (1981), G. Cohen (1979), Taub (1979), and Till and Walsh (1980).

G. Cohen (1979) compared young and elderly subjects in their abilities to derive inferences that are derivable from the content of a paragraph. In her study, well-educated subjects received a series of paragraphs presented by means of a tape recorder at a relatively slow rate (120 words per min). The following is representative of the paragraphs:

> Mrs. Brown goes to sit in the park every afternoon if the weather is fine. She likes to watch the children playing, and she feeds the ducks with bread crusts. She enjoys the walk there and back. For the past three days it has been raining all the time although it's the middle of the summer and the town is still full of people on holiday (G. Cohen, 1979, p. 416).

Following each paragraph, the subjects were asked two questions. One was a verbatim question that simply required recall of some factual information embedded within the paragraph (e.g., "What does Mrs. Brown give the ducks to eat?"). The other required an inference to be drawn from the factual content of the paragraph (e.g., "Did Mrs. Brown go to the park yesterday?"). The results, expressed as mean percentage of incorrect answers, are shown in Figure 8.4. Although the age difference was slight and statistically nonsignificant for verbatim questions, it was much larger and statistically significant for inference questions. Considerably deeper comprehension of the paragraph's content is surely needed to answer inference questions of this kind than to recall simply a factual bit of information.

Taub (1979) also found a modest age difference in comprehension of a paragraph's content, whereas Belmore (1981) found little age difference when subjects were tested with inferential questions immediately after reading a paragraph. Most important, Taub (1979) also found no age difference in memory for the ideas of a paragraph when his young and elderly subjects were equated in their ability to comprehend the content of that paragraph.

The importance of comprehension as a potential age-sensitive process was nicely demonstrated by Till and Walsh (1980). Memory was tested following various orienting tasks, such as giving a pleasant/unpleasant rating to each study-list sentence. Each sentence carried with it an implication that had to be inferred

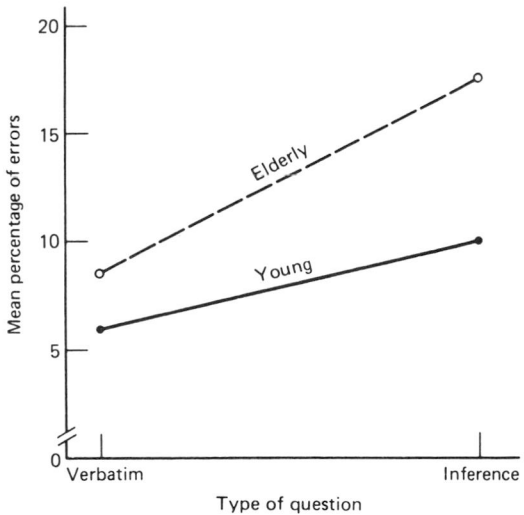

FIGURE 8.4 Age differences reflected in response to verbatim and inference questions that test comprehension of aural messages. (Adapted from G. Cohen, 1979, Table 1.)

from its content. For example, one sentence was, "The chauffeur drove on the left side." The implication is that the action took place in England. Full comprehension of the sentence would include this implication as well as knowledge of who did the driving. Following the study list, subjects received either a noncued recall test or a cued recall test for sentence content. The retrieval cue for each sentence in the cued recall condition was a single word relevant to the implication of that sentence. Thus, *England* was the retrieval cue for the previously given sentence. Young adult subjects recalled more sentences than elderly subjects in both recall conditions. More important, however, the magnitude of the age-related deficit was greater in the cued-recall condition than in the noncued condition. In fact, the young subjects had higher scores when cued than when noncued, whereas the opposite was true for elderly subjects. The implication of each sentence was seemingly comprehended to a greater degree by young than by elderly subjects, which is in agreement with G. Cohen's conclusion regarding the inferential content of sentences. Consequently, the implications were more likely to be represented in the memory traces of young subjects than in the memory traces of elderly subjects. Without such storage of implications, the retrieval cues could not be effective, in agreement with the general principles of encoding specificity.

In a second experiment, Till and Walsh (1980) demonstrated that the age-related deficit found in their first experiment could be overcome by giving their subjects an appropriate orienting task during the study trial. Subjects now had to write down for each sentence a single word that summarized the implication of that sentence. When then tested by implication retrieval cues, elderly subjects recalled as many sentences as did young subjects. These results suggest that the failure to comprehend the deeper meanings of sentences by many elderly people may be a production deficit rather than a true deficit in the ability to comprehend the deeper meanings. They also suggest, in agreement with Taub's (1979) results, that once comprehension is assured, the age-related deficit in memory for content may disappear. However, in a later extension of this study by Till (1985), an age-related deficit in recall was found even when a comprehension task was given and the elderly subjects' responses on the task were comparable to those of young subjects. This outcome suggests that elderly subjects may experience a retrieval problem, and therefore recall less than young subjects, even when initial comprehension has been assured for the elderly subjects.

The importance of retrieval as a probable cause, at least in part, for elderly subjects' difficulty in making use of inferred information in sentences was demonstrated further in a study by Hess and Arnould (1986). Their subjects received sentences, such as, "She had swept the garage floor that morning," that allowed an inference about the involvement of an instrument of some kind. They also received other sentences in which the instrument was explicitly stated (e.g., "with a broom" added to the previous sentence). A recognition test followed in which both implicit (or inferred) and explicit instruments were listed along with a number of distractors. Both young and elderly subjects had higher mean d' scores for explicit instruments than for implicit instruments. Most important, the elderly subjects were as accurate in recognizing old implicit instruments as were the young subjects (but not in recognizing old explicit instruments). The absence of an age difference in recognition memory for the implied instruments clearly suggests that the age difference in memory for implied information disappears when the heavy retrieval demand of a recall test is removed by the use of a recognition test.

There have been a number of other recent studies concerned with age differences in comprehension that have employed a variety of tasks that require reasoning and inferring from a paragraph's content in order to assure full comprehension. Light, Zelinski, and Moore (1982) found age-related deficits only when the informational load given to subjects appeared to exceed the working-memory capacity of elderly subjects, but not that of young subjects. The importance of an age difference in working-memory capacity in determining the presence of age-related deficits in inferring implicit information and other difficult content components that may exceed the working memory's capacity for elderly adults was also emphasized by Zacks, Hasher, Doren, Hamm, and Attig (1987) and Morrow, Altieri, and Leirer (1992). Light and Capps (1986) discovered the absence of an age difference in comprehending anaphoric referents for such sentence pairs as "Henry spoke at a meeting while John drove to the beach. He brought along a surfboard" (i.e., to whom does the "he" refer) when the second sentence followed immediately after the first. Both age groups made more errors when intervening sentences separated the two relevant sentences, but the error rate was greater for elderly subjects. The age-related deficit here appears to be a memory problem rather than a comprehension problem. That is, elderly subjects simply remember less of the factual information from the preceding sentence than do young subjects. Finally, Rebok, Montaglione, and Bendlin (1988) found no age difference in implying information from statements included in fictitious advertisements.

There are alternatives to testing for age differences in comprehension by means of inferences and understanding implicit information. Perhaps the most direct is by assessing on-line reading time for sentences. With this technique, Stine (1990) found some important age differences in the way reading time is allocated to organizational and integration operations, differences presumably attributable to an age difference in working memory's capacity. The implication is that the age difference in allocation yields an age difference in the quality of information that is encoded from each sentence. An intriguing alternative procedure was employed by Radvansky, Gerard, Zacks, and Hasher (1990). Consider the sentences "The girl was given a complete pedicure at the podiatrist" and "The girl was given a complete pedicure by the podiatrist" in which only one of the two had been part of a prior study list but both are given on a subsequent recognition test in which the old sentence is to be identified. Confusion errors are likely to be high in that the two sentences have the same mental or imaginal representation. By contrast, such confusion errors are likely to be much lower for the sentence pair "The girl had her handbag stolen at the podiatrist's" and "The girl had her handbag stolen by the podiatrist." Here the mental representations are quite different for the two sentences. Exactly this differential pattern of errors was found by Radvansky et al. (1990), and equivalently so for young and elderly subjects. This may be seen in Figure 8.5 for the percentages of errors for both "confusable" and "nonconfusable" sentence pairs. To the extent that constructing a mental representation of a sentence's content may be considered a comprehension or encoding process, these results imply that comprehension or encoding is largely age insensitive, at least when the constructive process does not place a strain on elderly adults' decreased working-memory capacity. Yet another procedure is to vary the distance between the major constituents within sentences. The age-related deficit in comprehension has been found to increase as the distance between constituents increases (Davis & Ball, 1989).

In general, these studies indicate that age differences in the comprehension of a paragraph's content are unlikely to be a major contributor to age-related deficits in paragraph memory unless the content of the paragraph places an unusually large strain on working memory's capacity. This is unlikely to be the case for most

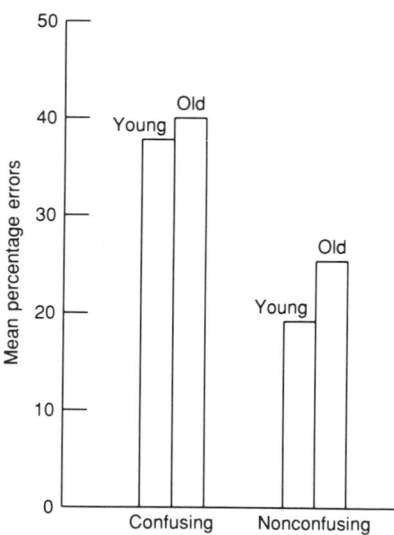

FIGURE 8.5 Mean percentages of errors for young and elderly subjects on confusable and nonconfusable sentence pairs. (Adapted from Radvansky, Gerard, Zacks, & Hasher, 1990, Table 1.)

paragraphs employed in memory research with elderly subjects. Nevertheless, age-related deficits in memory for a paragraph's content have often been reported even for paragraphs that are clearly comprehended by older adults. It seems likely that age-sensitive retrieval processes play a major role in determining these age-related deficits in paragraph memory.

Medical Information

There is one form of paragraph content that is likely to be especially difficult for elderly adults to comprehend—and it is a very important form. It consists of medical information intended either to inform individuals about a particular disease or to instruct individuals as to a medication or therapeutic regimen. Morrell, Park, and Poon (1989) demonstrated substantial age-related deficits in memory for medical information regardless of whether their subjects had unlimited time or limited time to study the information. Ley (1978; Ley et al., 1976) and Page, Versttraete, Robb, and Etzwiler (1981) also demonstrated a high negative correlation between age and memory for medical information. There has been great interest recently in finding ways to improve the communication of medical information to elderly adults. Some advances have been made in finding more effective ways of structuring medical text for elderly adults (Ley, 1976; Morrell et al. 1989; Morrow, Leirer, & Sheikh, 1988; Morrow, Leirer, & Tanke, 1991; Rice, Meyer, & Miller, 1989; Rice & Okun, 1991; see Park, 1992, for further review). One surprising outcome of these studies is the discovery by Morrell et al. (1990) that pictorial instructions on medication labels showed greater forgetting by elderly adults than did verbal instructions, although comprehension of the instructions was comparable for pictorial and verbal presentations.

Adult Age Differences in Memory for Longer Discourses

In the real world, memory for discourse usually involves sequences that are much longer than single paragraphs. The discourse is likely to be in the form of a story, novel, essay, newspaper or magazine article, and so on. Memory of individual ideas or propositions for this kind of material is less important than the ability to integrate the ideas together as a superordinate to subordinate hierarchy of propositions, or summary statements, about the material's content (Anderson & Bower, 1973). At the top of the hierarchy is a representation (or representations) of the material's central theme (or themes) (i.e., highest order propositions). Below it (or them) is an organization of interrelated subordinate propositions. We will begin our review of adult age differences in memory for longer discourses with a discussion of adult age differences in this integrative process.

Schema Abstraction

While reading or listening to, say, a story, an individual who is comprehending that story's content is abstracting various ideas and integrating them together. The final product of this abstraction process is a schematic representation, or *schema*, of the story's content that is stored in episodic memory as a complex memory trace. (The term "schema" is also used in reference to a preexisting knowledge system that is stored in generic memory; see pp. 238–239 and pp. 302–303). On retrieval of the schema from the store, the individual attempts to reproduce the story's content. However, the result is likely to be a reconstruction of the story rather than a true reproduction. Again a schema is only an abstraction. To fill in the details, the individual must tell the story in his or her own words. Moreover, the abstraction process itself may be influenced by the attitudes and beliefs of the individual reader or listener. The resulting schematic representation would then reflect those attitudes and beliefs rather than those of the story's author. Consequently, the individual's reconstruction of the story's content may well contain many distortions, inferences, and embellishments (Bartlett, 1932).

Unfortunately, little attention has been directed at adult age differences in the proficiency of schematic abstraction. Notable exceptions have been studies by Walsh and Baldwin (1977), Walsh, Baldwin, and Finkle (1980), Arenberg and Robertson-Tchabo (1985), Fullerton (1988), and Light, Zelinski, and Moore (1982). These studies are of great interest in that they suggest the possibility of little age change in the abstraction process. Walsh's studies were extensions of a well-known study by Bransford and Franks (1971). In that study, young adult subjects were exposed to a series of sentences that collectively communicated the four ideas shown in the bottom segment of Table 8.3 (i.e., the one-idea sentences). A number of sentences were exposed during a study trial, one sentence at a time. Some, but not all, of the one-idea sentences were included in the study phase. Similarly, some, but not all, of the two- and three-idea sentences were also included in the study phase. Collectively, the study-list sentences conveyed all four of the ideas shown in Table 8.3. The study phase was followed by a recognition memory test containing both old and new sentences, some from each class (i.e., one-, two-, and three-idea sentences). Most important, the four-idea sentence (top segment of Table 8.3) was shown in the test phase only, and it was, therefore, a new item. Nevertheless, there was a high false alarm rate for incorrectly recognizing this sentence as being old. Bransford and Franks (1971) reasoned that subjects abstract ideas from separate but interrelated (as in a story) sentences. These abstractions are integrated together and stored as a holistic representation (or schema) of the overall content. The four-idea sentence conforms to this holistic representation of the four ideas conveyed by the sentences actually exposed during the study phase. Consequently, this four-order sentence is readily but falsely identified as being old.

TABLE 8.3
Materials Used to Study the Abstraction Process in the Memory of
Connected Discourse[a]

Four-idea sentence
The ants in the kitchen ate the sweet jelly which was on the table. (Test only)
Three-idea sentences
The ants ate the sweet jelly which was on the table. (Study only)
The ants in the kitchen ate the sweet jelly. (Test only)
Two-idea sentences
The ants ate the sweet jelly. (Both study and test)
The sweet jelly was on the table. (Test only)
One-idea sentences
The jelly was on the table. (Study only)
The ants were in the kitchen. (Study only)
The jelly was sweet. (Test only)
The ants ate the jelly. (Test only)

[a] From: Bransford and Franks (1971), Table 1. (Used by permission of Academic Press and the author.)

Walsh and Baldwin (1977) found that this false recognition effect was as pronounced for their elderly subjects as for their young adult subjects. Later Walsh, Baldwin, and Finkle (1980) also discovered little sign of an age difference when abstract ideas (e.g., "the attitude was arrogant") substituted for the concrete ideas of the kind shown in Table 8.3. Elderly adults were as proficient as young adults in abstracting ideas and integrating them together into holistic representations. Whether or not the absence of an age-related deficit in abstraction and integration generalizes to more complex and longer materials, such as stories, is an important question. Here the diminished cognitive resources of elderly adults may result in decreased proficiency of the abstraction and integration process. There is also the question of whether or not age-related deficits are present when measures other than recognition are employed. Arenberg and Robertson-Tchabo (1985), Fullerton (1988), and Light et al. (1982) discovered young adults to be more accurate than elderly adults when inferences derived from linear order information (information about the comparative heights of paired individuals— e.g., sentences such as "Bill is taller than Sam") were needed to integrate that information and then reconstruct the order of all of the individuals named in the total series of sentences. There is also evidence to indicate an age-related deficit in another form of integration, namely one in which a picture's content is integrated with the content of a sentence relevant to that picture (Pezdek, 1980).

Levels of Propositions

Whether or not elderly adults are less proficient than young adults in abstracting and integrating information from longer discourse, the fact remains that there are age-related deficits in memory for the content of that discourse (e.g., G. Cohen, 1979; Gordon & Clark, 1974b). Research on the variables affecting the magnitude of these deficits and on the probable causes for the deficits has become very popular in recent years (see J. T. Hartley, 1989; J. T. Hartley, Harker, & Walsh, 1980; Hultsch & Dixon, 1984; Meyer & Rice, 1989; Zelinski & Gilewski, 1988, for further reviews). One probable reason for this popularity is the common assumption that such research has a high degree of ecological validity. That is, discourse memory, unlike memory for discrete words in a list, is a familiar form of everyday memory. This is undoubtedly true to some degree, but it is probably no more true than it is for memory for activities and actions, memory for sources of information, memory for spatial information, and so on, forms of memory that will be discussed in the following chapter. Moreover, everyday memory for such discourses as newspaper articles usually occurs incidentally rather than intentionally. Strangely, most research on age differences in discourse memory has nevertheless employed intentional memory conditions.

An important question concerns the levels of information within discourse at which age differences exist. That is, are age-related deficits found only for lower order propositions or are they also found for higher order propositions? Unfortunately, answers to this question have been quite conflicting. G. Cohen (1979), with a 300-word passage, found her young adult subjects to excel for both higher order and lower order propositions. With a still longer passage (over 600 words), Meyer, Rice, Knight, and Jessen (1979) and Meyer and Rice (1981) found a quite different outcome. There was little difference among age groups for higher order propositions, whereas older subjects recalled *more* lower order propositions than younger subjects. Zelinski, Gilewski, and Thompson (1980) also found no age difference in the recall of higher order propositions, but, in contrast to Meyer et al. (1979), they did find that their elderly subjects recalled fewer lower order propositions than their young subjects. Nor have later studies helped to clarify the ambiguities. Shown in Figure 8.6 are the outcomes obtained by Dixon, Simon, Nowak, and Hultsch (1982) (A) and by Spilich (1983) (B). Dixon et al. (1982) analyzed recall protocols for young, middle-aged, and elderly subjects at four propositional levels (1 = highest order; 4 = lowest order). Note that the magnitude of the age-related deficit was about the same at each propositional level, an outcome also reported by Petros, Tabor, Cooney, and Chabot (1983) and Zelinski et al. (1984). Spilich (1983) analyzed recall protocols for young adult subjects, normally aging elderly subjects, and memory-impaired elderly subjects also at four propositional levels. Note that young subjects and normally aging elderly subjects differed only at the lower propositional levels. Petros, Nor-gaard, Olson, and Tabor (1989) reported an outcome somewhat similar to that reported by Spilich (1983). That is, age-related deficits in recall were far more

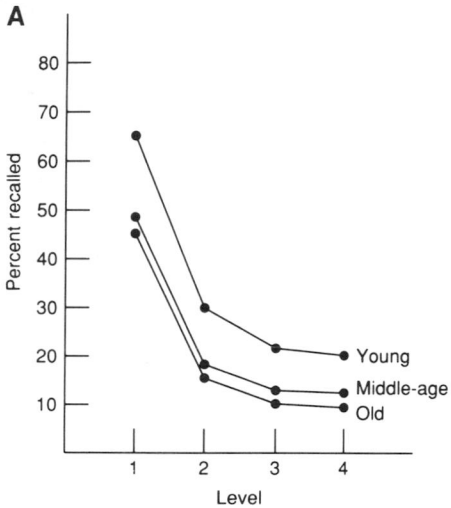

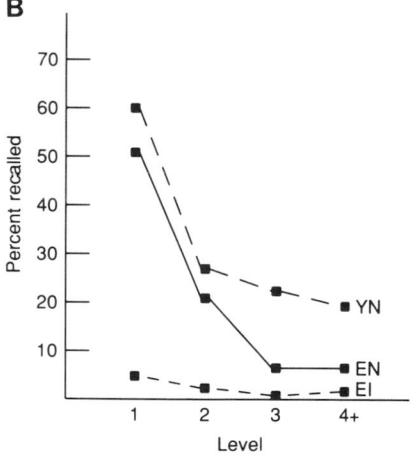

FIGURE 8.6 Age differences in percentages of propositions recalled at different levels in text structure. A: Young, middle-aged, and elderly subjects. (Adapted from Dixon, Simon, Nowak, & Hultsch, 1982, Figure 2.) B: Young normal (YN), elderly normal (EN), and elderly memory impaired (EI). (Adapted from Spilich, 1983, Figure 1.)

pronounced for lower-order propositions than for higher-order propositions. Similar results were obtained by Stine and Wingfield (1987b) for the propositions in single paragraphs (see Figure 8.3).

On the other hand, Zelinski et al. (1984) reported an outcome similar to that reported by Dixon et al. (1982)—that is, the age-related deficit was about the same at each propositional level. Added to the ambiguity of the results of these various studies is the peculiar pattern obtained by Byrd (1985). When subjects were asked to recall verbatim the content of a passage, the age-related deficit was greater for lower order propositions than for higher order propositions. However, when asked simply to summarize the content, the reverse outcome was found, that is, the deficit was greater for higher order than for lower order propositions.

Stine and Wingfield (1988) have suggested that the conventional propositional levels form of analysis may not be sensitive enough to detect age differences in the abstraction and integration of information within discourse. They proposed an alternative form of analysis, a relative memorability analysis, in which the probability of propositional recall for elderly subjects is determined as a function of the probability of recall by young subjects for the same propositions. However, it is difficult to believe that a standard propositional analysis is not sensitive to age differences. Age differences have been found in nearly every study using this form of analysis. The problem is in the different patterns of results obtained by different investigators. Of course, the means of presenting the discourse to subjects has varied greatly in these studies, as has the length and type of material presented. Conceivably, these are important variables that might affect the locus (i.e., propositional level) and the extent of age differences in discourse memory and contribute to our understanding of the reasons for age-related deficits in discourse memory. We will turn to these variables shortly.

Qualitative and Quantitative Age Differences in Discourse Memory

Recall of stories and other longer discourses often contain elaborations that were not in the original discourse. Elaborations may be either denotative or annotative. A denotative elaboration is one that is closely related to the content of the discourse and serves to fill in gaps within the discourse. An annotative elaboration is one that consists of evaluative and interpretive comments, often about the recaller's personal experiences. Gould, Trevithick, and Dixon (1991) found that denotative elaborations during recall of a story were produced equally by young adult and elderly subjects. Moreover, for both age groups, the number of these elaborations correlated significantly with gist recall. Significantly more annotative elaborations were produced by the elderly subjects than by the young subjects. For neither age group was the number of these elaborations correlated with gist recall. More annotative elaborations were also given by the elderly subjects than by the young adult subjects in Adams's (1991) study. This was the case for both a story and an essay, but especially so for the story. (See Stine and Wingfield, 1990, for a discussion of the assessment of qualitative age differences in the processing of discourse.)

Other qualitative changes in discourse memory are expected from the perspective of a life span developmental psychology (Labouvie, 1986; Labouvie-Vief & Blanchard-Fields, 1982; Labouvie-Vief & Schell, 1982; Mergler & Goldstein, 1983). From this perspective, what is encoded from discourse is information that has adaptive significance for the individual concerned. However, what is adaptive differs between younger and older adults. A primary cognitive task for younger adults is to acquire information and knowledge about their culture. Their focus during the encoding of discourse is therefore on the propositions it contains. Older adults, however, often have a different focus. Their interest may be more in the moral implications of the information they receive than in the propositional content of that information. Consequently, propositions are likely to be transformed into such forms as metaphors and morals. Evidence in support of this perspective comes from a study by Labouvie-Vief, Schell, and Weaverdyck (1982) in which subjects were asked to recall a fable either in detail or in summary form. In both conditions, the young adult subjects produced nearly verbatim reproductions of the fable's propositional content. When asked to recall in detail, the recall statements of the elderly subjects were much like those of the young subjects. However, when asked to summarize the fable, the recall protocols for many elderly subjects contained numerous statements about the moral meaning of the fable. By contrast, Adams, Labouvie-Vief, & Dorosz (1990) found that the fable recall protocols of their elderly subjects did not differ from those of their younger subjects. They discovered further the absence of an age-related deficit in the amount recalled from a fable (but a significant deficit for the amount recalled from a nonfable narrative).

Interestingly, Jackson and Kemper (1993) discovered that summary statements of expository texts were more succinct for their elderly subjects than for their young subjects. The elderly subjects needed only one sentence per central idea while the young subjects needed two or more. This finding contrasts with the usual picture of elderly adults being more verbose than young adults (Boden & Bielby, 1983; Gold, Andres, Arbuckle, & Schwartzman, 1988; Gould & Dixon, 1993; Pratt, Boyes, Robins, & Manchester, 1989) Greater verbosity for elderly adults has been reported in various situations, such as in normal conversations, in formal interviews, and in telling stories about personal experiences.

Procedural Variables

Procedural variables include the modality of presentation of the textual material, the rate of presentation of the material, and the orientation of the subjects to the material. G. Cohen's (1979) and Petros et al.'s (1989) subjects listened to their passages, Meyer et al.'s (1979) subjects read their passage, and Dixon et al.'s (1982) subjects either read or listened to their passage. As noted earlier, older subjects are especially likely to benefit from reading material relative to listening to material. Again, self-paced reading permits subjects to refer back to earlier content while they attempt to comprehend present content. However, conflicting results have been obtained between studies even when they have employed the same modality (e.g., contrast the outcomes for propositional recall in Cohen's (1979) study and Petros et al.'s (1989) study, even though material was presented aurally in each study). Petros et al. (1989) presented materials auditorily at different rates. Their young adult subjects recalled more with a slow rate (120 wpm) than with a fast rate (200 wpm), whereas their elderly subjects recalled no more with a slow rate than with a fast rate. Consequently, the magnitude of the age-related deficit in recall was actually greater with the slow rate than with the fast rate. This is somewhat surprising in that one would expect the slow rate to be especially beneficial for older subjects. By contrast, Riggs, Wingfield, and Tun (1993) found the expected outcome—the faster the rate, the greater the age-related deficit in memory as measured by free recall, cued recall, and a multiple-choice recognition test.

May, Hasher, and Stoltzfus (1993) discovered that the time of day in which subjects are tested greatly influences the magnitude of age differences in recognition memory of sentence content from a story. Pronounced age-related deficits were found when all subjects were tested in the late afternoon, but age differences were negligible when all subjects were tested in the morning. Elderly subjects appear to be more cognitively alert in the morning than later in the day, while young adults are at their best later in the day. This finding is important in that the majority of gerontological researchers test their subjects in the afternoon, and they may therefore overestimate the magnitudes of age-related deficits on memory tasks.

An especially important procedural variable would seem to be one that permits comparison of age differences under intentional- and incidental-memory conditions. In their study, E. W. Simon, Dixon, Nowak, and Hultsch (1982) obtained a strange outcome. Their young, middle-aged, and elderly incidental-memory subjects performed with three different orienting tasks during the presentation of a lengthy narrative passage. One of the tasks (making syntactic judgments) prompted shallow processing, whereas the other two tasks (making stylistic judgments and preparing to give advice based on the content of the passage) prompted deep processing. Other subjects at each age level received standard intentional-memory instructions. The young subjects recalled well under both deep-processing incidental-memory and intentional-memory conditions, but not under shallow-processing conditions, as might be expected. The two older groups, however, surprisingly recalled no more under deep-processing conditions than under shallow-processing conditions. Most surprisingly, if anything, the older groups recalled more under intentional-memory conditions than did the young subjects. Intentional-memory conditions have been employed in other studies that have usually found pronounced age-related deficits in the percentage of propositions recalled. A very different outcome was obtained by Arbuckle and Harsany (1985). The passage was one that described a moral dilemma. Young adult and elderly subjects in their intentional-memory condition were asked to listen to the passage and then recall as many of the main ideas and details as possible. Subjects in the incidental-memory condition were asked to listen to the passage in order to find alternative solutions to the dilemma described in it, without mention of the subsequent recall test. The elderly subjects recalled less verbatim information from the passage than did the young subjects. Most important, the amount of recall was greater for both age groups in the intentional-memory condition than in the incidental-memory condition, with a nonsignificant Age × Condition interaction effect.

The elderly adults in the incidental condition of Arbuckle and Harsany's (1985) study did recall a considerable amount of information, albeit less than elderly adults in the intentional condition. By contrast, Simon et al.'s (1982) elderly subjects recalled very little incidentally even though they were given a deep-processing orienting task comparable to that employed in Arbuckle and Harsany's (1985) incidental-memory condition. Clearly, this is an area of research that needs further investigation, given the likelihood that much of our everyday memory for discourse does occur under incidental-memory conditions.

An intriguing additional procedural variable was introduced in a study by McDaniel, Ryan, and Cunningham (1989). The objective of their study was to demonstrate a generation effect comparable to that found in word memory studies (see Chapter 7, p. 245). Some words in a passage had several letters deleted. Consequently, subjects had to generate these words. Ideas that were conveyed by sentences containing generated words were recalled better than ideas conveyed by sentences in which all of the words were intact. The generation effect was present for both young subjects (high school students) and elderly subjects. That is, recall was significantly greater for "deleted" ideas than for "intact" ideas. However, the magnitude of the age-related deficit in recall was as pronounced in the deleted condition as in the intact condition. Luszcz (1993), in one of her three conditions, also employed texts in which letters were deleted from some words. Subjects in another condition received the same sentences but the order of the words in each sentence was scrambled. The remaining subjects were in a control condition in which the sentences were in a normal typed form. The deletion and scrambled-order conditions were intended to facilitate item-information and relational information processing, respectively (McDaniel, Einstein, Dunay, & Cobb, 1986). Memory for textual material, like memory for catagorizable word lists, seemingly requires both forms of processing (see Chapter 7, p. 235). As may be seen in Figure 8.7, age-related deficits in recall occurred for expository texts in

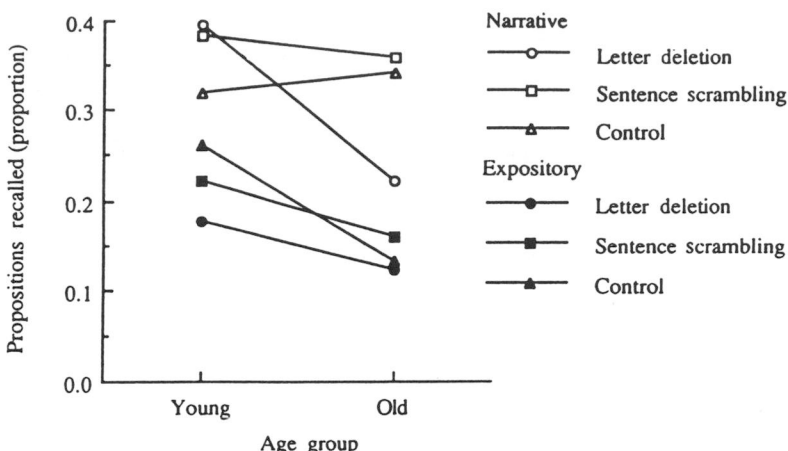

FIGURE 8.7 Recall of text under letter deletion, scrambled order, and control conditions during study. (Reprinted from Luszcz, 1993. Figure 1. Copyright 1993 by the American Psychological Association.)

all three conditions and in about equivalent amounts across conditions. However, with narrative texts, an age-related deficit was found only for the letter deletion condition. Luszcz (1993) concluded that focusing on item-information processing limits relational processing on narrative texts for elderly adults, but not for young adults, presumably due to the age difference in available processing resources. All of Luszcz's (1993) subjects performed under incidental-memory conditions. Of further interest would be the extent to which item-information and relational processing affects age differences in recall relative to the age difference for the same material studied under intentional-memory conditions and without an orienting task to perform.

Attributes of the Discourse

An important attribute of the discourse material itself is its genre, that is, whether it is narrative (describes actions and events that are related and occur over time; i.e., the text tells a story) or expository (describes actors or events in general terms; e.g., an encyclopedia article). The structure of a narrative text is more cohesive than that of an expository text. The cohesive structure should make processing of content easier, and it should therefore promote better memory. Research with young adult subjects only (e.g., Britton, Graesser, Glynn, Hamilton, & Penland, 1983) has frequently demonstrated higher levels of recall for narrative texts than for expository texts. Age-related deficits in recall have often been found to be greater with expository texts (e.g., Dixon et al., 1982;

Surber, Kowalski, & Pena-Paez, 1984) than with narrative texts (e.g., Mandel & Johnson, 1984; Smith, Rebok, Smith, Hall, & Alvin, 1983). However, for some forms of expository text, elderly subjects have been found to recall more central propositions than young adult subjects. This was the case for both the procedural expository texts (describing a sequence of steps needed to construct or prepare an object) and the descriptive expository texts (giving historical information about a topic) employed by Jackson and Kemper (1993). Their elderly subjects recalled nearly twice as many central propositions as did their young subjects and even slightly more noncentral propositions as well. Several studies have compared performances for the same groups of young and elderly subjects on both narrative and expository texts. However, the results have not been very satisfying. Both J. T. Hartley (1986) and Tun (1989) found that genre had little effect on the age-related deficit in recall, whereas Petros et al. (1989) and Luszcz (1993) found that the deficit was less for narrative texts than for expository texts. In fact, in her control condition, Luszcz (1903) found her elderly subjects to recall slightly more propositions than her young subjects. In addition, both Tun (1989) and Petros et al. (1989) found the interaction among age, genre, and propositional level to be negligible. That is, the age difference in differential recall of high- and low-level propositions was similar for narrative and expository texts.

As noted earlier (p. 289), alteration of text structure has been found to enhance elderly subjects memory for pertinent medical information (e.g., Rice, Meyer, & Miller, 1989). Rice et al. (1989) accomplished this by assuring that the most important information became main points in the organization of textual material about hypertension and arthritis. Similarly, underlining of particularly relevant information in a text seems to enhance memory for that information by elderly subjects by enabling them to ignore largely more irrelevant information (Taub, 1984; Taub, Sturr, & Monty, 1985). However, it is known that young adults benefit similarly in their text recall from such highlighting (Glynn & Muth, 1979). Consequently, it is unlikely that underlining would serve to reduce markedly the magnitude of age-related deficits in the recall of a text's content.

Prior Knowledge

Another important task attribute is the extent to which a discourse taps prior factual knowledge and therefore enhances both the comprehension and the ease of encoding its content. We know from free-recall research that preexperimental knowledge benefits recall for both young and elderly subjects. For example, Bäckman, Herlitz, and Karlsson (1987) found that elderly adult subjects recalled more famous names in a free-recall list when the names were "old" ones (i.e., people famous during the 1930s) than when they were new ones (i.e., people famous during the 1980s), presumably because of their greater knowledge of the older names. The reverse was true for their young adult subjects. A similar effect occurs

for discourse memory. Hultsch and Dixon (1983) demonstrated that elderly subjects recalled more of passages that were biographies of famous people with whom
they were very familiar than of passages about other famous people with whom
they were not familiar. However, Arbuckle, Vanderleck, Harsany, and Lapidus
(1990) found preexperimental knowledge to be no more effective in enhancing
text memory for elderly subjects than for young adult subjects.

There is another less obvious way in which generic knowledge may interact
with new episodic information. It is through the utilization of what memory
theorists call scripts (Schank & Abelson, 1977) and (see Hess, 1990, for further
review). As we discovered in Chapter 7 (p. 259), a script is a representation in
generic memory of a stereotyped activity, such as going to an Italian restaurant.
We expect this activity to include reading the menu, ordering an Italian special-
ity, and paying the bill. In a passage about someone going to eat at an Italian
restaurant, we would expect to encounter these typical actions. We wouldn't
expect to encounter, however, someone ordering sauerbraten. Basic research has
revealed that young adults have a high hit rate for typical actions when they are
contained in a passage and a high false alarm rate when they are not. They also
have a high hit rate for atypical actions when they are contained in the passage
and a low false alarm rate when they are not (e.g., Graesser, Woll, Kowalski, &
Smith, 1980). Presumably, older adults rely more on generic information than do
young adults while encoding episodic events that are relevant to scripted actions.
Consequently, relative to younger subjects, elderly subjects are expected to have
a higher hit rate for recognizing old typical actions as old, a higher false alarm
rate for recognizing new typical actions as old, and a lower hit rate for recognizing
old atypical actions as old. However, the false alarm rate for recognizing new
atypical actions as old should be negligible for both age groups.

Light and Anderson (1983) presented their young adult and elderly subjects
with passages that contained both typical and atypical actions. Their elderly
subjects displayed the same basic pattern of hits and false alarms for typical and
atypical actions as did their young subjects (see Figure 8.8). Note, for example,
for both age groups the high false alarm rate for typical actions and the low false
alarm rate for atypical actions that were not embedded in the passage. Contrary
to our expectations, however, the elderly subjects had a lower hit rate than the
young subjects for typical actions, and the age difference in hit rates for atypical
actions was negligible. Overall recognition memory scores (d' scores) were significantly higher for the young subjects. Other investigators (Hess, 1985; Hess,
Vandermaas, Donley, & Snyder, 1987; Reder, Wible, & Martin, 1986; Zelinski &
Miura, 1988) have reported somewhat different outcomes, but outcomes also
contrary to our predictions based on the principle that elderly subjects would rely
more on generic scripted information than would young subjects. For example,
in Hess's (1985) study, the false alarm rate for atypical actions was much higher
(.18) for his elderly subjects than for his young subjects (.07). Zelinski and Miura

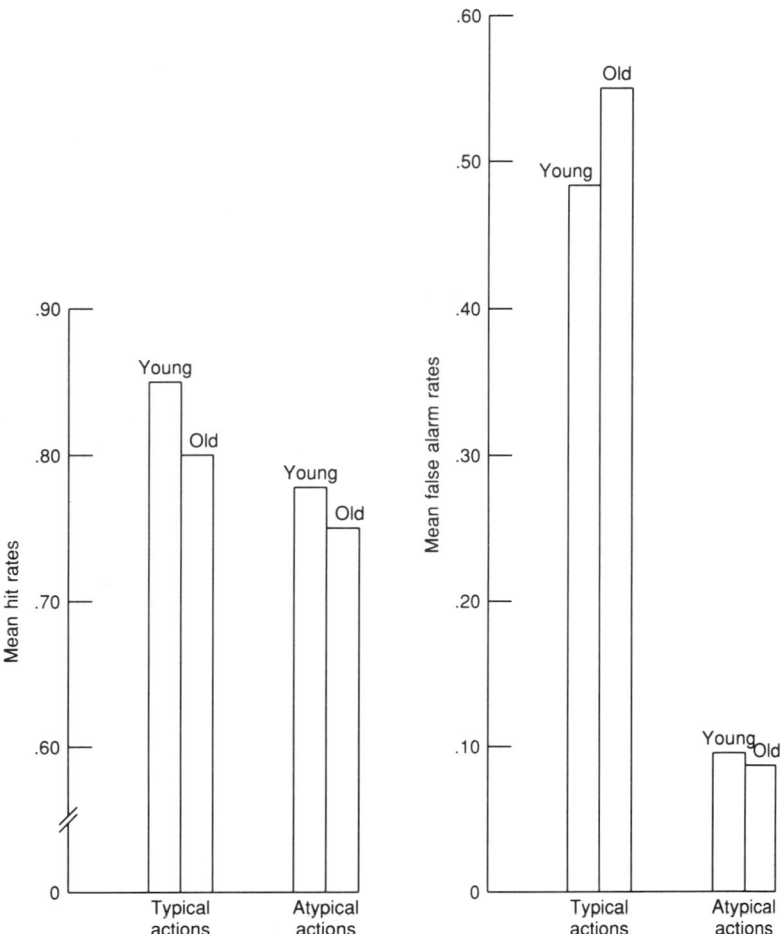

FIGURE 8.8   Age differences in hit rates and false alarm rates for recognition of typical and atypical scripted actions. (Adapted from Light & Anderson, 1983, Table 4.)

(1988) did discover, however, that elderly subjects were as capable as young subjects in utilizing background thematic information to integrate what would otherwise be atypical actions (i.e., atypical in the absence of the background information) into their episodic encodings of a passage. In addition, Hess, Donley, and Vandermaas (1989) found the magnitude of the age-related deficit in both recall and recognition to be less for typical actions than for atypical actions, an outcome that is suggestive of a greater dependency on scripts for elderly adults than for young adults in the encoding of scripted events.

A schema is another knowledge-based system that exists in an individual's generic memory (Brewer & Nakamura, 1984). The system consists of world knowledge other than that of scripted actions. The role played by a preexisting schema was nicely described by Hess and Flannagan:

> There is much evidence that memory for prose is partly determined by the conceptual relationship between the to-be-remembered information and those cognitive structures (e.g., schemas) activated during both encoding and retrieval. With respect to encoding, the speed with which information is processed and the manner in which it is represented in memory are influenced by expectations based on the individual's schematic knowledge" (c.f., Brewer & Nakamura, 1984), 1992, p. 52).

For example, one may have a schema about houses that would provide information on what to look for when shopping for a new home. The existence of that schema could influence what information is encoded when reading a text that includes information about a house. Hess and Flannagan (1992) reasoned that age differences in discourse memory should decrease as the relevance and consistency of the to-be-remembered information in the discourse to schema-based knowledge increases. In other words, as with scripts, elderly adults are expected to be more dependent on schema for encoding and retrieving new information than are young adults and are therefore expected to gain a greater benefit when a schema is highly relevant to the content of a new discourse. However, Hess and Flannagan's (1992) study provided little support for this position. That is, young adult and elderly adult subjects were found to be very similar in dependence on schema-driven encoding and retrieval processes.

Our concern thus far has been with what may be considered to be schema involving general knowledge (e.g., knowledge about houses). Such schema are likely to be possessed to some degree by adults of all ages. Of further concern are schema for specific knowledge domains that are possessed by experts in such areas as biology, medicine, physics, psychology, and so on. We would surely expect an expert in experimental psychology to comprehend and recall more information from an article in the technical journal *Memory & Cognition* than a layman or even a clinical psychologist. To what extent does expertise compensate for age-related declines in discourse memory? Relevant to this issue is a study by Morrow, Leirer, and Altieri (1992). They compared younger (late 20s and early 30s and older (mid and late 60s) pilots and nonpilots on their recall of both aviation-related and nonaviation-related narrative discourses. The percentages of propositions recalled for the aviation-related discourse were 26% for the younger pilots, 18% for the older pilots, 20% for the younger nonpilots, and 12% for the older nonpilots. Comparable percentages for the nonaviation-related discourse were 21%, 16%, 20%, and 14%. Note that expertise enhanced memory for the older pilots on the relevant material relative to the irrelevant material. Nevertheless,

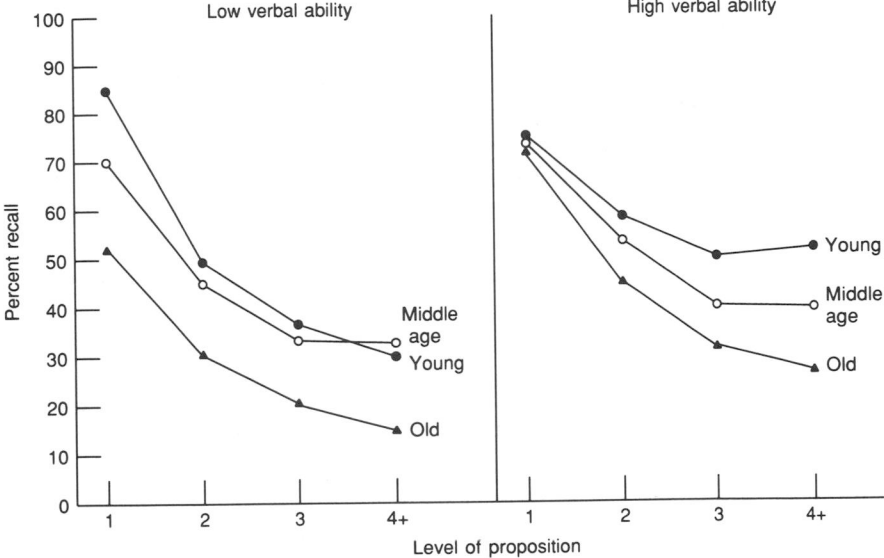

FIGURE 8.9   Percentage recall as a function of age, verbal ability, and level of proposition. (Adapted from Dixon, Hultsch, Simon, & Von Eye, 1984, Figure 1.)

the age-related deficit in memory was as large for the relevant material as it was for the irrelevant material.

Individual Differences Variables

Collectively, studies that have manipulated procedural and content variables have yielded relatively little in furthering our understanding of age differences in memory for longer discourses. Far more promising have been those studies that have examined the effects of individual differences variables on age differences in discourse memory (see J. T. Hartley, 1989, and Meyer and Rice, 1989, for further review). Foremost among these variables has been verbal ability as assessed by a vocabulary test. B. J. F. Meyer and Rice (1983) found age-related deficits in recall scores to be greater for low verbal ability subjects than for high verbal ability subjects. Although Rice and Meyer (1986) found a significant age-related deficit in text recall, they also found verbal ability to be a better predictor of recall than age per se. Especially intriguing are the results obtained by Dixon, Hultsch, Simon, and Von Eye (1984). They analyzed the interaction between verbal ability and propositional level for young adult, middle-aged, and elderly subjects. As may be seen in Figure 8.9, there was indeed a significant interaction. Low verbal ability elderly subjects clearly recalled fewer propositions than younger low verbal ability subjects at all propositional levels, but the age-related deficit was greatest for the highest order propositions. By contrast, high verbal ability elderly subjects were equivalent to high verbal ability younger subjects in recall of high order propositions. Age-related deficits for these elderly subjects were present only for lower order propositions, and the magnitude of the deficit increased as the thematic significance of the propositions decreased. Most important, it may be seen in Figure 8.9 that high verbal ability elderly subjects were as proficient in recall at all propositional levels as lesser ability younger subjects. Conceivably, many of the conflicting results on the interaction between age and propositional level in recall reviewed earlier may have resulted from differences among studies in the verbal abilities of the subjects entering into those studies. It is also conceivable that differences among these studies in the overall intelligence of the subjects entering into them accounts in part for the conflicting results. Hultsch, Hertzog, and Dixon (1984) found that age-related deficits in recall of a narrative text were greatly attenuated (but not eliminated) when recall scores were adjusted for individual differences in intelligence. Holland and Rabbitt (1990, 1992) discovered further that less intelligent older adults differed from more intelligent older adults in the amount of detail recalled from a text, but not in the recall of main points in the text.

Individual differences in other cognitive variables have been examined in studies by Hultsch and his colleagues (e.g., Hultsch, Hertzog, & Dixon, 1984; Hultsch, Hertzog, & Dixon, 1990). Especially impressive results were obtained in Hultsch et al.'s (1990) study. Individual differences in verbal speed (e.g., as assessed by reaction times on a lexical decision task) and working memory (e.g., as assessed by scores on a sentence construction task similar to the reading-span task of Daneman and Carpenter (1980; see Chapter 6, p. 215) accounted for a large segment of age differences in text recall scores. J. T. Hartley (1986) also found a large segment of age differences in text recall to be accounted for by individual differences in both simple abilities (e.g., verbal speed) and complex abilities (e.g., reading comprehension). An even more complex mental ability, reasoning (e.g., as measured by tests of inductive reasoning), accounted for another fairly large segment of the individual differences in text recall for subjects ranging in age from 55 to 84 yr (Zelinski, Gilewski, & Schaie, 1993).

A different kind of variable, namely student status, was discussed briefly in Chapter 6 (pp. 226–227). There we discovered evidence suggesting both its importance in determining age differences in text recall (Ratner et al., 1987) and its lack of importance (J. T. Hartley, 1986). The role played by current degree of mental activity (as exemplified, for example, by student status) in determining age differences in discourse memory remains poorly understood, and a topic that should receive considerable future attention.

Not surprisingly, the individual difference variable of greatest interest in current aging research on discourse memory is undoubtedly that of working-memory capacity (see G. Cohen, 1988, and Kemper, 1988, for further review). Hultsch et al. (1990) were able to find a large proportion of age differences in discourse memory for long texts to be accounted for by individual differences in working-memory capacity as measured psychometrically (see also Tun, Wingfield, Stine, and Mecaas, 1992). We discovered in Chapter 6 that Stine and Wingfield (1987a) had comparable success with age differences in memory for shorter passages (paragraphs). We also discovered there that other investigators (e.g., Light & Anderson, 1985) have been less successful, but that their measure of working-memory capacity was probably inadequate. In addition, an age-related decline in working capacity, as measured psychometrically, has been found to be correlated with age-related declines in comprehension of discourse on a limited-time reading test and with reading rate on an unlimited-time reading test (Norman, Kemper & Kynette, 1992; Norman, Kemper, Kynette, Cheung, & Anagnopoulus, 1991).

CHAPTER 9

Long-Term Episodic Memory: Automaticity and Rehearsal Independence

Introduction

Research on age differences in episodic memory began to move in an exciting new direction following the distinction made by Hasher and Zacks (1979, 1984) between effortful and automatic encoding processes. We discovered in Chapter 6 (p. 212) that automatic encoding processes are presumably unaffected by an individual's limited cognitive resources. The usual position is that they function independently of working memory's limited capacity (see Figure 6.16). According to Hasher and Zacks, "Automatic processes function at optimal levels, continuously and independently of intention . . . and these processes require only that the event be attended to. . . . The information encoded in this way is no different than it is when intention is activated" (1984, p. 1373). From this perspective, automatic forms of episodic memory should be *rehearsal independent* in the sense that rehearsal activity initiated by the intent to memorize should have little effect on subsequent memorability (Kausler & Lichty, 1988). By contrast, cognitively effortful forms of memory, as represented by traditional free-recall tasks, are *rehearsal dependent.* That is, memory performance is dependent on the quality and/ or quantity of the rehearsal the to-be-remembered events receive. When translated to laboratory conditions, rehearsal independency means that memory performances should be no better under incidental-memory conditions than under intentional-memory conditions. The null effect for intentionality is, in fact, a primary criterion for determining whether or not memory for specific kinds of events is truly automatic. Hasher and Zacks (1979) reasoned that automaticity of encoding occurs for information that is essential for maintaining continuity with the everyday world. Presumably, automaticity is ensured either by being innately programmed in the human organism or by being the end product of years of frequent practice during childhood (Hasher & Zacks, 1979).

Rehearsal independency is only one of the phenomena identified by Hasher and Zacks (1979, 1984) as being characteristic of automatic memory. The phenomenon of greatest concern to us is that of the expected absence of age effects on the proficiency of automatic memory. The automatic encoding of episodic events bypasses the limitations of working memory's capacity, and should therefore be unaffected by its diminished capacity in late adulthood. A form of memory supposedly unaffected by normal aging—no wonder automaticity became a focal point of aging memory research in the past twelve or so years! What kinds of episodic information are suspected of being encoded automatically? In general, they have been noncontent attributes of episodic events (Underwood, 1969). The prototype of automaticity for Hasher and Zacks (1979, 1984) is the encoding of the frequency with which specific events occur. However, the possibility that many other noncontent attributes (e.g., their temporal sequencing, their spatial location) are also encoded automatically has received widespread investigation, much of it conducted in gerontological laboratories.

Adult Age Differences in Memory for Noncontent Attributes of Episodic Events

Frequency-of-Occurrence Memory

Which commercials on television did you encounter more often in the past month, those for a particular brand of athletic shoes or those for a particular brand of beer? You probably have reasonable accuracy in judging one to have occurred more frequently than the other. Our attention to the content of events does seem to assure some degree of registration of the frequency with which they occur, presumably because each occurrence registers a separate memory trace in the long-term store (LTS) (Hintzman & Block, 1971; Hintzman & Stern, 1978). Your judgment about the shoe and beer commercials would undoubtedly be based on your incidental memory of their frequencies. But according to automaticity theory, your accuracy probably wouldn't be any greater if you had intended to memorize the frequency information. Nor should it be any less accurate if you are an average elderly adult than if you are an average young adult (or a child— children usually are as accurate in frequency judgments as are young adults; Hasher & Chromiak, 1977). Laboratory tests of the predictions derived from automaticity theory have to find substitutes for the kinds of events that vary in their everyday frequencies. The usual procedure is to present a lengthy series of words qua episodic events, with some of the words being seen once, some three times, some five times, and so on. Subjects performing under intentional-memory conditions are told in advance that they will subsequently be tested for their memory of the frequency with which the words occurred; subjects performing under incidental-memory conditions are usually told only that they will receive a later memory test, without identifying the nature of the test. The test itself may take various forms. For example, subjects may be asked to estimate for each word how often it occurred in the list (an absolute frequency-judgment test), or they may be given pairs of prior items and asked to judge for each pair which member had occurred more often (a relative frequency judgment test).

In recent years there has been an eroding of confidence in the true automaticity of frequency-of-occurrence memory. A number of basic researchers have discovered that several of the criteria established by Hasher and Zacks (1979) to define automaticity do not hold up well in the laboratory (e.g., Greene, 1984; Jonides & Naveh-Benjamin, 1987; Maki & Ostby, 1987; Naveh-Benjamin & Jonides, 1986; Sanders, Gonzalez, Murphy, Liddle, & Vitina, 1987). For example, evidence has emerged to indicate that intentionality can improve the accuracy of frequency judgments (Greene, 1984; Kausler, Wright, & Hakami, 1981; Naveh-Benjamin & Jonides, 1986; Sanders et al., 1987), that practice effects for accuracy of frequency judgments are present when subjects receive a series of lists (but in the direction of decreasing performance scores over successive lists; Greene, 1989c), and that subjects are adversely affected in accuracy of frequency judgments while performing under dual-task conditions (Kausler et al., 1981; Naveh-Benjamin & Jonides, 1986; Sanders et al., 1987). Each of these outcomes conflicts with one of the criteria for automaticity established originally by Hasher and Zacks (1979). What is surprising is that it took so long before the erosion began. It was known for some years before the advent of automaticity theory that variation in the depth of processing of study-list items produced by different orienting tasks affects the accuracy of frequency judgments (e.g., Rowe, 1974). This shouldn't be the case if frequency information is fully automatically encoded. However, confidence in the immunity of frequency-of-occurrence memory proficiency to major decrements from early to late adulthood has had little reason to erode, although the moderate age-related deficit consistently found on frequency-judgment tests does add to our doubts that the encoding of frequency information is always fully automatic (see Kausler, 1990b, for an extensive review).

Early studies on age differences in frequency-judgment test scores generally revealed either a statistically nonsignificant effect for age variation when a relative frequency-judgment test was used (Attig & Hasher, 1980; Kausler & Puckett, 1980a) or a modest age difference when an absolute judgment test was used (Attig & Hasher, 1979; Freund & Witte, 1978; Warren & Mitchell, 1980). Illustrative of these modest age differences with an absolute test are those reported by Freund and Witte (1978). The tested items had occurred either zero, one, two, three, or five times in the study list. Their results, expressed as mean judged frequencies as a function of actual frequency, are plotted in Figure 9.1 (perfect accuracy is indicated by the straight line). Note the absence of age differences for words with

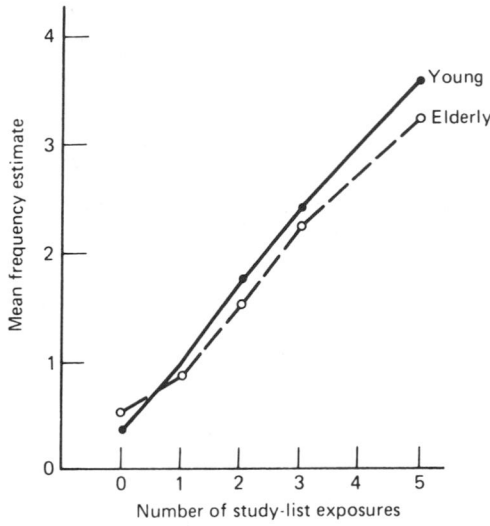

FIGURE 9.1 Age differences in absolute frequency judgment scores as a function of number of study-list exposures. (Adapted from Freund & Witte, 1978, Figure 1.)

low frequencies of occurrence, and the presence of only slight age differences for words with higher frequencies.

However, it is true that statistically significant age differences have been found in some studies even with a relative judgment test (e.g., Freund & Witte, 1986). Moreover, they have also been found under conditions which seem truly to involve incidental memory. The incidental-memory condition usually employed in frequency-judgment research is not, strictly speaking, incidental. Subjects are told to expect a memory test, even if they don't know what kind it will be. Conceivably, there is an age differential in the extent to which items are rehearsed under such conditions, sufficiently so to mask any age difference in the proficiency of frequency-of-occurrence memory. To avoid this problem, subjects need to encounter the to-be-tested words without any awareness of a forthcoming memory test. This was accomplished in a study by Kausler, Lichty, and Hakami (1984) through the use of a modified Brown-Peterson task introduced by Glenberg, Smith, and Green (1977). The to-be-remembered items are strings of digits, and the distracting task during the short-term retention intervals consists of pronouncing words. Over a number of trials, these words in Kausler et al.'s (1984) study varied in their frequencies of appearing in the distractor activity. At the end of the digit recall trials, all of the subjects were given a surprise relative frequency-judgment test for the previously encountered words. Although the age difference in test scores favoring young adults attained statistical significance in each of two experiments, it was, nevertheless, rather moderate in amount (about 8% in one experiment, and about 9% in the other). In a later study, Sanders, Wise, Liddle, and Murphy (1990) also avoided the problem created by standard incidental-memory conditions by having their subjects perform on a cover task (a word-searching task) that nicely disguised the frequency variation and the eventual administration of a memory test. This time the age difference failed to attain statistical significance. In fact, if anything, their elderly subjects scored slightly higher on a relative frequency-judgment test than did their young adult subjects. The studies cited thus far have all involved words as the episodic events varying in frequency. In a later section we will consider adult age differences in frequency-of-occurrence memory for another kind of episodic event, namely activities and actions performed in the laboratory.

It seems reasonable to conclude that there probably is a slight decrement in frequency-memory proficiency from early to late adulthood, but that the decrement is so slight that it will be detected in some small sample studies (e.g., Kausler et al., 1984), but not in others (e.g., Ellis, Palmer, & Reeves, 1988; Ozekes & Gilleard, 1989). This conclusion is based on the large sample study by Salthouse et al. (1988a) discussed in earlier chapters. One of the many tasks their subjects received was a relative frequency-judgment task. Shown in Figure 9.2 are mean scores for their 40–59 yr-old and their 60–79 yr-old subjects expressed as a percentage of loss relative to the mean score obtained by subjects in the 20–39 age range (see Kausler, Salthouse, and Saults, 1987, for additional analyses of these scores). The overall age difference in scores was statistically significant, but note

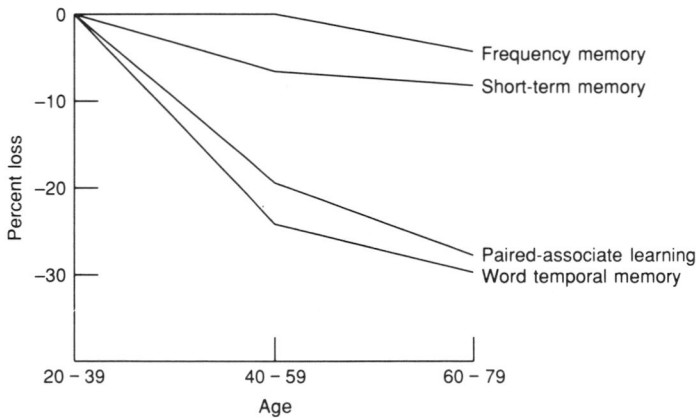

FIGURE 9.2 Percent loss for middle-aged and elderly subjects on several tasks, expressed relative to the scores of younger subjects. (Adapted from Salthouse, Kausler, & Saults, 1988a, Table 1.)

the absence of any decline by middle age, and the presence of only a 5% decline by late adulthood. For comparison sake, loss scores for three other tasks included in their study are also included in Figure 9.2. The age-related decrement for frequency memory may be seen to be even less than that found for a short-term memory task, and certainly far less than that found for either a temporal memory task or a paired-associate learning task. The modest decline could be attributable either to a slight age-related decline in the proficiency of the automatic encoding of frequency information or to an age-related decline in the retrieval of the multiple traces entering into frequency judgments. The theory of Hasher and Zacks (1979) stipulates only that the encoding of frequency information is automatic. Retrieval of that information is an effortful process, even on a relative frequency-judgment test. It may be only an age-sensitive retrieval process that accounts for the modest age sensitivity of frequency-of-occurrence memory.

Elderly adults may actually be as proficient as young adults in memory for frequency information when only truly automatic encoding processes are involved. Sanders et al. (1990) proposed what they call a nonoptimal model for frequency memory. According to this model, the encoding of frequency information requires only minimal effort, and little of working memory's capacity, to occur and to produce memory scores above chance values. When task conditions are such that only these automatic processes are activated, age differences in frequency-memory test scores are expected to be negligible. The task conditions employed in their own study (incidental memory, a word-searching cover task) presumably activates only age insensitive automatic processes. As noted earlier, they did find a negligible aging effect. The model also stresses the involvement of effortful encoding processes under various conditions, such as intentional-memory conditions, that may embellish the amount of information encoded and be utilized to enhance the accuracy of frequency judgments. For example, deeper processing of item information is likely under intentional-memory conditions, conceivably resulting in more durable multiple-memory traces of the items than would be possible with the shallow processing occurring under truly incidental memory conditions. These additional processes are effortful and therefore susceptible to the constraints placed on them by working memory's limited capacity, a capacity assumed to diminish with aging. Consequently, age-related deficits in performance may (but not necessarily) be the result (see Kausler, 1990b, for an extended discussion).

In the everyday world, our knowledge about frequencies of occurrence often pertains to categorical knowledge rather than to knowledge about discrete events. For example, you may be asked if you have seen more comedies or more dramas this year on television. Here the discrete events (individual comedies or individual dramas) convey frequency information in terms of their roles as instances of superordinates, with the instances themselves not being repeated (unless you watch summer reruns). To simulate this everyday situation, Kausler, Hakami, and

Wright (1982) employed a relative frequency-judgment task in which instances of taxonomic categories were presented with varying frequencies in a study list. For example, there may have been five men's first names, three names of states, and only one name of a religion. Judgments were then made in terms of which category of a pair (e.g., men's names versus state's names) had more representations within the study list. A statistically significant age difference, favoring young adults, in test scores was found, but, as with discrete item judgments, the absolute size of the age-related deficit was relatively slight.

Frequency judgments in the everyday world are also likely to involve judgments about relevant information that was accompanied by potentially distracting irrelevant information. Kausler and Hakami (1982) found a statistically significant age-related deficit in accuracy of frequency judgments for relevant events (words) that varied in their numbers of occurrences and were accompanied by irrelevant events (also words). Presumably, elderly adults are distracted to a greater degree than are young adults by simultaneously present irrelevant information, and they are therefore even less likely than young adults to engage in the effortful processing of the relevant events (see Chapter 6, p. 207). Interestingly, Kausler and Hakami (1982) also found the absence of an age effect for the accuracy of judging the frequencies of the irrelevant events (i.e., words paired with the relevant words). Presumably, the irrelevant events were encoded only by age-insensitive automatic processes.

Frequency judgments for words that were either generated or read were evaluated by Brown, Niinikoski, and Duke (1993). They found comparable effects for their young adult and elderly subjects. The slope of the line relating judged frequency to actual frequency was greater for generated words than for words that were read. The only significant effect of age resulted from the elderly subjects giving higher frequency estimates overall than did the young subjects.

Temporal Memory

Episodic events obviously take place over time. On Monday you watched a movie, on Tuesday you read a short novel, on Wednesday you played tennis, and so on. At the end of the week, how well do you remember when each of these events occurred? Would you be able to reinstate the order in which they occurred? Did you play tennis before you watched the movie? These questions all apply to your temporal-memory proficiency, that is, your proficiency in remembering the temporal sequencing of a series of episodic events. Hasher and Zacks (1979) postulated that temporal information is essential for maintaining continuity in our everyday lives, and that temporal information is therefore encoded automatically. If so, then temporal memory should satisfy the criteria of automaticity, including those of rehearsal independency and age insensitivity. There is some evidence with young adult subjects to indicate that at least some of these criteria are satisfied. For example, several studies have demonstrated comparable temporal-memory scores under intentional- and incidental-memory conditions (e.g., Azari, Auday, & Cross, 1989; Kausler, Lichty, & Davis, 1985; McCormack, 1981; Toglia & Kimble, 1976). However, other criteria have not been satisfied (e.g., the absence of nonspecific transfer; Zacks, Hasher, Alba, Sanft, & Rose, 1984). Most important, the criterion of greatest concern to us, the absence of age differences in temporal-memory proficiency, has not been satisfied.

To assess temporal-memory proficiency in the laboratory, words again serve as the usual source of episodic events. After the presentation of a series of words, subjects are given a test that calls upon their knowledge of the temporal sequencing of those words. One form of a test consists of presenting pairs of words and asking which member of each pair occurred more recently in the study list. Both McCormack (1982a) and Perlmutter, Metzger, Nezworski, and Miller (1981) employed this test format. McCormack (1982a) found a significant age-related deficit in test scores, whereas Perlmutter et al. (1981) found an absence of a statistically significant age difference. Another test format calls for presenting study-list items individually and asking subjects for each where it occurred in the input sequence (e.g., first tenth of the series, second tenth, and so on). A significant age-related deficit was found with this method by McCormack (1981). In a variation of this procedure, and with picture fragments as the episodic events rather than words, Russo and Parkin (1993) had their subjects identify which of two sequentially presented sets of pictures contained each test picture (i.e., the first or the second set). The percentage of correct temporal discriminations was significantly greater for their young subjects (67%) than for their elderly subjects (53%—a value that did not exceed chance expectancy). Yet another testing format calls for subjects "to keep track" of a series of categorical instances (e.g., instances of flowers, instances of metals, and so on) presented in a lengthy series. The series is interrupted at various points, and subjects are asked questions such as "What was the last *flower* you saw?" Zacks (1982) found her elderly subjects to be far less accurate than her young adult subjects on this temporal monitoring task.

In our opinion, the most sensitive test, and probably the most reliable (e.g., Kausler, Salthouse, and Saults, 1988, reported an interlist reliability coefficient of .55 for their elderly subjects), is one in which subjects are given a list of the previously studied words presented in a random order and they are asked to reconstruct the order in which they appeared. A subject's temporal-memory score is the correlation coefficient between the true order and the reconstructed order. This method was used by Salthouse et al. (1988a; see also Kausler et al., 1988) in their large-scale multipe-task study. Shown in Figure 9.3 are the mean correlation coefficients for their young, middle-aged, and elderly subjects (16 words in the list; intentional memory conditions). Note that a pronounced deficit was already apparent by middle age, with relatively little further deficit by late adulthood.

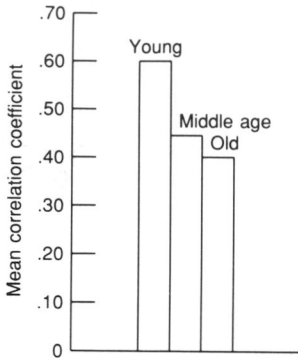

FIGURE 9.3   Mean temporal memory scores (correlations between true and recon-structed orders of words). (Adapted from Salthouse, Kausler, & Saults, 1988a, Table 1.)

This pattern differs greatly from that found with the same subjects for frequency-of-occurrence memory (see p. 310 and Figure 9.2). A very similar age-related deficit with the correlational method was found by Naveh-Benjamin (1990). The mean correlation coefficient for his young adult subjects (college students) was .51; the mean correlation coefficient for his elderly subjects (median age of 70 yr) was .36. His subjects also performed under intentional-memory conditions, with a slightly longer word list (20 words) than the one employed by Salthouse et al. (1988a). From Figure 9.3 it may also be seen that not only is the magnitude of the age-related deficit much greater for temporal memory than for frequency-of-occurrence memory, but also the age period in which the decline begins seems to be much earlier.

There is little question as to the pronounced age sensitivity of temporal memory. As we will discover later in this chapter, large age-related deficits in temporal-memory scores also occur when activities or actions serve as the episodic events rather than words. Why temporal memory is so affected by aging is largely unknown. The basic mechanism underlying temporal memory is itself poorly understood. One possibility is that temporal memory is mediated by the strength of memory traces—the stronger the trace of an episodic event, the more recent the event (Hinrichs, 1970). There are many problems with this model, however. A more popular current view is what is called a study-phase retrieval model or a reminding model (Tzeng & Cotton, 1980; Winograd & Soloway, 1985). According to this model, a second episodic event may remind someone of an earlier event. This reminding then becomes part of the memory of the second event and enables the individual to determine that the second event occurred more recently. How the reminding process enters into the age sensitivity of temporal memory is an unexplored issue. What is known is that frontal lobe dysfunctioning has been linked to temporal-memory impairments in amnesic patients (e.g., Schacter, 1987). Conceivably, the impairments in temporal memory found with normal aging are the consequence of some atrophy of the frontal lobes that occurs in aging.

The age sensitivity of temporal memory undoubtedly has many important implications for the everyday memory performances of elderly adults. It seemingly accounts for the problems many elderly people have in dating both personal events and world events. At a more esoteric level, it also has important implications for explaining age-related deficits in serial learning. Contemporary theories of serial learning often identify memory for temporal order as a component process, along with the availability for recall of the individual items (see Chapter 3, p. 103 and Crowder, 1976). When young adult subjects are tested for the ordinal position of items in a just practiced serial learning list, they are able to identify their positions fairly accurately (except for midlist items) (Schulz, 1955). Awareness of ordinality presumably provides the kind of contextual information that needs to be encoded along with event information in order to make reasonably accurate temporal discriminations among those events (Glenberg & Swanson, 1986). Ordinality and event information are conjointed independent environmental features that seemingly demand effortful encoding processes in order to become components of a common memory trace (Johnson, Peterson, Yap, & Rose, 1989; see Kausler, 1990b, for elaboration). Not surprisingly, the effortful nature of this form of encoding means that elderly adults are less proficient in accomplishing it than are younger adults.

Spatial Memory

"I remember seeing your keys, but I don't remember where in the house it was." The reference is to spatial, or location, memory, memory for another non-content attribute of episodic events that many psychologists at one time believed to be automatically encoded (e.g., Hasher & Zacks, 1979). However, a large amount of evidence from basic research has accumulated in recent years to indicate that spatial memory requires cognitive effort and that it scarcely qualifies for consideration as a form of automatic memory (e.g., Naveh-Benjamin, 1987, 1988). In general, the evidence on age differences in spatial memory is in support of this conclusion. That is, the majority of the evidence indicates that memory for spatial information is age sensitive (see Kirasic & Allen, 1985, and West, 1986, for further review).

Researchers in this area have been highly inventive in the tasks they have used to assess age differences in spatial memory proficiency. Both age differences in short-term memory and long-term memory for spatial information have been investigated.

Age differences in short-term memory for spatial information were tested by Schear and Nebes (1980) and Salthouse et al. (1988a) by means of a matrix of squares exposed briefly. Some of the squares are filled by distinctive markers, and subjects are asked to recall where the markers were located. Schear and Nebes (1980) found an age-related deficit for spatial location, but the deficit was no greater than the one they found for verbal short-term memory. The short-term location memory task was one of the multiple tasks included in Salthouse et al.'s (1988a) study. Subjects were presented a matrix of 25 squares (5 × 5 array), with seven of the squares made visually distinctive for 3 s on each of four trials. A subject's score consisted of the average number of target positions (i.e., the distinctive boxes) correctly recalled across the four trials. Mean recall scores (percent of targets correctly positioned) are shown in Figure 9.4. In contrast to the results obtained by Schear and Nebes (1980), scores on the spatial task were well

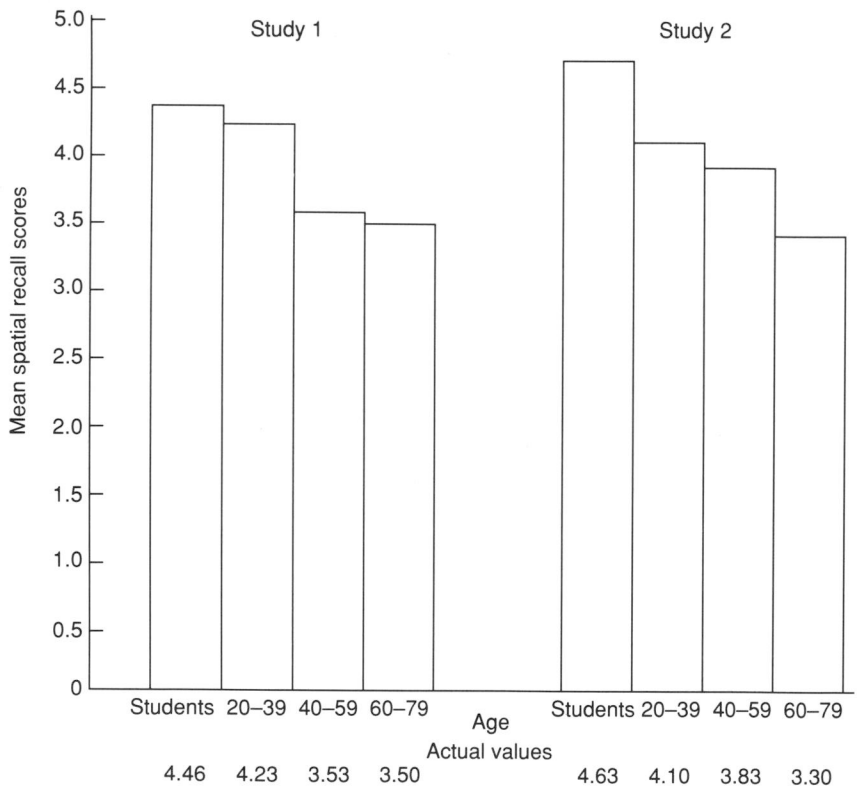

FIGURE 9.4 Short-term memory for spatial information. (Adapted from Salthouse, Kausler, & Saults, 1988a, Table 1.)

below those for the verbal short-term memory task included in the same study (see Chapter 5, p. 153 and Figure 5.8). However, for both tasks, there was only a modest decline in mean scores from young adulthood to middle age, and another modest decline from middle age to late adulthood.

One of the simplest procedures for testing age difference in long-term spatial memory is to present words or pictures at different locations on a page or on a screen, and then test for memory of where they had been placed (e.g., left or right half of the screen). McCormack (1982b) found no age difference for memory of location of words aligned vertically on cards, and Ozekes and Gilleard (1989) for pictures on a display board. Their results seem to be exceptions, however. Statistically significant age-related deficits in memory for locations of pictures projected on a screen were reported in two studies by Park (Park, Puglisi, & Lutz, 1982; Park, Puglisi, & Sovacool, 1983) and in a study by Denney, Dew, and Kihlstrom (1992). In Denney et al.'s (1992) study, words were presented in different quadrants of a computer screen. In one condition, subjects were asked to remember only the words, in a second condition to remember both the words and their locations on the screen, and in a third condition to remember neither the words nor their locations (an orienting task required subjects to process each word and answer a question about it). The second condition approximated an intentional-memory condition, the first condition approximated a modified incidental-memory condition (i.e., a memory set was activated, but not specifically for spatial location), and the third condition approximated a true incidental memory condition (i.e., no memory set at all was activated). For the young adult subjects, the percentage of correct quadrant identifications was 49% in the second condition (intentional memory), 39% in the first condition, and 38% in the third condition. Comparable percentages for the elderly subjects were 31%, 30%, and 29%. There was clearly an Age × Condition interaction effect. The young subjects displayed more intentional memory for spatial location than incidental memory. By contrast, intentionality had no beneficial effect for the elderly subjects. In fact, the elderly subjects scored close to chance expectancy in each condition.

A modified version of this kind of task, and one somewhat comparable to Salthouse et al.'s (1988a) short-term memory task, was employed by Pezdek (1983). Her subjects were given a matrix of 36 squares, 16 of which had either small household objects or small toys placed on top of them. After the objects had been removed, the subjects attempted to place each object on the square where it had been previously located. Young adult subjects were significantly more accurate than elderly subjects. A three dimensional matrix of 64 compartments entered into Cherry, Park, and Donaldson's (1993) study. Subjects had to remember in which compartments 24 red poker chips had been placed. Young adult subjects were again more accurate than elderly subjects, and elderly subjects benefited more from landmark cues (household objects) placed in eight of the compartments than did the young subjects.

The most frequently used test for long-term spatial memory, and one with seemingly greater ecological validity than picture/object/word location tests, is one in which memory for location of objects or places on a map is tested. Perlmutter et al. (1981) had their subjects study a map containing pictures of buildings at different locations. Their young subjects subsequently relocated correctly a significantly higher proportion of the pictures (.58) than their elderly subjects (.47). Especially informative are the map memory studies by Light and Zelinski (1983) and Zelinski and Light (1988). In Light and Zelinski's (1983) study, subjects studied a map showing the locations of 12 different structures (e.g., a church, a statue). They were then asked to identify from a list of 18 structures the 12 that had been on the map and to indicate on a blank map where each had been located. Of particular importance is the inclusion of a comparison of performances under intentional- and incidental-memory conditions. Intentional-memory subjects knew in advance that their memory for both the names of the structures *and* their locations would be tested. Incidental-memory subjects were informed in advance only that their memory for the names of the structures would be tested, thus making memory for locations incidental. Mean location memory scores (proportion of correct locations for correctly identified structures) are shown in Figure 9.5 under both conditions. Their elderly subjects scored well below the level of their young subjects under both intentional- and incidental-memory conditions. Moreover, regardless of age, subjects in the intentional-memory condition scored substantially higher than subjects in the incidental-memory condition. Zelinski and Light (1988) extended this study by comparing age differences in location memory when the structures were exposed on the map either simultaneously (as in Light and Zelinski's, 1983, study) or successively (two structures placed on each of six different blank maps). A pronounced age difference was found in each condition. Although the successive condition was more difficult overall than the simultaneous condition, the variation in condition did not interact significantly with age. Significant age differences in placing objects in their correct locations under a variety of conditions have also been found by Bruce and Herman (1983; variation in perspective while viewing objects), Bruce and Herman (1986; distinctive structures versus undifferentiated structures), Read (1987; location of real grocery items in a simulated supermarket display), Cherry and Park (1989; location of objects in a three-dimensional array), Moore, Richards, and Hood (1984; tactually presented objects), and J. L. Thomas (1985; cumulatively presented to-be-remembered structures and locations).

A real-world setting provided the context for a study by Uttl and Graf (1993). Young adult and elderly subjects spent over an hour in a novel office containing 40 target objects (e.g., a phone book and a stapler) placed in various locations. All of the subjects were asked to perform a series of secretarial tasks under the pretense that they were being tested for their ability to cope with a novel environment. In addition, half of the subjects in each age group were informed in

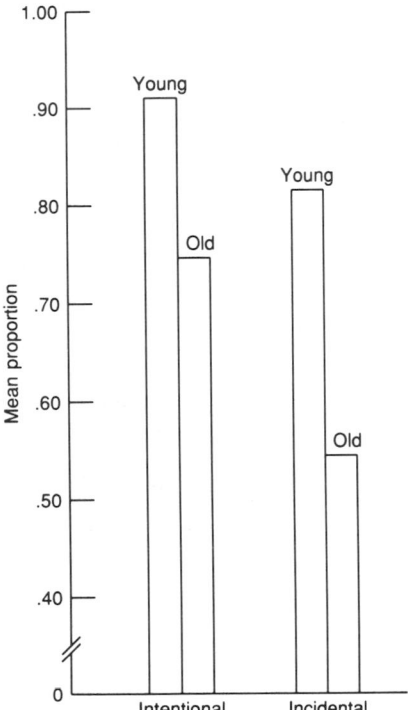

FIGURE 9.5 Age differences in spatial memory for objects on a map under intentional- and incidental-memory condition. (Adapted from Light & Zelinski, 1983, Table 1.)

advance that their memory for the locations of the objects would be tested later (intentional memory). The other subjects were told only that their memory would be tested later but without specification of the kind of test. Two forms of memory test were administered to all of the subjects, each test involving 20 of the objects in the office. The first was a map test, much like that of Light and Zelinski (1983), in which pictures of the objects were to be placed where they belonged on the map. The second was a relocation test in which the objects themselves were scattered on the desk in the office and were to be placed where they had been located previously. Spatial memory was significantly better for the young than for the elderly subjects, but the age-related deficit was greater for the map test than for the relocation test. The age-related deficit was also greater for intentional memory than for incidental memory. The percentages of correct locations for the young subjects were about 80%, 78%, 73%, and 71% in the relocation/intentional, relocation/incidental, map/intentional, and map/

incidental conditions, respectively. Comparable percentages for the elderly subjects were about 70%, 60%, 59%, and 45%.

There have been studies, however, in which age-related deficits have not been found for spatial memory of objects. Waddell and Rogoff (1981) compared middle-aged and elderly subjects in memory for the locations of such objects as a miniature mountain and a miniature church when the objects were placed either randomly in the cubicles of a box or in an organized manner that presented a three-dimensional scenic panorama. A typical age difference, favoring the younger subjects, was found for memory of locations of the randomly ordered objects, in agreement with Cherry, Park, and Donaldson's results (1993) when the objects were nondistinctive poker chips. However, this age difference disappeared for memory of the objects in the organized scene. Unfortunately, young adult subjects were not included in their study, making it impossible to determine if memory for organized spatial memory is age insensitive over the entire adult life span.

Sharps and Gollin (1987) also found typical age differences, favoring young adults over elderly adults, when objects were placed on a map, as in Light and Zelinski's (1983) study. However, the age difference disappeared when the same objects were placed at different locations in a large room (locations identical to those shown in the map for the other group) and subjects toured the room to discover these locations. They argued that the "visual distinctiveness" of spatial information is a critical factor in determining the presence or absence of age-related deficits in spatial memory, and concluded that "the spatial memory of elderly adults may be considerably better in the visually distinctive surroundings of their everyday life than has been indicated by many laboratory and clinical tests, which have generally used much more visually homogeneous task contexts" (Sharps & Gollin, 1987, p. 340). In support of their distinctiveness hypothesis, they (Sharps & Gollin, 1988) later replicated the finding of no age difference in the free recall of objects when those objects were placed in a visually distinctive context, such as at various locations in a room, in contrast to a nondistinctive context, such as on a black and white map of the room. Unfortunately, Park, Cherry, Smith, and Lafronza (1990) failed to replicate some of the negligible age differences found by Sharps and Gollin (1987). A possible explanation for the discrepant findings between the Sharps and Gollin (1987) and Park et al. (1990) studies was offered by Sharps (1991). He observed that the objects used by Park et al. (1990) had a greater categorical commonality than the objects used by Sharps and Gollin (1987). In his own study, Sharps (1991) replicated the procedure of the earlier study twice, once with objects that seem to be difficult to group into common categories (e.g., a jar, a rock, a compass) and once with objects more readily identified with the same category (a wrench, a hammer, and a screwdriver as members of the category *tools*). The results obtained with the low commonality objects replicated those of Sharps and Gollin (1987), while the results obtained with the high commonality objects replicated those of Park et al. (1990).

Memory for the locations of objects involves the perception and subsequent encoding of conjointed independent environmental features (i.e., the content of the object *and* its location). As noted in conjunction with temporal memory, the encoding of conjointed features is likely to be an age-sensitive cognitively effortful process. In fact, the encoding of conjointed features is much like learning paired associates, a form of learning we know to be highly age sensitive.

Source Memory

Do you know that there is a connection between Ronald Reagan and actress Jodie Foster? If you do, did you acquire the information in school or outside of school? If you don't remember which, you are manifesting what is called *source amnesia*. You probably remember that you acquired it originally from one of the media outside of school—but which one? If you don't remember, you are manifesting what is called *source forgetting*. The source of remembered episodic events is another important noncontent attribute that contributes greatly to the imperfections of everyday memory. Some events, however, seem to have virtually perfect source memory (what is commonly called "Flashbulb memory") For those of us who heard the news about President Kennedy being shot, we are likely to remember the source of that news (i.e., hearing it on the radio, hearing it from a friend, and so on), as well as remembering where we were at the time the news was heard (see Linton, 1975; but see also Chapter 10, p. 350).

Source amnesia and source forgetting were brought under laboratory control initially in a study by Schacter, Harbluk, and McLachlan (1984). Their subjects were organic amnesics and control subjects. They were presented with a series of factual questions about famous and nonfamous people, and they were provided with the answers when they did not know them. Half of the facts were read by one experimenter, the other half by a different experimenter. On a later test, they were asked the same questions, and, when they gave the correct answer, they were asked for the source of the knowledge. Relative to the control subjects, the amnesic subjects were far less certain that they had acquired the knowledge in the laboratory. That is, the amnesics were more prone to source amnesia than were the control subjects. Moreover, when the amnesics did remember acquiring the information in the laboratory, they were far less accurate than the control subjects in remembering which experimenter had been the source. That is, the amnesics were also more prone to source forgetting than were the control subjects.

Using a procedure patterned after that of Schacter et al. (1984), McIntyre and Craik (1987) compared young and elderly subjects in accuracy of a form of source memory. In this case, trivia questions were presented either by the experimenter or by an overhead projector. When presented later with the same questions, they were asked if they had acquired each answer in the laboratory or outside of the laboratory (source amnesia), and, if acquired in the laboratory, whether it had been presented by the experimenter or by the projector (source forgetting). Scores for source amnesia clearly revealed greater forgetting of source by elderly than by young subjects. Scores for source forgetting were largely obfuscated by floor effects and revealed no consistent pattern favoring young adults. In a follow-up study, Craik, Morris, Morris, and Loewen (1990) evaluated source memory proficiency for a group of elderly adults ranging in age from 60–84 yr, and found significant correlations between source amnesia scores and both age ($r = .49$— the greater the age, the greater the amount of source amnesia) and scores on a verbal fluency test ($r = -.38$—the greater the fluency, the less the amount of source amnesia). A verbal fluency test (naming words beginning with a designated letter for a fixed amount of time) is commonly assumed to be a measure of frontal lobe functioning. Old-old individuals appear to be especially susceptible to source amnesia, presumably because of their greater frontal lobe dysfunctioning, relative to younger individuals.

An intriguing phenomenon that is closely linked to source memory is the *false fame effect* (Jacoby, Kelley, Brown, & Jasechko, 1989). At stake is the probability of identifying on a test trial a nonfamous name as being a famous name when it had been encountered on a prior study phase, relative to other nonfamous names not previously encountered. During a study phase, Dywan and Jacoby (1990) had their subjects read a list of 40 nonfamous names under incidental-memory conditions (i.e., they had a nonmemory orienting task to perform). They then received a list of famous and nonfamous names and decided for each name whether or not it was famous. Of the nonfamous names in the test phase, half had been part of the names in the study phase. The probability of calling prior nonfamous names "famous" was .20 for their elderly subjects and .14 for their young adult subjects. Comparable probabilities for calling new nonfamous names "famous" were .14 and .25. The elderly subjects apparently had greater difficulty than the young subjects in monitoring the source of familiarity they had for those nonfamous names previously encountered in the study phase. That is, knowing they were familiar, but not remembering the source of where they encountered them before, they erroneously believed them to be famous. The young subjects were able to discount most of these names because they remembered their inclusion in the study phase.

Source memory has also entered heavily into research on memory for one's own actions. For example, how accurately do you remember which words in a list you passively read and which ones you actively generated? We will return to source memory in our later coverage of age differences in activity or action memory. It should be noted further that remembering the sex of voice conveying prior information may be interpreted as being a form of source memory, as it was in studies by Ferguson, Hashtroudi, and Johnson (1992) and Schacter, Kaszniak, Kihlstrom, and Valdiserri (1991) (1992) that will be reviewed shortly.

Other Noncontent Attributes

The principles of automaticity of encoding have been applied to several additional noncontent attributes of to-be-remembered items. Sex of voice for auditorily presented information is one such attribute. Consider, for example, the memory trace of the student who says, "In my psych class yesterday I heard this male voice behind me whisper, 'Shut up—I can't hear the lecture.'" Encoding of the episode obviously included the sex of the complainer as well as the content of the complaint. But did the encoding occur automatically? Would elderly students remember the sex of voice as well as young students?

The improbability of memory for sex of voice being a form of automatic memory has been amply demonstrated in basic memory research. Specifically, memory for sex of voice is significantly better under intentional memory conditions than under incidental-memory conditions (e.g., Geiselman & Bellezza, 1976). Moreover, memory for sex of voice is highly age sensitive. Kausler and Puckett (1981a) gave their young and elderly subjects successive tasks, each requiring memory of the content in 20 sentences. For each task, half of the sentences in the list were read in a man's voice, half in a woman's voice (randomly ordered). The tasks differed in one fundamental way. The first was administered with incidental-memory instructions, the second with intentional-memory instructions. The incidental–intentional distinction refers only to the sex of voice attribute. For both tasks, memory of sentence content was intentional. The content memory test involved cued recall in which the verb of each sentence served as the retrieval cue for recalling the two nouns (subject and object of the sentence) linked with it. For the first task (incidental memory), subjects did not know in advance that they would be tested for recognition of sex of voice of each sentence. For the second task, they knew they would be tested for both content and sex of voice.

Mean sentence recall scores (maximum = 40) are plotted in part A of Figure 9.6, while mean sex of voice recognition scores (maximum = 20) are plotted in part B. An age-related deficit was clearly present for sex of voice scores as well as for sentence recall scores, regardless of instructional condition. In addition, voice identification scores were higher at both age levels in the intentional condition than in the incidental condition. In fact, voice identification by the elderly subjects did not exceed chance expectancy (10 out of 20) in the incidental condition. On the other hand, sentence recall was poorer in the intentional condition than in the incidental condition. The disparity between conditions, however, was considerably more pronounced for the elderly subjects than for the young subjects. This pattern suggests a trade-off effect between the encoding of content and the encoding of noncontent information accompanying that content

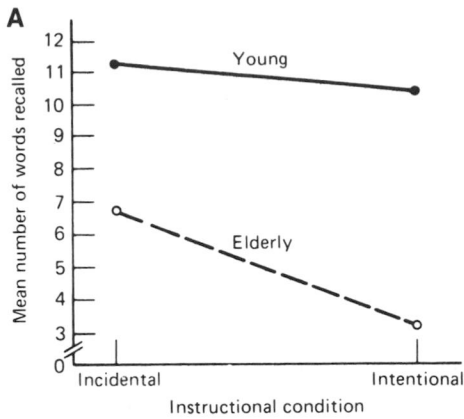

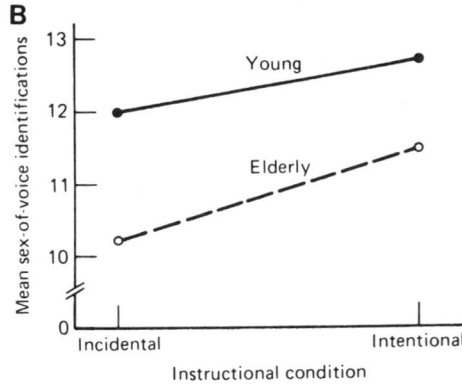

FIGURE 9.6 Age differences in recall of sentence content (A) and in recognition of sex of voice of those sentences (B). (Adapted from Kausler & Puckett, 1981a.)

(Light, Berger, & Bardales, 1975). When informed of a forthcoming test for memory of a noncontent attribute (i.e., the intentional condition), subjects utilize a segment of their processing capacity for encoding that attribute. The resulting exertion of cognitive effort enhances memory of that attribute relative to memory found when subjects are tested incidentally. At the same time, processing capacity available for the effortful encoding of item content is reduced. Consequently, content scores decrease from the incidental- to the intentional-memory condition, whereas noncontent attribute scores increase across conditions (i.e., a trade-off occurs). Given the relatively large processing capacity of the young adult, the adverse effect of the trade-off on content memory is slight for young subjects. Given the reduced capacity of the elderly adult, the magnitude of the trade-off effect is far more pronounced for elderly subjects (see A, Figure 9.6).

Ferguson et al. (1992) discovered that the age-related deficit in sex of voice (i.e., male or female) memory is less than the age-related deficit in memory for who of two people of the same sex (i.e., both male or both female) delivered the content conveyed by the voices. They also discovered that their young adult subjects benefited more from an additional cue than did their elderly subjects. The additional cue consisted having the male and female speakers be widely separated in the laboratory room. Relative to having the speakers close together, the young subjects' probability of correct source identification increased from .71 to .83. By contrast, the probability for the elderly subjects increased only slightly (from .67 to .69). The elderly subjects, however, made greater use of spatial cues when both voices were of the same sex than when they were of different sexes.

Generalizability of the age sensitivity of sex of voice memory may be somewhat limited, however. In a study by Schacter et al. (1991), young adult and elderly subjects received 40 fictitious facts about well-known people, half read in a male voice and half in a female voice. There was another important variable besides sex of voice. In one condition, the voice was randomized over the 40 facts. For the other condition, sex of voice was blocked, that is, male voice presentations occurred consecutively as did female voice presentations. Only in the blocked condition was the age-related deficit in voice identification statistically significant. The absence of an age difference in the random condition conflicts with the results obtained by Kausler and Puckett (1981a). Here an age-related deficit in voice identification scores was found when a random order of sex of voice was employed.

Age-related deficits in memory for a number of other noncontent attributes have also been reported. One of these attributes is for the case of words in a visually presented study list. Half of the words are presented in uppercase, half in lowercase, with subjects being tested for their accuracy of case identification. Young adults are clearly superior over elderly adults in their case identification scores (Kausler & Puckett, 1980b, 1981b). A study list may also be presented such that half of the words are presented visually, the other half auditorily. Non-content memory for modality of presentation may then be tested. In agreement with the automaticity principle, incidental memory for modality of presentation seems to be as proficient under incidental-memory condition as under intentional-memory conditions, both for elderly subjects and for young adult subjects (Lehman & Mellinger, 1984, 1986). However, there also appears to be a moderately large difference in accuracy of modality identification, favoring young adults (Lehman & Mellinger, 1984, 1986; Mellinger, Lehman, Happ, & Grout, 1990). Mellinger et al. (1990) had their subjects recall modality information with or without a secondary task (detecting the presence of a light). They found no difference between their young and elderly subjects in recalling with the added effort from the detection task. From this outcome, they concluded that the retrieval of modality information is no more effortful for elderly adults than for young adults. Finally, age-related deficits have also been reported for the memory of the color of pictures (Park & Puglisi, 1985) and memory of the lateral orientation of pictures (Bartlett, Till, Gernsbacher, & Gorman, 1983).

In summary, a vast amount of evidence has been accumulated to suggest that the encoding of noncontent attributes, whatever their nature, is cognitively effortful, and therefore susceptible to the reduced resources of elderly adults. However, several caveats are in order. First, the range of age-related deficits in memory for different noncontent attributes is considerable, with frequency memory and temporal memory apparently anchoring the extremes of slight and large deficits. Conceivably, effortful memory and automatic memory fall on a continuum, rather than into discrete forms, such that memory for some noncontent attributes are less effortful (or more automatic) than memory for other attributes. Alternatively, task conditions may determine if information about a noncontent attribute is encoded automatically or effortfully via strategic processes (Sanders et al., 1990). If task conditions discourage the use of rehearsal strategies, the resulting memory traces would have to be the products of automatic encoding processes. Here age-related deficits may not occur. However, if strategic encoding processes are activated, more relevant attribute information is likely to be encoded by young than by elderly subjects, leading to age-related deficits in attribute memory. Second, basic research presents a somewhat confusing picture. We have indicated that many recent studies with young adult subjects have provided evidence that seemingly refutes the automaticity of encoding a number of different noncontent attributes. However, it is also true that some recent studies have provided evidence firmly in agreement with the tenets of the automaticity principle. For example, Ellis and Rickard (1989) found no difference between intentional and incidental memory for either spatial or picture color memory, and Ellis (1990, 1991) found little, if any, enhancement of spatial memory with the intent to remember spatial information. Finally, automaticity refers only to encoding processes. What enters the episodic store must eventually be retrieved. Thus, even if the relevant information regarding a noncontent attribute is encoded equally by adults of all ages, age differences in effortful retrieval processes may result in age-related deficits in performance. Once more, the difficulty of separating the contributions of encoding and retrieval processes to age differences in performance scores is quite apparent.

Adult Age Differences in Memory for Activities and Actions

In the everyday world, we perform many activities—working on a crossword puzzle, repairing a broken appliance, writing a letter, balancing a check book, and so on. Memory of an activity usually persists even though there was no apparent attempt to commit it to memory and therefore little likelihood of rehearsing it either during or after its performance. Many of our other everyday memories seem to be characterized similarly by such rehearsal independency. That is, as with activity memory, memory occurs incidentally, and therefore in the absence of deliberate rehearsal. For example, we have memories, at least partial, of the contents of our conversations with other people and of the television programs we have watched. It seems highly unlikely that participating in a conversational exchange or watching a television program is accompanied by rehearsal of the content of the conversation or the content of the program. To the extent that the processes of activity memory are representative of the processes of rehearsal independent memory in general, our knowledge of adult age differences in activity memory should have important implications for adult age differences in other forms of rehearsal independent memory" (Kausler & Lichty, 1988, p. 94).

Memory for the Content of Activities and Actions

We do have memory of our everyday performances, usually in the absence of both the intent to remember and deliberate rehearsal. In fact, memory for one's own performed activities seems to be far more essential for maintaining continuity with the everyday world than memory for such noncontent attributes as frequency-of-occurrence, and it should therefore be a much stronger candidate for "wired in" automaticity of encoding. However, our everyday experiences tell us that activity memory is imperfect—we do fail to remember at times whether or not we turned off the stove when we left our residence, whether or not we turned off the lights of our parked automobile, and so on. Such memory failures are among the problems elderly people list when they complain about their memory problems. Despite its apparent rehearsal independency, activity memory may well be age sensitive.

An early study on what could be called activity memory was reported by Bromley (1958). The activities consisted of taking the subtests of the Wechsler intelligence test. Following completion of the series of subtests, his young adult and elderly subjects were given an unexpected incidental memory test of the content of their activities. The young subjects recalled an average of 75.1% of the subtests, the elderly subjects an average of 61.8%. Other researchers also found an age-related deficit in the recall of tests performed in the laboratory or clinic under incidental-memory conditions (Peak, 1968, 1970; Randt, Brown, & Osborne, 1980). After a hiatus of a several years, there have been a number of studies comparing age groups in their recall of the content of activities performed in the laboratory under either incidental- or intentional-memory conditions. The age-related deficit in recall has been found to approximate closely that reported by Bromley (1958).

Activity memory refers to memory of having performed activities that are continuous over a period of time, usually for several minutes (e.g., balancing a checkbook). In the laboratory it is simulated by having subjects perform for several minutes each on a series of tasks, such as solving anagrams and working on arithmetic problems, and then having them recall verbally what tasks they had been performing after the series is completed. Action memory refers to memory of having performed discrete, brief actions (e.g., picking up a coin from the sidewalk). In the laboratory it is simulated in the same way activity memory is simulated, only now subjects perform a series of brief actions (e.g., putting a cup on a saucer and closing a safety pin). This procedure was introduced only with young adult subjects by R. L. Cohen (1981; Cohen refers to memory of actions as memory for subject-performed tasks or SPTs). The outcomes of aging research on activity memory and action memory have been virtually identical. Both imply strongly that memory is rehearsal independent, but at the same time highly age sensitive.

Kausler and his associates have reported a number of studies on age differences in memory for the content of performed activities (i.e., remembering having solved anagrams, having worked on arithmetic problems, and so on) (Kausler & Hakami, 1983a; Kausler Lichty, & Davis, 1985; Kausler, Lichty, Hakami, & Freund, 1986; Kausler & Wiley, 1990a; Lichty, 1986; Lichty, Kausler, & Martinez, 1986; see Engelkamp & Cohen, 1991; Kausler & Lichty, 1988; and Norris & West, 1990, for further reviews). The standard procedure calls for comparing recall scores of young adult and elderly subjects performing on a series of tasks (ranging from 12 to 16 across studies) under incidental and intentional-memory conditions. The incidental-memory condition is especially effective in that no hint of a forthcoming memory test is given. Subjects are simply asked to perform the tasks for the purpose of providing normative information about scores on each task for people of different ages. Intentional-memory subjects are given the same information, but, in addition, they are told that their memory for the tasks will be tested at the end of the series. Shown in Figure 9.7 are representative outcomes of two of these studies. Note first that intentional memory is no better than incidental memory for either young or elderly subjects. Despite this apparent rehearsal independency (thereby satisfying one of the major criteria of automaticity), there is a substantial age-related deficit in recall scores, a deficit found in the other studies as well. Overall, the young subjects in these studies have averaged recalling about 75% of the tasks they performed, the elderly subjects about 60%. Again, these average scores are very comparable to those found in Bromley's pioneering study, thus providing convincing evidence that the age differences is not the result of a cohort effect (i.e., equivalent outcomes in a time-lag comparison; see Chapter 3, p. 70).

The fact that activity memory differs greatly from rehearsal-dependent forms of episodic memory, such as free recall of a word list, is also apparent when the percentage of subjects recalling tasks is plotted for serial positions within the list. The serial-position curves obtained in one of the activity memory studies are plotted in part A of Figure 9.8. Note for both young and elderly subjects the

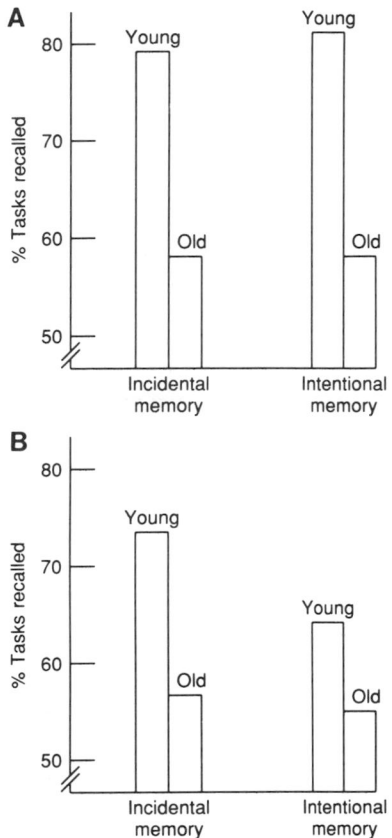

F I G U R E 9.7 Age differences in recall of activities under incidental- and intentional-memory conditions. (A: Adapted from data in Kausler & Hakami, 1983a. B: Adapted from data in Kausler, Lichty, Hakami, & Freund, 1986; reprinted from Kausler & Lichty, 1988, Figure 4.2.)

absence of a primacy effect and the presence of a pronounced recency effect found after a single trial. The same pattern has been found repeatedly in the other studies on activity memory. This pattern contrasts sharply with that found for a single free-recall word list where a pronounced primacy effect and a modest recency effect is the usual outcome (see Chapter 6, p. 176).

A number of task, subject, and procedural variations have been employed in the studies on activity memory. In general, task variables have been found to have little effect on the magnitude of the age-related deficit in recall. For example, Lichty et al. (1986) found the age-related deficit in recall to be as pronounced

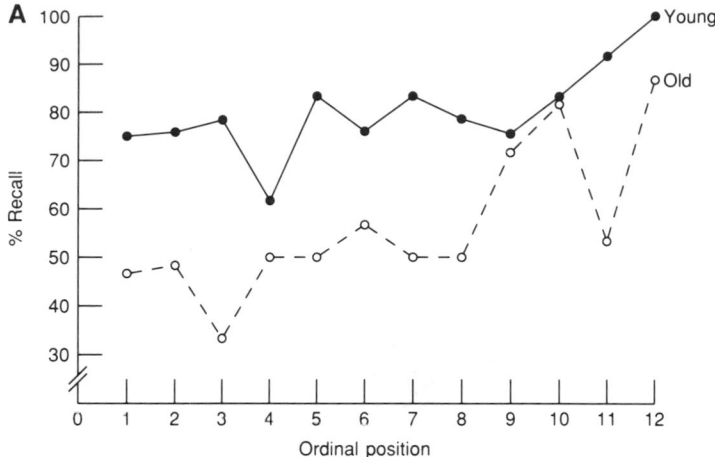

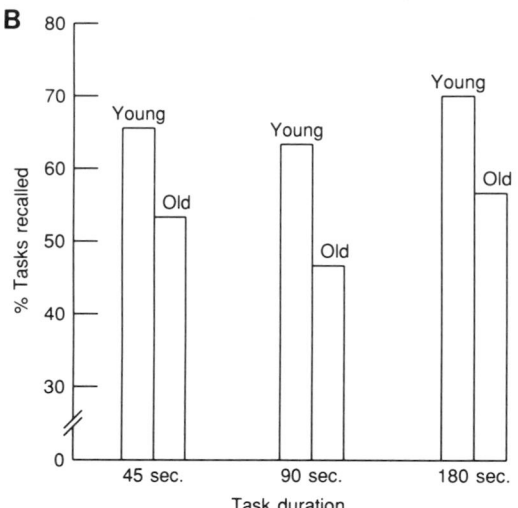

F I G U R E 9.8   A: Serial-position effects for recall of a series of activities. (Adapted from data in Kausler & Hakami, 1983; reprinted from Kausler & Lichty, 1988, Figure 4.3). B: Age differences in recall of activities as a function of task duration (Adapted from data in Kausler, Lichty, Hakami, & Freund, 1986; reprinted from Kausler & Lichty, 1988, Figure 4.6.)

for motor activities (e.g., putting rubber bands on a tube) as for cognitive activities (e.g., anagram solving), although recall overall was moderately higher for motor activities. Nor is a generation effect apparent for either young or elderly

TABLE 9.1

Recall Scores for Young and Elderly Subjects on 12 Different Cognitive Tasks[a]

Task	Recall score[b]		Age difference
	Young	Elderly	
Identical pictures	100	75	25
Word search	100	83	17
Estimation of length	83	75	8
Hidden patterns	83	50	33[c]
Anagrams	83	75	8
Instances of categories	83	50	33[c]
Cube comparison	75	50	25
Incomplete words	75	58	17
Vocabulary	75	83	−8
Nearer point	67	58	9
Calendar	58	33	25
Digit symbol	33	58	−25

[a] From data in Lichty, Kausler, and Martinez (1986). Reprinted by permission from Kausler and Lichty, 1988, Table 4.2.
[b] Percentage of subjects recalling a task performance.
[c] $p < .05$, (χ^2 test).

subjects (Lichty, Bressie, & Krell, 1988). That is, generated actions are remembered no better than actions performed at the request of the experimenter. This outcome also differs greatly from that found for rehearsal-dependent forms of memory (see Chapter 7, pp. 244–245). Especially intriguing is the outcome found when the duration of task performance is varied. Kausler et al. (1986) had their subjects perform for either 45 s, 90 s, or 180 s. Mean recall scores are plotted in part B of Figure 9.8. Note first that the magnitude of the age-related deficit was about the same for each duration. Note further that duration of performance on an activity had little, if any, effect on eventual recallability for both young and elderly subjects. Surprisingly, a subject's level of performance on a given task has little relatedness to subsequent recallability of that task, whether the subject be young or old (Kausler & Lichty, 1988). Nor does organizational ability appear to affect the recallability of activities. In Lichty et al's (1986) study, half of the activities performed in the laboratory were cognitive in nature (e.g., solving anagrams), the other half were motor in nature (e.g., moving a disk along a wire). No evidence of clustering based on cognitive and motor categories was found for either the young or the elderly subjects.

Although an overall age-related deficit in recall is evident, it is also true that there is considerable variability in the age differences manifested in recall for specific activities. For example, listed in Table 9.1 are the 12 different cognitive activities employed by Lichty et al. (1986) in their study. Also listed are the percentages of young and elderly subjects recalling each of the tasks. It may be seen that the tasks varied greatly in their subsequent recallabilities for both young and elderly subjects. Moreover, for only two of the tasks was the age difference in percentage statistically significant, and for two of the tasks there was a reverse nonsignificant age difference favoring elderly subjects. Comparable variability in recall was also found for the motor tasks employed by Lichty et al. (1986; see Kausler & Lichty, 1988). As observed by Kausler and Lichty, "Determining why some activities yield more distinctive memory traces than other activities and why some activities show less pronounced age deficits than other activities are important objectives of our future research on activity memory" (1988, p. 106).

Despite the pronounced age-related deficit in recall of activities, there is essentially no age difference when a recognition test replaces a recall test. For example, Lichty et al. (1986) found the hit rate for recognizing prior activities as old to be nearly 1.00 and the false alarm rate for recognizing new activities as new to be nearly zero for both their young and elderly subjects. The marked contrast in the magnitude of the age difference between recall and recognition memory tests is striking, and it suggests that the low scores of elderly subjects on a recall test may be largely a retrieval problem rather than a problem in the initial encoding and long-term storage of activity memory traces. Conceivably, any condition that enhances the retrieval of activity memory traces from the long-term episodic store should improve the recallability of activity information and may even reduce the magnitude of the age-related deficit in recall. One such condition is that of the "retrieval practice" procedure employed by Rabinowitz and Craik (1986) with verbal information (see Chapter 7, p. 269). This procedure was used in a study by Kausler and Wiley (1990a). After a varying number of activities had been performed, their subjects attempted a short-term retrieval of the just-performed activities. This procedure continued until all 12 activities had been performed. At the end of the series, the subjects recalled as many of all 12 activities as they could. Kausler and Wiley (1990a) found that short-term recall after every four activities resulted in better long-term recall for both young and elderly subjects than either no interpolated short-term recall or short-term recall after every two activities. However, the magnitude of the age-related deficit was about the same regardless of the retrieval practice condition. This outcome closely parallels that found by Rabinowitz and Craik (1986) with verbal materials.

Age differences in recall of a series of discrete actions performed in the laboratory have been investigated in a number of studies. A sample of these studies and their outcomes is given in Table 9.2. It is obvious that age-related deficits are as apparent for the recall of discrete actions as they are for the recall of continuous activities. However, it may be seen that the magnitude of the age-related deficit varied greatly across these studies, being highly statistically significant in some

TABLE 9.2

Summary of Studies on Adult Age Differences in Recall of Actions

		Recall (%)	
Study	Condition	Young	Elderly
Bäckman & Nilsson (1984)	Immediate recall	69	60
	Delayed recall	56	45
Bäckman & Nilsson (1985)	Immediate recall	56	45
	Delayed recall	53	47
Bäckman (1985b)	Immediate recall	53	47
	Delayed recall	51	50
R. L. Cohen, Sandler, & Schroeder (1987)	Immediate recall (14 actions)	66	59
R. L. Cohen, Sandler, & Schroeder (1987)	Immediate recall (37 actions)	45	34
Guttentag & Hunt (1988)	Immediate recall	89	68
Knopf & Neidhardt (1989a)	High-familiarity actions	68	48
Knopf & Neidhardt (1989a)	Medium-familiarity actions	61	44
Knopf &Neidhardt (1989a)	Low-familiarity actions	53	34
Lichty (1986)	Brief delay of recall	63	48

studies (e.g., Guttentag & Hunt, 1988; Knopf & Neidhardt, 1989a) but not significant in other studies (e.g., Bäckman & Nilsson, 1984; R. L. Cohen, Sandler, & Schroeder, 1987; Dick, Kean, & Sands, 1989). Of considerable importance, is the identification of conditions that may possibly minimize the magnitude of the age-related deficit in recall of actions. From Table 9.2, it is apparent that the age-related deficit is unaffected by the familiarity of the actions (Knopf & Neidhardt, 1989a; see also Knopf, 1992, and Lichty, 1986). Both young adult and elderly subjects recall more highly familiar actions (e.g., turning on a light) than unfamiliar actions (e.g., powdering a light bulb), but the magnitude of the age-related deficit is about the same for each (Knopf & Neidhardt, 1989a). The age-related deficit is less for shorter lists of actions performed in the laboratory than for longer lists, but the disparity is relatively small (Brooks & Gardiner, 1994; R. L. Cohen et al., 1987; see Table 9.2). Nor does the presence of categorizable actions markedly alter the magnitude of the age-related deficit in recall. This is true whether the categories consist of actions without external objects (e.g., making a fist) and actions with external objects (e.g., bouncing a ball; Bäckman & Nilsson, 1984, 1985) or actions based on the part of the body involved (e.g., arms, torso; Norris and West, 1993). In both cases, little clustering by category has been found for either young adults or elderly adults. The age-related deficit remains about the same whether actions are performed only once in a series or if they are performed twice, although, not surprisingly, recall is greater for actions performed twice than for actions performed once, regardless of the subjects' age (Cohen et al., 1987; Kausler, Wiley, & Phillips, 1990). The age-related deficit in recall has also been found to be greater when the actions involve external objects than when they do not and when the pacing of the actions is fast rather than slow (Norris & West, 1991).

In general, there is considerable similarity between activity memory and action memory. For example, there is convincing evidence (R. L. Cohen, 1981, 1983; Lichty, 1986) that action memory, like activity memory, is rehearsal independent. Moreover, serial-position curves found for action memory closely resemble those found for activity memory in the sense of an absence of a primacy effect and the presence of a recency effect (R. L. Cohen, 1983; Helstrup, 1986). Specific actions, like specific activities, show considerable variability in their recallabilities and in the magnitudes of their age differences (Kausler & Lichty, 1988).

In addition, age-related deficits in action memory, like those in activity memory, are much less with a recognition test than with a recall test (Kausler & Wiley, 1990b; Knopf & Neidhardt, 1989a), with hit rates for identifying old actions as old being nearly 1.00 for both young and old subjects. For example, Kausler and Wiley's (1990b) subjects performed a series of actions long enough to expect probability of recall to be well below 1.00 regardless of the subjects' age, and yet the hit rates were 0.96 for their young subjects and 0.91 for their elderly subjects. Furthermore, Norris and West (1991) discovered that the age difference is greatly diminished when external cues are present during recall to provide retrieval support (e.g., looking at a foot to cue recall of the prior action of tapping the foot).

Norris and West (1993) also found the age-related deficit to be less pronounced when subjects enacted their previously performed actions rather than described them verbally. Brooks and Gardiner (1994) also had their subjects enact the to-be-recalled actions rather than describe them verbally. However, in their study, only the verbal commands for actions were given during the initial study phase (i.e., subjects heard the commands but did not act them out). Enactment in this case was considered by the investigators to be a form of prospective memory. With a relatively long series of actions, the age-related deficit in enacted recall was as pronounced as it was for verbal recall of the actions following their performances during the initial study phase (i.e., the usual performance verbal recall sequence—what Brooks and Gardiner referred to as retrospective action memory).

Overall, the evidence from research on age differences in action memory suggests that much of the difficulty elderly adults have in recalling their own actions rests in age-sensitive retrieval processes. However, it is clear that retrieval processes alone cannot account for the age-related deficit in the recall of actions. Kausler and Wiley (1991) provided their subjects with the same kind of "retrieval practice" given earlier with verbal materials and activities. That is, their subjects received short-term recall trials after every few actions had been performed, and they then received a long-term recall test of all of the actions. As with verbal material and activities, short-term recall increased moderately later long-term recall, but in equivalent amounts for young adult and elderly subjects. The net effect was an age-related deficit in long-term recall following short-term recall that was as pronounced as the deficit without prior short-term recall. It does appear that elderly adults are less proficient in encoding their own actions than are younger adults. Consequently, enough information is encoded to permit recognition of previously performed actions, but not enough information to permit substantial amounts of free recall of those actions.

Encoding of Activity and Action Information

Given the commonality of functional relationships with independent variables, it seems reasonable to conclude that activity memory and action memory appear to be regulated by the same basic mechanisms. Kausler and Lichty (1988) have proposed a two-stage sequence of encoding processes that determines memorability of either activities or actions, one patterned after the two stages postulated to govern memorability following maintenance rehearsal of the kind given to words when their reading serves as the distractor task for a Brown-Peterson short-term memory task (see Chapter 5, p. 163). Naveh-Benjamin and Jonides (1984) reasoned that for maintenance rehearsal the first stage consists of the activation of a program for pronouncing the words. It is this activation that transmits memory traces of the words to the episodic store. The second stage consists of maintaining the extant program for successive rehearsals of these words. Continuation of the pronunciation program is assumed to yield little further transmission of information to the episodic store. For activity and action memory, it is the operationalization of a program for performing each task (the first stage) that results in the transmission of a trace of that program to the episodic store. Continuation of that program via sustained performance on specific task elements (the second stage) results in little further transmission of information (see Figure 9.9). This, presumably, is why memory for activities performed for 180 s is no better than memory for activities performed for 45 s (see B, Figure 9.8). The prolonging of duration serves only to extend the second stage proposed in the model. The critical first stage is affected only by the initial activation of the program.

In further support of Kausler and Lichty's (1988) model is the finding that repeating actions enhances memory of the content of those actions for both young and elderly subjects, relative to single performances of the same actions, but only when the repetitions are distributed (i.e., other actions intervene between the first and second performances) (Kausler, Wiley, & Phillips, 1990).

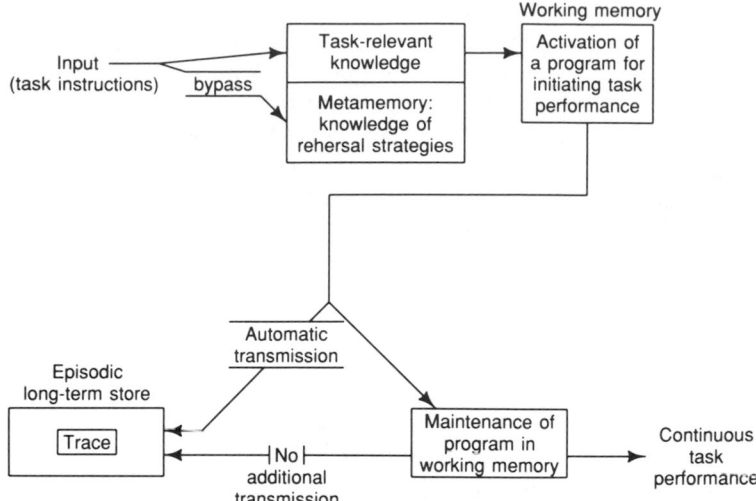

FIGURE 9.9   Two-stage model of activity and action memory. (Adapted from Kausler & Lichty, 1988, Figure 4.10.)

Massing the repetitions in the sense of performing them consecutively (e.g., putting two cups on two saucers, one after the other) was found to yield no better recall than performing each action only once. When actions are distributed, their programs must be separately activated, thus assuring multiple traces of that activation. Multiple traces, in turn, provide additional opportunity for retrieval at the time of recall, particularly if different kinds of contextual information are encoded at the time of activation and stored along with the trace of an action's program.

Why then age-related deficits in recall of either activities or actions if the first, and critical, stage occurs automatically? Kausler and Lichty (1988) suggested that contextual information present at the time a motor program is activated, such as thoughts about the nature of the activity or action or the verbal command given by the experimenter to initiate an activity or action, may be encoded along with the trace of the program, but more thoroughly by young subjects than by elderly subjects. That is, dual encoding involving both motor and verbal information may take place to a greater degree for young than for elderly adults. Consequently, the resulting memory traces for a series of activities or actions may be more distinctive, and therefore more accessible for retrieval, for young than for elderly subjects. Alternatively, the distinctive contextual information could be encoded during the second stage, and added to the traces of the motor program established automatically during the first stage (Sanders et al., 1990). However, this possibility seems unlikely. Presumably, prolonging the duration of an activity should enhance the opportunity for such encoding, thereby increasing the memorability of that activity. As we discovered earlier, variation in duration of the second stage seems to have little effect on memorability.

The nature of the memory trace created by performing an activity or action has been tested further by means of an interference paradigm. R. L. Cohen (1989) found that the recency effect for the recall of a series of actions was eliminated when his young adult subjects performed a series of interfering and rehearsal-preventing actions that differed from those in the to-be-remembered series. That is, recall of the last few actions in the series decreased to the level of recall for the earlier actions in the same series. The implication is that motor program information for each action is indeed stored, and it is this information that is interfered with by the other actions interpolated between the end of the to-be-remembered series and the signal to recall that series. Interestingly, Cohen (1989) found an equivalent interference effect when his subjects merely watched the experimenter perform the interpolated actions rather than perform them themselves. Apparently, observing an action being performed is sufficient to activate the same program in the observer, thus assuring its transmission to the LTS as a memory trace.

An extension of the interference paradigm to include verbal material as the source of interference made it seem highly unlikely that verbal memory traces are stored along with motor program traces, and to a greater degree by young adults than by elderly adults. If verbal information is encoded while performing an activity or action, then a subsequent verbal task should interfere partially with the retention of the overall activity or action memory trace. In a study by Kausler, Wiley, and Lieberwitz (1992), both verbal and motor interference conditions were employed, but with the interference occurring for the short-term memory of a triad of actions rather than at the end of the to-be-remembered series. Their subjects performed eight triads of actions, and subsequently recalled each triad. For four of the triads, recall occurred immediately after the third action had been performed (i.e., a zero-s retention interval). For the other four triads, recall was delayed for 15 s. During the 15-s retention interval, the subjects either did nothing to prevent verbal rehearsal of the prior actions (unfilled condition) or they performed one of three interfering tasks. Some subjects performed other actions unrelated to the to-be-remembered actions (as in R. L. Cohen's, 1989, study), other subjects observed the experimenter perform the unrelated actions (also as in Cohen's study), and still other subjects counted backwards by threes from a given number (the familiar verbal interference task used in short-term memory research with verbal materials) (see Chapter 5, p. 163). Means for the number of actions recalled in each condition and each age group are given in Table 9.3 (maximum score = 12 in each cell). Note the presence of a pronounced Interference Condition × Retention Interval interaction and the absence of an Age ×

TABLE 9.3

Means and Standard Deviations for Short-Term Memory Recall at 0- and 15-s Retention Intervals under Varying Interference Conditions[a,b]

	Interference condition			
Age group	Unfilled	Subject performed	Experimenter performed	Counting
		0-s interval		
Young				
M	11.83	11.33	11.44	11.78
SD	0.39	0.77	0.78	0.55
Elderly				
M	11.00	11.06	11.56	11.39
SD	1.28	0.87	0.62	0.61
		15-s interval		
Young				
M	11.61	8.72	9.56	10.94
SD	0.61	2.09	1.65	1.06
Elderly				
M	10.61	6.61	7.33	9.44
SD	1.58	2.43	2.33	1.54

[a] Reprinted from Kausler, Wiley, & Lieberwitz, 1992, Table 1. Copyright 1992 by the American Psychological Association.
[b] M, mean; SD, standard deviations.

Interference Condition × Retention Interval interaction. For both young and elderly subjects (and equally so), there was significant interference produced by interpolated motor actions, whether performed by the subjects or by the experimenter, but not for the interference produced by interpolated verbal activity. Given this outcome, it seems unlikely that verbal information enters into the memory traces of actions regardless of the performer's age. Whatever advantage younger performers have over elderly performers remains undetermined. It could be argued that memory for activities performed in the laboratory has little resemblance to memory for the kinds of activities performed in the everyday world. Consequently, the age-related deficits found in the laboratory may grossly exaggerate the deficits found outside of the laboratory. However, many of us do work on word puzzles at home, and we perform other activities that aren't far removed from those employed in activity memory research. Studies that have employed seemingly "real-world" tasks have yielded conflicting results. Fairly substantial age-related deficits in content memory have been found in one study when the laboratory activities were components of an integrated series that could just as readily be performed in the everyday world (making clay; Padgett & Ratner, 1987). However, little in the way of an age-related deficit was found when the series of laboratory activities simulated those entering into the preparation for travel (Norris & West, 1988). Obviously, the processes of activity and action memory remain less than fully identified, including the specific process or processes responsible for age-related deficits in recall.

Memory for Noncontent Attributes

Activities or actions within a series may vary in their frequencies of occurrences just as words in a series may vary in their frequencies. Age differences in memory for the frequencies with which activities were performed were tested by Kausler, Lichty, and Freund (1985). Activities, such as working on arithmetic problems, were performed either 0, 1, 2, 3, or 4 times, with repetitions of the same activity being widely separated in the total series. Half of the subjects at each age level (young adult and elderly adult) performed under intentional-memory conditions, half under incidental-memory conditions. After completing the series, subjects were given a list of descriptions of the activities, and they were asked how often they had performed on each. In agreement with the rehearsal-independent nature of activity memory, accuracy of frequency estimates was as high incidentally as intentionally at both age levels. In addition, as may be seen in the top part of Figure 9.10, age differences in accuracy of frequency estimates were fairly negligible, just as they are for age differences in frequency judgments for words in a series (see p. 310). On the other hand, a more pronounced age-related deficit in frequency judgments was found for actions by Liu and Kausler (1993). Half of the actions in a lengthy series were performed once and the other half twice. Subjects were then asked for each old action the number of times it had been performed. For once-performed actions, hit rates were .91 and .77 for their young and elderly subjects, respectively. For twice-performed actions, comparable values were .93 and .88. The elderly adults obviously had greater difficulty than the young subjects in discriminating between once-performed actions and actions that were not performed at all (zero-occurrence actions were included in the frequency-judgment test).

Age-related deficits in temporal memory for when activities were performed within a series are quite pronounced, just as they are for word temporal memory (see p. 314). Kausler, Lichty, and Davis (1985) had their subjects rank the 16 activities they had performed in the order they had been performed. Mean correlation coefficients between the true order and the reconstructed order of the activities are shown in part B of Figure 9.10 for young and elderly subjects performing under incidental- and intentional-memory conditions. Although the age difference in temporal memory scores was large, the difference in scores under incidental and intentional-memory conditions was negligible, again in agreement with the position that activity memory, in general, is a rehearsal-independent form of memory that is, nevertheless, highly age sensitive. The age sensitivity of

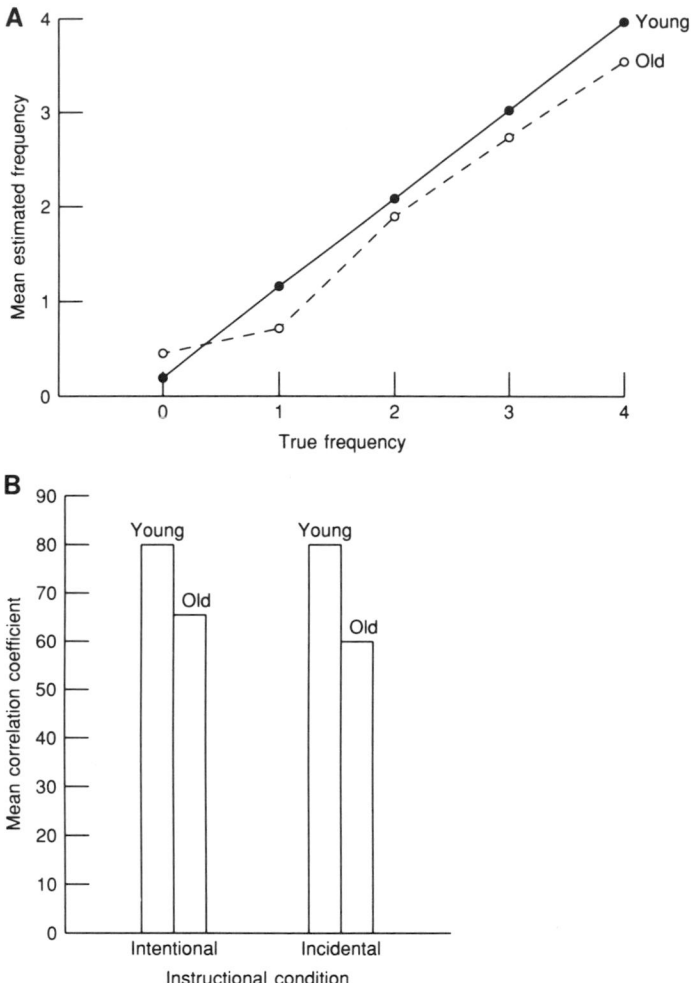

FIGURE 9.10   A: Covariation between true and estimated frequencies of activities. (Adapted from data in Kausler, Lichty, & Freund, 1985; reprinted from Kausler & Lichty, 1988, Figure 4.8.) B: Age differences in correlation coefficients between true order and reconstructed order of activities under intentional and incidental memory conditions. (Adapted from data in Kausler, Lichty, & Davis, 1985.)

activity temporal memory was also demonstrated in Salthouse et al.'s (1988) multiple-task study. After completing each of two separate series of activities (i.e., cognitive tasks), their subjects ranked the activities in each series in the order performed. The correlation coefficient between true order and reconstructed order again served as the measure of activity temporal memory. For the first and second series of activities the correlation coefficients between age (range of 20 to 79 yr) and temporal memory scores were $-.25$ and $-.31$, respectively. The commonality between action memory and activity memory is illustrated further by the pronounced age-related deficit in temporal memory for a series of actions found by Kausler and Wiley (1990b).

Interestingly, Kausler and Phillips (1988) found that temporal memory correlational scores for a series of activities were markedly increased for elderly subjects, approximating those of young subjects, when subjects were stopped after performing each triad of activities and were asked to recall those just-performed tasks. That is, subjects had to recall, after a short retention interval, three activities they would later be asked to recall after a longer retention interval. For a series of 12 tasks, they had four short-term memory tests (i.e., one after every three tasks), followed eventually by a recall test for the content of all 12 tasks and a temporal memory test (reconstructed order). Although the "retrieval practice" (see Chapter 7, p. 269) had little effect on the age-related deficit in content memory scores, (see p. 332) it nearly eliminated the age-related deficit in temporal memory scores.

There is another form of temporal memory for actions that has considerable importance in the everyday world. In the everyday world, many actions are bipolar in the sense that they occur in cycles. For example, we lock a door and later unlock the same door. The memory task here is not to remember the content of the action but rather to remember which pole of the cycle (e.g., locking or unlocking) was performed more recently. The temporal discrimination is made difficult by the fact that a given cycle is likely to have been performed many times, and it requires a discrimination only in terms of which pole had been performed last. It is this kind of temporal memory that is of great concern to many elderly adults (e.g., "I have trouble remembering if I locked my apartment door when I left this morning"). Surprisingly, in a laboratory simulation of cyclic temporal memory, Wiley and Kausler (1993) found it to be age insensitive. Their subjects performed such actions as turning on a switch (or turning off a switch) and then later in the series performed the other pole of turning off the switch (or turning it on). On a subsequent temporal-memory test, a hit was defined as correctly identifying which action had been performed more recently. The hit rates were .76 for the young subjects and .75 for the elderly subjects. In addition, the hit rate for each age group was as high under incidental-memory conditions as under intentional-memory conditions, thus indicating the rehearsal-independent nature of this form of temporal memory. In a second experiment, Wiley and Kausler (1993) discovered that the hit rate for both young and elderly subjects decreased significantly (and to the same degree for the two age groups) when the bipolar cycles were repeated three times in a lengthy series, with the temporal discrimination involving only the third and final cycle, relative to one-cycle hit rates. Although these results suggest that this form of temporal memory may be age insensitive, Wiley and Kausler warned about the generalizability of their results to the everyday world. As they observed, in the everyday world the lags are undoubtedly likely to be much greater than those entering into their study. Moreover, in the everyday world, bipolar actions commonly occur over many cycles. As the number of cycles increases beyond three, interference effects may indeed increase at a faster rate for elderly adults than for young adults, and the extent of an age-related deficit in temporal memory may increase accordingly.

Reality Monitoring and Source Memory

"Did I take the trash out—or did I just think about doing it?"

Activities and actions are often planned in advance of doing them, and at times it may be difficult to remember if the plan was actually executed. Discriminating between planning and execution corresponds to what Johnson (e.g., Johnson & Raye, 1981) has labeled *reality monitoring*. It refers to our ability to distinguish between an imagined event and a perceived event, that is, between internally derived and externally derived memories. Basically, reality monitoring is a form of source memory, only the discrimination is between internal and external sources rather than between two external sources (see p. 325). In this case, the imagined event is the planning of an activity. Age differences in the ability to discriminate between planned-only and planned-plus-executed activities were investigated by Kausler, Lichty, and Freund (1985) in their frequency-judgment study. Some of their tasks were planned once but were never really performed; others were planned twice and were performed either once or not at all. At stake was the extent planning without execution would inflate frequency estimates of how often the tasks were actually performed. Both young and elderly adults were quite capable of discriminating accurately between planning and performing. For example, frequency estimates of how often a task had actually been performed were no greater for tasks planned twice, but performed only once, than for tasks both planned and performed only once.

In somewhat related studies, Guttentag and Hunt (1988) and G. Cohen and Faulkner (1989) had their subjects perform some discrete actions and only imagine performing other actions. Guttentag and Hunt's (1988) young subjects recalled more of both the performed actions (89%) and the imagined actions (76%) than their elderly subjects (68% and 60%, respectively). Their subjects were also to judge for each action if it had been performed or imagined (i.e., reality monitoring). Although the age difference, favoring young subjects, in accuracy of these judgments was statistically significant, the moderate difference was attributable to just a few of the elderly subjects. By contrast, G. Cohen and Faulkner (1989) found that their elderly subjects had considerably more difficulty than their young subjects in discriminating between imagined and performed actions.

Other investigators have employed different tasks for evaluating age differences in reality monitoring and have found fairly pronounced age-related deficits. For example, Koriat, Ben-Zur, and Sheffer (1988) developed a laboratory task to investigate adult age differences on a familiar form of everyday memory failure. The phenomenon in question is failing to remember that you already told this story or joke to your audience. Repetition of the story could lead to personal embarassment and a bored audience. The failure seemingly results from impaired output monitoring. For their laboratory task, they simply determined the frequency on a free-recall task with which subjects repeated in the recall trial words that had already been recalled earlier in the trial. Their elderly subjects not only repeated substantially more words during the trial than their young subjects, they also misidentified many more previously recalled words as being unrecalled. The implication is that elderly adults are likely to experience greater difficulty in monitoring their verbal outputs than young adults in the everyday world, and they are therefore more likely to repeat previously emitted statements. J. C. Rabinowitz (1989b), in his generation effect study (see Chapter 7, p. 245), found accuracy of identifying which words were read and which were generated to be far greater for his young than for his elderly subjects. Hashtroudi, Johnson, and Chrosniak (1989) discovered their elderly subjects to be less accurate in distinguishing the external and internal source of memories (saying or listening to words) under some conditions but not under other conditions. They concluded appropriately that elderly adults do not experience a general deficit in reality monitoring. The deficit seems to occur under conditions in which elderly adults have difficulty inhibiting personal thoughts while imagining events (see Chapter 6, p. 222), thoughts that add to the resulting memories and make them resemble memories resulting from perceived events (Hashtroudi, Johnson, & Chrosniak, 1990). Overall, the results of these various studies indicate that age differences in the efficacy of reality monitoring are modest, if they exist at all.

Adult Age Differences in Other Forms of Rehearsal-Independent Memory

As noted in the beginning of this chapter, many of our everyday memory experiences other than activity and action memory appear to be rehearsal independent. We do have memory for the contents of conversational exchanges, albeit often imperfectly, usually without the intent to remember and without the activation of rehearsal processes. Although there have been a number of studies with young adults dealing with memory for conversations (see G. Cohen, 1989b, for a review), there has been little research directed at age differences in memory for conversational content. Laboratory simulations of memory for conversations were employed in aging studies by Kausler and Hakami (1983b) and Hauge (1987). In both studies memory for topics of conversation was tested under both incidental (no memory test expected) and intentional (memory test expected) conditions. For each of a series of topics (e.g., the presidency of the United States) young and elderly subjects were asked to respond "yes" or "no" to three questions (e.g., "Do you believe presidents should be limited to one six-year term?") and then to elaborate on their answer. In both studies, all subjects were asked subsequently to recall the topics that had just been discussed. The outcomes of these studies were conflicting regarding rehearsal independency. In support of rehearsal independency, Kausler and Hakami (1983b) found a null effect for the incidental and intentional variation at both age levels. However, contrary to the independency principle, Hauge (1987) reported significantly higher recall intentionally than incidentally, again for both young and elderly subjects. In addition, young adults recalled a significantly higher percentage of topics (66.7% in Kausler and Hakami's study, 80.8% in Hauge's study) than elderly subjects (54.9% in Kausler and Hakami's, 1983b study, 75.5% in Hauge's, 1987, study). Hauge (1987) also discovered that young subjects recalled significantly more specific questions than did elderly subjects. The presence of an age-related deficit clearly fails to satisfy one of the major criteria established by Hasher and Zacks (1979) for automaticity. However, the reason for the deficit may well rest in the effortful retrieval processes required to recall topics. In agreement with this possibility, elderly subjects in both studies did not differ from young subjects in hit rates (nearly 1.00 for each age group) for recognizing prior questions as having been asked (as with recognition of prior activities or actions, a ceiling effect present for both age groups limits interpretation of this null effect).

Age-related deficits in remembering conversational content can have serious implications in everyday living. For example, remembering what the physician told you determines how effectively you carry out the treatment program prescribed for you. There is evidence available indicating that elderly patients remember less of that content than do young adult patients (Ley, 1978, 1979). There is also evidence indicating that elderly individuals remember less about the topics discussed in an interview situation than do younger individuals (Herzog & Rodgers, 1989).

Rehearsal-independent memory also would seem to be involved in our memories of the contents of movies and television programs watched. We watch movies and television programs with the objective of simply comprehending them—and not remembering them. Several early studies (H. S. Conrad & Jones, 1929; Jones, Conrad, & Horn, 1928) reported that young adults remembered more content of a movie than elderly subjects. In recent years, the focus has shifted to adult age differences in memory for the content of television programs. Several studies have compared young and elderly subjects in their memory for the thematic content of short television programs watched in the laboratory, as well as for the content of commercials interspersed within the programs (Cavanaugh, 1983, 1984; Cavanaugh & Perlmutter, 1980; Levin, Petros, & Filippi, 1980), and for the content of simulated news programs watched in the laboratory (Hill, Crook, Zadek, Sheikh, & Yesavage, 1989; Stine, Wingfield, & Myers, 1990). Age differences in memory scores for these materials tend to be slight. An age difference in the recall of medical advice while watching a videotaped consultation was also found to be negligible (McGuire, 1993). Unfortunately, only intentional memory conditions were employed in these studies, thereby limiting the information they provide regarding rehearsal independency. In general, however, these studies indicate that age-related deficits are not very pronounced. Most important, they suggest that they are particularly negligible for high verbal (i.e., having high vocabulary test scores) elderly individuals; Cavanaugh, 1983; Cavanaugh & Perlmutter, 1980). Interestingly, Kausler and Hakami (1983b) reported a rather large positive correlation ($r = .76$) between vocabulary test scores and recall of topics scores. Conceivably, high verbal ability assures comprehension of either a conversation or the content of a television program. As with connected discourse, one cannot have memory unless the to-be-remembered material has been comprehended adequately.

CHAPTER 10

Long-Term Episodic Memory: Retention and Forgetting

Introduction

Episodic memory's contributions to the overall adaptability of the human organism are hindered by one of life's inevitabilities—forgetting. Once material is encoded, stored, and retrieved shortly after its presentation, there is no assurance of its permanent retrievability. Consider, for example, a paired-associate list that has been practiced to the point where every response is given correctly to its paired stimulus item. If the same stimuli are presented again a day later, a week later, or a year later, how many of the correct responses have been retained and how many forgotten at each retention interval? Similarly, how many of the words in a free-recall list that were successfully recalled after a single study trial will continue to be recalled successfully long after that trial? Forgetting many previously remembered episodic events is seemingly inevitable. Whether forgetting is the result of an actual loss of information from the long-term store (LTS) or simply the inability to gain access to still available information is usually unknown. Our concern, of course, is with possible age differences in the rate of forgetting, and, if there are such difference, what accounts for them. We will begin our review with attempts to evaluate age differences in real-life forgetting, and we will then turn to studies in which age differences in forgetting have been investigated by means of traditional laboratory simulations.

Adult Age Differences in Real-Life Forgetting

Impersonal Events

A popular notion about human aging is that recently acquired material is poorly retained by elderly people, while material acquired years earlier is remarkably preserved. Support for this notion has come from both clinical studies of senile individuals (Ribot, 1882; Shakow, Dolkart, & Goldman, 1941) and anecdotes provided by elderly people themselves. A good example of the latter is a comment made by composer Aaron Copland in describing the problems he encountered while writing his autobiography: "I have no trouble remembering everything that happened 40 or 50 years ago—dates, places, faces, music. But I'm going to be 90 my next birthday, Nov. 14th, and I find I can't remember what happened yesterday" (*Time*, 1980, p. 57). Our faith in Copland's analysis of his difficulties with retaining current events is enhanced by the fact that he would really be only 80 years old on his next birthday.

In this section, we will review research studies that have attempted to test for the retention of events, names, and so on acquired in real-life situations. Obviously, research of this kind has to rely on methods other than controlled laboratory assessments. Our first objective is to discover what truth there is to the notion that episodic events experienced early in life are remarkably preserved as one gets older. Very long-term memory is sometimes referred to as either *remote memory* or *tertiary memory* (as distinguished from secondary long-term memory of the kind tested shortly after material has been studied; Poon, 1985).

One of the first studies on this topic was by Schonfield (1969b). Adults ranging in age from their 20s to their 70s were simply asked to recall the names of all of their grade school and high school teachers. Acquiring the names of our teachers is an experience shared by all of us. By the time his subjects had reached their 20s, they had already forgotten a third of the names of their teachers. Beyond that age, forgetting began to slow down considerably. Nevertheless, for people age 70 and beyond, more than half of the names had been forgotten. Fairly comparable rates of forgetting over the years were found later by Bahrick, Bahrick, and Wittlinger (1975) for names of high school classmates, by Bahrick (1979) for names of streets in the city housing the college attended by the subjects, by Bahrick (1984b) for Spanish vocabulary acquired in high school Spanish classes, and by Bartlett and Snelus (1980) for titles of songs. For example, the retention-time function observed by Bahrick (1979) for names of streets is plotted in Figure 10.1. The independent variable in this case is the number of years passing since graduation from college. Retention scores were adjusted, or corrected, for the number of visits made to the city in question during the intervening years. The similarity to the retention-time (expressed as age) function obtained by Schonfield (1969b) is striking. Again, the rate of forgetting is rapid for the first few years following acquisition of the to-be-remembered in formation, followed by a general leveling off for the amount retained. Similar functions have been found for several other kinds of material that have been similarly tested.

A general representation of this function is shown in Figure 10.2. Note that forgetting is quite rapid for the first few years after acquisition. After 4 to 6 yr it levels off, and retention remains rather stable for the rest of one's lifetime. Somewhere between 20 to 40% of the original material is seemingly retained in what Bahrick (1984b) calls a *permastore*. The information in permastore is probably

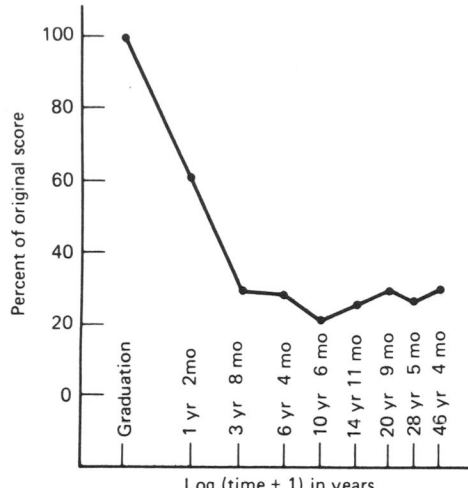

FIGURE 10.1   Retention of names of streets in the city housing in the college attended, plotted as a function of years intervening since graduation. (Adapted from Bahrick, 1979, Figure 1.)

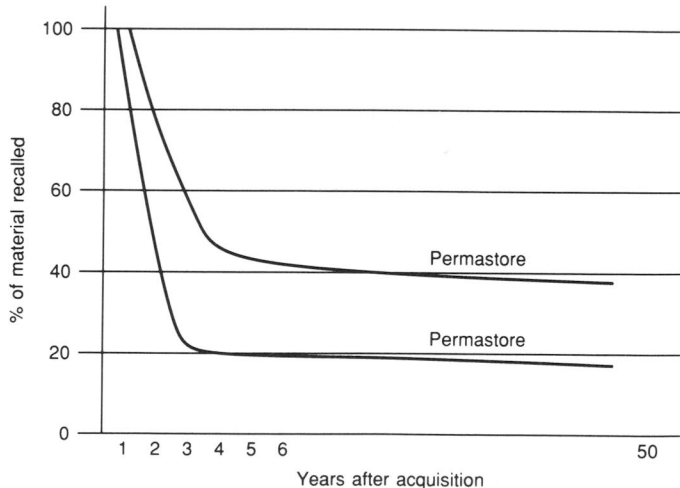

FIGURE 10.2   General time-forgetting function for such material as foreign language vocabulary acquired in high school. (Adapted from Kausler, 1989b, Figure 2.9.)

that portion of the original material that was highly "overlearned" at the time of acquisition. Of course, there are some exceptions, with trivia experts remembering virtually all of the names of television shows from 30 yr ago and becoming champions on the game show *Jeopardy*. However, Squire's studies (Squire, 1989; Squire & Slater, 1975) of the long-term retention of the names of television programs that were on the air for only one year have yielded results that seem to question the generalizability of a permastore. Over a period of 15 yr forgetting seems to be gradual and progressive (i.e., fairly linear), rather than negatively accelerated with a leveling off after 4 to 6 yr. However, his results (Squire, 1989) do suggest that the amount of forgetting for names of these programs during the period of 6 to 15 yr after they were on television is, in absolute sense, quite small (about 5%, compared to a 20% loss from the first through sixth year). Nor do the faces of a professor's students appear to attain a permastore status. Bahrick (1984a) tested the recognition memory of faces in professors' introductory course classes (about 40 students per class) at several retention intervals extending over 8 yr. Recognition memory scores were moderately high (about 65%; each student's picture was tested with four foils) 11 days after the end of the 10-wk term, but they were close to chance (about 25%) after 8 yr. The degree of original acquisition, of course, was undoubtedly much less than that occurring for students' acquisition of their classmates' names or their teachers' names. These results attest further that a high degree of overlearning is surely required before information enters a permastore.

Generalizing from these studies, the notion that remote or tertiary memories of long ago events are remarkably immune to forgetting does not appear to be true. Of course, it is still remarkable that retention does hold up as well as it does in late adulthood. However, as noted by Salthouse (1982), there is a problem in interpreting the results of studies in which retention of information acquired at age 20 (say for names and locations of streets in one's college town) is compared for individuals now 60 yr old and individuals now 30 yr old. Age of the memory (40 yr and 10 yr for 60- and 30-year-old individuals) is obviously confounded with the actual ages of those individuals. Nevertheless, the confounding seems to be tolerable in that neither variable (age of memory and age of individuals) has an effect on the amount apparently retained. By the time 10 yr have passed there is little further forgetting regardless of the individual's increasing age. That is, 30-yr-old and 60-yr-old individuals are expected to show equivalent amounts of retention and forgetting.

A somewhat different strategy for studying age differences in remote memory was developed by Warrington and Silberstein (1970), one that has been employed in a number of later studies (see Erber, 1981, 1987, for additional review). Instead of testing for the retention of episodic events shared with relatively few individuals, such as teachers' names, they tested the retention of newsworthy events, that is, events shared by virtually all of us. Their procedure has the advantage of studying the effect on retention of the age of an event as well as the effect of the age of the individuals being tested for retention (both at acquisition and at the time of testing). At the same time, the procedure is loaded with methodological problems that confound possible age changes in retention with changes linked to other potentially causative factors.

In the original study by Warrington and Silberstein (1970), remoteness of events extended only to 18 mo prior to the time of testing. No adult age differences in retention were found within this limited degree of remoteness. In a more comprehensive study by Warrington and Sanders (1971), individuals ranging in age from 40 to 80 yr were tested for the retention of events occurring during 2-yr periods, beginning with 1967–1968 and ending with 1930–1931. The popular notion mentioned earlier predicts that the oldest members of the total group should excel for retention of the most remote events (those of 1930–1931), whereas the youngest members should excel for retention of the most recent events (1967–1968; remember the study was conducted around 1970). Contrary to this notion, Warrington and Sanders (1971) discovered that retention decreased progressively with increasing age for all degrees of remoteness. That is, their oldest subjects retained less of early events as well as more recent events. These results were subsequently replicated by Squire (1974). Relatively poor retention of early events seemingly applies to even so-called "flashbulb" memories (e.g., remembering where you were when you heard about Pearl Harbor or the assassination of President Kennedy; see also Chapter 9, p. 321), memories that are often viewed as being immune to forgetting. Yarmey and Bull (1978) discovered that a number of their elderly subjects had difficulty remembering what they were doing when they heard about President Kennedy's assassination.

Other studies that followed soon after Warrington's pioneering research, however, reported highly conflicting results. Botwinick and Storandt (1974a, 1980) found no overall age differences for events occurring from the 1890s to the 1960s, and others have found small or unsystematic age differences over a long historical time period (Howes & Katz, 1988; Perlmutter, Metzger, Miller, and Nezworski, 1980; Storandt, Grant, & Gordon, 1978). Perlmutter (1978a) found significantly superior retention overall (i.e., combining all the time periods being tested) by her older subjects, and Poon, Fozard, Paulshock, and Thomas (1979) found no age differences for the retention of relatively recent events and superior retention by elderly adults for more recent events! The most recent study was by Howes and Katz (1988). They used a skillfully crafted assessment procedure with demonstrated sound psychometric properties. Their results indicated that middle-aged subjects remembered more than elderly subjects about historical events all of the subjects had lived through, both remote and recent. These results are largely in agreement with those obtained earlier by Warrington and Sanders (1971).

The absence of pronounced age differences in the retention of relatively recent events (Poon et al., 1979; Warrington & Silberstein, 1970) should not be surprising, despite the fact that this outcome conflicts with the popular notion about aging's effects on the retention of recently acquired material. As we shall see in a later section, the relative absence of an aging effect is in agreement with the negligible aging effect generally found in laboratory studies of age differences in retention. The implication is that elderly adults study current events as thoroughly as young adults. Having acquired as much (if not more) information, they also retain the events as well over retention intervals that are of the same duration for each age level. What is surprising is that some studies (e.g., Speakman, 1954; Warrington & Sanders, 1971) found inferior retention for relatively recent events by elderly subjects. In Speakman's study (1954) retention was assessed for the incidental memory of the colors of postage stamps that had been discontinued relatively recently; in Warrington and Sanders's study (1971) retention was assessed for relatively recent newsworthy events. It seems likely that the elderly subjects in these studies suffered more from an initial acquisition deficit than from a subsequent retention deficit. Given poorer acquisition, poorer retention is the expected consequence. This is the probable reason why elderly adults recognize famous faces from an earlier era (e.g., Greta Garbo) more easily than more recent famous faces (e.g., Stefan Edberg) (Bäckman & Herlitz, 1990; Wahlin et al., 1993). That is, they simply learned less about recent famous people than they did about famous people earlier in their adulthood.

Interpretation of whatever age differences exist in the retention of truly newsworthy events is especially difficult. Given the potential presence of causative factors other than age level at the time retention is assessed, it is little wonder that some investigators have found an age difference in retention favoring elderly subjects (Poon et al., 1979), whereas other investigators have found age differences favoring younger subjects (e.g., Howes & Katz, 1988; Warrington & Sanders, 1971). A potentially critical factor is the age of individuals at the time a newsworthy event occurs. Consider, for example, a retention test conducted in 1990 for events that occurred in 1960. Subjects who are 80 yr old at the time of the test were 50 yr old at the time the events happened, whereas subjects who are 50 yr old at the time of the test were only 20 yr old at the time the events happened. To the extent that initial acquisition may be greater at age 20 than at age 50, the events of 1960 were acquired initially more thoroughly by present 50-year-old subjects. (Actually, the reverse could be true—better acquisition by the older than by the younger individuals, assuming the former are more interested in newsworthy events.) Consequently, differences in retention between 50- and 80-yr-old subjects may actually be an irrelevant factor. What really matters is the degree of initial acquisition of the to-be-remembered material, a factor laboratory studies consistently identify as a critical one influencing the subsequent course of retention. There is, in fact, some evidence to indicate, at least for some kinds of real-life events, that age at the time of occurrence does greatly influence the amount retained years later (Storandt et al., 1978).

Another complicating factor is the historical time period in which remote events took place. Events taking place in some years, or periods of years, are far more dramatic and worthy of attention than the events taking place in other years. Consider, for example, the world events transpiring in 1941–1942 versus those in 1961–1962. To those individuals who lived through them as young adults, the years 1941–1942 included unique events that are likely to be retained forever. The events occurring during 1961–1962 were not nearly as unique. A retention test conducted years after these events should reveal superior recall scores for 1941–1942 than for 1961–1962. Consider the likely outcome of a retention study designed to measure retention of 40-year-old events. Scores are likely to be higher if the test had been administered in 1981–1982 (therefore, assessing retention of events during 1941–1942) than if it is administered in 2001–2002 (therefore, assessing retention of events during 1961–1962). Our conclusion regarding the effects of aging on remote retention is certain to be influenced strongly by this variation in time of measurement. There is also the distinct possibility that elderly adults' memories of early events is based on memories derived from recollections of those events over the years, and therefore receive further rehearsal (Schonfield & Stones, 1979; Welford, 1958), rather than on memories of the original event per se.

These complications do not enter into assessments of retention of names of teachers, names of streets in one's college town, and so on. Regardless of their age at the time retention is assessed, all subjects were about the same age at the time the to-be-retained material was learned. Moreover, there is no reason to expect age differences in retention to be affected greatly by the historical time period in which events occurred. Neither teachers nor streets are likely to have been more distinctive in, say, the 1940s than in the 1930s or 1950s. Consequently, the course of forgetting over years of living for these kinds of events provides a more reliable picture of real-life forgetting than does the course of forgetting for so-called newsworthy events. That picture indicates diminishing retention as the cumulative effects of intervening events increases. Most important, it is essentially the same picture revealed by laboratory studies for adults of all ages.

Personal Idiosyncratic Events: Autobiographical Memory

Do you remember the events that happened on your first date? How you spent your first paycheck? What you did on your vacation trip in 1985? These are examples of personally experienced events, events that are unique to you. Remote memory of this kind is often called *autobiographical memory*. Assessment of autobiographical memory obviously presents a number of methodological problems.

Accuracy of the content of the memory may be questioned, even when it is seemingly verified by another individual, such as a spouse. Especially questionable is accuracy of the time the remembered event occurred, as it is identified by the subject. Despite these problems, there have been a number of studies that have examined age differences in autobiographical memory (e.g., G. Cohen & Faulkner, 1988; Crovitz & Quina-Holland, 1976; Crovitz & Schiffman, 1974; Fitzgerald & Lawrence, 1984; Franklin & Holding, 1977; Fromholt & Larsen, 1991; Holding, Noonan, Pfau, & Holding, 1986; Hyland & Ackerman, 1988; MacKinnon & Squire, 1989; McCormack, 1979; Rubin, 1982; Sagar, 1990; Sperback, Whitbourne, & Hoyer, 1986) (see Rubin, Wetzler, and Nebes, 1986, for further review).

The standard procedure is one introduced years ago by Galton (1911). Subjects are presented with a series of words (e.g., book, machine, sorry, surprised) and are asked to associate freely to each word with a personal memory. After the last memory is recalled, they are then asked to date when the remembered event occurred. In general, studies using this method have indicated that more recent memories are recalled more frequently than are more remote memories, regardless of a subject's age (e.g., Hyland & Ackerman, 1988), although a U-shaped function has also been reported (MacKinnon & Squire, 1989; McCormack, 1979). That is, both remote and recent events are recalled more frequently than temporally intermediate events. (Interestingly, organic amnesics appear to report about as many remote memories as age-matched control subjects, but they recall far fewer recent memories, that is, memories for events that occurred after the onset of their memory disorder). Shown in Table 10.1 is the distribution of

TABLE 10.1

Distribution of Memories in Percentages across Subjects' Lives[a]

Age of memories (in yrs)	Participant groups (by age)				
	17 to 22 (n = 24)	45 to 49 (n = 11)	50 to 55 (n = 13)	61 to 66 (n = 12)	67 to 73 (n = 12)
0 to 10	95.4	79.8	57.3	44.0	47.2
11 to 20	4.6	6.6	11.1	7.9	12.5
21 to 30		6.6	12.4	7.4	6.0
31 to 40		6.0	12.8	12.5	7.9
41 to 50		1.0	6.4	15.3	10.2
51 to 60				9.7	13.9
61 to 70				3.2	2.3

[a]From Hyland and Ackerman, 1988, Table 3. Copyright 1988 by the Gerontological Society of America. Adapted by permission.

memories found by Hyland and Ackerman (1988) for subjects ranging in age from 17 to 73 yr. Note that for each age group the most frequently recalled events were those that had occurred in the past 10 yr. This outcome suggests that more recent memories of older adults are not especially vulnerable to forgetting, although many more events that occurred within the past month were recalled by young adults (56% of the total events recalled) than by elderly adults (18%). Of course, young adults have had little opportunity to experience remote salient events that are particularly memorable. Interestingly, Rabbitt and McInnis (1988) discovered that more intelligent older people recall earlier memories from childhood than do less intelligent older people. There is also evidence to indicate that at all age levels emotional words evoke more recent memories than do nonemotional words (Fitzgerald & Lawrence, 1984).

Another procedure is to have subjects recall their especially vivid memories and then attempt to date them. With this procedure, G. Cohen and Faulkner (1988) found that adults of all ages recalled most frequently memories from the first decade of their lives and that the frequency of memories recalled declined steadily for each decade beyond the first. This outcome is, of course, quite different from that found with the word-prompt method, but the focus here is on especially vivid memories and not just any memory. A somewhat different outcome was reported by Fitzgerald (1988) with older subjects (62–75 yr) only. The peak frequency occurred for memories of events that occurred when the subjects were from 11 to 25 yr old. Beyond that age the distribution of memories was about the same for each further decade of life. A variation of this procedure calls for subjects to recall the events that were most important in their lives. Here the distribution of memories is like the U-shaped distribution sometimes found with the word-prompt procedure (Holt & Larsen, 1991). That is, both remote and recent events are recalled more frequently than are midlife events.

Why Forgetting?

Proactive and Retroactive Interference

Why do we forget the names of some of our teachers, the names or locations of streets in our college town, the names of people in the news, and so on? The probable reason was identified years ago by Müller and Pilzecker (1900). There is interference produced by the acquisition of similar events both prior to and after the designated to-be-remembered event. Interference from prior events was labeled *proactive interference*, and interference from events interpolated between the acquisition and the retention test for the to-be-remembered events was labeled *retroactive interference*. Consider, for example, a college student who attended the University of Missouri-Columbia. One of the streets bordering the campus is Elm Street, a street running east-west. The student's hometown may also have had a street named after a tree, but it may have been Maple Street rather than Elm. Even if the hometown had an Elm Street, it may have run north-south rather than east-west. Proactive interference would be the likely consequence in either case. After leaving the university, the former student may live in various cities that have streets named Oak, Locust, and Poplar—but no Elm. Here retroactive interference is the likely consequence. As a result of the combined interference, the former student may quickly "forget" the name of the street bordering the campus.

Interference Proneness

As noted in Chapter 4 (p. 123), a familiar theme in the experimental psychology of aging is that elderly adults are more interference prone than are younger adults. Consequently, they are expected to be more susceptible to the adverse effects on retention of proactive and retroactive interference than are younger adults, just as they are expected to be more susceptible to negative transfer under interference conditions. If true, elderly adults should manifest faster forgetting of recently acquired information than do younger adults—thus accounting for the notion that elderly people have particular difficulty in remembering relatively recent events. The notion that an age difference in interference proneness is responsible for whatever age difference exists for long-term episodic forgetting apparently originated in Welford's (1958) review of early studies contrasting retention between young and elderly subjects. Illustrative of these early studies is one by Cameron (1943). A three-digit number was read three times to both young and elderly subjects. A 1-min retention interval then followed. During this interval, experimental subjects of both ages performed another task (backward spelling), while control subjects simply rested. No age difference in retention was found for control subjects. By contrast, a pronounced age difference, favoring young adults, was found for experimental subjects. The age-related deficit in retention supposedly resulted from the greater interference produced by the interpolated task (i.e., retroactive interference) for the elderly subjects than for the young subjects. However, the interpolated material was highly dissimilar to the to-be-remembered material, making pronounced retroactive interference unlikely. More probable is the proactive interference exerted by other three-digit numbers familiar preexperimentally to the subjects.

Problems in Testing the Interference Proneness Hypothesis

There is an important problem inherent in Cameron's (1943) study and in other early studies on age differences in retention that limit the validity of their test of the hypothesis that elderly adults are more prone to interference than are

younger adults. It is the failure of the investigator to equate age groups in acquisition of the to-be-remembered material. Young adults are almost certain to have
acquired more information than elderly adults after a fixed number of exposures
to the to-be-remembered material. Thus, after three readings of a number, young
adults are likely to be able to recall immediately more of that number than are
elderly adults. Of all of the variables that could affect retention, the most important may be the degree to which the material has been acquired before the onset
of the retention interval—the more thoroughly the material has been acquired,
the more resistant it is to forgetting (Underwood, 1954). Consequently, unless
age differences in amount of original acquisition are eliminated, an age difference
in rate of forgetting may be the anomalous consequence. Whether or not differential degrees of initial acquisition have differential effects on rate of forgetting
has been hotly debated by basic memory researchers (Bogartz, 1990; Loftus, 1985;
Slamecka, 1985; Slamecka & McElree, 1983). Nevertheless, the best strategy for
evaluating the effects of aging per se on rate of long-term forgetting would seem
to be to equate age groups as closely as possible in degree of original acquisition.

More recent studies of age differences in retention have been cognizant of this
problem, and they have involved a valiant effort to equate age groups in degree
of original acquisition. The standard solution has been to take all subjects to the
same criterion of mastery. For example, practice continues over trials until an
errorless trial occurs (or, perhaps, two consecutive errorless trials). The mean
number of trials needed to attain this criterion is likely to be somewhat greater
for elderly subjects than for young subjects. Just how satisfactory this procedure is
for equating age groups in degree of original acquisition is debatable (Kausler,
1970). A potential problem exists in the possibility of an age difference of overlearning received by the easiest components of the material. These are the components of the total task acquired early in practice. Because elderly adults usually
take more trials to master the total material, they have more opportunity than
young subjects to overlearn these initially acquired components. In general, overlearning serves to increase resistance to forgetting. Consequently, greater overlearning by elderly subjects than by young subjects could lead to an underesti-
mation of the true extent of an age-related deficit in retention. There are other
methods available for equating groups in degree of original acquisition (Underwood, 1964), but, unfortunately, these methods have yet to be applied in experimental aging research.

Even if age groups could be equated for degree of original acquisition, there is
a related issue to be considered. Young adults are more likely than elderly adults
to acquire material through the use of elaborative rehearsal (e.g., the use of
imagery and verbal associations to list items). This presents a problem in evaluating age differences in retention in that there is convincing evidence with young
adult subjects to indicate that material acquired elaboratively is more resistant to
forgetting than material acquired rotely (e.g., Adams & Montague, 1967; Bugel-

ski, 1968). Consequently, elderly adults might be expected to forget more than young adults simply because the products of initial acquisition differ between the two groups. If elderly adults could be prodded to rehearse elaboratively to the same extent as young adults, then whatever age-related deficit exists may disappear or, at least, be greatly ameliorated.

Laboratory Studies: Retention of Successive Lists

Most of the studies that have compared young and elderly subjects in susceptibility to retroactive or proactive inhibition or interference have been guided by the formal interference theory described in Chapter 4 (p. 122). The procedure employed in these studies calls for the use of consecutively practiced paired-associate lists that bear the A–B, A–C interference relationship indigenous to research on negative transfer. (Note that we are assuming that a learned paired associate is actually an episodic memory.) Experimental subjects practice initially on an A–B list, followed, usually immediately, by practice on an A–C list (which, therefore, functions much like the interpolated task in Cameron's, 1943, study—but in a known, interference-producing role). Recall of A–B content is then tested after some specified retention interval. Practice on A–C pairs (e.g., A_1–C_1) is assumed to encounter interference from the associations acquired from their A–B counterparts (e.g., A_1–B_1). This interference produces some degree of unlearning or weakening of each A–B association (see part A of Figure 10.3). Unlearning is one of the two main processes postulated by interference theory to produce retroactive inhibition or interference (Melton & Irwin, 1940). The other process is competition at recall (see A, Figure 10.3). At the time of recall each A stimulus element has entered into two associations, one with a B response element, the other with a C response element. The stronger A–C associations compete with the weakened A–B associations for recall, in effect inhibiting the recall of the A–B associations. Control subjects learn only the A–B list, therefore, bypassing the unlearning and competition at recall (see top, Figure 10.3) produced by the interpolated A–C list. These subjects are also tested for recall of A–B content following the retention interval. Inferior recall of the A–B content by experimental subjects relative to control subjects defines the phenomenon of *retroactive inhibition*. Its presence presumably results from the interference processes (unlearning and competition at recall) operating only in the experimental condition or, at least, to a greater extent in the experimental condition than in the control condition (retention is usually less than perfect in the control condition as we will see shortly).

Alternatively, as illustrated in part B of Figure 10.3, an investigator may be interested in the retention of the A–C, or second, list content manifested by subjects in the experimental condition. In this case, subjects in the control

Condition	Learn List 1	Sequence Learn List 2		Recall List 1
			(Retention interval)	
Experimental	$A_1 \rightarrow B_1$	$A_1' \xrightarrow{\nearrow B_1 \text{ (some} } C_1 \text{ unlearning)}$		$A_1' \xrightarrow{\nearrow C_1 \text{ (competition at}} B_1 \text{ time of recall)}$ $\left.\right\}$ Difference favoring control condition =
Control	$A_1 \rightarrow B_1$	(Retention Interval)		$A_1 \rightarrow B_1$ Retroactive inhibition

B Time

Condition	Learn List 1	Sequence Learn List 2		Recall List 1
			(Retention interval)	
Experimental	$A_1 \rightarrow B_1$	$A_1' \xrightarrow{\nearrow B_1 \text{ (some}} C_1 \text{ unlearning)}$		$A_1' \xrightarrow{\nearrow B_1 \text{ (competition at}} C_1 \text{ time of recall)}$ $\left.\right\}$ Difference favoring control condition =
Control	$A_1 \rightarrow C_1$	(Retention Interval)		$A_1 \rightarrow C_1$ Proactive inhibition

Time

FIGURE 10.3 Schematic representation of the procedures defining retroactive inhibition (A) and proactive inhibition (B).

condition receive only the A–C list (i.e., a list identical in content to the second list received by experimental subjects). Recall of A–C content is then tested following the retention interval for subjects in both conditions. Inferior recall by experimental subjects, again relative to control subjects, defines the phenomenon of *proactive inhibition*. Its presence is also presumed to result from interference processes present to a greater extent in the experimental condition than in the control condition. The primary source of interference is competition at recall between A–B and A–C associations present in the experimental condition, but not in the control condition.

Interference may also occur for the single list learned by control subjects. Here the interference comes from associations learned outside of the laboratory that form an A–B, A–C relationship with the associations acquired in the laboratory. These interfering associations may be acquired either prior to practice on the laboratory list, or they may have been acquired during the retention interval. Of course, similar extraexperimental associations may be involved for subjects in both the retroactive and proactive experimental conditions, thereby contributing additional sources of interference for these subjects.

Our interest is in aging studies that have made use of these standard procedures to determine the presence or absence of age differences in interference proneness and, therefore, in the rate of forgetting. The popular choice in these studies has been to use the sequence defining retroactive inhibition. A factorial design is employed in which age variation is combined with variation in list sequence (i.e., a control condition receiving only an A–B list and an experimental condition receiving successive A–B, A–C lists). If elderly adults are indeed more interference prone than young adults, then an outcome of the general kind shown in Figure 10.4 is expected. The critical component of this hypothetical outcome is a statistically significant interaction between age and the list-sequence condition. The age difference in the control condition should be slight, whereas the age difference for subjects in the experimental condition should be pronounced (with greater forgetting of the first list being manifested by the elderly subjects). In other words, a multiplicative relationship, one implying the age sensitivity of the processes varied by the manipulable independent variable. These processes, of course, are those postulated by interference theory to be produced by the interpolated A–C list.

A number of tests of age differences in the amount of retroactive inhibition have been reported in which young and elderly subjects were taken to the same criterion of learning on the A–B list (see also Chapter 4, pp. 128–129, for studies employing other than the A–B, A–C list sequence). In studies by Gladis and Braun (1958), Wimer and Wigdor (1958), and Hulicka (1967a) the age difference in amount of retroactive inhibition was not statistically significant. The results for two of these studies are plotted in Figure 10.5. Part A shows the outcome of Wimer and Wigdor's (1958) study. Their experimental subjects, both

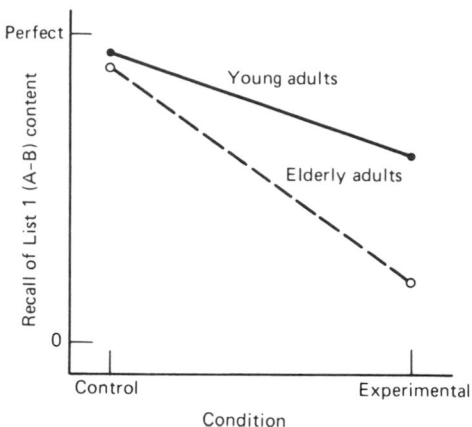

F I G U R E 10.4 Outcome of a hypothetical study on age differences in retroactive inhibition based on the principle that elderly adults are more interference prone than young adults.

young and elderly, practiced on a four-pair A–B list to a criterion of one errorless trial; next they practiced on a four-pair A–C list to a criterion of two successive errorless trials. Then 15 min after learning the first list (with much of this time being spent practicing on the second list), they were tested for recall of the B responses when cued by their A elements. Their control subjects, both young and elderly, also practiced on the A–B list to a criterion of one errorless trial, and 15 min later (the time being filled by performance on a nonlearning task to prevent further rehearsal of the A–B pairs), they, too, were tested for recall of B responses. Note in part A of Figure 10.5 that pronounced retroactive inhibition occurred at both age levels. That is, for each age group, recall in the experimental condition was well below recall in the control condition (even with a single list and no laboratory-induced interference, some forgetting occurred in the control condition; see part A of Figure 10.5), as predicted by interference theory. Most important, however, the amount of retroactive inhibition was certainly no greater for elderly subjects than for young subjects. Thus, there was no hint of the interaction effect predicted on the basis of greater interference proneness for elderly adults than for young adults. In fact, if anything, the amount of retroactive inhibition was slightly greater for their young subjects than for their elderly subjects (see A, Figure 10.5).

Part B of Figure 10.5 shows the outcome of Hulicka's (1967a) study. Although the age difference in amount recalled, favoring young adults, was greater in the experimental condition than in the control condition, the disparity was not large enough to permit rejection of the null hypothesis for the interaction effect. Of

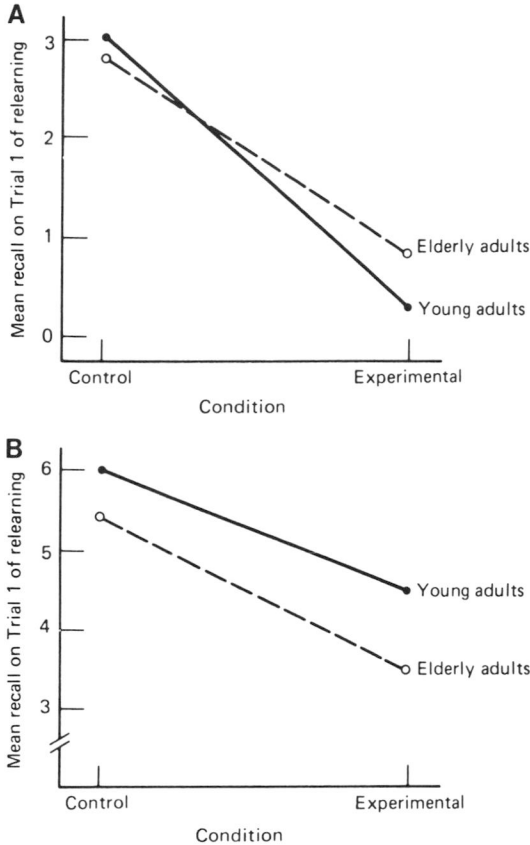

FIGURE 10.5 Results obtained in tests of age differences in amount of retroactive inhibition. (A: Adapted from Wimer & Wigdor, 1958, Table 2.) B: Adapted from Hulicka, 1967a, Table 3.)

further interest is a study by Arenberg (1967b) employing a partial retroactive inhibition design in which only the experimental condition (A–B, A–C) was included. Significantly poorer retention of the A–B list was found for elderly subjects but only with a fast rate of item presentation for the content of the two lists. With a slower rate of presentation, the age difference did not reach statistical significance.

These studies suggest that there does not appear to be a pronounced adult age difference in rate of forgetting, at least as far as forgetting is studied under the conditions yielding retroactive inhibition. Of course, the age equality in rate of forgetting occurred only when the age groups were taken to the same criterion of

mastery on the to-be-retained material. To achieve this equality, the elderly subjects in both Wimer and Wigdor's (1958) study and Hulicka's (1967a) study
required nearly twice as many trials as the young subjects. As indicated earlier,
the additional study opportunity given elderly subjects probably results in considerable overlearning for some components of the to-be-retained pairs. Given this
overlearning, the retention found for elderly adults appears to approximate that
of young adults. It is a different matter, however, when the same amount of
limited practice on the first list is given to both age groups. This condition was
included in a second experiment by Hulicka (1967a). All of her subjects received
the same number of practice trials on the A–B list (six), with experimental
subjects then practicing on the second list to a criterion of one one errorless trial.
Here the interaction effect was clearly statistically significant, with the age difference, favoring young adults, being more pronounced in the experimental condition than in the control condition.

   Any conclusion that there is no age difference in retroactive inhibition is
complicated by the fact that several studies have reported a greater amount for
elderly subjects than for young subjects even when the first list is learned to the
same criterion by both age groups (Arenberg, 1968b; Kay, 1951; Suci, Davidoff,
& Brown, 1962; Traxler, 1973). The picture is complicated further by the conflicting results obtained with a free-recall task. Query and Megran (1983) gave
their subjects five study-test trials on a free-recall list, followed by a single study-
test trial on a different list. The amount of retroactive inhibition produced by the
new list was assessed by giving their subjects another study-test trial on the original list. The decline in recall from the fifth trial to the last trial on the original
list was about the same for their young and elderly subjects. However, with a
similar procedure, Worden and Meggison (1984) found the decline in recall for
the original list to be greater for elderly than for young subjects. Complicating
the picture even more is the fact that the age groups in these studies differed in
amount of recall on the trial preceding the interpolation of the new list.

   A final resolution of the issue of adult age differences in the amount of retroactive inhibition must await new studies in which the methodological problems
inherent in these studies have been solved. In the meantime, our best estimate is
that if age differences exist in the amount of retroactive inhibition, they are likely
to be moderate.

Laboratory Studies: Single-List Retention

   Of additional interest is the possibility of an age difference in the forgetting of
a single list's content. Retention of a single list is required of control subjects in a
study on retroactive inhibition. Note again in Figure 10.5 that the control sub-

jects, whether young or elderly, in both retroactive inhibition studies exhibited some forgetting. That is, recall of that list was less than maximum (4 in part A, 7 in part B), even though the retention interval lasted only minutes and there was no interpolated interfering list. We discovered earlier that interference theorists (Underwood, 1957; Underwood & Postman, 1960) view such forgetting as resulting from interference by material acquired in the everyday world that is similar in content to the to-be-retained laboratory material, sufficiently so to generate an A–B, A–C sequence. An age difference in interference proneness again leads to the prediction of greater forgetting of a single list's content by elderly subjects than by young subjects. This does not seem to be true, at least when the retention interval spans only minutes. In both of our retroactive inhibition studies, the amount of forgetting for the single list (control condition) was about the same for young and elderly subjects (see Figure 10.5). But what about longer retention intervals? Are age differences still absent when retention of a single list is tested after hours have lapsed? Weeks? Years? The situation is akin to that in the real world when we master the names of a new president's first appointments of cabinet members. Remembering those names becomes increasingly difficult as resignations occur, and new names replace the original members. That is, retroactive interference during the retention interval adds to the proactive interference from the names of other cabinet members who preceded the to-be-remembered ones (i.e., proactive interference comparable to the kind identified by Underwood in single-list retention). These interference processes are simulated in the laboratory with single lists of verbal or pictorial material, but within a time-compressed framework.

Early studies on age differences in the forgetting of single lists over prolonged retention intervals reported conflicting evidence. Hulicka and Weiss (1965) evaluated age differences in retention after intervals of 20 min and one week. Surprisingly, their elderly subjects (mean age, 68 yr) retained more than their younger subjects (mean age, 38 yr). In addition, Desroches, Kaiman, and Ballard (1966) reported no age differences in the rate of forgetting over a 1-wk retention interval. Their "younger" subjects, however, were middle-aged adults who were equivalent in their rate of learning the original list with their elderly subjects. On the other hand, significantly greater forgetting by elderly subjects was found by both Davis and Obrist (1966) and Harwood and Naylor (1969). In the study by Davis and Obrist (1966), paired associates made up the single list and the retention interval was 48 hr. In the study by Harwood and Naylor (1969), free recall of names of common objects made up the single list and the retention interval was 4 wk. Although a statistical age difference in amount retained was found in both studies, the absolute magnitude of the age difference was actually fairly small. Greater forgetting by elderly than by young subjects was also found by Wimer (1960) for word pairs over a 1-mo retention interval, Belbin and Downs

(1965) for word pairs over a 3-d interval, Hulicka and Rust (1964) for nonsense equations over a 1-wk interval, and by Bruning, Holzbauer, and Kimberlin (1975) for a word list over a 1-d interval.

More recent studies have also yielded conflicting evidence. Harker and Riege (1985) compared rates of forgetting for young and elderly subjects over retention intervals of 2, 20, and 200 min. Their items included both words and designs, and their recognition memory test was conducted for different subsets of items at each retention interval. Despite the higher recognition scores for their young subjects at the 2-min retention interval, especially for words as items, the Age × Retention Interval interaction effect was negligible for both words and designs. The implication is that there was little age difference in rate of forgetting. However, this interpretation is complicated by the fact that accuracy in recognition was greater for young subjects after 200 min than it was for elderly subjects after 20 min (see Loftus, 1985, for a discussion of this problem). Much longer retention intervals (extending over 3 wk) were employed by Mitchell, Brown, and Murphy (1990) for the recognition memory of pictures of common objects. They too found no significant Age × Retention Interval interaction effect, even though the age groups were not equated for degree of initial acquisition. However, interpretation is again complicated by the fact that accuracy of recognition at 1 wk for their elderly subjects had been reduced to a level that was not reached until after 3 wk by their young subjects. A similar problem exists in a study by Hultsch, Hertzog, and Dixon (1984) in which the rate of forgetting of propositions in a narrative discourse was about the same for young and elderly subjects. However, immediately after presentation of the discourse the young subjects averaged 24% of the propositions recalled and the elderly subjects only 11% (after a 1-mo retention interval the percentages of recalled propositions were reduced to 12% and 3% for young and elderly adult subjects, respectively).

By contrast, several other recent researchers have reported significantly greater losses for elderly subjects than for young subjects. A variety of verbal and pictorial materials have entered into these studies, as well as a variety of retention intervals. Both word pairs and picture pairs were employed by Howe and Hunter (1986) with a 1-wk retention interval, a word list with a 1-wk interval by Light, Singh, and Capps (1986), pictures and line drawings by Park, Puglisi, and Smith (1986) with a 1-mo interval, and prose by G. Cohen and Faulkner (1984) with a 1-wk interval. As is usually the case, there is no assurance in these studies of equal acquisition by young and elderly subjects after presentation of the to-be-remembered material, again making their outcomes difficult to interpret.

There have been two other recent studies dealing with age differences in retention over lengthy intervals that have the advantage over the other studies in their tighter control over the equality of initial mastery of the material by young and elderly subjects. Rybarczyk, Hart, and Harkins (1987) employed a lengthy list of pictures of common objects. The pictures were exposed for about half a second longer for their elderly subjects than for their young adult subjects, a procedure that resulted in approximately equal performance scores shortly after (10 min) the entire list had been presented. For this test a subset of the total number of pictures was presented along with new or distractor pictures for a recognition memory test. Other subsets of previously untested list pictures and new distractor pictures were presented for additional recognition memory tests after 2 hr and after 48 hr. Test scores at each retention interval, expressed as d' values, are shown in part A of Figure 10.6 for both age groups. It may be seen that the rate of forgetting was about the same for the elderly subjects as for the young subjects. A similar procedure was employed by Park, Royal, Dudley, and Morrell (1988) with line drawings of complex scenes composing the single list. Different subsets of old and new pictures were given a recognition memory test at retention intervals of 48 hr, 1 wk, 2 wk, and 4 wk after the immediate recognition memory test. Their results (with scores expressed as hits minus false alarms, scores comparable to d' scores) are shown in part B of Figure 10.6. Note that no age difference in forgetting was observed through 48 hr, as in Rybarczyk et al.'s (1987) study. However, beyond 48 hr it is apparent that there was a moderate age difference in rate of forgetting, sufficiently so to yield a significant Age × Retention Interval interaction effect. Nevertheless, note that after 4 wk the two groups were essentially equal in amount retained.

Possible exceptions to equivalent rates of forgetting for young and elderly subjects were reported by Brainerd, Reyna, Howe, and Kingma (1990), Giambra and Arenberg (1993), and Huppert and Kopelman (1989). Huppert and Kopelman's study list consisted of 120 pictures taken from magazines (e.g., pictures of people and pictures of scenes). Recognition memory tests for subsets of 40 old and 40 new pictures were given 10 min after the study list (filled with conversation), 24 hr later, and 1 wk later. Huppert and Kopelman (1989) identified two subgroups of young adult and elderly subjects who had equivalent mean recognition hit rates on the 10 min test (85%). Despite the matching of performance shortly after study, the subgroups differed considerably on the later recognition memory tests. At 24 hr the mean hit rates were 80% and 70% for the young and elderly subgroups, respectively: comparable values after 1 wk were 75% and 60%. Of course, it may be argued that matching age groups 10 min after study does not necessarily equate the groups in initial acquisition. Brainerd et al. (1990) reported greater forgetting of paired associates over a two week interval for their elderly subjects than for their young subjects, and Giambra and Avenberg (1993) reported the same for sentences, even though the age groups were presumably equated for initial acquisition in each study.

Our conviction that adult age differences in rate of forgetting, given age group equivalence in initial acquisition, are slight remains unshaken, even though some researchers (Howe & Hunter, 1986) have reported substantially greater forgetting by elderly subjects than by young subjects when recall rather than recognition is

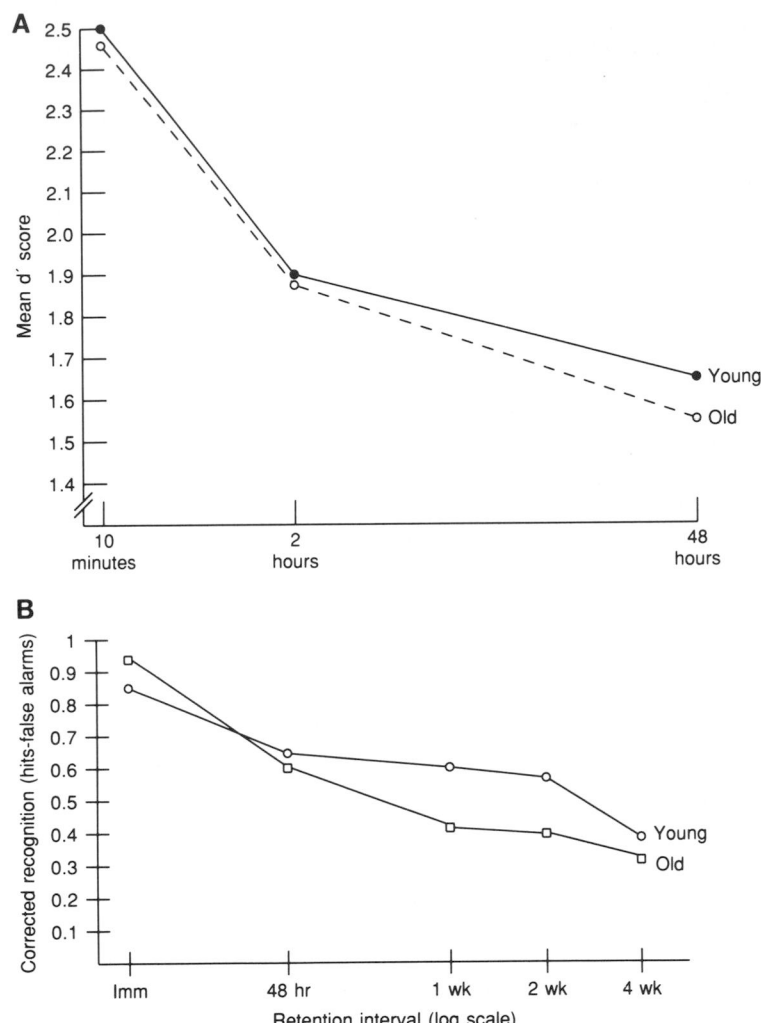

FIGURE 10.6   Forgetting curves for pictorial materials. A: Pictures of objects (Adapted from Rybarczyk, Hart, & Harkins, 1987, Table 1.) B: Pictures of complex scenes (Reprinted from Park, Royal, Dudley, & Morrell, 1988, Figure 1. Copyright 1988 by the American Psychological Association.)

required. It is true, of course, that our evidence is from laboratory simulations of forgetting with lists of items as the to-be-retained material. Our confidence in the generalizability of the results found for laboratory-induced forgetting to everyday forgetting is bolstered by the striking similarity between the forgetting curves for list materials (e.g., Figure 10.6) and forgetting curves with everyday materials, such as names of college town streets (Figure 10.1). In both cases, most of the forgetting occurs shortly after acquisition, and it eventually levels off with the remaining material residing in a permastore state. The difference between laboratory forgetting and much of the forgetting occurring in the real world rests largely in the time compressed nature of the former—that is, forgetting occurs over weeks rather than years. Moreover, in Bahrick's (1984b) study of professors' retention of the faces (and names) of their students (see Chapter 7, p. 260), the rate of forgetting was no greater for professors in their 60s at the time of the original classes than it was for younger professors.

Laboratory Studies: Retention of Activities and Actions

Our focus thus far has been entirely on the forgetting of content information when words, pictures, or verbal propositions serve as the to-be-remembered information. What about age differences in the rate of forgetting of activities or actions? Here we find surprisingly little information on what should be important topics of investigation. There have been, however, four recent studies on age differences in the forgetting of actions performed in the laboratory and one on the forgetting of activities.

Two of the studies involved a recall test both shortly after performance of a single series of actions and after one or more retention intervals. Knopf and Neidhardt (1989b) had their young and elderly subjects recall a lengthy series of actions shortly after the completion of the series, and several times later at retention intervals through 3 wk. Recall scores were far from perfect for both age groups (but significantly higher for the young subjects) at the immediate retention test. Amazingly, however, neither age group manifested any further decline in recall scores throughout the lengthy retention period. That is, there was no indication of forgetting by either young or elderly subjects. There is a problem in interpreting this outcome, however. Successive recall tests, in effect, provide additional performances of those actions (even if they are only verbal reinstatements) that could be remembered on the immediate recall test. As we discovered earlier, repeated actions tend to be recalled far better than actions performed only once (see Chapter 9, p. 335). To circumvent this problem, Phillips and Kausler (1992) gave their subjects only one recall trial, with half of the subjects recalling 10 min after the last action had been performed and the other half 24 hr after the last action. Recall scores were clearly lower after 24 hr than shortly after performance for both young and elderly subjects. However, the Age × Retention Interval interaction effect fell far short of statistical significance, implying equivalent rates of forgetting for young and elderly subjects. Acceptance of equal forgetting rates is again complicated by the presence of a large age difference in recall at the short retention interval. Phillips and Kausler (1992) discovered further that rate of forgetting was unaffected by a shift in the physical environment from time of original performance to time of recall (i.e., a context shift; see Chapter 7, p. 264). This was the case for both young and elderly subjects.

In the third study, Kausler and Wiley (1990b) employed a recognition test rather than a recall test. To avoid the problem of testing every action at each retention interval, half of the actions in a lengthy series were tested shortly after the completion of the series and the other half 24 hr later. In agreement with Knopf and Neidhardt's (1989b) results, their young adult subjects showed no forgetting. That is, their recognition test scores indicated nearly perfect recognition at both times of measurement. However, Kausler and Wiley's (1990b) elderly subjects did show a modest, but statistically significant, amount of forgetting over 24 hr. There seems to be little loss of content information for actions over 24 hr for both young and elderly adults as revealed by a recognition test. What does seem to happen is that this information becomes increasingly difficult to recall regardless of a subject's age, as indicated in Phillips and Kausler's (1992) study.

In the fourth study (Nyberg, Nilsson, & Bäckman, 1992), the subjects performed on 6 successive series of actions (12 actions per series). Each of the series was followed by an immediate recall test. On these immediate tests, the young subjects recalled significantly more actions than the elderly subjects. Fifteen minutes after the immediate recall test for the last list, the subjects received a final recall test in which they attempted to recall all of the 72 actions previously performed. The young subjects again recalled significantly more than the elderly subjects. However, the Age × Retention Interval (i.e., immediate versus final recall) interaction was not statistically significant. The implication is that proactive interference produced by preceding series of actions and retroactive interference produced by following series of actions were no greater for the elderly subjects than for the young subjects. However, the presence of an age difference on the immediate recall tests again complicates any conclusion of no age difference in rate of forgetting. More firmly established is another outcome of this study. Forgetting of actions over 15 min was much less pronounced than was forgetting of sentences describing those actions (these sentences were the to-be-remembered items for other groups in the study). This was true for both the young and the elderly subjects. Regardless of age, susceptibility to proactive and retroactive interference seems to be less pronounced for actions than for verbal materials.

Finally, Earles and Coon (1994) assessed retention over a 6-mo interval of a series of activities performed in the laboratory (e.g., digit copying, letter comparison). The assessments were made by telephone calls in which subjects were asked to describe the activities performed days, weeks, or months earlier. The Age × Retention Interval interaction was not significant, implying again an age equivalence in rate of forgetting activities. However, the age-related deficit in recall after a short retention interval suggests that the age groups differed in amount recalled immediately after completing the activities, thus again complicating any interpretation of the Age × Retention Interval interaction.

Laboratory Studies: Retention of Noncontent Attributes

It seems unlikely that forgetting would be restricted to the content of material. Noncontent attributes of that material surely suffer forgetting as well. Little is known, however, about adult age differences in the rate of forgetting of frequency-of-occurrence information, temporal information, spatial information, source information, and so on. The little research that has been done has focused on noncontent attributes of actions performed in the laboratory. In a study discussed earlier (see Chapter 9, p. 339), Liu and Kausler (1993) had their subjects give frequency judgments 24 hr after performance as well as shortly after performance. To avoid testing the same actions twice, half of the actions at each frequency level were tested immediately after performance and the other half 24 hr later. Both the young and the elderly subjects displayed moderate amounts of forgetting over 24 hr, but the Age × Retention Interval interaction was not statistically significant. Any conclusion about equal rates of forgetting of frequency information by young and elderly adults is again complicated by the age-related deficit in frequency memory scores shortly after performance. The other noncontent attribute tested for an age difference in rate of forgetting is that of temporal information. Kausler and Wiley (1990b) tested their subjects for their temporal memory of the order in which actions were performed (as well as testing for memory of their content; see Chapter 9, p. 341). Temporal memory scores were, as expected, much higher for the young than for the elderly subjects at the short retention interval. More important, both groups had significantly lower scores 24 hr later—and the Age × Retention Interval interaction effect was not significant. This outcome suggests that temporal information may be forgotten at equivalent rates for young adults and elderly adults. However, we once more have the problem created by unequal test scores for the two age groups at the time of initial testing. We greatly need other studies examining age differences in rates of forgetting for such noncontent attributes of actions and activities as spatial location information and source information as well as additional studies on age differences in forgetting of frequency and temporal information for words as well as actions. Especially needed are studies in which the researchers have found ways of equating young and elderly subjects in initial acquisition of the attributes.

CHAPTER 11

Long-Term Episodic Memory: Implicit Memory

Nature of Implicit Memory

An intriguing phenomenon associated with Korsakoff's syndrome is the relative sparing of several forms of memory and learning from the amnesic symptoms that otherwise characterize this disease. It is the long-term memory of episodic events of the kind discussed in previous chapters that is largely impaired with the disease (see, for example, Squire and Butters, 1984). Generic memory (see Chapter 12) is relatively spared as is procedural learning (see Chapter 2). Nor does the sparing of memory loss with amnesia end here. Warrington and Weiskrantz (1968, 1970) discovered yet another form of memory that is left relatively untouched by the disease. Their amnesic and control subjects received a word list to study for either a recall test or a recognition test. Not surprisingly, the amnesics scored well below the control subjects on both episodic-memory tests. What was surprising was the outcome of a different kind of memory test administered to all of the subjects. They first received a study list containing a number of to-be-remembered words. On a later test the subjects received either fragmented words (e.g.,—h a——; a fragment-completion test) or the first three letters of a word (e.g., sha____; a stem-completion test), and they were asked to produce a word that conformed to the partial information given. Some of the words had been part of the prior study list, others had not. Suppose, for example, that *shape* had been a study-list word for half of the subjects. The probability of it being produced was much greater than the probability of other words that also matched the partial information given (e.g., *shark*), but had not been in the study list. Most important, the probability of *shape*'s production was much greater for this half of the subjects than for the other half who did not have this word in the study list (but who received the same partial information on the word production test). The structures of study and implicit-memory test lists for a stem completion task are illustrated in Table 11.1. Note that both subgroups receive the same stems on the test list, but only half of them are the stems of study-list words received by a

TABLE 11.1

Sample Target Words and Baseline Words for a Study List and an Implicit-Memory Test List (Stem-Completion Test)

Study list		Test list	
Subgroup 1	Subgroup 2	Subgroup 1	Subgroup 2
shade	chair	sha____ (target)	cha____ (target)
print	trade	pri____ (target)	tra____ (target)
		cha____ (baseline for)	sha____ (baseline for)
		tra____ (baseline for)	pri____ (baseline for)

given subgroup. The other half are stems for words received only by the other subgroup, and they provide baselines for estimating guessing rates for target words when they were not in the study list). The amnesic and control subjects did not differ in their production probabilities, even though the amnesics recalled or recognized far fewer of the produced words on the overt episodic-memory test. Numerous other researchers (e.g., Graf & Schacter, 1985; Graf, Squire, and Mandler, 1984) have since replicated the basic outcome of Warrington and Weiskrantz's (1968, 1970) pioneering studies with amnesic subjects.

The phenomenon discovered by Warrington and Weiskrantz (1968, 1970) finally entered the basic memory laboratory in a series of experiments by Jacoby and Dallas (1981). Their supplementary test, however, differed from that of Warrington and Weiskrantz (1968, 1970). Young adult subjects were subjected to brief exposures (around 30 ms) of words, and were asked to identify each word. The proportion of words correctly identified was much greater for those words that had been included in a prior study list than for words that had not been included—whether or not the study-list words were episodically memorable. The prior occurrence of a word gives it an advantage over other words, regardless of the format of the test employed (i.e., fragment completion, stem completion, or perceptual identification). In effect, prior occurrences "prime" the relevant words for later memorability. However, the form of the memory test needed to demonstrate the "lingering memory" of the primed words differs from an episodic-memory test in that no reference is made to the episodic event. Most important, retrieval of the primed words appears to be automatic in the sense that conscious recollection plays no role in its operations. Conscious recollection is seemingly equally unnecessary when memory is assessed by either a word-fragment test, a stem completion test, or a perceptual identification test. By contrast, recall or recognition of previously studied words requires conscious recollection in the form of some kind of active and intentional retrieval process.

Memory in the absence of conscious recollection has often been called *procedural memory* (Squire, 1986). However, our preference is to avoid confusion with what we have earlier called procedural learning (Chapter 2, p. 59), and to refer to it by its other common name, *implicit memory* (Graf & Schacter, 1985). Recollective episodic memory of the same events involved in implicit memory is then commonly referred to as *explicit memory* or *declarative memory*. The two forms of episodic memory have also been known as *indirect* (for implicit) and *direct* (for explicit) memory. Research on implicit memory became one of the "hot" areas of research in the 1980s (see Richardson-Klavehn & Bjork, 1988, for a detailed review), and the heat has persisted into the 1990s. Interest was stimulated by the apparent dissociations between implicit memory and episodic memory. The initial dissociation involved the diagnostic category of subjects, that is, amnesic versus normal, as the critical independent variable. Individuals diagnosed as amnesic manifested performance decrements for standard episodic-memory tasks, but not for implicit-memory tasks. Research with young adult subjects expanded the dissociations to include various manipulable independent variables. For example, Jacoby and Dallas (1981) discovered that variations in task orientation that were designed to vary the level of processing of study-list words had a pronounced effect on explicit memory tests for those words, but no effect on implicit-memory tests of the same words. An especially intriguing dissociation was reported by Tulving, Schacter, and Stark (1982). A critical independent variable in their study was the duration of the retention interval, either for 1 hr or for 1 wk after the presentation of the study list. The dramatic difference in rate of forgetting they found for their explicit-memory test (word recognition) and their implicit-memory test (fragment completion) may be seen in Figure 11.1. Note that considerable forgetting occurred for episodic events—but not for implicitly remembered events.

On the surface, it is tempting to view implicit memory as simply a phenomenon of semantic (or lexical) memory (see Chapter 12). A simplistic view is that study-list words activate their lexical representations, and that this activation persists until partial information is presented on the implicit-memory test. Recently activated representations are more immediately accessible than are representations for other words sharing this partial information, but they were not primed during study phase. However, as noted by Tulving et al. (1982), there is a problem here:

> It is worth noting that although the priming effects of interest in this article were demonstrated in what is clearly a semantic-memory task, it is not clear that they can be regarded as a phenomenon of semantic memory. The matter has been discussed elsewhere (Tulving, 1983). For instance, the fact that there was no reduction

in the size of the priming effect over a 7-day interval does not encourage the view of priming as a temporary activation of relevant information in the lexical or conceptual network (Collins & Loftus, 1975). (p. 341).

Activation of a node is likely to persist for seconds, not for days. Then what is the nature of implicit memory? Here is Tulving et al.'s (1982) answer:

> Since the priming effects described in this article clearly are independent of episodic memory, and since there are problems with their interpretation in terms of modifications of semantic memory, we are tempted to think that they reflect the operation of some other, as yet little understood, memory system (p. 341).

Many memory psychologists, however, have been reluctant to accept further proliferation of the total-memory system into yet a third separate system to join the generic and explicit episodic systems. A popular alternative instead is to conceptualize implicit memory as being governed by data-driven perceptual processes or procedures (Jacoby, 1983; Nelson, Keelean, & Negrao, 1989; Roediger & Blaxton, 1987). Thus implicit memory is viewed in terms of the involvement of perceptual skills similar to those involved in some forms of procedural learning (e.g., mirror reading; see Chapter 2, p. 59). By contrast, explicit memory is

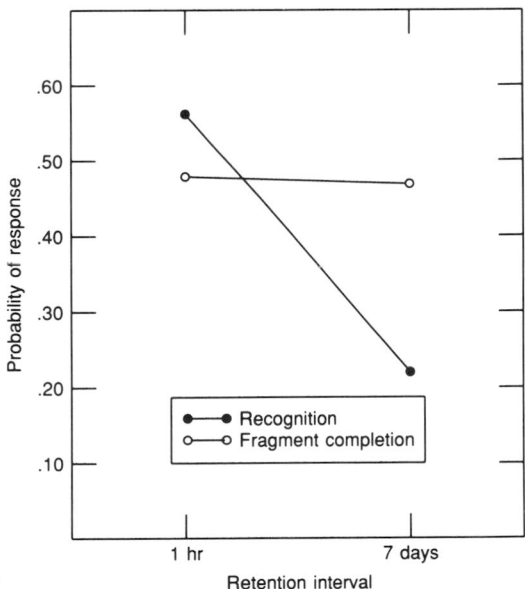

FIGURE 11.1 Time course of priming effects in word-fragment completion and recognition over an interval from 1 hour to 7 days. (Reprinted from Tulving, Schacter, & Stark, 1982, Figure 1. Copyright 1982 by the American Psychological Association.)

conceptually driven in the sense of being governed by higher order processes. The distinction between data-driven and conceptually driven was nicely summarized by Roediger and Blaxton: "On an implicit memory test such as perceptual identification in which subjects are to identify isolated words from brief glimpses, processing should depend heavily on characteristics of the data display and the match of such perceptual features during study and test" (p. 380). The match of features during study and test is viewed as being critical to the manifestation of implicit memory. For example, Jacoby and Dallas (1981) found no facilitation of visual word identification on their implicit-memory test when the prior study list was presented auditorily. That is, there was no match between the auditory feature analytic processes operating during study and the visual feature analytic processes operating during the test. Similarly, Roediger and Blaxton (1987) found the degree of implicit memory to be greater with a word fragment test when both study-list words and word fragments were in the same visual format (e.g., both hand-printed or both typed) rather than in different formats (e.g., hand-printed study-list words and typed word fragments). Here too there should be greater commonality between study-test processes in the former than in the latter.

Adult Age Differences in Implicit Memory

Our main concern, of course, is with adult age differences in implicit memory phenomena (see Howard, 1988a, in press, and Light, 1988b, for additional reviews). The absence of age-related deficits for implicit-memory phenomena, in combination with pronounced age-related deficits for explicit-memory phenomena, could be viewed as a dissociation in support of implicit memory's status as a separate memory system. Alternatively, the absence of age-related deficits for implicit memory could simply indicate that data-driven processes are far less age sensitive than are conceptually driven processes.

The first study on adult age differences in implicit memory was by Light, Singh, and Capps (1986). Their study was essentially a replication of Tulving et al.'s (1982) study, extended to include elderly subjects as well as young adult subjects. Young and elderly subjects received a lengthy study list in which the words were later tested for explicit memory (old-new recognition) and implicit memory (fragment completion). The tests were administered either shortly after study or 7 d later, and they were administered either in the order of explicit test first, implicit test second, or in the reverse order. As expected, an overall age difference, favoring young adults, was found for the explicit-word recognition test. For the fragment completion implicit-memory test, the overall mean score (proportion of fragments completed with words from the prior study list) was slightly, but not significantly, greater for the young subjects (.518) than for elderly subjects (.476). For both age groups, the mean scores for these experimental words were significantly greater than the mean scores for the same words when they had not been included in the prior study list (i.e., control words). Two subgroups were employed at each age level in order to permit an experimental word-control comparison while holding constant the content for the two subsets of words. The experimental words in the study list for Subgroup 1 served as control words for Subgroup 2, and the experimental words in the study list for Subgroup 2 served as control words for Subgroup 1 (see Table 11.1).

Two other results obtained by Light et al. (1986) are of interest. In contrast to the negligible decline in implicit-memory test scores over a 7-d interval reported by Tulving et al. (1982), Light et al. (1986) found a moderate, but significant, decline in implicit-memory test scores over the same retention interval. The amount of the decline was about the same for young and elderly subjects. There was an important difference between the two studies, however. Light et al.'s (1986) initial test was given shortly after the study list had been presented, whereas Tulving et al.'s (1982) initial test was given about 1 hr after study-list presentation. Other investigators (Sloman, Hayman, Ohta, Law, & Tulving, 1988) have found that forgetting on the fragment-completion task occurs rapidly for a few minutes after study, but then its rate slows down considerably (with some retention still apparent after several months!). Where retention intervals are set seems to be a critical factor in determining the extent of forgetting observed in any study of fragment completion. In addition, Light et al. (1986) found stochastic independence between performance on the two tests (i.e., no difference in fragment completion scores between old words correctly recognized as old and old words incorrectly recognized as new)—but only for subjects, young and elderly, receiving the explicit-memory test first.

Light and Singh (1987) tested for the generalizability of the age insensitivity of implicit memory to other kinds of implicit-memory tests. One of the other tests they employed was a stem-completion test in which subjects were given the three initial letters of a to-be-produced word. In addition, a cued-recall test served as the explicit-memory test. The cues here were the same initial letters given for the to-be-produced words on the implicit-memory tests. Shown in Figure 11.2 are the results obtained for young and elderly subjects on the two kinds of tests. Note the pronounced age-related deficit on the explicit cued-recall test, and the modest age difference (but again favoring the young subjects) on the implicit-memory test. In another experiment, a perceptual identification test replaced the word completion test as the measure of implicit memory, but the outcome was much the same. Given the consistent pattern of results obtained with different measures, Light and Singh (1987) concluded that "These results, similar to those observed in amnesics, suggest that older adults are impaired on tasks which require conscious recollection but that memory which depends on automatic activation processes is relatively unaffected by age" (p. 531).

Our confidence in Light and Singh's (1987) conclusion is shaken somewhat by the fact that a consistent finding in Light's (Light et al., 1986; Light & Singh, 1987) studies has been the presence of a moderate age difference in implicit-

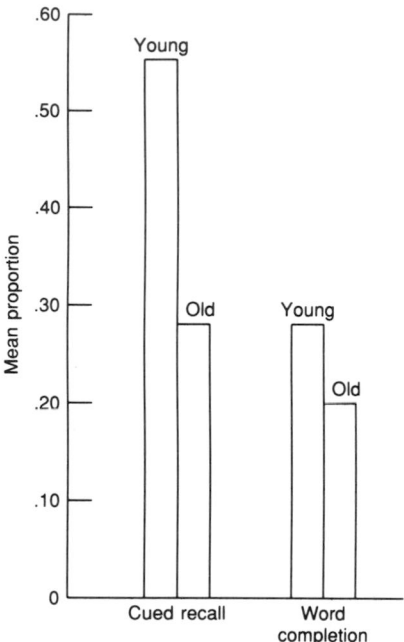

FIGURE 11.2   Age differences for explicit-memory (cued recall) and implicit-memory (stem completion) tests. For the implicit test, means are for the difference between experimental and baseline words. (Adapted from Light & Singh, 1987, Table 2.)

memory test scores, even though the differences were never large enough to attain statistical significance. They were large enough, however, to attain statistical significance in a study by Chiarello and Hoyer (1988) with the stem-completion task. In fact, larger stem-completion scores were found for their young subjects at each of three different retention intervals. H. P. Davis et al. (1990) found a statistically significant age effect for scores on stem-completion task with subjects ranging in age from 20 to 80 yr. However, the age-related deficit was apparent only for subjects 70 yr old and older. They argued that the age-related deficit may have attained statistical significance at younger ages if larger sample sizes had been employed.

The importance of sample size in testing an expected null effect for age variation on implicit-memory test scores was revealed in a study by Hultsch, Masson, and Small (1991). The samples entering into most studies on implicit memory have been rather small. In their study, Hultsch et al. (1991) employed large samples at each of three age levels (19–36, 55–69 and 70–89 yr), and they did find the moderate age-related deficit in implicit-memory test scores to attain statistical significance for both of the two older groups of subjects. Their subjects received 30 nouns on a lexical decision task. This task was followed by a stem-completion test involving words from the prior task as well as new words. Mean stem-completion scores (target minus baseline proportions of critical words constructed) were .078, .055, and .055 for the 19–36, 44–69, and 70–89 age groups, respectively. Not surprisingly, Hultsch et al. (1991) also found significant age-related deficits for three tests of explicit memory given to the same subjects. For example, the proportion of words recalled from a free-recall study list composed of words from several taxonomic categories were .668, .614, and .545 for the three age groups. Note, however, that the magnitude of the age-related deficit did not differ greatly from that found for the implicit test. The similarity in outcomes raises questions about the existence of a true dissociation between implicit and explicit memory and the likelihood of the two forms of memory involving grossly different processes. On the other hand, other evidence from this study does provide support for the notion that different processes mediate implicit memory, at least as tested by a stem-completion test, and explicit memory. Clustering scores for the word-recall task were found to correlate significantly at each age level with the number of words recalled but not with stem-completion scores. Several other individual-differences tests were also administered to the same subjects. They included a verbal ability test and a working-memory test. Hultsch et al. (1991) discovered that the individual-differences variables that correlated highly with implicit-memory test scores differed greatly from those that correlated highly with explicit-memory test scores. This outcome again suggests different processes for implicit and explicit memory—but it doesn't rule out the possibility that the processes of implicit memory, like the processes of explicit memory, are age sensitive.

Is implicit memory truly age insensitive? The studies reviewed thus far have clearly not resolved this important issue. Needed in addition to data from larger samples are data on age differences with other presumed tests of implicit memory. In fact, there seems to be a nearly infinite number of ways of testing implicit memory, and a fairly large sample of those tests has already appeared. Thus, the flow of data on adult age differences in novel tests of implicit memory has been steadily increasing—but, alas, the outcomes have continued to be inconsistent.

The differential effects of variation in depth of processing on explicit and implicit memory tests reported by Jacoby and Dallas (1981) were replicated by Park and Shaw (1992) for both young and elderly subjects. That is, for each group, a deep orienting task yielded greater recall (explicit memory) than a shallow orienting task. Stem completion (implicit memory) scores, however, were no higher after deep processing than after shallow processing. Most important, there was a pronounced age-related deficit on the explicit test but not on the implicit test. The dissociation for age as the variable provides firm support for the age insensitivity of implicit memory in contrast to the pronounced age sensitivity of explicit memory. In addition, the priming effect for stem completion increased equally in amount for the two age groups as the number of initial letters given in the stem increased from 2 to 4.

An intriguing novel implicit-memory test is one employed initially by Jacoby and Witherspoon (1982) and later applied to aging research by Howard (1988) and Rose, Yesavage, Hill, and Bower (1986). The procedure requires having subjects answer questions that bias the less frequent meaning of a homophone (words that are pronounced alike, but have different spellings and different meanings; e.g., *read* as the more frequent meaning, *reed* as the less frequent meaning), such as "Name a musical instrument that employs a *reed.*" After all questions have been answered, subjects are given a spelling test in which homophones are among the auditorily presented words, some from the prior questions, others that were not included in those questions. The measure of implicit memory is the extent to which subjects spell the previously encountered homophones with the less frequently occurring word (e.g., *reed* to "read"). Howard's (1988) evidence regarding age differences for this kind of an implicit-memory test is somewhat ambiguous. In several different experiments, young adults appeared to be more biased toward spelling the infrequent words than were elderly adults (i.e., greater implicit memory scores for young subjects), an outcome also reported by Rose et al. (1986). However, Howard (1988) argued that her young subjects had greater explicit memory of the prior sentences than did her elderly subjects, and that memory of these sentences influenced their spellings. In a clever variation of the standard procedure in another experiment, Howard's (1988) procedure seemingly minimized the extent of explicit memory's involvement, and by so doing largely eliminated the advantage of young subjects on the implicit-memory test.

Age differences were also missing in a study by Mitchell, Brown, and Murphy (1990). Their procedure utilized a variation of Jacoby and Dallas's (1981) perceptual priming procedure in which pictures replaced words. The pictures were drawings of common objects that subjects had to name as quickly as possible. Implicit memory was measured by the faster naming time on a second presentation of the pictures, relative to naming time on their first presentation. Age differences in the magnitude of the priming effect were found to be negligble. Moreover, the priming effect for both young and elderly subjects was as robust for pictures that had been forgotten as for pictures that were correctly recognized on the explicit-episodic-memory test (i.e., stochastic independence). In addition, the magnitude of the priming effect declined considerably for both age groups over a 24-hr retention interval, but it remained stable thereafter through a 3-wk retention interval. By contrast, episodic memory of the pictures dropped greatly for both age groups from one day to three weeks (see Chapter 10, p. 364). On the other hand, greater implicit-memory scores for young adult than for elderly subjects were reported by Russo and Parkin (1993) when fragments of pictures of common objects rather than whole pictures were presented for identification. Implicit memory was again measured by faster naming time on the second exposure to each picture fragment.

Another kind of implicit-memory test is one in which subjects are asked to generate instances of a category following exposure to those instances in a prior list (Light & Albertson, 1989). The young and elderly subjects initially encountered a lengthy word list for which they were to rate each word on a pleasant–unpleasant dimension. Embedded in the list were 18 target words, three instances (of relatively low frequency in taxonomic norms) of each of six different categories. After varying retention intervals, subjects were given the names of different categories, and they generated eight instances of each. The probabilities of generating target words from the study list are shown in Figure 11.3, along with the probabilities of generating the same words when they were baseline items (i.e., had not been part of the study list). Note that a modest, and statistically nonsignificant, age-related deficit existed in the magnitude of the priming effect (probability of target words minus probability of baseline words). On the other hand,

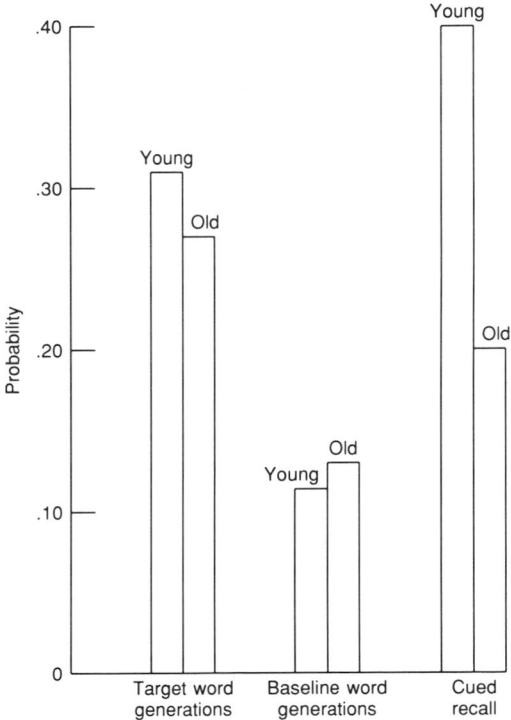

FIGURE 11.3   Age differences for explicit-memory (cued recall) and implicit-memory (category-instance generation) tests. (Adapted from data in Light & Albertson, 1989.)

the age-related deficit in explicit memory, measured by the cued recall (category names as the cues) of target instances, was much greater, and statistically significant.

An especially informative test was one conducted by Light, LaVoie, Valencia-Laver, Owens, and Mead (1992). In their first experiment, they employed an incidental-memory procedure in which a shallow orienting task was performed for half of the 80 words presented and a deep orienting task for the other half. In addition, half of the words at each level of processing were presented aurally and half visually. In their first experiment, each of the prior study-list words was then exposed briefly (visually) along with a number of new words not previously seen or heard, and the subjects were asked to identify each one. Mean proportions of words identified correctly are given in Table 11.2 for each category of words (i.e., prior aurally presented words, prior visually presented words, and new words at each level of processing and for young and elderly subjects). It may be seen that the magnitudes of priming effects (old words minus new words: a measure of implicit memory) were about the same for their young and elderly subjects, implying the absence of an age difference in implicit-memory proficiency. It may also be seen that at each age level the magnitude of the priming effect was much greater for previously seen words than for previously heard words.

The outcome of Light et al.'s (1992) first experiment is in agreement with Roediger and Blaxton's (1987) position that the proficiency of processing on an

TABLE 11.2

Proportions Correct and Standard Deviations of Perceptual Identification as a Function of Age and Item Status in Experiments 1 and 2[a]

Experiment[b]	Young			Older		
	Saw	Heard	New	Saw	Heard	New
Experiment 1						
Syllable count						
P	**.606**[c]	.509	.427	**.693**	.630	.540
SD	.189	.170	.189	.137	.131	.131
Pleasantness						
P	**.703**	.594	.471	**.658**	.578	.503
SD	.219	.201	.170	.140	.141	.144
Experiment 2						
P	.457	**.495**	.397	.443	**.498**	.378
SD	.193	.152	.166	.122	.112	.134

[a] Reprinted from Light, LaVoie, Valencia-Laver, Owens & Mead, 1992, Table 1. Copyright 1992 by the American Psychological Association.
[b] P, proportion; SD, standard deviation.
[c] Test modalities are in bold.

implicit-memory test is contingent on the match between perceptual features present during study and test. In this case, the match was for visual features during study with visual features during test. Even stronger support for this position would be gained if the reverse could be demonstrated—that is, a greater priming effect when the match is between aural features. And it was indeed demonstrated in Light et al.'s (1992) second experiment. The procedure approximated that of their first experiment except that the perceptual identification of the words now consisted of hearing them embedded in noise. The magnitude of the priming effect was now greater for previously heard words than for previously seen words (see Table 11.2). Most important, the priming effect for both sets of words was slightly greater for their elderly subjects than for their young subjects. This was the case, even though their young subjects outscored the elderly subjects on tests of explicit memory for the same words. For anyone keeping a box score on the age sensitivity versus age insensitivity game, add two firm points for insensitivity.

Other points for the age insensitivity of implicit memory when accompanied by age sensitivity of explicit memory (i.e., a dissociation) were added in a unique study by Schacter, Cooper, and Valdiserri (1992). They found no age difference in a priming effect for drawings of objects that could either exist or not exist in three-dimensional form. Subjects were first asked to view each drawing and judge if the object depicted faced primarily left or right. Then on separate tests the subjects were asked to decide if each drawing was old or new (i.e., a standard recognition test of explicit memory) and to decide if each object could or could not exist in the real world (a test of implicit memory). Their young subjects clearly scored higher than their elderly subjects on the explicit test but not on the implicit test. On the implicit test, the priming effect was defined as the difference in proportions of objects correctly identified (i.e., could exist or could not exist in the real world) between those previously seen in the left-right task and those not previously seen. That difference was .12 for young subjects and .19 for elderly subjects when the objects could exist and zero for each group when they could not exist.

Age insensitivity of the priming of perceptual identification was demonstrated by Hamberger and Friedman (1992) for a different kind of dependent variable as well as for the standard savings in identification time. The new dependent variable was event-related potentials (ERP). Rugg, Furda, and Loriat (1988) had proposed earlier that, unlike behavioral manifestations of the repetitions of words, ERP manifestations are influenced strongly by the level of processing required by task demands. In agreement with this position, Hamberger and Friedman (1992) found that identification of words was faster on their second presentation whether the prior processing of those words was shallow or deep and equally so for young and elderly subjects. By contrast, ERP amplitude increased on the second presentation, and equally so for young and elderly subjects, only when prior processing had been deep.

On the other hand, points for the age sensitivity of implicit memory accumulated in the first of two experiments by Howard, Fry, and Brune (1991), but not in their second experiment. In the first experiment, subjects listened to simple sentences containing unrelated nouns, and they were asked to expand each sentence by adding words and phrases (an orienting task for later incidental-memory tests). For example, one of the sentences was "The queen fell down the stairs." Stem completion provided the implicit-memory test. The first noun of a given sentence was paired with the first three letters of the second noun (e.g., *queen— sta*), with subjects asked to complete the stem with whatever word first came to mind. The proportion of young subjects completing the stems with the prior nouns was substantially greater than that of elderly subjects, implying greater implicit memory for the former age group. However, equivalent implicit-memory scores for young and elderly subjects were found in their second experiment in which noun pairs (e.g., *queen—stairs*) rather than sentences were presented before the implicit memory, and subjects made up their own sentence incorporating the two nouns. A stem-completion test like that of the first experiment provided the measure of implicit memory.

Why Age Sensitivity on Some Tasks and Not Other Tasks?

It seems likely that whether or not age-related deficits exist for implicit memory is contingent on the kind of task and test used to evaluate implicit-memory proficiency. However, even when they do exist, the magnitude of the deficit is much less than that found for virtually any test of explicit memory. In fact, in his review of the research literature, Graf (1990) concluded that there is, on the average, only a 4% age difference in performance on implicit-memory tests. There must indeed be important differences in the processes mediating implicit memory and explicit memory to account for the vast disparity in the age sensitivity of the two forms of episodic memory. There is factor-analytic evidence (Mitchell, 1989) indicating that implicit-memory tasks and episodic-memory tasks load on different factors, and equivalently so for young and elderly subjects, and, as noted earlier, a different pattern of correlations with individual differences variables exist for scores on explicit- and implicit-memory tasks. Light and Albertson (1989) concluded that the critical factor determining the presence or relative absence of age-related deficits is whether or not the memory task requires deliberate or conscious recollection of particular events. Explicit-memory tasks clearly call upon such recollection. In principle, implicit-memory tasks do not require such recollection—nor do some lexical memory tasks (see Chapter 12, p. 396) and at least some procedural learning tasks (see Chapter 2, p. 65). Performance on implicit-memory tests should therefore be guided by unconscious, automatic processes that are relatively spared from impairment with normal aging. The implication is that implicit memory is a separate memory system, at least one that exists somewhat apart from a highly age-sensitive episodic-memory system. More generally, it may be part of a broader procedural memory system that incorporates both motor and verbal skill information. The critical age-insensitive process, retrieval without deliberate recollection, is one that should be shared by performance on all implicit-procedural-memory tasks.

If this perspective is correct, then it would be reasonable to argue that it shouldn't matter which specific test is used to assess the proficiency of the implicit-memory system. Stated differently, the scores earned on different implicit-memory tests (e.g., fragment completion, perceptual identification, instance generation) administered to the same subjects should be highly intercorrelated. This may not be true, however, at least for young adult subjects. Witherspoon and Moscovitch (1989) found stochastic independence between scores on fragment completion and perceptual identification. That is, the proportion of fragmented words from a prior study list that was completed with old words was no greater for perceptually identified old words than for unidentified old words. They reasoned that different memory tasks and tests tap different component processes, and that this is as likely to be true for implicit-memory tasks as it is for episodic-memory tasks. (But see also Rajaram and Roediger, 1993. They found very similar patterns of outcomes for four separate implicit-memory tests [young adults only]: fragment completion, stem completion, word identification, and anagram solution. The implication is that there is a high degree of commonality among the processes governing these various forms of implicit memory.) Some of these component processes are probably age sensitive, whereas others are age insensitive (Dunn & Kirsner, 1989; Howard, 1988a). Rather than accepting the view that implicit memory per se is age insensitive, we need to continue our research to discover which specific processes of its (probably) many component processes are age insensitive and which are not. There is also the strong possibility that explicit-memory processes (e.g., the use of encoding and retrieval strategies) may serve to enhance performance on some forms of implicit-memory tests, but especially so for young adults (Graf, 1990; Hamberger & Friedman, 1992). The net effect should be to inflate the magnitude of the age-related deficit found for those tasks.

Conscious Recollection versus Automaticity

Like research on memory for noncontent attributes, research on implicit memory has served to focus attention on automatic memory processes. However, in this case, the focus is on automaticity of retrieval rather than on automaticity of encoding. Performance on such implicit-memory tasks as stem completion may be governed solely by an automatic process that requires no conscious recollection of prior study-list words. However, some stems may provoke conscious recollection of words encountered earlier in a study list, thereby contributing to the completions of the stems with those prior words. Such recollection is presumably more likely to occur for young adults than for elderly adults. There is convincing evidence to indicate that this is indeed the case.

One procedure used to separate conscious recollection from automatic activation is one introduced by Gardiner (1988) and discussed earlier in Chapter 7. The procedure calls for a memory test in which subjects report for each word recalled or recognized as being in a prior study list whether they actually recollect that word's presence in the list or whether they merely "know" that it was in the list without recollecting its occurrence. In a series of studies, Gardiner and his associates (e.g., Gardiner & Parkin, 1990) have demonstrated that recollection scores and know scores are differentially affected by such variables as divided attention and levels of processing, as they are expected to be if one score is determined by a conscious process and the other by an unconscious process. The results of one aging study with this procedure (Parkin & Walter, 1992) were given in Chapter 7 (see p. 250 and Figure 7.7). This procedure was also employed in an aging study by Mäntylä (1993). Young adult and elderly subjects were given a lengthy list of words. For each word, they were asked to generate one association that gives a good description of the target word. On a subsequent memory test, they were given these prior associations as cues for recalling the words on the study list. For those words recalled, the subjects indicated whether they remembered (or recollected) their occurrences in the study list, as determined by their evoking particular images or associations, whether they knew of their occurrences without evoking any specific recollections of those occurrences, or whether they were simply guessing as to prior occurrences. The response probabilities of remember, know, and guessing responses are shown in Table 11.3. It may be seen that there was a pronounced age-related deficit in the proportion of remember responses but not in know responses. These results, along with those of Parkin

TABLE 11.3

Response Probabilities as a Function of Age in Experiment 1[a]

	Response Type						
	Remember		Know		Guess		Total
Condition[b]	M	SD	M	SD	M	SD	M
Young	.54	.22	.11	.12	.05	.04	.70
Old	.26	.21	.10	.14	.05	.05	.41

[a] Adapted from Mäntylä, 1993, Table 1.
[b] M, mean; SD, standard deviation.

and Walter (1992), provide support for the hypothesis that "aging selectivity impairs retention accompanied by recollective experience but has no effects on retention in the absence of recollective experience" (Mäntylä, 1993, p. 386).

Further strong support for this hypothesis comes from the use of the ingenious *process-dissociation procedure* introduced by Jacoby (1992; Jacoby, Toth, & Yonelinas, 1993; Jennings & Jacoby, 1993). In Jacoby's (1992) study, subjects were given two variations of a stem-completion test. On an inclusion test, they were instructed to complete stems with words from the prior study list (if unable to do so, they gave the first word that came to mind). On an exclusion test, they were instructed to complete stems with words that were not in the prior list. As noted by Jacoby et al., "If recollection were perfect, subjects would always complete stems with old words for the inclusion test and never complete stems with old words for the exclusion test; that is, responding would be under complete intentional control" (1993, p. 141). In the absence of recollection, subjects should be as likely to give an old word when trying not to do so (i.e., an exclusion test) as when trying to do so (i.e., an inclusion test). The two procedures enable an investigator to separate what is recalled from a list via conscious recollection and what is automatically recalled. With this procedure, Jacoby (1992) found elderly adults to show considerably less recollection than young adults, a result in agreement with that obtained by Mäntylä (1993) with a quite different procedure. Jennings and Jacoby (1993) had their subjects read a list of nonfamous names and were then given inclusion and exclusion tests. Elderly subjects were again less proficient than young subjects only for decisions requiring conscious recollection.

Future Research

Howard (1988) astutely noted that the concept of implicit memory carries with it a potentially important implication for the episodic memory of noncontent attributes, such as frequency-of-occurrence information and spatial location information. We discovered in Chapter 9 (p. 307) that memory for such information is often viewed as being governed by automatic encoding processes. Nevertheless, age-related performance deficits are commonplace for tests of noncontent attributes. These tests, however, have required retrieval processes that demand conscious recollection, and are therefore likely to be age sensitive. Thus, the performance deficits may be the consequence of these age-sensitive retrieval processes, and not age-sensitive encoding processes. Howard's suggestion is that implicit-memory tests replace explicit-memory tests of noncontent attributes, thereby eliminating the involvement of conscious recollection. Applications of ingenious new test procedures should have a high priority in future research on age differences in memory for noncontent attributes.

That such procedures are possible was demonstrated in studies by Wiggs and Martin (1993) and Wiggs (1993). In Wiggs and Martin's (1993) study, words that varied in their frequencies of occurrence were read by young and elderly subjects who subsequently received an absolute judgment test of frequencies of occurrence. Not surprisingly, the young subjects were more accurate than the elderly subjects on this direct test of frequency-of-occurrence memory. However, reading speed increased equally for the two age groups over the study trial as a function of frequency (i.e., words were read faster with each repetition in the list). This change in reading speed may be considered an indirect test of frequency-of-occurrence memory. Thus, when conscious recollection was not required, elderly subjects did not differ from young adult subjects in the proficiency of frequency-of-occurrence memory. Wiggs (1991) varied the frequency with which Japanese idiograms occurred in a study list. Young adult subjects were more accurate than elderly subjects in frequency judgments (explicit test). However, the age groups did not differ on an implicit test that involved what is known as the *mere exposure effect* (Zajonc, 1968). Briefly, the effect consists of an increasing likability expressed for a stimulus the more often subjects are exposed to that stimulus. Wiggs (1991) found likability ratings for the idiograms to increase equally for young and elderly subjects as their frequencies of exposure in the study list increased. Again, when conscious recollection was not required, there was no age difference in frequency-of-occurrence memory.

CHAPTER 12

Generic (Semantic) Memory and Metamemory

Introduction

"What does the word 'psychology' mean?" "What is the capital of Missouri?" The fact that we can answer such questions is a clear demonstration of our possession of a component of the human memory system Tulving (1972) called *semantic memory*. The reference is to a store, or repository, of our permanent knowledge of the universe, a knowledge we share with others. Access to that knowledge is usually gained rapidly and seemingly effortlessly. Tulving (1983, 1985) later proposed that semantic memory and episodic memory exist as separate, but interacting, memory systems, and he elaborated considerably on their distinguishing characteristics (1983, 1985). For example, semantic memory is postulated to have its origin earlier in childhood than does episodic memory. Most important is the distinction between the two systems in their "units" of memory. Semantic memory is viewed as the repository of facts, ideas, and concepts that are stored without reference to the temporal and spatial context present at the time of their storage. That is, the information is stored without personal reference. Thus, stored in semantic memory is knowledge about the thousands of words and facts we know, but with little, if any, information pertaining to when and where such words as *psychology* and such facts as "Jefferson City is the capital of Missouri" became part of our permanent knowledge. By contrast, episodic memory is viewed as the repository of memory traces of personally experienced events or episodes for which temporal and spatial contextual information is essential (e.g., memory of the where and when of your first bicycle spill—or memory for "apple" being one of the words included in the word list recently studied in the laboratory). The interaction between semantic memory and episodic memory was described in Chapter 5 where we discovered that the information encoded for transmission to the episodic store usually includes elements "copied" from semantic memory and that this information is often organized in a way that emulates organization within semantic memory.

Not all memory theorists believe that it is necessary to postulate separate long-term systems in order to accommodate semantic- and episodic-memory phenomena (e.g., McKoon, Ratcliff, & Dell, 1986). That is, both sets of phenomena can seemingly be explained within the constraint of a single long-term memory system. Whether or not this is true should have little impact on aging research. Age differences found for semantic-memory tasks have proved to be quite different than age differences found for episodic-memory tasks, and they clearly merit our detailed consideration regardless of one's theoretical position on the separate systems issue. In fact, these differential outcomes provide part of the evidence in support of separate semantic and episodic systems. When the same independent variables have quite different effects on semantic- and episodic-memory task performances, dissociations are said to exist, dissociations suggestive of different systems governing performances on those tasks (see Tulving, 1983, 1985 for elaboration). (Similar arguments may be made for procedural learning and implicit memory). Adult age variation is among the variables producing such dissociations. In contrast to the pronounced age differences commonly found for episodic-memory tasks, the age differences for semantic memory tasks are highly selective and often negligible.

Our preference is to use the term *generic memory* in place of semantic memory. The intent is to broaden the concept of a permanent knowledge system to include other components besides knowledge of words and facts. For example, it surely includes information that allows us to translate such verbal commands as "put the cup on the saucer" into an action that fulfills the command. Another important component consists of knowledge about our own personal memory system, including knowledge of its current effectiveness and, to some degree, knowledge of how the episodic-memory system operates (e.g., the more you rehearse, the better you will remember). Memory psychologists call this component of generic memory *metamemory*. Conceivably, many of the episodic-memory problems experienced by older individuals are derived not from deficiencies in the episodic-memory system per se, but rather from the ineffective operation of metamemory. The component of generic memory that has been most frequently investigated by both basic memory researchers and experimental aging psychologists is the *internal lexicon* or "mental dictionary." It is the large store of information we have about words and the concepts they represent. Our review will begin with age differences in the structure and the operations of the internal lexicon, and it will end with age differences in metamemorial processes.

Adult Age Differences in the Internal Lexicon

Age Differences in Structure

As you read the present material, note how rapidly and easily you identify each word being read. Word identification per se seems to be unaltered by age. An

excellent demonstration of the absence of an adult age difference in word identification was given by Wingfield, Aberdeen, and Stine (1991). Their young adult
and elderly subjects received increasing amounts of word-onset information for
each of a number of words until they were able to identify correctly each word.
Subjects at each age level were able to identify the spoken words after hearing
only 50 to 60% of their onsets.

Wingfield et al. (1991) also discovered that the amount of onset information
needed for the identification of spoken words was markedly reduced (hearing
only 20% to 30% of the words) when the words were embedded in meaningful
sentences. Such expediency could hardly be accomplished unless the information
stored in the internal lexicon is organized in some manner. That is, it seems
highly unlikely that information about the sensory features and the meanings of
thousands of words is stored haphazardly or randomly. Over the years a number
of different models or theories have been offered to represent the organizational
structure of the lexicon. For example, one form of organization is in terms of a
collection of lists (Landauer & Freedman, 1968) in which each list consists of a
specific category (e.g., *dogs*) and the instances of that category (e.g., *collie, poodle*).
Our choice, however, of the best model to guide research on aging's effects on the
lexicon and its operations is an associative network model patterned after a model
presented originally by Collins and Quillian (1969). Some of the model's basic
features are illustrated in Figure 12.1 for several different words (see Howard,

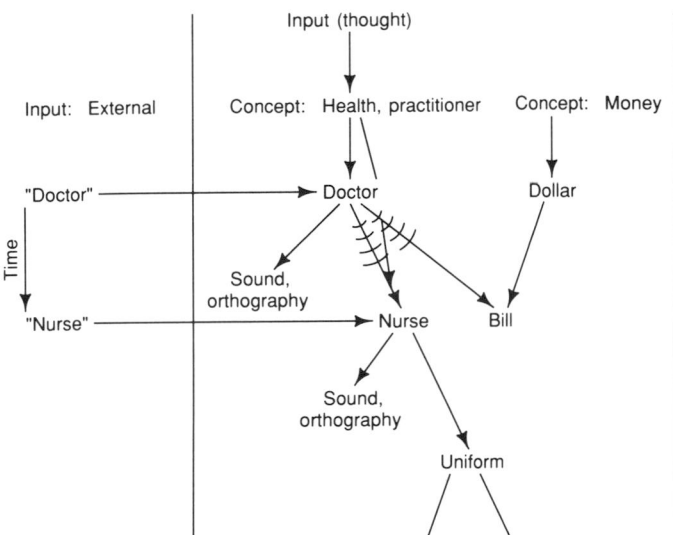

FIGURE 12.1 Network organization of the internal lexicon and its activation by either external input (visually presented words) or internal input (thought). Wavy lines
represent spreading activation.

1983a, for a more detailed description of associative network theory). Associative connections exist between a specific concept (e.g., "health practitioner") and the representations of words, commonly called *nodes*, that are instances or exemplars of that concept (e.g., *doctor, nurse*). They also exist between the representations of different words that are related to one another (e.g., *doctor* with both *nurse* and *bill* and *nurse* with *uniform*). These associative connections are important ingredients of a given word's meaning or semantic content. Note further that the "distance" between words varies as a function of their degree of relatedness—for example, *doctor* being located closer to *nurse* than to *bill*. One other kind of connection is basic to the model, namely that between a word's representation and the sensory information (orthographic and phonological) needed to spell and to pronounce that word. The remaining feature of the model is its hierarchical structure, as illustrated in Figure 12.2 for the superordinate of *birds*. That is, organization is assumed to follow a top-to-bottom structure from superordinates to subordinates to specific instances of the subordinates.

Our present interest rests in possible changes in the structure of the lexicon from early to late adulthood. One possible change is the loss of representations of individual words with normal aging. However, this seems unlikely based on such evidence as the stability, or even increases, in vocabulary test scores over the course of the adult life span (see Chapter 12 in Kausler, 1991, for a detailed review). For example, Berkowitz (1953) found scores on the Vocabulary subtest of the Wechsler Adult Intelligence Scale to be about the same for adults in their 60s and 70s as they are for adults in their 20s and 30s. This is true even though

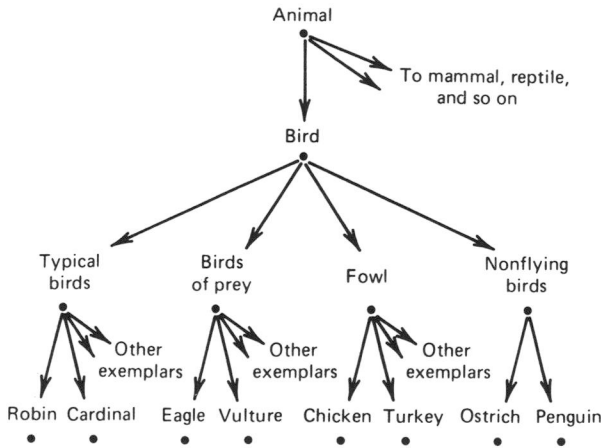

F I G U R E   12.2   Hypothetical organizational plan for storing information in an individual's lexicon. The hierarchical nature of the plan (from superordinate to subordinates to exemplars) is illustrated for the superordinate concept of birds.

the elderly subjects in this study, and most other cross-sectional studies of adult age differences in vocabulary, tend to have less formal education than the younger adults—and vocabulary test scores are known to correlate positively and highly with educational level (e.g., Birren & Morrison, 1961). In fact, when samples of young adult and elderly subjects are matched in educational level, the usual finding is that the elderly subjects outscore the young subjects (e.g., Kausler & Puckett, 1980a). The loss of representations of factual information is equally unlikely, given the overall stability of scores on general information components of intelligence tests from early to late adulthood (e.g., Berkowitz, 1953) and evidence indicating that elderly adults are as aware of what facts they know and what facts they do not know as are young adults (e.g., J. L. Lachman, Lachman, & Thronesbery, 1979; Perlmutter, 1978a). Moreover, elderly adults appear to be as proficient as young adults in inferring information from facts stored generically (e.g., answering such questions as "What U.S. president was the first to see an airplane fly?"; Camp, 1981).

However, other structural changes in the lexicon are possible. Connections between words could be altered or even lost, thus adversely affecting the lexicon's organization. Alternatively, the "distances" between related words could increase or decrease. The net effect would be changes in the meanings of various words. This possibility is suggested by evidence indicating that the definitions given by elderly subjects to words on a vocabulary test may be qualitatively inferior to those given by young adult subjects (Botwinick & Storandt, 1974b). However, such age differences could be the result of diminished access to information in the lexicon with increasing age, rather than the result of true structural changes—relevant information is still present, it simply can't be retrieved. The situation would be much like that occurring if you wished to obtain a book from the library. The book may be there, but, for whatever reason you are unable to take it out of the library. Nor is the fact that elderly individuals make moderately more errors in naming pictures of objects or actions (Albert, Heller, & Milberg, 1988; Bowles, Obler, & Albert, 1987) necessarily attributable to a "loss" from the lexicon of the representations of the words naming those pictures. Such errors probably result from diminished connections between separate nonverbal and verbal cognitive systems (Paivio, 1971). Moreover, the increased error rate in picture naming is limited largely to individuals in their 70s and beyond (e.g., Albert et al., 1988), and for individuals younger than age 70 there are no apparent age differences in the latencies of naming pictures of common objects (e.g., Poon & Fozard, 1978).

Not surprisingly, there are, in addition, generational differences in picture naming. G. B. Butterfield and Butterfield (1977) presented pictures of objects that were in use only recently, such as a felt-tip marking pen. Only one of their elderly subjects used the word "marker" to label the object, whereas nearly all of the young adult subjects assigned the correct name to the object. By contrast, we would expect many elderly adults, but few young adults, to apply the label "churn" to a picture of one. It has also been found that elderly adults respond faster to pictures of objects familiar to their generation than do young adults, whereas the opposite is true for pictures of objects of a more recent vintage (Poon & Fozard, 1978).

To investigate age-related changes in the lexicon's organizational structure we obviously need a better tool than simple word naming. The usual choice has been the familiar word-association test. On a word-association test the usual procedure is to give subjects a series of stimulus words (e.g., *table*) and ask them to give for each the first word that comes to mind. For *table*, the probability is high that you would give *chair* as your immediate response, the reason being that it is the most frequently given response (i.e., the *primary* association). From the perspective of the associative network model, the representation of *chair* is stored in proximity to the representation of *table*, and it is activated via the connection between the two representations. However, for a large group of individuals a number of other responses are also likely to be given (e.g., *eat* as a response to *table*) with varying frequencies. The second most common response is called the secondary association, the third most popular the tertiary, and so on. Our assumption is that the distance between stimulus word and response word representations in the network is greater as the frequency of the response decreases.

The number of different responses given offers one means of examining possible age differences in the lexicon's structure. Of interest is the possibility of greater variability (i.e., a greater number of different responses) in the word associations given by elderly subjects than by younger subjects. The presence of greater between-subjects variability would seemingly signal the presence of structural changes with aging. Another index of a structural change is provided by the proportions of subjects giving the most common responses. Decreased proportions for elderly subjects, relative to younger subjects, would again signal the presence of structural changes with aging. A third index is derived by giving the same subjects repeated presentations of the same stimulus words. Of interest in this case is within-subject variability, that is, the giving of different responses on the successive repetitions. A structural change with aging is suspected if elderly subjects are less likely than younger subjects to emit the same response to successive presentations of the same stimulus (i.e., they exhibit greater response variability). The final index rests in the qualitative nature of the associations given. Consider, for example, *hill* as a stimulus word. Two possible associations are *mountain* and *climb*. They are representative of two broad classes of associations, paradigmatic (*mountain*) and syntagmatic (*climb*). A paradigmatic association is a word of the same grammatical class as the stimulus word, and it may usually replace the stimulus word in any sentence containing it (e.g., I climbed the— —hill or mountain). A syntagmatic association is a word from a grammatical class that differs from the class of the stimulus word (e.g., a verb instead of a noun). Young adults' word associations are characterized by a large proportion of paradigmatic associations and a small proportion of syntagmatic associations (by contrast, children exhibit the opposite pattern). A major reduction in the proportion of paradigmatic associations given by elderly subjects, relative to younger subjects, would seem to indicate a structural change in the lexicon with aging.

A number of early studies on age differences in word associations reported evidence with each of these indices that appeared to indicate structural changes in the lexicon with aging. Riegel and Birren (1965, 1966), Tresselt and Mayzner (1964), and Perlmutter (1978b, 1979b) reported greater between-subject variability for elderly than for younger subjects. Lower proportions of subjects giving the most common responses were also observed by these same investigators, as well as by Riegel and Riegel (1964). Perlmutter (1979b) found within-subject variability with repeated stimulus words to be greater for elderly than for younger subjects, and Riegel and Riegel (1964) found the proportion of paradigmatic associations to be less for elderly than for younger subjects. However, more recent evidence gathered in three exceptionally thorough and well-controlled studies (Lovelace & Cooley, 1982; Burke & Peters, 1986; Scialfa & Margolis, 1986) strongly contradicts the outcomes of the above studies. Lovelace and Cooley (1982) analyzed the associations given to 56 stimulus words by both elderly subjects (mean age = 71.3 yr) and younger subjects (mean age = 34.5 yr). Among their analyses were comparisons between younger and older subjects on the primary associations and on the proportions of total associations that were paradigmatic. In both cases age differences were negligible (e.g., for 45 of the stimulus words the primary association was the same word for the two groups). The same comparisons, along with several additional ones, were made by Burke and Peters (1986) for over 100 stimulus words. The outcomes are shown in Figure 12.3. The age difference was negligible for the proportions of total responses that were paradigmatic, for the proportions of identical primary and secondary responses, and for the proportions of identical response on the original test and a retest several months later. Moreover, the two groups were very comparable in the mean number of different words given as response. Finally, Scialfa and Margolis (1986) found no age difference in either the commonality or the variability of associates to either high-frequency or low-frequency words.

It is puzzling why there were such different outcomes regarding age differences in word associations between the earlier and later studies. However, a likely reason was identified by both Lovelace and Cooley (1982) and Burke and Peters (1986). In each study, correlations between vocabulary test scores and various word-association scores were found to be moderately high. In fact, vocabulary test score proved to be a much better predictor than age for such subject scores as the percentage of associations that were paradigmatic. In the later studies the age groups were roughly comparable in verbal ability as assessed by a vocabulary test. The elderly subjects in the earlier word-association studies were probably less

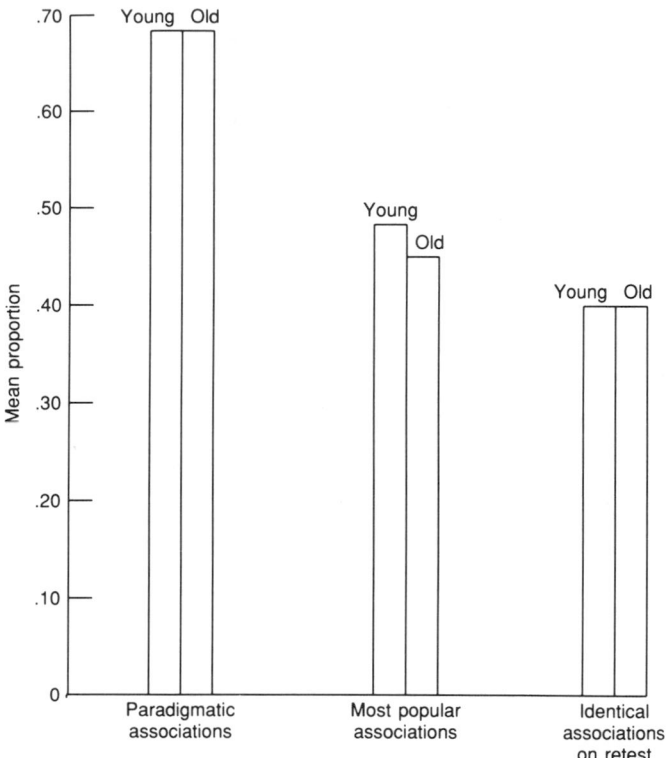

FIGURE 12.3   Proportions of associations that were paradigmatic, popular, and identical on retest. (Adapted from Burke & Peters, 1986, Tables 2, 3.)

verbally proficient than the young subjects. Further confirmation of the absence of age differences in word associations comes from Howard's (1980) study employing a constrained word-association test (in contrast to the *free* word-association procedure employed in the other studies—i.e., subjects are free to give whatever response word they wish). The constraint was to give *only* instances of a category to the name of that category as the stimulus word (e.g., "a *metal*"). As noted in Chapter 7 (p. 232), age differences in the content of the instances named were negligible. Negligible age differences in content were also found when subjects emitted continuously for several minutes instances of a designated category (Brown & Mitchell, 1991; Fitzgerald, 1983). However, Brown and Mitchell (1991) did discover that elderly adults are less consistent than young adults in the instances they name when retested a week or several weeks later. In addition, age differences in the word associations given in response to pictures of common objects as stimulus elements tend to be fairly negligible (Puglisi, Park, & Smith,

1987). Another form of a constrained association is one in which subjects are asked to give a response that describes each of a series of stimuli. Stine (1986) found negligible age differences in descriptive associations to common objects. However, Mäntylä (1993; Mäntylä & Bäckman, 1990) did find one interesting difference in descriptive associations given by young and elderly adults. Elderly subjects tended to give more schematic and typical associations (e.g., *fruit* to *apple*) than did young subjects, whereas young adults gave more idiosyncratic or distinctive associations (e.g., *computer* to *apple*). We discovered in Chapter 7 (p. 275) that atypical associations serve to enhance the distinctiveness of a memory trace, thereby giving young adults a memory advantage over elderly adults.

Overall, our best conclusion is that aging has little effect on the associative structure of the internal lexicon, a conclusion reached earlier by both Lovelace and Cooley (1982) and Burke and Peters (1986). On the other hand, cohort differences are present for word associations, especially for words that do not have strong primary associations (Bowles, Williams, & Poon, 1983).

Age Differences in Lexical Access for Words

Access to single words in the lexicon occurs automatically when that word is presented visually or auditorily. The sensory presentation of a word activates that word's representation (often called a logogen rather than a node; Morton, 1969), resulting in the recognition or identification of that word. When letter strings are presented to elderly subjects, they are slower than young adults in identifying them as words, but no slower than they are in identifying nonwords in terms of their orthographic characteristics (Madden & Greene, 1987). However, the process of gaining access to a given node can begin even before the word associated with that node is presented physically. The "head start" in access was clearly demonstrated in a classic study by Tulving and Gold (1963). They presented target words for visual recognition or identification. Some of the target words were presented alone, others were preceded by other words making up a sentence in which the targets were the last words of the sentences. Recognition thresholds (i.e., the time needed to identify the word) were much less when the targets were congruent with the preceding words (e.g., COLLISION preceded by "Three people were killed in a terrible highway") than when presented alone. On the other hand, recognition thresholds were much higher when the targets were incongruent with the preceding words (e.g., COLLISION preceded by "Far too many people today confuse communisim with"). Our first concern is with Tulving and Gold's (1963) congruent condition. Here the preceding words serve as a context for priming the activation of the target word's node in advance of the word itself, thus lowering the word's recognition or identification threshold. Such context effects account in part for the ease of reading normal sentences. The priming effect was later demonstrated to occur even when the context consists of only a single word that is related to the target word. The underlying process responsible for such facilitation was eventually labeled *spreading activation* (Collins & Loftus, 1975). Of further interest are the heightened threshold values observed by Tulving and Gold (1963) in their incongruent condition. They imply the existence of inhibitory mechanisms that, under certain conditions requiring attentional processes, serve to delay the recognition or identification of words.

Age differences in various attributes of spreading activation have become the primary tool for investigating age differences in lexical access. The nature of spreading activation may be understood with reference to Figure 12.1 (the curved lines). Consider *doctor* as a priming word temporally preceding the target word *nurse*. Once the node for *doctor* is activated, that activation spreads automatically to other nodes connected to it, including the node for *nurse*. If the wave of advance activation reaches that node before the word *nurse* is presented, then recognition of *nurse* should be enhanced. That is, its recognition or identification threshold is lower than it would be without such preactivation. The activation would also spread to other nodes connected with *doctor*'s node, but the "distance" to be traveled may be much greater (e.g., the node for *bill*). By contrast, if the priming word for *nurse* had been an unrelated word, such as *grass*, there should no advance activation of *nurse*'s node via spreading activation. Some evidence for the absence of age differences in spreading activation comes from the presence of a false recognition effect for elderly subjects as well as for young subjects. *Late* as a study-list item activates not only its own representations but also such related representations as that for *tardy*, leading to the frequent false recognition of *tardy* as a study-list item (see Chapter 6, p. 189). A number of more direct tasks have been introduced as a means of evaluating the various effects of spreading activation, most of which have found their way into experimental aging research.

One of the simplest tasks is to have subjects read the target word when it is presented, with the subject's pronunciation latency being measured by a voice key. This task was employed by Cerella and Fozard (1984) under standard priming conditions. That is, half of the to-be-pronounced target words were preceded by a related word, the other half by an unrelated word. Although their elderly subjects were moderately slower than their young adult subjects in pronouncing words regardless of their prior context word, they also exhibited a mean priming effect (defined as the mean latency for unrelated primes minus the mean latency for related primes) that was as large (27 ms) as that exhibited by the young subjects (28 ms).

A far more complex task is one that involves a modification of the basic Stroop test (R. E. Warren, 1972). This task was involved in a study by Howard, Lasaga, & McAndrews (1980). Briefly, on the Stroop test reaction time in identifying the name of a color is increased when the color is that of the ink a word is printed in relative to naming the same color in isolation. Reading the word occurs automatically, thereby competing with, and interfering with the identification of the color name. The competition is especially pronounced when the word is the name of a color other than that of its own print. Nevertheless, the interference is substantial when a neutral word, such as *bird*, is printed in the to-be-named color. This interference may be increased still more by the indirect activation, via spreading activation, of *bird*'s node prior to its exposure. To accomplish this objective, subjects are given a set of relevant instances, such as *canary*, *sparrow*, and *pigeon*, to hold in memory prior to their exposure to *bird*. The memory-set words are then recalled after naming the color ink of *bird*. The amount of interference created by spreading activation is determined by contrasting the reaction time for color naming in the relevant instance condition with reaction time in a control condition. The appropriate control condition is one in which subjects receive an irrelevant set of words (e.g., *valley*, *river*, and *canyon*) to hold in memory prior to their exposure to *bird*. In their use of this procedure, Howard et al. (1980) found that the increase in mean reaction time from irrelevant to relevant instances was as great for elderly subjects as for young adult subjects (see Figure 12.4).

The most popular task in this area of research is the lexical decision task. Here subjects are presented letter strings, and they are to decide whether or not each string makes up a meaningful word. Half of the strings conform to a real word, with "Yes" being the correct answer, and half conform to a nonword (e.g., *RIKE*), with "No" being the correct answer. Our interest rests in the word half of the trials. In most studies priming (or contextual) variation is extended to permit a

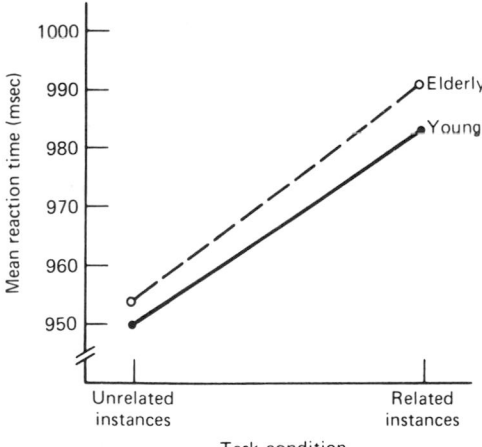

FIGURE 12.4 Age differences in reaction times for naming the print color of words that are either unrelated or related to words previously stored in memory. (Adapted from Howard, Lasaga, & McAndrews, 1980, Table 3.)

test of differential age differences for automatic activation of nodes and attentional activation of nodes (Posner & Snyder, 1975). The former is mediated by spreading activation, a cognitively effortless process, and therefore one that should be age insensitive. The latter is mediated by controlled effortful processes that may be age sensitive, given the presumed diminished attentional resources of elderly adults. The distinction between the two forms of activation is best made with reference to the two kinds of word primes that are standard in lexical decision research. The word preceding a target word is either related or unrelated to the target word (as was also true in Cerella and Fozard's, 1984, pronunciation study described previously), with subjects receiving equal numbers of each prime-target pair type. Thus, some of the pairs are of the *doctor-nurse* related type, others of the *inch-city* unrelated type. The presence of a number of related pairs means that subjects are likely to develop an expectancy of each word following the prime to be related to that prime. Consequently, attention is directed by primes such as *inch* to nodes representing related words in the lexicon (e.g., *ruler*) in advance of seeing the target word. However, the target word disconfirms this expectancy, and attention must be redirected to another segment of the lexicon containing the target word's (*city*) node in order to make the "Yes" decision. Attentional activation should be slower than automatic activation. As a result, faster decision times for related targets than for unrelated targets could be due to either the faster activation for the former or the slower activation of the latter—or, more likely, a combination of the two. What is needed is a neutral condition in which neither the facilitation provided by a confirmed expectancy nor the inhibition provided by a disconfirmed expectancy are involved. This neutral condition is accomplished by having a neutral prime precede a third of the real words in the many prime-target trials a subject received. That neutral prime is usually either the word *blank* or a series of X's. Reaction times for the words following neutral primes serve as the baseline for determining the facilitation that occurs with related word primes from both automatic and attentional processes and the inhibition that occurs with unrelated word primes from attentional processes only.

The results from several studies using the neutral prime control condition have yielded consistent evidence indicating the absence of age differences for the automatic component of activation, but conflicting evidence for the attentional component (Bowles & Poon, 1985; Chiarello, Church, & Hoyer, 1985; Howard, Shaw, & Heisey, 1986). Chiarello et al. (1985) found comparable facilitating and inhibitory effects in reaction times for young and elderly subjects. However, both Bowles and Poon (1985) and Howard, Shaw, and Heisey (1986) failed to find a significant inhibitory effect in the unrelated word prime condition, although in both studies there was a significant facilitation effect for both young and elderly subjects, and one equivalent in magnitude for the two age groups. An additional feature of Howard, Shaw, and Heisey's (1986) study is of particular importance. The investigators varied the time between the onset of the prime and the onset of the target word (i.e., the stimulus-onset asynchrony or SOA). In the other studies we have reviewed, the SOA was constant, and it was set at values of 500 ms or longer. This duration is probably long enough for the facilitation produced by spreading activation to be apparent for elderly subjects as well as for young adult subjects, even though spreading activation may progress more slowly for the former. The specific SOA values in Howard, Shaw, and Heisey's (1986) study were 150, 450, and 1000 ms. Shown in Figure 12.5 are mean reaction times at each interval for both targets preceded by related words and targets preceded by unrelated words. Note that a priming effect, defined as mean reaction time for unrelated pairs minus mean reaction time for related pairs, was evident for young adults, but not for elderly adults, at the SOA value of 150 ms. Apparently, 150 ms is not enough time for activation to reach related nodes in the older adult's lexicon. On the other hand, equivalent priming effects were observed for the two age groups at the longer SOAs. Although spreading activation occurs as automatically for elderly adults as for young adults, it also occurs more slowly for elderly adults, in agreement with the general slowing-down principle (see Chapter 6, p. 203). Several meta-analyses have indicated that the slope of the linear function relating mean reaction times for elderly subjects to mean reaction times for young adult subjects is about 1.5 for various lexical tasks, indicating that for

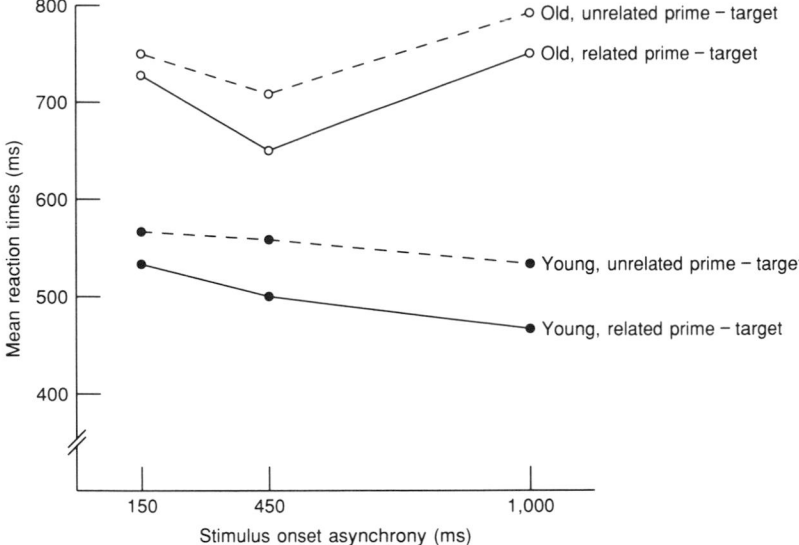

FIGURE 12.5 Age differences in mean reaction times for lexical decisions with three different intervals between the prime and the target. (Adapted from Howard, Shaw, & Heisey, 1986, Table 3.)

each process on a lexical task elderly subjects require about one and a half times the time needed by young adults to complete the process (Lima, Hale, & Myerson, 1991; Myerson, Ferraro, Hale, & Lima, 1992; Myerson, Hale, Wagstaff, Poon, & Smith, 1990).

There is a problem in the use of so-called neutral primes as the baseline for evaluating the effects of attentional activation processes, both for facilitation and inhibition. Howard, Shaw, and Heisey (1986) argued that such primes may not really be neutral in the sense of the absence of any advance activation of lexical nodes. Fortunately, a more effective procedure for testing the effects of attentional facilitation or inhibition was introduced by Neely (1977) and eventually applied to tests of age differences by Burke, White, and Diaz (1987) and Balota, Black, and Cheney (1992). The procedure calls for a number of conditions in which category names serve as primes for either expected or unexpected categorical instances as target words. For example, *tree* is the prime on most trials (expected condition) for the name of a tree as the target (e.g., *elm*), but on a few trials (unexpected condition) it is followed instead by an instance of a different category as the target (e.g., *fog*). Similarly, *vegetable* is the prime on most trials (expected condition) for instances from another category (e.g., *animals*), but on a few trials (unexpected condition) it is followed by an instance of its own category (e.g., *spinach*). By various comparisons of mean reaction times for these conditions, automatic and attentional components of activation may be separated. With this procedure, and with subjects performing on a lexical decision task, Burke et al. (1987) were able to demonstrate equivalent activation effects between young and elderly subjects not only for automatic activation processes, but for attentional processes as well. In a somewhat related study, Bowles and Poon (1988) found the activation effects to be even greater for elderly subjects. Balota et al.'s (1992) concern about the adequacy of neutral primes as a baseline for contrasting automatic and attentional activation effects with a lexical decision task led them to substitute a pronunciation task for the lexical decision task. Surprisingly, they found an interaction between relatedness, expectancy, and SOA that is inconsistent with the notion of independent automatic and attentional mechanisms in priming effects, regardless of the age of subjects.

Two other kinds of tasks have been employed in research on age differences in lexical activation. The first calls for presenting paired letter strings of various combinations, namely word-word pairs, word-nonword pairs, word-nonword pairs, and nonword-nonword pairs, and requiring subjects to respond "Yes" only if both intrapair strings are real words. With this task, Meyer and Schvaneveldt (1971) demonstrated faster times for young adults when word-word pairs consisted of related words than when they consisted of unrelated words. Howard et al. (1981) subsequently found an equivalent positive effect, and equal in magnitude, for elderly adults. Equivalent age effects were also found by Bowles and Poon (1981) with a modified version of this task. Word frequency replaced relatedness or unrelatedness as the variable distinguishing word pairs. Some word pairs for "Yes" decisions consisted of unrelated high-frequency words, others of unrelated low-frequency words. Considerable research with young adults (e.g., Scarborough, Cortese, & Scarborough, 1977) has revealed that the nodes for high-frequency words are accessed more rapidly than are the nodes for low-frequency words. Bowles and Poon (1981) found that the advantage for high-frequency words over low-frequency words was as pronounced for elderly subjects as for young subjects.

The final task we will consider is an expanded version of Tulving and Gold's (1963) sentence context task in which dependent variables other than recognition thresholds are employed. A number of aging studies (Burke & Yee, 1984: G. Cohen & Faulkner, 1983; Madden, 1986, 1988) have made effective use of this task. In Madden's studies the task conditions included sentences preceding the target word that were neutral in terms of relatedness to the target (e.g., CHILD preceded by "They said it was the") as well as congruent and incongruent relatedness (as in Tulving and Gold's, 1963, study). The subject was then asked to make a word or nonword decision (e.g., Madden, 1986b) regarding the target, with reaction time being measured. His evidence suggests an age equivalence for both automatic facilitation and attentional inhibition of nodal activation. Burke and Yee (1984) and G. Cohen and Faulkner (1983) also provided evidence for age equivalence in automatic facilitation for task conditions in which subjects decided whether or not the target word that preceded a complete sentence was related in some way to the sentence's content (e.g., "The cook cut the meat"— knife? for the related condition, key? for the unrelated condition), with reaction time again being measured. However, no inhibitory attentional effect was found by Burke and Yee (1984) for unrelated target words for either young or elderly subjects.

There is a great deal of converging evidence coming from many studies employing a wide range of paradigms and tasks to indicate the striking robustness of activation processes in the lexicon with normal aging. This is certainly true for automatic activation, and it is probably true for attentional processes as well, although the evidence here is somewhat less convincing, despite their apparent cognitive effortfulness. However, "robustness" here refers only to the qualitative attributes of activation. The same mechanisms determining facilitation and inhibition of activation seem to be operative for adults of all ages. Age equivalence in quantitative attributes is another matter. We know that elderly adults are slower overall in their lexical decisions than are young adults despite their comparability in activation processes (see, for example, Figure 9.5). At least part of this slower responding by older adults seems to be due to their slower activation of nodes per se, that is, in their activation either directly by a physically presented word or indirectly by spreading activation from a previously activated node (Balota & Duchek, 1988). This doesn't tell the whole story, however. As noted earlier, the results obtained by Howard, Shaw, and Heisey (1986) suggest that the time course of spreading activation differs for young and elderly individuals, requiring more time to travel from node to node for elderly than for young individuals. Is there any reason to expect automatic processes, such as spreading activation and nodal activation, to be exceptions to the general slowing of processes with normal aging?

There is an important corollary of the slower rate of spreading activation that accompanies normal aging. It should take more time for activation to spread to distant, but still related nodes (see Figure 12.1), for elderly adults than for young adults. Consequently, in a fixed period of time, the number of distant nodes activated by spreading activation should be greater for young than for elderly adults. The disparity in amount of spreading should affect the interaction between the generic and episodic memory systems. According to Burke et al. (1987), activation of a node may be viewed as initiating the encoding process necessary for forming an episodic trace of the word represented by that node. However, the mere activation of nodes gives no assurance that episodic memory for the words represented by those nodes will be equivalent for young and elderly subjects when memory is tested later by recall or recognition. Striking demonstration of the superior episodic memory of young adults was provided in several of the studies reviewed in this section in which an incidental memory test (recall and/or recognition) was given for the words encountered during the lexical task (Burke & Yee, 1984; Burke et al., 1987; Howard, Shaw, & Heisey, 1986; Madden, 1986). The results obtained by Howard, Shaw, & Heisey (1986) for recognition of both primes and targets from the prior lexical task are typical of the age deficits found in these studies (see Figure 12.6). Why such age deficits exist is unknown. However, one possibility is that young adults process both primes and target words more elaborately than do elderly adults, even when the only decision to be made involves whether or not the target word is indeed a word. Elaboration is viewed here in terms of the activation of nodes that are at various distances from the nodes for primes and targets. The faster spreading of activation for young subjects should assure the activation of more remote nodes than would be the case for elderly subjects, resulting in an enriched and more durable memory trace for young subjects than for elderly subjects.

Stimulus Degradation and Lexical Access

Stanovich (1980) reported evidence with young adult subjects to support what he called an interactive compensatory principle. The principle states that a reduction in the stimulus quality of a word in a lexical decision task demands an increase in the contextual support provided by a related preceding priming word. The net effect is to increase the magnitude of a priming effect relative to the magnitude found with unrelated or neutral primes. Ferraro and Kellas (1992)

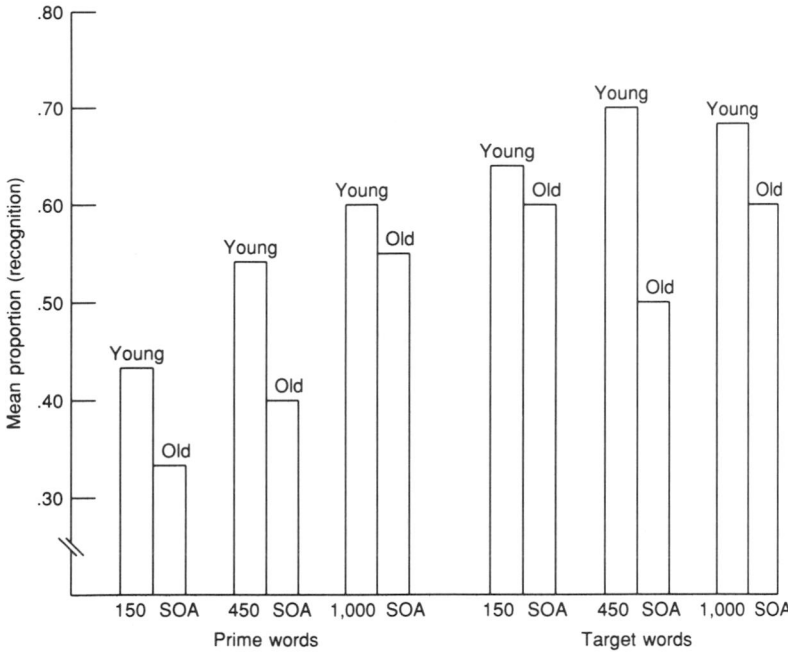

FIGURE 12.6 Mean proportions of prime and target words recognized following a lexical decision task with three different stimulus-onset asynchrony (SOA) values (150, 450, and 1000 ms). (Adapted from data in Howard, Shaw, & Heisey, 1986.)

found that the compensatory effect produced by degraded stimuli was considerably greater for their elderly subjects than for their young adult subjects. Variation in the degree of degradation was accomplished by having target words presented at different levels of orientation. The maximum degradation was produced by inverting them. For normally presented target words the magnitude of the priming effect was 28 ms for the young subjects and 40 ms for the elderly subjects. For inverted words the effects were 125 ms and 621 ms, respectively. Madden (1992) also found a greater compensatory effect for his elderly subjects than for his younger subjects when degradation was produced by inserting asterisks between successive letters of target words. However, the magnitude of the effect was much less than that found by Ferraro and Kellas (1992). In Madden's (1992) study, subjects in their 20s, 30s, 40s, 50s, 60s, and 70s were employed. Time to identify target words was found to slow down at a rate of 4 ms per year when the words were intact—and 10 ms per year when they were degraded. The greater slowing down for the degraded than for the intact words provides support for the complexity hypothesis associated with the general slowing-down model (see Chapter

6, pp. 204). Additional processes are required when words are degraded than when they are intact, thus increasing the complexity of word identification.

Verbal Fluency

Access to multiple words is at stake in a test of verbal fluency. Such tests are of particular interest in gerontology because they are commonly believed to serve as a measure of frontal lobe dysfunctioning. On most tests subjects are given a letter of the alphabet (e.g., "S") and a limited time (e.g., 60s) to write as many words beginning with that letter as possible.

Unfortunately, studies of age differences in verbal fluency test scores have yielded conflicting results. In some studies, young adult subjects have been found to elicit moderately, but statistically significant, more words than elderly subjects (Birren, 1955; Brown & Mitchell, 1991; McCrae, Arenberg, & Costa, 1987; Salthouse, 1993). For example, A. S. Brown and Mitchell (1991) gave their subjects 2 min to elicit words to a two-letter stimulus (e.g., words beginning with BE). Their young subjects averaged 14.1 words and their elderly subjects 12.8. However, in other studies, the age difference has been found to be slight or nonexistent (e.g., H. P. Davis et al., 1990). Salthouse (1993) did find that the age difference, favoring young adults, on his verbal fluency tests was much less pronounced than the age differences on several purely speed tests (e.g., letter copying). As noted by Salthouse (1993), verbal fluency test scores reflect both a knowledge base (i.e., a vocabulary) favoring elderly adults and a speed factor favoring young adults. He suggested that studies of age differences on verbal fluency tests yield different outcomes that are contingent on the extent of the knowledge base of the elderly subjects entering into those studies.

Age Differences in Lexical Access for Categorical Information

Thus far our focus has been only on the accessing of individual words within the lexicon. The lexicon, however, is the store for much more than just knowledge about individual words. It is also the store for higher order information, such as the organization of words into superordinate, subordinate, and coordinate structural representations.

Interest in possible age differences in access of categorical information began with a study by Eysenck (1975). Eysenck's tasks were ones used earlier by Freedman (Freedman & Loftus, 1971; E. F. Loftus, Freedman, & Loftus, 1970) with young adult subjects. The first task calls for presenting a series of category names and having subjects generate an instance beginning with a letter that is presented simultaneously with each category name. For example, given *fruit* as the category, the letter might be either A or K. With young subjects, reaction time is considerably faster for the A than for the K. The letters are selected deliberately to be cues for retrieving instances of the category that vary in their familiarity. Thus, *A* is a cue for retrieving *apple*, a high-dominance (i.e., high-familiarity) instance of *fruit*, from the lexicon, whereas *K* is a cue for retrieving *kumquat*, a low-dominance (i.e., low-familiarity) instance. Eysenck (1975) found relatively little disparity in speed of generation between high- and low-dominance instances for either younger or older subjects (see part A of Figure 12.7). Most important, he also found no age difference in reaction time for either kind of cue (but see Byrd, 1984, for a different outcome when a procedural modification had been made). On the other hand, Eysenck (1975) did find that elderly subjects were significantly slower than young subjects on a second task in which decisions were made as to whether or not paired words were related to one another (see part A of Figure 12.7). However, variation in dominance had little effect on response speed for either age group. For related words, one member of the pair was the name of a category, the second an instance of that category (e.g., *fruit apple*) or *fruit-kumquat*); for unrelated pairs, the second word was not an instance of the category represented by the first word (e.g., *fruit sofa*).

Eysenck's (1975) study provides mixed evidence regarding the age sensitivity or insensitivity of access to categorical information. What is especially surprising is the pattern of his results, with the age deficit appearing for the less cognitively effortful recognition task than for the more effortful response-generation task. There have been a number of later studies that have offered converging evidence from various task on the extent of age differences in access to categorical information (see also evidence on the flanker effect, p. 189).

In three of these studies (Madden, 1985; Mueller, Kausler, & Faherty, 1980; Petros, Zehr, & Chabot, 1983) a modification of Posner's chronometric task (Posner & Mitchell, 1967: see Chapter 5, pp. 161–162) was employed in which

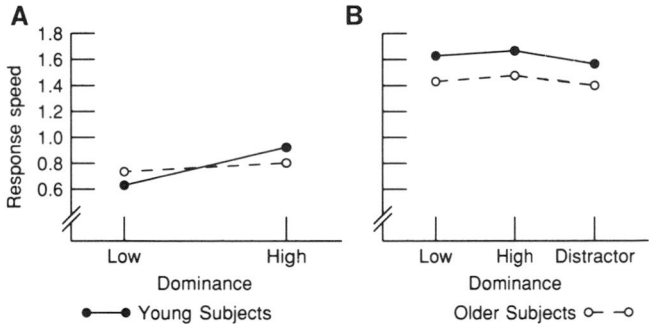

FIGURE 12.7 Mean response speed by young and old subjects of recall (A) and recognition (B) for high- and low-dominance exemplars of a category. Values on the ordinate are reciprocals of observed response latencies. (Adapted from Eysenck, 1975, Figure 1.)

same or different decisions had to be made about the physical or name identity of paired words rather than paired letters. In one of the conditions entering into Mueller, Kausler, and Faherty's (1980) study, the paired words were either coordinates (i.e., instances of the same taxonomic category; e.g., *deer elk*), in which "same" was the correct response, or they were semantically unrelated words, in which case "different" was the correct response. In another condition, the paired words were either physically identical (e.g., *DEER DEER*; "same") or physically different (e.g., *DEER deer*; "different"). Age differences in mean reaction times for same decisions under these two conditions are graphed in Figure 12.8. Clearly, the elderly subjects were much slower overall than the young subjects, and categorical decisions were slower overall than physical identity conditions. Most important, however, the magnitude of the age difference was only slightly greater (13 ms) for categorical identity decisions than for physical identity decisions. Thus, the mean reaction time for the elderly subjects was proportionally no greater for categorical decisions than for physical identity decisions, relative to the mean reaction times of young subjects. Categorical decisions involve a central (or cognitively higher order) process, matching in terms of categorical memberships, that is clearly missing for physical decisions. The absence of an Age × Decision interaction effect suggests that this matching process is age insensitive. A similar outcome was reported by Madden (1985) when same meaning decisions were based on synonymity rather than common categorical membership. From this evidence it is tempting to conclude that access to categorical information occurs as proficiently for elderly subjects as for young subjects. Moreover, there is evidence from a factor-analytic study by Hertzog,

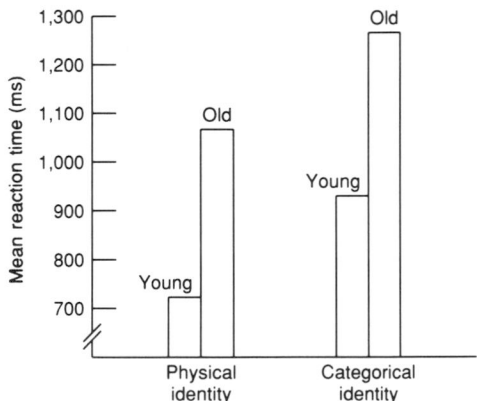

FIGURE 12.8 Age differences in mean reaction times for same decisions on word pairs containing either physically identical words or words from the same taxonomic category. (Adapted from Mueller, Kausler, & Faherty, 1980, Table 1.)

Raskind, and Cannon (1986) that the kinds of tasks employed by Eysenck (1975) measure the same factors in late adulthood as in early adulthood. These conclusions are tempered, however, by the fact that in a study similar to that of Mueller et al. (1980), Petros et al. (1983) did find disproportionately slower mean reaction times under the same category condition, relative to the physical identity condition.

Further evidence for the comparability between young and elderly adults in the processes mediating the accessing of categorical information comes from studies by Howard (1983b) with the lexical decision task and by Balota and Duchek (1988) with the priming and pronunciation task. In Howard's (1983b) study two letter strings were presented together (top-bottom) on a computer screen, and subjects responded "Yes" only if both strings composed real words. For word-word pairs the top word was a category name and the bottom word an instance of either that category (related condition) or an instance of a different category. In addition, in the related condition half of the instances were high in dominance and half were low in dominance. Examples of these various conditions are *bird robin* (related, high dominance), *bird duck* (related, low dominance), and *bird linen* (unrelated). Assuming that subjects read word pairs in a top-to-bottom order, the category name served as a prime for activation of the instance's node in the related word conditions. Howard (1983b) found a significant priming effect (i.e., faster reaction times for related word pairs than for unrelated word pairs)—an effect that was as great for her elderly subjects as for her young subjects. However, the magnitude of the priming effect was found to be no greater when the instances were high in dominance than when they were low in dominance.

Dominance was also varied for successively presented category name-instance name pairs by Balota and Duchek (1988), as was the SOA interval (200, 350, 500, and 800 ms). Thus, as in Howard's (1983b) study, the category name served as a prime for activating the related instance's node. Subjects were required to read silently the first word of each pair and to pronounce outloud the second word as quickly as possible. Mean pronunciation latencies for these pairs were contrasted with mean latencies for neutral pairs of words. The facilitation in latencies produced by priming is shown in Figure 12.9 for both young and elderly subjects under all conditions. There were several important findings. First, the extent of priming was, if anything, slightly greater for elderly subjects than for young subjects, in agreement with the general age insensitivity of categorical access. Second, contrary to Howard's (1983b) results, facilitation from priming was restricted largely to high-dominance categorical instances for both young and elderly subjects. Third, facilitation from priming was restricted to SOAs greater than 200 ms, again for both young and elderly subjects.

Collectively, the results obtained in these studies strongly imply that the processes mediating access to categorical information (e.g., category-instances relatedness) are comparable to the processes mediating individual word recognition

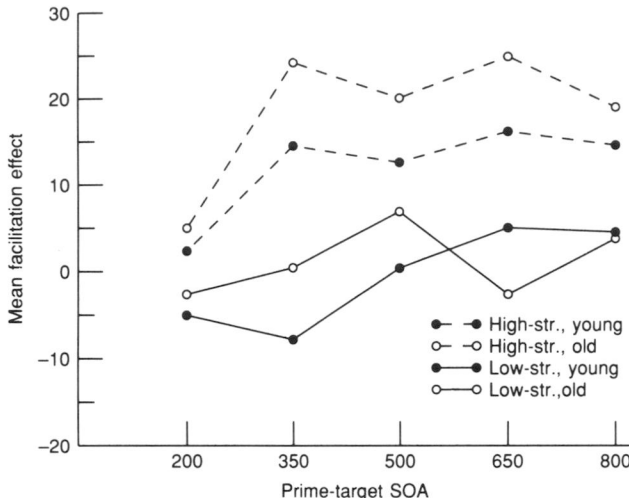

FIGURE 12.9 Mean facilitation effect (neutral minus related prime condition) in the semantic priming task as a function of age, strength (str), and stimulus-onset asynchrony (SOA). (Reprinted from Balota & Duchek, 1988, Figure 2. Copyright 1988 by the American Psychological Association.)

or identification. In particular, spreading activation appears to be a primary process in facilitating access to categorical information. Most important, there appear to be no qualitative changes with aging in its basic operation. Unresolved, however, are two other important issues. The first concerns the existence of age differences in the time course of spreading activation. Balota and Duchek (1988) found virtually no facilitation via priming for either young or elderly subjects with an SOA of 200 ms. Their outcome differs from that of Howard, Shaw, and Heisey (1986). Remember that they found a significant priming effect on a lexical decision task with an even briefer SOA (150 ms), but only for young subjects. However, it should be noted that Madden (1989) found a significant priming effect at 100 ms for his elderly subjects as well as his young subjects for word or nonword decisions when a sentence context provided the prime. A significant priming effect was observed for both age groups in Balota and Duchek's (1988) study with an SOA of 350 ms. Conceivably, spreading activation does progress from category node to instance node more rapidly for younger than for older individuals, in agreement with the slowing-down principle, but it requires, on the average, between 200 and 350 ms to reach the related node for young adults and at least 350 ms for elderly adults. Replications of Balota and Duchek's (1988) study that include SOAs between 200 and 350 ms are needed to resolve this issue. However, as noted by Balota and Duchek (1988), there is another possible reason for the disparity in outcome of their study and that of Howard, Shaw, and

Heisey (1986). The studies differed in the task performed and the responses required—"Yes"/"No" decisions about words versus the simple pronunciation of words. Balota and Duchek (1988) suggested that the lexical decision task of Howard, Shaw, and Heisey (1986) may require an additional process (a postaccess checking) that is absent in the pronunciation task. They suggested further that it may be this added process that is slower for elderly adults, thus accounting for their absence of a priming effect at 150 ms.

The second issue concerns "distance" within the lexicon that must be "traveled" to promulgate spreading activation. The distance analogy implies that facilitation by a category name should be greater for high-dominance instances than for low-dominance instances in that high-dominance nodes are stored in closer proximity to category nodes than are low-dominance nodes. Moreover, if the rate of spreading activation slows down with aging, the distance effect should be more pronounced for elderly than for young subjects. That is, the rate should determine how far distant nodes can be in order to benefit from spreading activation in a fixed time interval. This distance effect received partial support in Balota and Duchek's (1988) study where little facilitation was found for low-dominance instances—but for young subjects as well as for elderly subjects. Further partial support was obtained in Mueller, Kausler, Faherty, and Oliveri's (1980) study with category name-instance name pairs and "Yes/"No" decisions regarding intrapair relatedness. Facilitation was found for pairs containing typical instances (e.g., *animal dog*), and to a greater magnitude for elderly than for young subjects, but not for atypical instances (e.g., *animal tadpole*). In fact, an inhibitory effect was found for the latter (i.e., in mean decision time, relative to unrelated word pairs), and for both young and elderly subjects. The issue is complicated further by the fact that Howard (1983b, 1988b) found no effect of dominance on reaction times for either young or elderly subjects, an outcome clearly at odds with both the distance principle and the slowing-down principle. Hopefully, future studies employing finer grained variations in relatedness than in past studies will be able to provide the kind of evidence needed to resolve this important issue.

Separate Memory Systems?

To complete the picture, we need to return to the issue of whether or not generic memory and episodic memory are separate memory systems. We have discovered that, in general, age differences in lexical processes are modest, and largely quantitative in nature. This basic age insensitivity contrasts sharply with the more pronounced age sensitivity found for episodic-memory processes. This dissociation provides support for Tulving's (1972) contention that they are indeed separate systems. However, aging research has also provided support for the contention that generic-memory and episodic-memory phenomena are governed by a single long-term memory system. The rationale involved here is that if the same phenomena are manifested for both lexical tasks and episodic-memory tasks, then the same memory system is involved in each set of phenomena. The one phenomenon that has been of particular interest is that of priming effects. We already know that they occur on lexical decision tasks. However, episodic priming effects have also been clearly demonstrated for young adults (McKoon & Ratcliff, 1979, 1980), and for elderly adults as well (Balota & Duchek, 1989; Howard, Heisey, & Shaw, 1986; Rabinowitz, 1986). The procedures employed to demonstrate episodic priming will be described in our review of the aging research on this topic.

In Rabinowitz's (1986) study young and elderly subjects received a lengthy study list of paired words for subsequent cued recall (the first word, A, in each pair serving as the cue for recall of the second word, B). Before receiving the cued-recall test, they were given an individual item recognition test in which words from the prior study list were included, along with a number of new words. Some of the old items were B words that were preceded on the recognition test by the A words that had been paired with them in the study list (the subjects were not informed of this arrangement). Other old items were also B words, but they were preceded by old A items that had not been paired with them in the study list. Thus, there was the equivalent of related and unrelated pairs of the kind found on lexical decision tasks. In effect, the A word for a related pair serves as a prime for the recognition of B as an old item. Most important, this procedure permits the separation of priming effects (mean reaction times for unrelated A-B sequences minus mean reaction time for related sequences) for B items later recalled to A cues and B items that were not so recalled. The resulting priming effects may be seen in Figure 12.10 for both young and elderly subjects. They were present for both young and elderly subjects and for both recalled and non-recalled B words. Moreover, the magnitude of the priming effect for nonrecalled words was greater for elderly subjects (about 150 ms) than for young subjects (about 50 ms). However, for recalled words the direction was reversed, that is, the priming effect was greater for young subjects (about 250 ms) than for elderly subjects (again, about 150 ms).

Significant priming effects were also found by Howard, Heisey, and Shaw (1986) when sentences served as the study-list items for a later cued-recall memory test. In this case, the individual items on a recognition test were nouns from the prior sentences that were preceded either by a noun from the prior sentence (related pair condition) or by a noun from a different sentence (unrelated pair condition). The priming effect (again defined as the difference in mean reaction times for unrelated and related pairs) was about the same for young subjects (88 ms) and elderly subjects (101 ms) when sentences were presented twice in the study list, and it was as apparent for nouns later recalled on the cued-recall tests as for nouns that were not recalled, regardless of age level. However, some age difference were observed. When sentences were presented only once, the amount

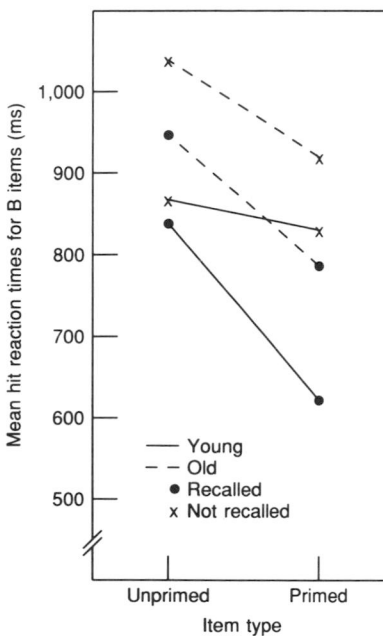

FIGURE 12.10 Hit reaction times for unprimed and primed items as a function of age and subsequent recall. (Adapted from Rabinowitz, 1986, Figure 3.)

of priming was greater for young than for elderly subjects. In addition, an asymmetry was found in priming for elderly subjects, but not for young subjects. That is, "backward" priming (object of a sentence as the prime, subject of the sentence as the target) was significantly less than "forward" priming (subject as prime, object as target) for elderly subjects, whereas they were equivalent for young subjects.

Minor age differences in episodic priming effects were also found by Balota and Duchek (1989), but the overall pattern was much the same for young and elderly subjects. As noted by Howard, Heisey, and Shaw (1986), the episodic priming task seems to offer a means of testing the amount of information acquired in a study phase that is more sensitive than either a cued recall test or a traditional recognition memory test (i.e., one in which test words are ordered randomly). In effect, an episodic priming effect is very similar to, if not identical with, what we earlier called implicit memory (Chapter 11).

The issue of separate memory systems or a single long-term system is likely to remain unresolved for some time. It is an issue that should be the subject of many basic research studies in the future. It is also an issue in which aging research should continue to bask in the glory of being able to contribute to the eventual resolution of the issue.

When Lexical Access Fails

When he was in his 70s, Donald Hebb, a brilliant physiological psychologist, wrote an article describing what he believed to be the adverse consequences of aging on his own cognitive functioning (Hebb, 1978). One of the problems he noted was an increased number of incidences in which he couldn't find the right word to express a particular thought, even though he knew he knew the word. That is, access to the word in the lexicon was blocked for whatever reason. This is a problem known to all of us. At the time it occurs we are in a "tip-of-the-tongue" (TOT) state. R. Brown and McNeill (1966) discovered that when we are in that state we often have some knowledge about the word, such as its initial letter and perhaps the number of syllables it has, but not enough to assure retrieval of the total word. However, when given a multiple-choice recognition test, we usually recognize the word immediately. TOT states are failures to gain access to an appropriate word (or name) in the lexicon. Access begins in this case with a thought we wish to express (see Figure 9.1). Ordinarily, thought (i.e., a concept we are experiencing; e.g., "coldness") is successful in activating rapidly the right word or words—but not always (e.g., "I feel—pause for several seconds—"frigid"). We now have evidence to indicate that Hebb's observation about himself has generalizability to the elderly population overall. TOT states do seem to occur more often in late adulthood than in early adulthood, and they represent what seems to be an important exception to the overall robustness of lexical processes with aging. (See Burke and Laver, 1990, for further review and elaboration of the retrieval processes underlying TOT states).

One form of evidence consists of having adults of different ages keep a diary in which they record each occurrence of a TOT state for a period of several weeks. With this procedure Burke, Worthley, and Martin (1988) discovered that elderly adults report about twice as many TOT states per month as do young adults. Elderly adults also report on memory questionnaires a frequency of TOT states that is about twice that of young adults (G. Cohen & Faulkner, 1986). When asked in a controlled setting to answer such questions as "What is the name for a person who collects postage stamps?" elderly subjects were found to experience more TOT states than young adult subjects in attempting to respond with "philatelist" (Burke, MacKay, Wothley, & Wade, 1991). However, it has also been reported that their success rate in gaining eventual access to the blocked word or name can be fairly high, provided they exert sufficient cognitive effort in an attempt to retrieve the information (Finley & Sharp, 1989), but it is likely to be less than that of younger adults (M. Martin, 1986; Maylor, 1990c).

There is evidence (Maylor, 1990a) to indicate that elderly adults are less likely than younger adults to experience a "blocker" (a word similar to the target word that persists in interfering with retrieval of the target word; e.g., "frugal" instead of "frigid") while in a TOT state, and they are also less likely to report partial information about the target word, such as the initial letter, the number of syllables in the target word, or semantic information about the target word (Maylor, 1990a, 1990b).

In addition, Bowles and Poon (1985) provided convincing laboratory evidence of an adult age difference in gaining access to words that satisfy a momentary need (see Bowles, Obler, and Poon, 1989, for elaboration). Their procedure reversed that of a standard vocabulary test, and it is, in effect, comparable to the kind of test used to induce TOT states in controlled settings. Instead of being given words and asked to define each, subjects were given definitions and asked to name the word fitting that definition. Providing a definition, such as "A mythical animal with one straight horn on its head," is comparable to "thinking out loud" about a specific concept. They also included with each definition one of six different kinds of word primes that was available while the subjects attempted to find the right word. One prime consisted of the correct word itself (e.g., *unicorn* for the above definition), another of a semantically related word (e.g., *dragon*), another of an orthographically similar word (e.g., *uniform*), and so on. The number of correct words (out of 20) to the definitions are shown in Figure 12.11 for both young and elderly subjects under all six priming conditions. The age difference, favoring young subjects, in the number of correct responses was significant in all but the correct word and letter prime conditions. The absence of an age difference for the correct prime condition clearly indicates that the presence of the age difference in other conditions resulted from an age-related access or retrieval problem, and not from loss of the relevant information in the lexicon (the age difference for these other conditions was later replicated with the same materials by Bowles, 1989). The correct words in these two studies were all of relatively low frequency in the English language. Interestingly, Rissenberg and Glanzer (1987) found no age-related deficit in giving correct words to match definitions when the words were higher in their frequency of occurrence and therefore of greater familiarity to adults of all ages. Failure to access appropriate words, in general, is likely to be inversely related to their frequency of use. It is perhaps only with relatively infrequently used words that older adults experience increased difficulty in word finding. However, Heller and Dobbs (1993) found an age-related deficit in word naming on a task in which subjects simply described the events they observed in a video cartoon.

Age differences on a definition-to-word task contrast sharply with age differences on a word-to-definition task (i.e., a standard vocabulary test). If anything, elderly adults score higher on vocabulary tests than do young adults. There seems to be some degree of asymmetry between thought-to-word and word-to-thought

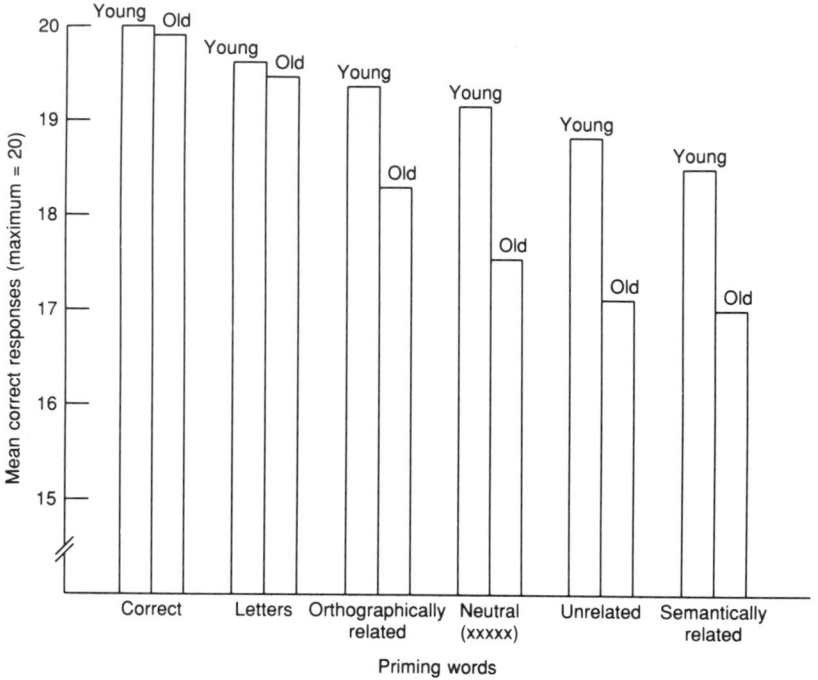

FIGURE 12.11   Correct words named to definitions with various priming conditions. (Adapted from Bowles & Poon, 1985, Table 2.)

access processes. That is, the former appear to be more susceptible to age-related decrements in proficiency than the latter.

Adult Age Differences in the Use of Syntax

Also stored generically is our knowledge of the rules of grammar, that is, the syntax of our language. Although there is no evidence to suggest that people become "ungrammatical" as they grow older with normal aging, there is evidence to indicate more subtle age differences in syntactical production and comprehension (e.g., Emery, 1985; Kemper, 1986, 1987a, 1987b; Kynette & Kemper, 1986; see Kemper, 1992, for a detailed review). For example, Kemper (1986) had young and elderly subjects repeat or paraphrase sentences of varying lengths and syntactical complexities. Age-related deficits were found only when complex sentences (e.g., those containing embedded clauses) were encountered. A unique longitudinal study was conducted by Kemper (1987a) in which the diaries of the same individuals were analyzed over a number of years. The syntactical structure of the sentence productions recorded in the diaries were generally less complex when the diary-keepers were old than when they were young. Bromley (1991) also found elderly adults to write less complex sentences than younger adults when writing self-descriptions (but there was no age difference in either sentence length or sentence readability). Nevertheless, Kemper concluded that "Although studies of adults' speech production (Kemper, Kynette, Rash, Sprott, & O'Brien, 1989; Kynette & Kemper, 1986) and writing (Kemper, 1987a) reveal that older adults are unlikely to produce complex grammatical forms spontaneously, their speech does not evidence a progressive degeneration into 'baby talk'" (1992, p. 221). The changes in syntactic complexity do seem to be large enough, however, to alert researchers in the area of prose memory to be cautious about syntactic complexity in their selection of material for tests of age differences in discourse memory. Most important, communications involving information about diseases, medications, self-care, and other important everyday topics for elderly people should avoid unnecessary syntactic complexities.

Adult Age Differences in Metamemory

Metamemory is another part of the generic-memory system. It means knowing about remembering, that is, knowing what one's own memory system can and cannot accomplish. Through such knowledge, we are able to assess somewhat realistically just how much new episodic information we can assimilate in a given time period, we are able to evaluate somewhat realistically just how likely previously encoded information is retrievable, we are able to know what memory strategies we have available and how to deploy those strategies contingent on the requirements of various tasks, and so on. Developmental research began with studies of children of different ages. This research demonstrated that self-knowledge about memory increases dramatically from early to late childhood (see Flavell & Wellman, 1977). An important remaining question is, "Does metamemory decrease dramatically from early to late adulthood?" If it does, the implications for the memory performances of older adults are considerable.

Research on adult age differences in metamemorial functions has become a highly visible component of aging research in recent years. In our review of these age differences, we will distinguish among three forms of metamemory. The first is *off-line evaluation* of memory proficiency. By this we mean how people evaluate their memory proficiency in their everyday lives. How good (or bad) is it? How does it compare with your proficiency when you were a young adult? Of particular interest is how well these self-assessments, or self-perceptions, usually conducted by means of a memory questionnaire, correlate with actual memory performances. The second is *on-line evaluation* of memory proficiency. Here subjects are asked to perform on a specific memory test, and are asked to evaluate how well they will do on it, which specific items of to-be-remembered information will actually be remembered, and so on. The third is *monitoring* of memory performances in the sense of knowing what strategies should be most effective in enhancing memory performance for a designated task.

Age Differences in Off-Line Evaluation of Episodic Memory

In their excellent review of memory questionnaires, Gilewski and Zelinski (1986) cited four reasons why self-assessments of memory proficiency are important. First, there is some evidence for a reliable correlation between the frequency and intensity of elderly adults' complaints about their memory system's functioning and performance on laboratory tests of memory (e.g., Riege, 1982; Zelinski, Gilewski, & Thompson, 1980). Presumably, scores on a soundly constructed memory questionnaire provide a means of identifying the components of memory that are the primary sources of such complaints (e.g., prospective memory, memory for names). Moreover, Gilewski and Zelinski (1986) believe that "for many older people, memory questionnaires appear to be less threatening than laboratory tests, and the greater face validity of questionnaires compared with memory tests may increase cooperation during assessment" (1986, p. 93). If true, questionnaires could offer a valuable means of identifying those normally aging individuals who might benefit from a memory training program. Perhaps—but there is also considerable evidence that community-dwelling elderly subjects recruited specifically because of their complaints about having memory problems perform no worse than noncomplaining elderly subjects on such laboratory memory tasks as the free recall of a word list (e.g., Scogin, Storandt, & Lott, 1985; Zarit, Cole, & Guider, 1981; see also Chapter 4, p. 113). In addition, memory training for "complainers" may improve their performances on laboratory tasks of memory, but it seems to leave unaltered the extent of their complaints (Scogin et al., 1985) (see Chapter 4, p. 113).

The second reason identified by Gilewski and Zelinski (1986) is that assessment of memory problems with questionnaires "provide valuable information for detecting dementia" (p. 93). However, given the pronounced differences in performance between normally aging individuals and SDAT individuals (see, for example, Poon, 1986) on both episodic and lexical laboratory memory tasks, one wonders what self-assessments via questionnaires can add diagnostically. The third reason is the potential value self-assessments have in differentiating between depression and dementia as the sources of everyday memory problems and complaints. This may prove to be true, at least for distinguishing between cognitively normal elderly adults with depression and individuals in the early stage of dementia. Gilewski and Zelinski's (1986) description of the fourth reason is the following:

Memory complaints are important phenomena on their own right. Complaints provide useful information about how people view their general cognitive functioning as they age. Their perception of their memory capabilities may influence their performance on memory tasks (Poon, Fozard, & Treat, 1978). Therefore it is useful to have self-assessment data to control for this influence" (1986, p. 93).

Questions may also be raised about this reason. To what does "memory tasks" refer? Performance on laboratory tasks? Memory performances in the everyday world? At stake is the validity of self-assessments as a predictor of memory task performances, wherever they may occur. As we will see later, the evidence for their validity is somewhat limited. (See also Rabbitt & Abson, 1990).

This reviewer's admittedly pessimistic perspective about memory questionnaires and self-assessments undoubtedly reflects his bias toward experimental psychology and the use of laboratory tasks as the best means of assessing memory performances of elderly adults. The fact remains that there are many memory questionnaires in existence, and a large amount of information has been gathered about their psychometric attributes and the covariations between scores on these questionnaires and various kinds of memory performances. Our review will attempt to be as fair and unbiased as possible.

In their review of metamemory questionnaires, Gilewski and Zelinski (1986) identified 10 different questionnaires then in existence. Summary information about these questionnaires is given in Table 12.1 (see Dixon, 1989, for further review). As may be seen there, they differ greatly in the number of items they contain, the number of different scales (dependent measures), and the availability of psychometric information (e.g., reliability and internal consistency). Other questionnaires have appeared since Gilewski and Zelinski's (1986) review, and other new ones will undoubtedly appear in the future. One of the new questionnaires is called the Memory Assessment Clinics Self-Rating Scale (the MAC-S; Crook & Larrabee, 1990; Winterling, Crook, Salama, & Gobert, 1986). It contains 45 items that assess the ability to remember information, the frequency-of-occurrence of memory failures, and such global factors as a comparison of one's overall memory proficiency relative to other people. The MAC-S joins that select group of questionnaires that have well-established psychometric properties, including the identification of its factor structure (five different ability-to-remember factors and five frequency-of-occurrence factors; Crook & Larrabee, 1990). Another new questionnaire was introduced by McEvoy and Moon (1988). Its questions cover 10 different areas of everyday forgetting, such as forgetting names and faces, forgetting to keep appointments, and forgetting to perform routine tasks.

Our emphasis will be on the two most widely used questionnaires. The first was originally known as the Metamemory Questionnaire (Zelinski, Gilewski, & Thompson, 1980). It has since been shortened from 92 items to 64 items, and it has been renamed the Memory Functioning Questionnaire (MFQ; Gilewski,

TABLE 12.1

Descriptive Features of Ten Memory-Assessment Questionnaires[a]

Author(s)	Questionnaire	Number of items	Items published?	Scaling	Dependent measure(s)
Psychometric properties not examined					
Perlmutter (1978a)	Memory Questionnaire	60	Yes	4 & 10 pts.	5 composite scores
Zarit, Cole, & Guider (1981)	Memory Complaints Questionnaire	12	No	3–11 pts.	Total score
Niederehe et al. (1981)	Metamemory Questionnaire	134	No	varies	—
Hulicka (1982)	Self-Assessment of Memory Questionnaire	45+	No	—	Total score
Psychometric properties examined					
Herrmann & Neiser (1978) and	Inventory of Memory Experiences (IME)	72	Yes	7 pts.	Part F: 8 factor scores & total score
Herrmann (1979)	Short Inventory of Memory Experiences (SIME)	32	No	7 pts.	Part R: 3 section scores / Pat F: 8 factor scores / Part R: 2 section scores
Zelinski et al. (1980) and	Metamemory Questionnaire	92	Yes	7 pts.	9 scale scores
Gilewski et al. (1983)	Memory Functioning Questionnaire (MFQ)	64	No	7 pts.	7 scale scores
Goldberg et al. (1981)	Wadsworth Memory Questionnaire (WMQ)	35	No	5 pts.	—
Riege (1982)	Memory Self Report	30	Yes	4 pts.	4 category scores
Sunderland et al. (1983)	Everyday Memory Questionnaire	35	Yes	5 pts.	Total score
Dixon & Hultsch (1983a)	Metamemory in Adulthood	120	No	5 pts.	8 factor scores

[a] Adapted from Gilewski and Zelinski, 1986, Table 11.1. (Copyright 1986 by the American Psychological Association. Adapted by permission.)

Zelinski, & Schaie, 1990; Gilewski, Zelinski, Schaie, & Thompson, 1983; Zelinski, Gilewski, Anthony-Bergstone, 1990). Shown in Table 12.2 are the nine scales included in the original questionnaire, along with a sample item for each scale. Two of the scales (Reliance on Memory and Effort Made to Remember) have been eliminated in the shorter MFQ version of the questionnaire. The MFQ has been factor analyzed, and the factor structure appears to be invariant for adults of different ages (Gilewski et al., 1990). There appear to be four factors, General Frequency of Forgetting, Seriousness of Forgetting, Retrospective Functioning, and Mnemomic Usage, that account for nearly 37% of the variance in response to the 64 items. The internal consistency of the MFQ has been

TABLE 12.2

Scales and Sample Items from the Metamemory Questionnaire[a]

Scale	Sample item
1. General rating	1. How would you rate your memory in terms of the kinds of problems you have?
2. Reliance on memory	2. How often do you need to rely on your memory without the use of remembering techniques, such as making lists, when you are engaged in . . . (a) social activities?
3. Retrospective functioning	3. How is your memory compared to the way it was . . . (b) one year ago?
4. Frequency of forgetting	4. How often do these present a memory problem for you . . . (a) names?
5. Frequency of forgetting when reading	5. As you are reading a novel, how often do you have trouble remembering what you have read . . . (a) in the opening chapters once you have finished the book?
6. Remembering past events	6. How well do you remember things which occurred . . . (a) last month?
7. Seriousness	7. When you actually forget in these situations, how serious of a problem do you consider the memory failure to be . . . (a) names?
8. Mnemonics	8. How often do you use these techniques to remind yourself about things . . . (a) keep an appointment book?
9. Effort made to remember	9. How much effort do you usually have to make to remember in these situations . . . (a) names?

[a] Adapted from Gilewski and Zelinski, 1986, Table 11.7. (Copyright 1986 by the American Psychological Association. Adapted by permission.)

demonstrated to be high, making the test a reliable one for evaluating memory self-appraisals. The second is known as the Metamemory in Adulthood questionnaire (MIA; Dixon & Hultsch, 1983a). As noted in Table 12.1, it contains 120 questions that have been identified through factor analysis as measuring eight different primary factors (see Table 12.3 for a description of the factors and a sample item for each factor). Additional analyses (Hertzog, Dixon, Schulenberg, & Hultsch, 1987; Hertzog, Hultsch, & Dixon, 1987) have revealed that these eight factors may be subsumed under two higher order, or secondary, factors. The first involves beliefs about self-efficacy in using memory, that is, belief's about one's overall memory competence; the second combines knowledge about memory and affect (e.g., anxiety) about its operations.

Age differences in large samples of subjects ranging in age from 20 to 78 yr were examined by Hultsch, Hertzog, and Dixon (1987) for scores on both the MFQ and MIA. Significant age difference were found for the General Rating and Retrospective Functioning scales of the MFQ (see Table 12.2), with the difference being especially pronounced between subjects in the youngest (20–26 yr) and oldest (69–78 yr) age ranges tested. Significant age differences were also found for the Strategy, Capacity, Change, and Locus dimensions of the MIA (see Table 12.3). Loewen, Shaw, and Craik (1990) also found lower scores on the Capacity dimension of the MIA for their elderly subjects than for their young adult subjects. Most important, there appear to be progressive declines with increasing age in beliefs about one's own memory capacity and about the stability of memory as one gets older.

The more negative view of their own memory capability expressed by elderly individuals is also characteristic of their view of other elderly individuals' memory capabilities. Erber (1989; Erber, Szuchman, & Rothberg, 1990a, 1990b) had young and elderly subjects read vignettes describing someone identified as being either young or old having problems with a specific form of memory (e.g., remembering a telephone number). Both young and elderly subjects were more likely to evaluate the fictitious individuals as having "mental difficulty" and in need of memory training when they were identified as being old than they were identified as being young. Failures of memory by elderly adults were viewed as being due to lack of ability, whereas failures by young adults were viewed as being due to lack of effort (Erber & Rothberg, 1991). The subjects, and especially the young adults, in Erber et al.'s (1990b) and Erber and Rothberg's (1991) studies tended to perceive very long-term memory failures (e.g., forgetting an old recipe) as being more indicative of mental difficulty and the need for evaluation than they did short-term (e.g., forgetting a to-be-dialed telephone number) or long-term (e.g., forgetting items on a shopping list). Physicians have also been found to perceive very long-term memory failures to need more urgent care than other forms of memory failures (Erber, Rothberg, Szuchman, & Etheart, 1993). Ryan (1992), in a sample ranging in age from 18 to 74 yr, also found beliefs about memory functioning to

TABLE 12.3

The Eight Dimensions of the Metamemory in Adulthood (MIA)[a] Instrument

Dimension	Description	Sample item
Strategy	Knowledge and use of information about one's remembering abilities such that performance in given instances is potentially improved (+ = high use).	Do you write appointments on a calendar to help you remember them?
Task	Knowledge of basic memory processes, especially as evidenced by how most people perform (+ = high knowledge).	For most people, facts that are interesting are easier to remember than facts that are not.
Capacity	Knowledge of memory capacities as evidenced by predictive report of performance on given tasks (+ = high capacity).	I am good at remembering names.
Change	Perception of memory abilities as generally stable or subject to long-term decline (+ = stability).	The older I get the harder it is to remember things clearly.
Activity	Regularity with which respondent seeks and engages in activities that might support cognitive performance (+ = high regularity).	How often do you read newspapers?
Anxiety	Knowledge of reciprocal influence of emotional state and cognitive performance (+ = high knowledge).	I find it harder to remember things when I'm upset.
Achievement	Perceived importance of having a good memory and performing well on memory tasks (+ = high achievement).	It is important that I am very accurate when remembering names of people.
Locus	Perceived personal control over remembering abilities (+ = internality).	Even if I work on it my memory ability will go downhill.

[a] Adapted from Dixon and Hultsch, 1983a, Table 2. (Copyright 1983 by the Gerontological Society of America. Adapted by permission.)

be more positive for young adults than for older adults, especially adults over age 65. Moreover, Ryan and See (1993) discovered that the belief about memory decline with normal aging applies to oneself as well as to the "typical" older adult. Other researchers have found that this negative impression of older adults applies to other cognitive tasks as well, such as the reasons for having difficulty in academic performances (B. D. Bell & Stanfield, 1973; Reno, 1979) and for succeeding in a computer course (Ryan, Szechtman, & Bodkin, 1992).

Our main concern is with the relationship between self-evaluation of episodic-memory proficiency and performance on episodic-memory tasks. Are low self-evaluations, whether expressed by low scores on formal questionnaires or by simple complaints about memory problems, reflected accurately in low performances on laboratory tasks? The evidence is decidedly mixed (see Gilewski & Zelinski, 1986, and Zelinski, Gilewski, and Anthony-Bergstone, 1990, for further reviews). On the positive side, Dixon and Hultsch (1983b) found positive relationships between recall scores for prose passages and scores on the knowledge of memory capacity dimension, scores on the task knowledge dimension, and scores on the strategy dimension of the MIA for both young and middle-aged subjects. For their elderly subjects, prose recall scores were found to be correlated significantly with scores on the task dimension, the achievement dimension, and the locus of control dimension. An implication of this outcome is that the affective state associated with one's view toward one's own memory proficiency is especially important in determining performance level for elderly adults. Cavanaugh and Poon (1989) found task and capacity scores to be better predictors of prose recall scores than age per se. Zelinski et al. (1990) reported modest, but significant correlation coefficients, between scores on several scales of the MFQ (e.g., frequency of forgetting) and scores on both word-list recall and word-list recognition tests.

On the negative side, West, Boatwright, and Schleser (1984) found little relationship between scores on several scales derived from Perlmutter's (1978a; see Table 12.1) questionnaire, presumably measuring the same dimensions as the capacity, strategy, and task dimensions of the MIA, and scores on free-recall tasks for their elderly subjects. Sunderland, Watts, Baddeley, and Harris (1986) also reported little in the way of positive relationships between scores on their questionnaire (see Table 12.1) and scores on several laboratory memory tasks for their older subjects. Taylor, Miller, and Tinklenberg (1992) correlated self-reports of 30 elderly adults, all of whom had expressed complaints about their memory proficiency, with declines in word-recall scores over a 4-yr period—and reported essentially a zero correlation. A weak relationship between self-report scores and laboratory memory performance was also found by O'Hara, Hinrichs, Kohout, Wallace, and Lemke (1986). Symbolic of the ambiguities surrounding research on self-evaluations is the mixed results obtained when self-evaluations are taken both before and after elderly subjects complete a formal memory training course.

McEvoy and Moon (1988) discovered moderate changes in expressions of complaints about memory problems for their elderly subjects, whereas Scogin et al. (1985) reported no change (see Chapter 4, p. 113).

Of course, validation studies of questionnaires have focused solely on performances on laboratory memory tasks as the external criterion for determining the predictive validity of those questionnaires. The ultimate criterion is performance on everyday memory activities. A familiar argument is that many laboratory memory tasks have little relevance for memory performances outside of the laboratory. It is interesting that the strongest evidence for the validity of self-evaluation questionnaires comes from studies employing prose recall as the laboratory task (Dixon & Hultsch, 1983b; Cavanaugh & Poon, 1989), a task often argued to have greater ecological validity than most other laboratory tasks. It should be noted that, although their results were generally negative, Sunderland et al. (1986) did find modest support for a positive covariation between self-evaluation and task performance only with prose recall.

There are other problems with memory questionnaires as well. Conceivably, adults of all ages may not be the best judges of their own memory shortcomings. Of interest here is the fact that Sunderland, Harris, and Baddeley (1983) found for both severely head-injured subjects and matched control subjects that ratings of memory proficiency given by significant other persons (e.g., spouses) are better predictors of subjects' performances on laboratory memory tasks than were the subjects' self-evaluations. Another problem may lie in the strategy applied in the construction of questionnaires. It seems to rely heavily on an empirical approach in which many questions are included, and scales are then derived by means of factor analysis or cluster analysis. Missing is any guidance provided by memory theory, such that scores may be derived separately for memory functioning as it involves effortful episodic memory, automatic episodic memory, prospective memory, lexical memory, and so on. Not surprisingly, clinical assessments of memory proficiency seem to be moving in the direction of providing profiles based on scores on a theoretically oriented battery of laboratory memory tasks (e.g., Wilson, Cockburn, & Baddeley, 1985) or in the direction of employing computerized simulations of everyday memory tasks (Crook & Larrabee, 1988). Finally, the effective use of questionnaires is challenged by the apparent fact that some normally aging individuals perceive themselves as not really being handicapped by everyday memory problems (Cavanaugh & Morton, 1988; Sunderland et al. 1986). Interestingly, Cavanaugh's (1986–87) elderly subjects' self-rating of their memory proficiency was as high as that of young adults—even though they viewed their proficiency as having declined with aging! On the other hand, several authors (e.g., Perlmutter et al., 1987; Cavanaugh, Morton, & Tilse, 1989) have argued that many elderly people have stereotyped views about the inevitability of large declines in memory proficiency in late adulthood. As noted by Ryan (1992), these views may be based on falsely optimistic beliefs about the great accuracy of memory in earlier adulthood, thus making any age-related declines in memory proficiency greatly exaggerated.

Age Differences in On-Line Evaluation of Episodic Memory

As a subject in a memory experiment, you are told that you will be given a list of 20 words to study for as long as you wish, and you will then be asked to recall as many of the words as possible. You are given the further information that *apple*, and *table* are representative of the kinds of words included on the list. How many of the 20 words do you predict you will actually recall? A prediction of "18" would surely be an expression of your confidence in your episodic-memory system's high level of proficiency. By contrast, a prediction of "3" would seemingly express the pessimistic faith you have in your episodic-memory proficiency. This simple procedure was followed in an innovative study by Bruce, Coyne, and Botwinick (1982) as a means of evaluating age differences in the accuracy of on-line self-evaluation of memory proficiency. Each subject was given as much time as needed to study the word list and then completed the recall test. They found that young adult subjects were fairly accurate in their predicted recall scores. Elderly subjects predicted approximately the same amount of recall as did the young subjects, but they also recalled significantly fewer words than did the young subjects. Consequently, they had overestimated their episodic-memory proficiency. As observed by Bruce et al. (1982), "The present finding of no age differences in predicted recall, coupled with the finding of age differences in actual recall, suggests that memory knowledge does not keep pace with changes in memory performance" (1982, p. 357).

A further demonstration of this aberrant pace for elderly individuals was provided by Lovelace and Marsh (1985). The procedure, however, departed considerably from that of Bruce et al. (1982). The materials in the study list consisted of 60 paired associates (unrelated words). After each pair had been presented, the subjects were asked to rate how likely they would be able to match correctly the two elements on a later memory test. Ratings were done on a five-point scale (1 = quite sure I will *not* recall; 5 = quite sure I will recall). For the memory test, the subjects received the stimulus elements of the pairs randomly arranged in one column and the response elements randomly arranged in another column, with their task being to match stimulus–response (S-R) pairs as they had appeared in the study list. For each match they were asked to rate their confidence in its correctness on a three-point scale (1 = a guess, 3 = sure it is correct). The nature of the age differences in predictive ability may be seen in Figure 12.12. Plotted there are the mean proportions of items correctly matched for each subclass of prediction ratings (i.e., pairs rated "1," pairs rated "2," and so on). Note that both young and elderly subjects displayed considerable accuracy in knowledge about their memory proficiency. For both groups of subjects the proportion correctly

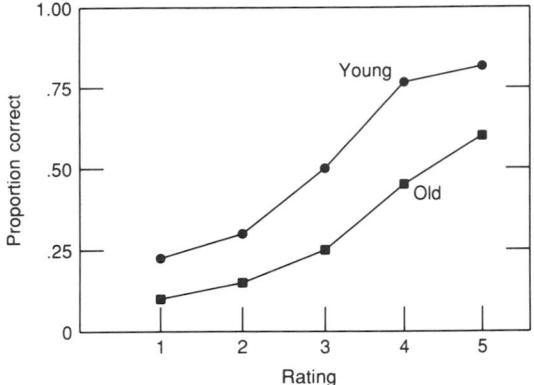

FIGURE 12.12 Proportion correct associative matches for young and old adults conditional on the rating the pairs received during study. (Adapted from Lovelace & Marsh, 1985, Figure 1.)

matched increased progressively from those pairs rated "1" to those pairs rated "5." However, it is also quite evident that the elderly subjects overestimated their memory proficiency to a greater degree than the young subjects. For those pairs rated "5" (sure I will remember), the elderly subjects matched correctly only about 60%, the young subjects about 85%. On the other hand, the age difference in the accuracy of evaluating the correctness of the matches on the memory test was negligible, with both groups being correct more than 90% of the time. Other researchers (e.g., Brigham & Pressley, 1988; Perlmutter, 1978a) have also found elderly subjects to give predictions of amount recalled comparable to those of young subjects, even though the amount actually recalled is less than that of young adults. In addition, elderly subjects tend to have greater confidence in the correctness of their recalls than do middle-aged subjects despite the higher level of recall of the latter (Perfect & Stollery, 1993).

There is also evidence available (Devolder, Brigham, & Pressley, 1990; Hertzog, Dixon, & Hultsch, 1990) indicating that the tendency of elderly subjects to overestimate their subsequent memory performances applies to some memory tasks, but not to other tasks. The nature of the task is indeed likely to be a potent determiner of how well adults of any age are able to predict their memory performance. The importance of the kind of task performed was clearly demonstrated with young adults in a study by R. L. Cohen (1988). His subjects were quite accurate in predicting which words in a study list they would be able to recall. However, their predictions regarding which performed actions would later be recalled amounted essentially to nothing but guesses. Our knowledge concerning the proficiency of our effortful episodic-memory processes is, not surprisingly, greater than our knowledge concerning the proficiency of our automatic episodic-memory processes. Of interest here is another component of the study by Bruce et al. (1982). Their subjects actually received four different kinds of word lists (effortful memory), one containing only high-imagery words, a second only low-imagery words, a third only high-frequency words, and the fourth only low-frequency words. We know that subjects can recall more high-imagery words than low-imagery words, and more high-frequency words than low-frequency words (Kausler, 1974; see also Chapter 7, pp. 252–255). Apparently both young and elderly subjects know that these disparities in recall should apply to their own memory performances. The number of words predicted to be recalled was greater for the high-imagery list than for the low-imagery list, and greater for high-frequency words than for low-frequency words (Bruce et al., 1982). Similarly, both young and elderly subjects were quite accurate in predicting the effect of increasing study time on the number of words that can be recalled on a free-recall task—that is, the longer the study time allowed, the greater the number of words recalled (Coyne, 1985).

However, our knowledge about our own effortful memory processes seems to have its limitations too, regardless of one's age. One such limitation was nicely demonstrated in a study by Rabinowitz, Ackerman, Craik, and Hinchley (1982). They asked their young and elderly subjects to rate the likelihood of recalling paired associates that were studied either under standard learning instructions or instructions that stress the use of interactive imagery to link together the S-R elements of each pair. Although recall of the paired associates was much higher in the interactive imagery condition, the predicted ratings of recall were no higher than in the standard learning condition. Apparently, neither young nor elderly subjects were aware of the mnemonic advantage of using imagery, even though they appeared to make use of it.

An even more dramatic illustration of our general unawareness of how our memory system operates was provided by Shaw and Craik (1989). Their subjects received a lengthy study list in which each word was presented with one of three types of cues. For example, given *ice* as a study-list word, it could be accompanied by a letter cue ("starts with ic: ice"), a rhyme cue ("rhymes with dice: ice"), or a category cue ("something slippery: ice"). The cues were intended to vary the level of processing (shallow to deep) the words received. Category cues should promote deeper processing than either letter (orthographic sensory processing) or rhyme (phonological sensory processing) cues, and therefore greater memorability. In addition, phonological cues were expected to yield deeper processing and greater memorability than letter cues. As may be seen in Figure 12.13, these predictions were fully confirmed for both young and elderly subjects on a cued-recall test (the cues for recall were the cues presented with the words on the study list). The young subjects excelled in recall with letter and rhyme cues, but, surprisingly, not for category cues. Our main interest, however, is in the predictions

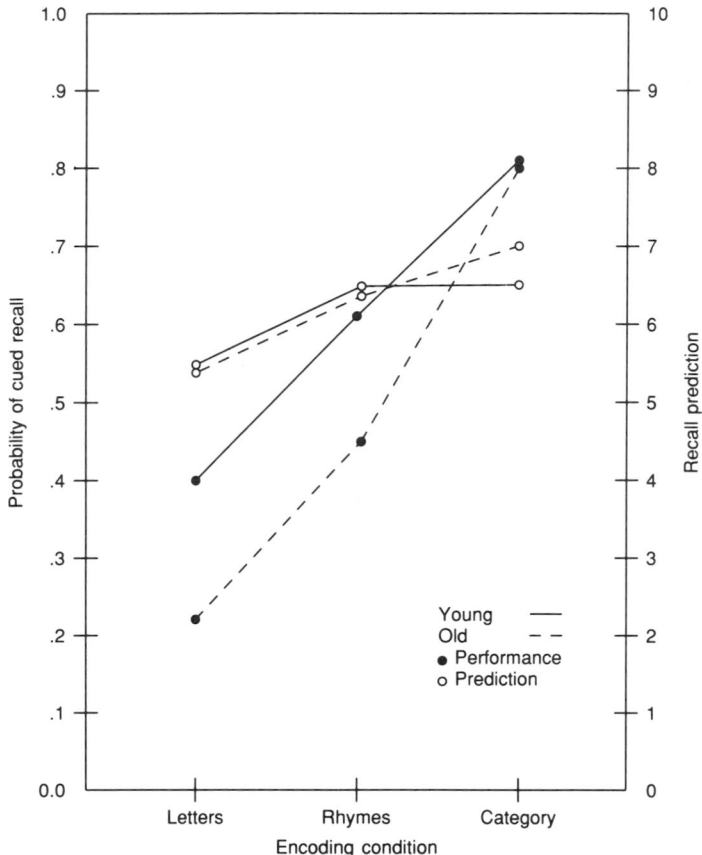

FIGURE 12.13 Probability of cued recall and recall predictions as a function of encoding cues extant at study. (Reprinted from Shaw & Craik, 1989, Figure 1. Copyright 1989 by the American Psychological Association.)

of later recall the subjects gave after encountering each cue-target word pair in the study list. The predictions were given on a 0 (certain *not* to recall) to 10 (certain to recall) scale. Mean prediction scores are also given in Figure 12.13. Note first that young and elderly subjects were virtually identical in their mean predictions. Of course, since recall was higher overall for the young subjects, this means that the elderly subjects, as in Bruce et al.'s (1982) study and in Lovelace and Marsh's (1985) study, overestimated their memory proficiency to a greater extent than did young subjects. Note further that for both age groups there was only a modest increase in predicted recall from the letter cue to the category cue condition. Unlike memory researchers, subjects of all ages are seemingly unaware of the advantage deep processing has over shallow processing in promoting sub-sequent memorability. In fact, it was only with deep processing that both young and elderly subjects tended to underestimate their memory proficiency. Young and elderly adults also appear to be equivalent in their limited knowledge not only about encoding processes but also about retrieval processes (Annoshian, Mammarella, & Hertel, 1989).

Of further interest are age differences in how young and elderly subjects eval-uate their own memory performances after the memory performance is completed (i.e., postdiction rather than prediction). Hanley-Dunn and McIntosh (1984) discovered that their elderly subjects rated their free-recall performances more poorly than did their young adult subjects, even though the two age groups, surprisingly, did not differ in their recall scores. Thus, the elderly subjects were less accurate postdictively than the young subjects. In addition, the correlation between rated performance and actual recall scores was moderately high for the elderly subjects ($r = .62$) as well as for the young subjects ($r = .70$). Devolder et al. (1990), however, found their elderly subjects to be as accurate as their young adult subjects in evaluating their memory performances on a variety of memory tasks. Additional research on age differences in postdictions is clearly needed.

Finally, research on on-line evaluation should be aided greatly by the recent development of a self-efficacy questionnaire (Memory Self-Efficacy Question-naire (MSEQ); Berry, West, & Dennehey, 1989). Self-efficacy in this context refers to "people's judgments of their capabilities to organize and execute courses of action required to attain designated types of performances" (Bandura, 1986, p. 391). Subjects are asked to evaluate how well they would expect to do on 10 different memory tasks (e.g., remembering telephone numbers and memory for locations in a room). The test has been demonstrated to have adequate reliability, and it shows clear age differences in self-evaluations. Most important, scores on the test have been found to correlate moderately well with on-line evaluations given for performance on actual laboratory task (Berry et al., 1990). Moreover, there is evidence from factor analysis (Hertzog, Hultsch, & Dixon, 1989) indicat-ing that both the MIA and the MFQ measure a higher order factor of self-efficacy. Surprisingly, however, other investigators (Rebok & Balcerak, 1989) have found that a memory training program has no effect on self-efficacy ratings for either young adults or elderly adults.

Age Differences in Episodic-Memory Monitoring Skills

Our concern here is with knowledge regarding the skills needed to store infor-mation episodically. In an interesting study by Murphy, Sanders, Gabriesheski, and Schmitt (1981), young and elderly subjects were given a series of pictures of common objects to study with the objective being to recall the names of the objects in serial order. Some of the series were of memory-span length, others of subspan length (two items less), and others of supraspan length (two items more). Most important, the subjects were allowed as much time as they wanted to study each string before they felt ready to recall it without error. The results are plotted in Figure 12.14 for both the proportion of strings recalled at each length and the mean time spent studying each type of string. Note that the elderly subjects spent considerably less time than the young subjects in studying both the span-length and supraspan-length strings and that the adverse effects are clearly reflected in the poorer recall performance of the elderly subjects for each length. Apparently, the elderly subjects failed to assess realistically the strain placed on their episodic-memory systems by the longer series of items, and they, therefore, failed to spend sufficient time rehearsing those series. Stated somewhat differently, the elderly subjects were less cautious than the young subjects in evaluating their readiness for recalling without error. As with other aspects of performance on memory tasks (see Chapter 7, p. 250), this evidence conflicts with the generally held notion that elderly adults are more cautious than young adults. However, it should be noted that other researchers have found negligible age differences in study time

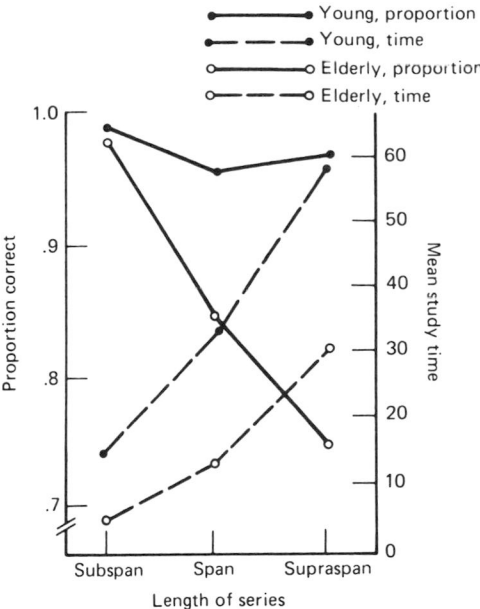

FIGURE 12.14 Age differences in proportion of serial strings recalled and mean time spent in studying the strings before feeling readiness to recall without error. (Adapted from Murphy, Sanders, Gabriesheski, & Schmitt, 1981, Figure 1, Table 1.)

when subjects are allowed as much time as they need to master a list of materials (e.g., Bruce et al., 1982; McDowd & Botwinick, 1984; Perlmutter, 1978a; Rabinowitz, 1989a).

An outcome similar to that of Murphy et al.'s (1981) study was obtained by Bruce et al. (1982) in their free-recall study. As noted earlier, their subjects were allowed as much time as they needed to study the list before attempting recall. Although the young and elderly subjects did not differ significantly in the mean time spent studying, they did differ significantly in the number of words recalled. The elderly subjects did not attempt to compensate for their diminished episodic-memory proficiency by allotting additional time for rehearsing the to-be-remembered words.

In a second experiment, Murphy et al. (1981) employed a forced time condition in which elderly subjects had to spend at least as much time studying to-be-recalled strings as the young adults averaged studying those length strings in the first experiment. Thus, for span-length and supraspan-length strings, they had to spend at least 32 and 59 s, respectively (i.e., the mean times observed in the first experiment; see Figure 12.14). With these expanded study periods, their elderly subjects recalled as many strings without error as did the young subjects in the first experiment.

Another form of a memory skill was investigated in a follow-up study by Murphy, Schmitt, Caruso, and Sanders (1987). Young and elderly subjects were again allowed to take as much time as needed to study strings of pictures for serial recall. This time, however, they were required to rehearse out loud. As in the earlier study (Murphy et al., 1981), the young subjects spent more time rehearsing span-length and supraspan-length strings. The overt verbalization of rehearsal also allowed the investigators to examine age differences in the number of re-hearsals (i.e., item name repetitions) per list. Young subjects conducted significantly more rehearsals than did elderly subjects—and, of course, they recalled significantly more supraspan-length strings than elderly subjects. Moreover, they found that young subjects were more likely than elderly subjects to "test themselves" (i.e., recall the series subvocally) spontaneously as a means of determining their readiness for correct overt recall. Most important, additional elderly subjects who were instructed to study longer and to test themselves before attempting overt recall were found to approach the level of recall manifested by young adults. When given additional strings, but without instructions to test themselves, these elderly subjects continued to do so anyway, resulting in the maintenance of a high level of recall.

These studies have important implications for interpreting age deficits found in both the laboratory and real-life settings. For example, in the laboratory, we discovered in Chapter 3 that elderly subjects perform less proficiently than younger subjects on paired-associate learning tasks even when practice is self-paced. We also discovered a similar phenomenon in the present chapter for serial free recall. Conceivably, elderly subjects simply overestimate their own competence and, therefore, fail to allow themselves the full amount of extra rehearsal time and self-testing time they really need to master such tasks. Similarly, in the real world, many elderly people may have the tendency to terminate their rehearsal of to-be-remembered information too soon. With a little more time and effort devoted to rehearsal activity and self-testing, they may well discover considerable increments in their memory proficiency. From this perspective, it is to the advantage of elderly people to stress to them the existence of moderate declines in the proficiency of memory processes with aging. Once they confront this knowledge realistically, they may be better prepared to work harder to enhance the memorability of episodic information. They may also be willing to participate in memory training courses. The results obtained by Murphy et al. (1987) suggest that such memory skills as self-testing can be acquired, and once acquired are capable of being maintained for future use. Hill, Sheikh, and Yesavage (1987) discovered further that elderly subjects become more accurate predictors of their own memory test performances after they have had mnemonic training. At the same time, we must realize that there are obvious limitations to what can be accomplished by training memory skills. Much of our everyday memory occurs incidentally, and without conscious awareness of what memory skills are being applied. In fact, for many forms of memory, such as automatic episodic memory, we aren't even in the position of knowing fully what processes are responsible for the encoding and transmission of information to the long-term episodic store.

Age Differences in Self-Evaluation of Factual Knowledge Memory Proficiency

"What is the capital of Lebanon?" This is the type of question included on subtests of global intelligence tests that measure general knowledge. Scores on such subtests generally show little, if any decline, from early to late adulthood (see p. 391 and Camp, 1989a, 1989b, for further review). Such factual questions may also be viewed as testing information in the generic stores, as may questions requiring inferences to answer them (e.g., "What piece of playground equipment would be most useful in weighing a sack of potatoes?"; Camp & Pignatiello, 1988). Camp and Pignatiello (1988) found that elderly subjects were as confident as younger subjects in their own ability to answer such factual and inferential questions. However, the elderly subjects also believed that the ability to retrieve factual information is, in general, less proficient in late adulthood than in early adulthood. On the other hand, they also believed that the ability to engage in the inferential reasoning needed to answer questions is stable with aging, and may even increase from early to late adulthood. A number of other researchers have found no age differences in the relationship between the "feeling-of-knowing" answers to factual questions and the accuracy of those answers (Bäckman & Karlsson, 1985; Butterfield, Nelson, & Peck, 1988; J. L. Lachman, Lachman, & Thronesbery, 1979; R. Lachman & Lachman, 1980; and R. Lachman, Lachman, & Taylor, 1982).

REFERENCES

Adamowicz, J. K. (1976). Visual short-term memory and aging. *Journal of Gerontology, 31*, 39–46.

Adamowicz, J. K. (1978). Visual short-term memory, age, and imaging ability. *Perceptual and Motor Skills, 46*, 571–576.

Adamowicz, J. K., & Hudson, B. R. (1978). Visual short-term memory, response delay, and age. *Perceptual and Motor Skills, 46*, 267–270.

Adams, C. (1991). Qualitative age differences in memory for text: A life-span developmental perspective. *Psychology and Aging, 6*, 333–336.

Adams, C., Labouvie-Vief, G., & Dorosz, M. (1990). Adult age group differences in story recall. *The Journals of Gerontology: Psychological Sciences, 45*, P17–27.

Adams, J. A. (1971). A closed-loop theory of motor learning. *Journal of Motor Behavior, 3*, 111–149.

Adams, J. A., & Montague, W. E. (1967). Retroactive inhibition and natural language mediation. *Journal of Verbal Learning and Verbal Behavior, 6*, 528–535.

Adams-Price, C. (1992). Eyewitness memory and aging: Predictors of accuracy in recall. *Psychology and Aging, 7*, 602–608.

Adelson, E. H. (1978). Iconic storage: The role of rods. *Science, 201*, 544–546.

Albert, M. S., Heller, H. S., & Milberg, W. (1988). Changes in naming ability with age. *Psychology and Aging, 3*, 173–178.

Albert, M. S., & Kaplan, E. (1980). Organic implications of neuropsychological deficits in the elderly. In L. W. Poon, J. L. Fozard, L. S. Cermak, D. Arenberg, & L. W. Thompson (Eds.), *New directions in memory and aging: Proceedings of the George Talland Memorial Conference.* Hillsdale, NJ: Erlbaum.

Allard, F., & Burnett, N. (1985). Skill in sport. *Canadian Journal of Psychology, 39*, 294–312.

Allen, G. A., Mahler, W. A., & Estes, W. K. (1969). Effects of recall tests on long-term retention of paired associates. *Journal of Verbal Learning and Verbal Behavior, 9*, 463–470.

Allen, G. L., Siegel, A. W., & Rosinski, R. R. (1978). The role of perceptual context in structuring spatial knowledge. *Journal of Experimental Psychology: Human learning and Memory, 4*, 617–630.

Allen, P. A. (1990). Influence of processing variability on adult age differences in memory distribution of order information. *Cognitive Development, 5*, 177–192.

Allen, P. A. (1991). On age differences in processing variability and scanning speed. *The Journals of Gerontology: Psychological Sciences, 46*, P191–201.

Allen, P. A., & Coyne, A. C. (1988a). Age differences in primary organization or processing variability? Part I: An examination of age and primary organization. *Experimental Aging Research, 14,* 143–149.

Allen, P. A., & Coyne, A. C. (1988b). Age differences in primary organization or processing variability? Part II: Evidence for processing variability. *Experimental Aging Research, 14,* 151–157.

Allen, P. A., & Coyne, A. C. (1989). Are there age differences in chunking? *The Journals of Gerontology: Psychological Sciences, 44,* P181–183.

Allen, P. A., & Crozier, L. C. (1992). Age and ideal chunk size. *The Journals of Gerontology: Psychological Sciences, 47,* P47–51.

Allen, P. A., Madden, D. J., Weber, T., & Crozier, L. C. (1992). Age differences in shortterm memory: Organization or internal noise? *The Journals of Gerontology: Psychological Sciences, 47,* P281–288.

Allen, P. A., Madden, D. J., Weber, T. A., & Groth, K. E. (1993). Influence of age and processing stage on visual word recognition. *Psychology and Aging, 8,* 274–282.

Allen, P. A., Namazi, K. H., Patterson, M. B., Crozier, L. C., & Groth, K. E. (1992). Impact of adult age and Alzheimer's disease on levels of neural noise for letter matching. *The Journals of Gerontology: Psychological Sciences, 47,* P344–349.

Amberson, J. L., Atkeson, B. M., Pollack, R. H., & Malatesta, V. J. (1979). Age differences in dark-interval threshold across the life-span. *Experimental Aging Research, 5,* 423–433.

Amrhein, P. C., & Morris, J. C. (1989). Movement plan preparation is impaired in elderly persons who fall. *Society for Neuroscience Abstracts, 15,* 1199.

Amrhein, P. C., Stelmach, G. E., & Goggin, N. L. (1991). Age differences in the maintenance and restructuring of movement preparation. *Psychology and Aging, 6,* 451–456.

Amrhein, P. C., & Theios, J. (1993). The time it takes elderly and young individuals to draw pictures and write words. *Psychology and Aging, 8,* 197–206.

Amrhein, P. C., Von Dras, D., & Anderson, M. (1993). Evidence of direction loss in elderly movement preparation is not due to spatial orienting effects. *Experimental Aging Research, 19,* 71–95.

Anders, T. R., & Fozard, J. L. (1973). Effects of age upon retrieval from primary and secondary memory. *Developmental Psychology, 9,* 411–415.

Anders, T. R., Fozard, J. L., & Lillyquist, T. D. (1972). Effects of age upon retrieval from short-term memory. *Developmental Psychology, 6,* 214–217.

Anderson, D. C., & Borkowski, J. G. (1978). *Experimental psychology.* Glenview, IL: Scott, Foresman.

Anderson, J. R. (1974). Retrieval of propositional information from long-term memory. *Cognitive Psychology, 6,* 451–474.

Anderson, J. R. (1980). *Cognitive psychology and its implications.* San Francisco: W. H. Freeman.

Anderson, J. R., & Bower, G. H. (1973). *Human associative memory.* Washington, D.C.: Winston.

Ankus, M., & Quarrington, B. (1972). Operant behavior in the memory disordered. *Journal of Gerontology, 27,* 500–510.

Anooshian, I. J., Mammarella, S. L., & Hertel, P. T. (1989). Adult age differences in the knowledge of retrieval processes. *International Journal of Aging and Human Development, 29,* 39–52.

Anschutz, L., Camp, C. J., Markley, R. P., & Kramer, J. J. (1985). Maintenance and generalization of mnemonics for grocery shopping by older adults. *Experimental Aging Research, 11*, 157–160.

Anschutz, L., Camp, C. J., Markley, R. P., & Kramer, J. J. (1987). A three-year follow-up on the effects of mnemonics training in elderly adults. *Experimental Aging Research, 13*, 141–143.

Anshel, M. H. (1978). Effect of aging on acquisition and short-term retention of a motor skill. *Perceptual and Motor Skills, 47*, 993–994.

Arbuckle, T. Y., & Gold, D. P. (1993). Aging, inhibition, and verbosity. *The Journals of Gerontology: Psychological Sciences, 48*, P225–232.

Arbuckle, T. Y., Gold, D. P., & Andres, D. (1986). Cognitive functioning of older people in relation to social and personality variables. *Psychology and Aging, 1*, 55–62.

Arbuckle, T. Y., Gold, D. P., Andres, D., Schwartzman, A. E., & Chaikelson, J. (1992). The role of psychosocial context, age, and intelligence in memory performance of older men. *Psychology and Aging, 7*, 25–36.

Arbuckle, T. Y., & Harsany, M. (1985). Adult age differences in recall of a moral dilemma under intentional, incidental and dual task instructions. *Experimental Aging Research, 11*, 175–178.

Arbuckle, T. Y., Vanderleck, V. F., Harsany, M., & Lapidus, S. (1990). Adult age differences in memory in relation to availability and accessibility of knowledge-based schema. *Journal of Experimental Psychology: Learning, Memory, and Cognition, 16*, 305–315.

Arenberg, D. (1965). Anticipation interval and age differences in verbal learning. *Journal of Abnormal Psychology, 70*, 419–425.

Arenberg, D. (1967a). Regression analyses of verbal learning on adult age differences at two anticipation intervals. *Journal of Gerontology, 22*, 411–414.

Arenberg, D. (1967b). Age differences in retroaction. *Journal of Gerontology, 22*, 88–91.

Arenberg, D. (1968a). Input modality in short-term retention of old and young adults. *Journal of Gerontology, 23*, 462–465.

Arenberg, D. (1968b). Retention of time judgment in young and old adults. *Journal of Gerontology, 23*, 35–40.

Arenberg, D. (1976). The effects of input condition on free recall in young and old adults. *Journal of Gerontology, 31*, 551–555.

Arenberg, D. (1977). The effects of auditory augmentation on visual retention for young and old adults. *Journal of Gerontology, 32*, 192–195.

Arenberg, D. (1978). Differences and changes with age in the Benton Visual Retention Test. *Journal of Gerontology, 33*, 534–540.

Arenberg, D. (1982). Estimates of age changes on the Benton Visual Retention Test. *Journal of Gerontology, 37*, 87–90.

Arenberg, D., & Robertson-Tchabo, E. A. (1977). Learning and aging. In J. E. Birren & K. W. Schaie (Eds.), *Handbook of the psychology of aging, 1st ed.* New York: Van Nostrand Reinhold.

Arenberg, D., & Robertson-Tchabo, E. E. (1985). Adult age differences in memory and linguistic integration revisited. *Experimental Aging Research, 11*, 187–191.

Atkinson, R. C., & Juola, J. F. (1973). Factors influencing speed and accuracy of word recognition. In S. Kornblum (Ed.), *Attention and performance IV*. New York: Academic Press.

Atkinson, R. C., & Raugh, M. R. (1975). An application of the mnemonic keyword method to the acquisition of a Russian vocabulary. *Journal of Experimental Psychology: Human Learning and Memory, 1*, 126–133.

Atkinson, R. C., & Shiffrin, R. M. (1968). Human memory: A proposed system and its control processes. In K. W. Spence & J. T. Spence (Eds.), *The psychology of learning and motivation. Vol. 2.* New York: Academic Press.

Attig, M., & Hasher, L. (1979, April). *Differences in memory processes among adults: Deterioration or response bias?* Paper presented at the annual meeting of the Eastern Psychological Association, Philadelphia.

Attig, M., & Hasher, L. (1980). The processing of frequency of occurrence information by adults. *Journal of Gerontology, 35*, 66–69.

Axelrod, S. (1963). Cognitive tasks in several modalities. In. R. H. Williams, C. Tibbitts, & W. Donahue (Eds.), *Processes of aging. Vol. 1.* New York: Atherton.

Ayllon, T., & Azrin, N. H. (1965). The measurement and reinforcement of behavior of psychotics. *Journal of Experimental Analysis of Behavior, 8*, 357–383.

Azari, N. P., Auday, B. C., & Cross, H. A. (1989). Effects of instructions on memory for temporal order. *Bulletin of the Psychonomic Society, 27*, 203–205.

Babcock, R. L., & Salthouse, T. A. (1990). Effects of increased processing demands on age differences in working memory. *Psychology and Aging, 5*, 421–428.

Bäckman, L. (1985a). Compensation and recoding: A framework for aging and memory research. *Scandinavian Journal of Psychology, 26*, 193–207.

Bäckman, L. (1985b). Further evidence for the lack of adult age differences on the recall of subject performed tasks: The importance of motor action. *Human Learning, 4*, 79–87.

Bäckman, L. (1986). Adult age differences in cross-modal recoding and mental tempo, and older adults' utilization of compensatory task conditions. *Experimental Aging Research, 12*, 135–140.

Bäckman, L. (1989). Varieties of memory compensation by older adults. In L. W. Poon, D. C. Rubin, & B. A. Wilson (Eds.), *Everyday cognition in adulthood and late life.* Cambridge: Cambridge University Press.

Bäckman, L. (1991). Recognition memory across the adult lifespan: The role of prior knowledge. *Memory & Cognition, 19*, 63–71.

Bäckman, L., & Herlitz, A. (1990). The relationship between prior knowledge and face recognition memory in normal aging and Alzheimer's Disease. *The Journals of Gerontology: Psychological Sciences, 45*, P94–100.

Bäckman, L., Herlitz, A., & Karlsson, T. (1987). Pre-experimental knowledge facilitates episodic recall in young, young-old, and old-old adults. *Experimental Aging Research, 13*, 89–91.

Bäckman, L., Josephsson, S., Herlitz, A., Stigsdotter, A., & Vitanen, M. (1991). The generalizability of training gains in dementia: Effects on face-name retention. *Psychology and Aging, 6*, 489–492.

Bäckman, L., & Karlsson, T. (1985). The relation between level of general knowledge and feeling of knowing: An adult study. *Scandinavian Journal of Psychology, 26*, 249–258.

Bäckman, L., & Larsson, M. (1992). Recall of organizable words and objects in adulthood: Influences of instructions, retention interval, and retrieval cues. *The Journals of Gerontology: Psychological Sciences, 47*, P273–278.

Bäckman, L., & Mäntylä, T. (1988). Effectiveness of self-generated cues in younger and older adults: The role of retention interval. *International Journal of Aging and Human Development, 26*, 241–248.

Bäckman, L., Mäntylä, T., & Erngrund, K. (1984). Optional recall in early and late adulthood. *Scandinavian Journal of Psychology, 25*, 306–314.

Bäckman, L., Mäntylä, T., & Herlitz, A. (1990). The optimization of episodic remembering in old age. In P. B. Baltes & M. M. Baltes (Eds.), *Successful aging: Perspectives from the behavioral sciences*. New York: Cambridge University Press.

Bäckman, L., & Nilsson, L-G. (1984). Aging effects in free recall: An exception to the rule. *Human Learning, 3*, 53–69.

Bäckman, L., & Nilsson, L-G. (1985). Prerequisites for the lack of age differences in memory performance. *Experimental Aging Research, 11*, 67–73.

Bacon, L. D., Wilson, R. S., & Kaszniak, A. W. (1982). Age differences in memory scanning? *Perceptual and Motor Skills, 55*, 499–504.

Baddeley, A. D. (1978). The trouble with levels: A reexamination of Craik and Lockhart's framework for memory research. *Psychological Review, 85*, 139–152.

Baddeley, A. D. (1981). The concept of working memory: A view of its current state and probable future development. *Cognition, 10*, 17–23.

Baddeley, A. D., & Hitch, G. (1974). Working memory. In G. H. Bower (Ed.), *The psychology of learning and motivation*. Vol. 8, New York: Academic Press.

Baddeley, A. D., Thomson, N., & Buchanan, M. (1975). Word length and the structure of short-term memory. *Journal of Verbal Learning and Verbal Behavior, 14*, 575–589.

Bahrick, H. P. (1979). Maintenance of knowledge: Questions about memory we forgot to ask. *Journal of Experimental Psychology: General, 108*, 296–308.

Bahrick, H. P. (1984a). Memory for people. In J. E. Harris & P. E. Morris (Eds.), *Everyday memory, actions and absent-mindedness*. London: Academic Press. (pp. 19–34).

Bahrick, H. P. (1984b). Semantic memory content in permastore: Fifty years of memory for Spanish learned in school. *Journal of Experimental Psychology: General, 113*, 1–29.

Bahrick, H. P., Bahrick, P. O., & Wittlinger, R. P. (1975). Fifty years of memory for names and faces: A cross-sectional approach. *Journal of Experimental Psychology: General, 104*, 54–75.

Balota, D. A., Black, S. R., & Cheney, M. (1992). Automatic and attentional priming in young and older adults: Reevaluation of the two-process model. *Journal of Experimental Psychology: Human Perception and Performance, 18*, 485–502.

Balota, D. A., & Duchek, J. M. (1988). Age-related differences in lexical access, spreading activation, and simple pronunciation. *Psychology and Aging, 3*, 84–93.

Balota, D. A., & Duchek, J. M. (1989). Spreading activation in episodic memory: Further evidence for age independence. *Quarterly Journal of Experimental Psychology, 41A*, 849–876.

Balota, D. A., Duchek, J. M., & Paullin, R. (1989). Age-related differences in the impact of spacing, lag, and retention interval. *Psychology and Aging, 4*, 3–9.

Baltes, M. M., & Zerbe, M. B. (1976). Re-establishing self-feeding in a nursing home resident. *Nursing Research, 25*, 24–26.

Baltes, P. B. (1987). Theoretical propositions of life-span developmental psychology: On the dynamics between growth and decline. *Developmental Psychology, 23*, 611–626.

Banaji, M. R. & Crowder, R. C. (1989). The bankruptcy of everyday memory. *American Psychologist, 44*, 1185–1194.

Bandura, A. (1986). *Social foundations of thought and action: A social cognitive theory.* Englewood Cliffs, NJ: Prentice-Hall.

Baron, A., & LeBreck, D. B. (1987). Are older adults generally more conservative? Some negative evidence from signal detection analyses of recognition memory and sensory performance. *Experimental Aging Research, 13*, 163–165.

Baron, A., & Mattila, W. R. (1989). Response slowing of older adults: Effects of time limit contingencies on single and dual task performances. *Psychology and Aging, 4*, 66–72.

Baron, A., & Menich, S. R. (1985). Age-related effects of temporal contingencies on response speed and memory: An operant analysis. *Journal of Gerontology, 40*, 60–70.

Baron, A., Menich, S. R., & Perone, M. (1983). Reaction times of younger and older men and temporal contingencies of reinforcement. *Journal of the Experimental Analysis of Behavior, 40*, 275–287.

Baron, R. A., & Byrne, D. (1977). *Social psychology: Understanding human interaction.* Boston: Allyn & Bacon.

Barrett, T. R., & Watkins, S. K. (1986). Word familiarity and cardiovascular health as determinants of age-related recall deficits. *Journal of Gerontology, 41*, 222–224.

Barrett, T. R., & Wright, M. (1981). Age-related facilitation in recall following semantic processing. *Journal of Gerontology, 36*, 194–199.

Bartlett, F. C. (1932). *Remembering: A study in experimental and social psychology.* Cambridge, England: Cambridge University Press.

Bartlett, J. C., & Fulton, A. (1991). Familiarity and face recognition: The factor of age. *Memory & Cognition, 19*, 229–238.

Bartlett, J. C., & Leslie, J. E. (1986). Aging and memory for faces versus single views of faces. *Memory & Cognition, 14*, 371–381.

Bartlett, J. C., Leslie, J. E., Tubbs, A., & Fulton, A. (1989). Aging and memory for pictures of faces. *Psychology and Aging, 4*, 276–283.

Bartlett, J. C., & Snelus, P. (1980). Lifespan memory for popular songs. *American Journal of Psychology, 93*, 551–560.

Bartlett, J. C., Strater, L., & Fulton, A. (1991). False recency and false fame of faces in old age. *Memory & Cognition, 19*, 177–188.

Bartlett, J. C., Till, R. E., Gernsbacher, M., & Gorman, W. (1983). Age-related differences in memory for lateral orientation of pictures. *Journal of Gerontology, 38*, 439–446.

Basden, B. H., Basden, D. R., & Bartlett, K. (1993). Memory and organization in elderly subjects. *Experimental Aging Research, 19*, 29–38.

Bashore, T. R., Osman, A., & Heffley, E. F., III (1989). Mental slowing in elderly persons: A cognitive psychophysiological analysis. *Psychology and Aging, 4*, 235–244.

Battig, W. F. (1968). Paired-associate learning. In T. R. Dixon & D. L. Horton (Eds.), *Verbal behavior and general behavior theory.* Englewood Cliffs, NJ: Prentice Hall.

Battig, W. F., & Montague, W. E. (1969). Category norms for verbal items in 56 categories: A replication and extension of the Connecticut category norms. *Journal of Experimental Psychology Monograph, 80* (3, Pt. 2).

Begg, I., & Paivio, A. (1969). Concreteness and imagery in sentence meaning. *Journal of Verbal Learning and Verbal Behavior, 8*, 821–827.

Belbin, E., & Downs, S. (1965). Interference effects from new learning: Their relevance to the design of adult training programs. *Journal of Gerontology, 20,* 154–159.

Bell, B. D., & Stanfield, G. G. (1973). Chronological age in relation to attitudinal judgments: An experimental analysis. *Journal of Gerontology, 28,* 491–496.

Bellezza, F. S. (1981). Mnemonic devices: Classification, characteristics, and criteria. *Review of Educational Research, 51,* 247–275.

Belmore, S. M. (1981). Age-related changes in processing explicit and implicit language. *Journal of Gerontology, 36,* 316–322.

Beres, C. A., & Baron, A. (1981). Improved digit symbol substitution by older women as a result of extended practice. *Journal of Gerontology, 36,* 591–597.

Bergquist, T. F., Duke, L. W., & Davis, G. (1989, November). *Cognitive/behavioral interventions for age-related memory decline.* Paper presented at the annual meeting of the Gerontological Society of America, Minneapolis, Minnesota.

Berkowitz, B. (1953). The Wechsler-Bellevue performance of white males past 50. *Journal of Gerontology, 8,* 76–80.

Bernbach, H. A. (1975). Rate of presentation in free recall: A problem for two-stage memory theories. *Journal of Experimental Psychology: Human Learning and Memory, 104,* 18–22.

Berry, J. M., West, R. L., & Dennehey, D. M. (1989). Reliability and validity of the Memory Self-Efficacy Questionnaire (MSEQ). *Developmental Psychology, 25,* 701–713.

Binks, M. G., & Sutcliffe, J. (1972). *The effects of age and verbal ability on short-term recognition memory.* Paper presented at the annual conference of the British Psychological Society, Nottingham.

Birren, J. E. (1955). Age changes in speed of response and perception and their significance for complex behavior. In *Old age in the modern world.* Edinburgh: Livingstone.

Birren, J. E. (1964). *The psychology of aging.* Englewood Cliffs, NJ: Prentice Hall.

Birren, J. E. (1965). Age changes in speed of behavior: Its central nature and physiological correlates. In A. T. Welford & J. E. Birren (Eds.), *Behavior, aging and the nervous system.* Springfield, IL: Charles C. Thomas.

Birren, J. E. (1974). Translations to gerontology—From lab to life: Psychophysiology and speed of response. *American Psychologist, 29,* 808–815.

Birren, J. E., & Botwinick, J. (1951). The relation of writing speed to age and to the senile psychoses. *Journal of Consulting Psychology, 15,* 243–249.

Birren, J. E., & Botwinick, J. (1955). Age differences in finger, jaw, and foot reaction time to auditory stimuli. *Journal of Gerontology, 10,* 429–432.

Birren, J. E., & Morrison, D. F. (1961). Analysis of the WAIS subtests in relation to age and education. *Journal of Gerontology, 16,* 363–369.

Birren, J. E., Riegel, K. F., & Morrison, D. F. (1962). Age differences in response speed as a function of controlled variations of stimulus conditions: Evidence of a general speed factor. *Gerontologia, 6,* 1–18.

Bjork, R. A. (1988). Retrieval practice and the maintenance of knowledge. In M. M. Gruneberg, P. E. Morris, & R. N. Sykes (Eds.), *Practical aspects of memory: Current research and issues. Vol. 1.* Chichester, England: John Wiley.

Blumenthal, J. A., Emery, C., Madden, D. J., Schiebolk, S., Walsh-Riddle, M., George, L. K., McKee, D. C., Higginbotham, M. B., Cobb, F. R., & Coleman, R. E. (1991). Long-term effects of exercise on psychological functioning in older men and women. *The Journals of Gerontology: Psychological Sciences, 46,* P352–361.

Blumenthal, J. A., & Madden, D. J. (1988). Effects of aerobic exercise training, age, and physical fitness on memory-search performance. *Psychology and Aging, 3,* 280–285.

Boden, D., & Bielby, D. D. (1983). The past as resource: A conversational analysis of elderly talk. *Human Development, 26,* 308–319.

Bogartz, R. S. (1990). Evaluating forgetting curves psychologically. *Journal of Experimental Psychology: Learning, Memory, and Cognition, 16,* 138–148.

Bolla-Wilson, K., & Bleecker, M. L. (1986). Influence of verbal intelligence, sex, age and education on the Rey Auditory Verbal Learning Test. *Developmental Neuropsychology, 2,* 203–211.

Bolles, R. C. (1979). *Learning theory (2nd. ed.).* New York: Holt, Rinehart, & Winston.

Borkan, G. A., & Norris, A. H. (1980). Assessment of biological age using a profile of physical parameters. *Journal of Gerontology, 35,* 177–184.

Borod, J. C., & Goodglass, H. (1980). Lateralization of linguistic and melodic processing with age. *Neuropsychologia, 18,* 79–83.

Bosman, E. A. (1993). Age-related differences in the motoric aspects of transcription typing skill. *Psychology and Aging, 8,* 87–102.

Botwinick, J. (1967). *Cognitive processes in maturity and old age.* New York: Springer.

Botwinick, J. (1970). Learning in children and in older adults. In L. R. Goulet & P. B. Baltes (Eds.), *Life-span developmental psychology.* New York: Academic Press.

Botwinick, J. (1971). Sensory-set factors in age differences in reaction time. *Journal of Genetic Psychology, 119,* 241–249.

Botwinick, J. (1978). *Aging and behavior (2nd. ed.).* New York: Springer.

Botwinick, J., & Birren, J. E. (1965). A follow-up study of card-sorting performance in elderly men. *Journal of Gerontology, 20,* 208–210.

Botwinick, J., Brinley, J. F., & Robbin, J. S. (1959). Maintaining set in relation to motivation and age. *American Journal of Psychology, 72,* 585–588.

Botwinick, J., & Kornetsky, C. (1960). Age differences in the acquisition and extinction of GSR. *Journal of Gerontology, 15,* 83–84.

Botwinick, J., Robbin, J. S., & Brinley, J. F. (1960). Age differences in card-sorting performance in relation to task difficulty, task set, and practice. *Journal of Experimental Psychology, 59,* 10–18.

Botwinick, J., & Storandt, M. (1974a). *Memory, related functions and age.* Springfield, IL: Charles C. Thomas.

Botwinick, J., & Storandt, M. (1974b). Vocabulary ability in later life. *Journal of Genetic Psychology, 125,* 303–308.

Botwinick, J., & Storandt, M. (1980). Recall and recognition of old information in relation to age. *Journal of Gerontology, 35,* 70–76.

Botwinick, J., & Thompson, L. W. (1966). Components of reaction time in relation to age and sex. *Journal of Genetic Psychology, 198,* 175–183.

Bousfield, W. A. (1953). The occurrence of clustering in the recall of randomly arranged associates. *Journal of General Psychology, 49,* 229–240.

Bower, G. H. (1970). Analysis of a mnemonic device. *American Scientist, 58,* 496–510.

Bower, G. H. (1981). Mood and memory. *American Psychologist, 36,* 129–148.

Bower, G. H., & Clark, M. C. (1969). Narrative stories as mediators for serial learning. *Psychonomic Science, 14,* 181–182.

Bowles, N. L. (1989). Age and semantic inhibition in word retrieval. *The Journals of*

Gerontology: Psychological Sciences, 44, P88–90.

Bowles, N. L., Obler, L. K., & Albert, M. L. (1987). Naming errors in healthy aging and dementia of the Alzheimer Type. *Cortex, 23*, 519–524.

Bowles, N. L., Obler, L. K., & Poon, L. W. (1989). Aging and word retrieval: Naturalistic, clinical, and laboratory data. In L. W. Poon, D. C. Rubin, & B. A. Wilson (Eds.), *Everyday cognition in adulthood and late life*. New York: Cambridge University Press.

Bowles, N. L., & Poon, L. W. (1981). The effect of age on speed of lexical access. *Experimental Aging Research, 7*, 417–425.

Bowles, N. L., & Poon, L. W. (1985). Aging and retrieval of words in semantic memory. *Journal of Gerontology, 40*, 71–77.

Bowles, N. L., & Poon, L. W. (1988). Age and context effects in lexical decisions: An age by context interaction. *Experimental Aging Research, 14*, 201–206.

Bowles, N. L., Williams, D., & Poon, L. W. (1983). On the use of word association norms in aging research. *Experimental Aging Research, 9*, 175–177.

Boyarsky, R. E., & Eisdorfer, C. (1972). Forgetting in older persons. *Journal of Gerontology, 27*, 254–258.

Brainerd, C. J. (1985). Model-based approaches to storage and retrieval development. In C. J. Brainerd & M. Pressley (Eds.), *Basic processes in memory development: Progress in cognitive development research*. New York: Springer-Verlag.

Brainerd, C. J., Reyna, V. F., Howe, M. L., & Kingma, J. (1990). Development of forgetting and reminiscence. *Monographs of the Society for Research in Child Development, Vol 1*, p. 55.

Bransford, J. D., (1979). *Human cognition: Learning, retention, and understanding*. Belmont, CA: Wadsworth.

Bransford, J. D., & Franks, J. J. (1971). The abstraction of linguistic ideas. *Cognitive Psychology, 2*, 331–350.

Braun, H. W., & Geiselhart, R. (1959). Age differences in the acquisition and extinction of the conditioned eyeblink response. *Journal of Experimental Psychology, 57*, 386–388.

Brewer, W. F., & Nakamura, G. V. (1984). The nature and function of schemes. In R. S. Wyer, Jr. & T. K. Srull (Eds.), *Handbook of social cognition*. Hillsdale, NJ: Erlbaum.

Brigham, M. C., Presseley, M. (1988). Cognitive monitoring and strategy choice in younger and older adults. *Psychology and Aging, 3*, 249–257.

Brinley, J. F. (1965). Cognitive sets, speed and accuracy of performance in the elderly. In A. T. Welford & J. E. Birren (Eds.), *Behavior, aging, and the nervous system*. Springfield, IL: Charles C. Thomas.

Britton, B. K., Graesser, A. C., Glynn, S. M., Hamilton, T., & Penland, M. (1983). Use of cognitive capacity in reading: Effects of some content features of text. *Discourse Processing, 6*, 39–57.

Bromley, D. B. (1958). Some effects of age on short-term learning and remembering. *Journal of Gerontology, 13*, 398–406.

Bromley, D. B. (1991). Aspects of written language production over adult life. *Psychology and Aging, 6*, 296–308.

Bronfenbrenner, U. (1977). Toward an experimental ecology of human development. *American Psychologist, 32*, 513–531.

Brooks, B. M., & Gardiner, J. M. (1994). Age differences in memory for prospective compared with retrospective subject-performed tasks. *Memory & Cognition, 22*, 27–33.

Brooks, D. N., & Baddeley, A. D. (1976). What can amnesic patients learn? *Neuropsychologia, 14,* 111–122.

Brown, A. S., & Mitchell, D. B. (1991). Age differences in retrieval consistency and response dominance. *The Journals of Gerontology: Psychological Sciences, 46,* P332–339.

Brown, J. A. (1958). Some tests of the decay theory of immediate memory. *Quarterly Journal of Experimental Psychology, 10,* 12–21.

Brown, J. C., Niinikoski, J., & Duke, L. W. (1993). Generation effect and frequency judgment in young and elderly adults. *Experimental Aging Research, 19,* 147–164.

Brown, R., & McNeill, D. (1966). The "tip of the tongue" phenomenon. *Journal of Verbal Learning and Verbal Behavior, 5,* 325–337.

Bruce, D. (1989). Functional explanations of memory. In L. W. Poon, D. C. Rubin, & B. A. Wilson (Eds.), *Everyday cognition in adulthood and late life.* New York: Cambridge University Press.

Bruce, P. R., Coyne, A. C., & Botwinick, J. (1982). Adult age differences in metamemory. *Journal of Gerontology, 37,* 354–357.

Bruce, P. R., & Herman, J. F. (1983). Spatial knowledge of young and elderly adults: Scene recognition from familiar and novel perspectives. *Experimental Aging Research, 9,* 169–173.

Bruce, P. R., & Herman, J. F. (1986). Adult age differences in spatial memory: Effects of distinctiveness and repeated experiences. *Journal of Gerontology, 41,* 774–777.

Bruning, R. H., Holzbauer, I., & Kimberlin, C. (1975). Age, words, imagery, and delay interval: Effects on short-term and long-term retention. *Journal of Gerontology, 30,* 312–318.

Bugelski, B. R. (1968). Images as mediators in one-trial paired-associate learning: II. Self-timing in successive lists. *Journal of Experimental Psychology, 77,* 328–334.

Bugelski, B. R., Kidd, E., & Segmen, J. (1968). Image as a mediator in one-trial paired-associate learning. *Journal of Experimental Psychology, 76,* 69–73.

Bunce, D. J., Warr, P. B., & Cochrane, C. J. (1993). Blocks in choice responding as a function of age and physical fitness. *Psychology and Aging, 8,* 26–33.

Burke, D. M., & Laver, G. D. (1990). Aging and word retrieval: Selective age deficits in language. In E. A. Lovelace (Ed.), *Aging and cognition: Mental processes, self-awareness and interventions.* Amsterdam: North Holland.

Burke, D. M., & Light, L. L. (1981). Memory and aging: The role of retrieval processes. *Psychological Bulletin, 90,* 513–546.

Burke, D. M., MacKay, D., Worthley, J., & Wade, E. (1991). On the tip of the tongue: What causes word finding failures in young and old adults? *Journal of Memory and Language, 30,* 542–579.

Burke, D. M., & Peters, L. (1986). Word associations in old age: Evidence for consistency in semantic encoding during adulthood. *Psychology and Aging, 1,* 283–292.

Burke, D. M., White, H., & Diaz, D. L. (1987). Semantic priming in young and older adults: Evidence for age constancy in automatic and attentional processes. *Journal of Experimental Psychology: Human Perception and Performance, 13,* 79–88.

Burke, D. M., Worthley, J., & Martin, J. (1988). I'll never forget what's-her-name: Aging and tip of the tongue experiences in everyday life. In M. M. Gruneberg, P. E. Morris, & R. N. Sykes (Eds.), *Practical aspects of memory: Current research and issues. Vol. 2. Clinical and education implications.* Chichester, England: John Wiley.

Burke, D. M., & Yee, P. L. (1984). Semantic priming during sentence processing by young and older adults. *Developmental Psychology, 20*, 903–910.

Buschke, H. (1974). Two stages of learning by children and adults. *Bulletin of the Psychonomic Society, 2*, 392–394.

Buschke, H. (1988). Memory for details in aging and dementia. In M. M. Gruneberg, P. E. Morris, & R. W. Sykes (Eds.), *Practical aspects of memory: Current research and issues.* Chichester: Wiley.

Buschke, H., & Macht, M. L. (1983). Explanation and conceptual memory. *Bulletin of the Psychonomic Society, 21*, 397–399.

Butterfield, E. C., Nelson, T. O., & Peck, V. (1988). Developmental aspects of the feeling of knowing. *Developmental Psychology, 24*, 654–663.

Butterfield, G. B., & Butterfield, E. C. (1977). Lexical codability and age. *Journal of Verbal Learning and Verbal Behavior, 16*, 113–118.

Byrd, M. (1984). Age differences in the retrieval of information from semantic memory. *Experimental Aging Research, 10*, 29–33.

Byrd, M. (1985). Age differences in the ability to recall and summarize textual information. *Experimental Aging Research, 11*, 87–91.

Byrd, M., & Moscovitch, M. (1984). Lateralization of peripherally and centrally masked words in young and elderly people. *Journal of Gerontology, 39*, 699–703.

Caird, W. K. (1964). Remembering activity and memory disorder. *Nature, 201*, 295–299.

Caird, W. K. (1966). Aging and short-term memory. *Journal of Gerontology, 21*, 295–299.

Cameron, D. E. (1943). Impairment at the retention phase of remembering. *Psychiatric Quarterly, 17*, 395–404.

Camp, C. J. (1981). The use of fact retrieval vs. inference in young and elderly adults. *Journal of Gerontology, 36*, 715–721.

Camp, C. J. (1989a). Facilitation of new learning in Alzheimer's Disease. In G. Gilmore, P. Whitehouse, & M. Wykle (Eds.), *Memory and aging: Research, theory, and practice.* New York: Springer.

Camp, C. J. (1989b). World-knowledge systems. In L. W. Poon, D. C. Rubin, & B. A. Wilson (Eds.), *Everyday cognition in adulthood and late life.* New York: Cambridge University Press.

Camp, C. J., Markley, R. P., & Kramer, J. (1983). Spontaneous use of mnemonics by elderly individuals. *Educational Gerontology, 9*, 57–71.

Camp, C. J., & McKitrick, L. A. (1992). Memory interventions in DAT populations: Methodological and theoretical issues. In R. L. West & J. D. Sinnott (Eds.), *Everyday memory and aging: Current research and methodology.* New York: Springer-Verlag.

Camp, C. J., & Pignatiello, M. F. (1988). Beliefs about fact retrieval and inferential reasoning across the adult lifespan. *Experimental Aging Research, 14*, 89–97.

Canestrari, R. E., Jr. (1963). Paced and self-paced learning in young and elderly adults. *Journal of Gerontology, 18*, 165–168.

Canestrari, R. E., Jr. (1964). Age differences in paired-associate learning as a function of response pretraining. Cited in J. Botwinick, *Cognitive processes in maturity and old age.* New York: Springer. (Unpublished, 1964).

Canestrari, R. E., Jr. (1968). The effects of commonality on paired-associate learning in two age groups. *Journal of Genetic Psychology, 108*, 3–7.

Canestrari, R. E., Jr. (1968). Age changes in acquisition. In G. A. Talland (Ed.), *Human aging and behavior.* New York: Academic Press.

Cavanaugh, J. C. (1983). Comprehension and retention of television programs by 20- and 60-year olds. *Journal of Gerontology, 38,* 190–196.

Cavanaugh, J. C. (1984). Effects of presentation format on adults' retention of television programs. *Experimental Aging Research, 10,* 51–53.

Cavanaugh, J. C. (1986–87). Age differences in adults' self-reports on memory ability: It depends on how and what you ask. *International Journal on Aging and Human Development, 24,* 271–277.

Cavanaugh, J. C., Grady, J. G., & Perlmutter, M. (1983). Forgetting and use of memory aids in 20 to 70 year olds everyday life. *International Journal of Aging and Human Development, 17,* 113–122.

Cavanaugh, J. C., & Morton, K. R. (1988). Older adults' attributions about everyday memory. In M. M. Gruneberg, P. E. Morris, & R. N. Sykes (Eds.), *Practical aspects of memory: Current research and theory. Vol. 1.* Chichester, England: John Wiley.

Cavanaugh, J. C., Morton, K. R., & Tilse, C. S. (1989). A self-evaluation framework for understanding everyday memory in aging. In J. D. Sinnott (Ed.), *Everyday problem solving: Theory and application.* New York: Praeger.

Cavanaugh, J. C., & Perlmutter, M. (1980, September). *Age differences in adults' recall of television program content.* Paper presented at the annual meeting of the American Psychological Association, Montreal.

Cavanaugh, J. C., & Poon, L. W. (1989). Metamemorial predictors of memory performance in young and older adults. *Psychology and Aging, 4,* 365–368.

Ceci, S. J., & Tabor, L. (1981). Flexibility and memory: Are the elderly less feeble? *Experimental Aging Research, 1,* 147–158.

Cerella, J. (1985). Information processing rates in the elderly. *Psychological Bulletin, 98,* 67–83.

Cerella, J. (1990). Aging and information processing rate. In J. E. Birren & K. W. Schaie (Eds.), *Handbook of the psychology of aging.* 3rd Ed. San Diego: Academic Press.

Cerella, J., & Fozard, J. L. (1984). Lexical access and age. *Developmental Psychology, 20,* 235–243.

Cerella, J., Poon, L. W., & Fozard, J. L. (1982). Age and iconic read-out. *Journal of Gerontology, 37,* 197–202.

Cerella, J., Poon, L. W., & Williams, D. M. (1980). A quantitative theory of mental processing time and age. In L. W. Poon (Ed.), *Aging in the 80s: Selected contemporary issues in the psychology of aging.* Washington, D.C.: American Psychological Association.

Cermak, L. S., Lewis, R., Butters, N. & Goodglass, H. (1973). Role of verbal mediation in performance of motor tasks by Korsakoff patients. *Perceptual and Motor Skills, 37,* 259–262.

Charness, N. (1981a). Aging and skilled problem solving. *Journal of Experimental Psychology: General, 110,* 21–38.

Charness, N. (1981b). Search in chess: Age and skill differences. *Journal of Experimental Psychology: Human Perception and Performance, 7,* 467–476.

Charness, N. (1981c). Visual short-term memory and aging in chess players. *Journal of Gerontology, 36,* 615–619.

Charness, N. (1983). Age, skill, and bridge bidding: A chronometeric analysis. *Journal of Verbal Learning and Verbal Behavior, 22,* 406–416.

Charness, N. (1987). Component processes in bridge bidding and novel problem-solving tasks. *Canadian Journal of Psychology, 41*, 223–243.

Charness, N. (1989). Age and expertise: Responding to Talland's challenge. In L. W. Poon, D. C. Rubin, & B. A. Wilson (Eds.), *Everyday cognition in adulthood and late life.* Cambridge: Cambridge University Press.

Charness, N., & Schumann, C. E., & Bovitz, G. M. (in press). Training older adults in word processing: Effects of age, training technique, and computer anxiety. *International Journal of Technology and Aging.*

Cherry, K. E., & Park, D. C. (1989). Age-related differences in three-dimensional spatial memory. *The Journals of Gerontology: Psychological Sciences, 44*, P16–22.

Cherry, K. E., Park, D. C., & Donaldson, H. (1993). Adult age differences in spatial memory: Effects of structural context and practice. *Experimental Aging Research, 19*, 333–350.

Cherry, K. E., Park, D. C., Frieske, D. A., & Rowley, R. L. (1993). The effect of verbal elaborations on memory in young and older adults. *Memory & Cognition, 21*, 725–738.

Chiarello, C., Church, K. L., & Hoyer, W. J. (1985). Automatic and controlled semantic priming: Accuracy, response bias, and aging. *Journal of Gerontology, 40*, 593–600.

Chiarello, C., & Hoyer, W. J. (1988). Adult age differences in implicit and explicit memory: Time course and encoding effects. *Psychology and Aging, 3*, 358–366.

Clancy, S. M., & Hoyer, W. J. (1988, August). *Effects of age and skill on domain-specific visual search.* Paper presented at the meeting of the Cognitive Science Society, Montreal.

Claparede, E. (1911). Recognition et moiite. *Archives de Psychologie (Genève), 11*, 79–90.

Clark, J. E., Lanphear, A. K., & Riddick, C. C. (1987). The effects of videogame playing on the response selection processing of elderly adults. *Journal of Gerontology, 42*, 82–85.

Clarkson-Smith, L., & Hartley, A. A. (1989). Relationships between physical exercise and cognitive abilities in older adults. *Psychology and Aging, 4*, 183–189.

Clarkson-Smith, L., & Hartley, A. A. (1990). The game of bridge as an exercise in working memory. *The Journals of Gerontology: Psychological Sciences, 45*, P233–238.

Clifton, J. (1986). *Cognitive components of music reading and sight reading performance.* Doctoral Dissertation, University of Waterloo.

Cockburn, J., & Collin, C. (1988). Measuring everyday memory in elderly people: A preliminary study. *Age and Aging, 17*, 265–269.

Cockburn, J., & Smith, P. T. (1988). Effects of age and intelligence on everyday memory tasks. In M. M. Gruneberg, P. E. Morris, & R. N. Sykes (Eds.), *Practical aspects of memory: Current research and issues. Vol. 2: Clinical and educational implications.* Chichester: Wiley.

Cockburn, J., & Smith, P. T. (1991). The relative influence of intelligence and age on everyday memory. *The Journals of Gerontology: Psychological Sciences, 46*, P31–36.

Cohen, G. (1979). Language comprehension in old age. *Cognitive Psychology, 11*, 412–429.

Cohen, G. (1988). Age differences in memory for text: Production deficiency or processing limitations? In L. L. Light & D. M. Burke (Eds.), *Language, memory, and aging.* New York: Cambridge University Press.

Cohen, G. (1989). *Memory in the real world.* Hove and London: Erlbaum.

Cohen, G. (1990). Recognition and retrieval of proper names: Age differences in the fan effect. *European Journal of Cognitive Psychology, 2,* 193–204.

Cohen, G., & Faulkner, D. (1983). Word recognition: Age differences in contextual facilitation effects. *British Journal of Psychology, 74,* 239–252.

Cohen, G., & Faulkner, D. (1984). Memory in old age: "Good in parts." *New Scientist, 104,* 49–51.

Cohen, G., & Faulkner, D. (1986). Memory for proper names: Age differences in retrieval. *British Journal of Developmental Psychology, 4,* 187–197.

Cohen, G., & Faulkner, D. (1988). Life span changes in autobiographical memory. In M. M. Gruneberg, P. E. Martin, & R. N. Sykes (Eds.), *Practical aspects of memory: Current research and issues. Vol. 1.* Chichester: Wiley.

Cohen, G., & Faulkner, D. (1989). Age differences in source forgetting: Effects on reality monitoring and on eyewitness testimony. *Psychology and Aging, 4,* 10–17.

Cohen, N. J., & Squire, L. R. (1980). Preserved learning and retention of pattern-analyzing skill in amnesia: Dissociation of knowing how and knowing that. *Science, 210,* 207–210.

Cohen, R. L. (1981). On the generality of some memory laws. *Scandinavian Journal of Psychology, 22,* 267–281.

Cohen, R. L. (1983). The effects of encoding variables on the free recall of words and action events. *Memory & Cognition, 11,* 575–582.

Cohen, R. L. (1988). Metamemory for words and enacted instructions: Predicting which items will be recalled. *Memory & Cognition, 16,* 452–460.

Cohen, R. L. (1989). The effects of interference tasks on recency in the free recall of action events. *Psychological Research, 51,* 176–180.

Cohen, R. L., Sandler, S. P., & Schroeder, K. (1987). Aging and memory for words and action events: The effects of item repetition and list length. *Psychology and Aging, 2,* 280–285.

Collins, A. M., & Loftus, E. F. (1975). A spreading activation theory of semantic processing. *Psychological Review, 82,* 407–428.

Collins, A. M., & Quillian, M. R. (1969). Retrieval time from semantic memory. *Journal of Verbal Learning and Verbal Behavior, 8,* 240–247.

Conrad, H. S., & Jones, H. E. (1929). Psychological studies of motion pictures: III. Fidelity of report as a measure of adult intelligence. *University of California Publications in Psychology, 3,* 245–276.

Conrad, R. (1964). Acoustic confusions in immediate memory. *British Journal of Psychology, 55,* 75–84.

Coppinger, N. W., & Nehkre, M. F. (1972). Discrimination learning and transfer of training in the aged. *Journal of Genetic Psychology, 120,* 93–102.

Corkin, S. (1968). Acquisition of motor skill after bilateral medial temporal-lobe excision. *Neuropsychologia, 6,* 255–265.

Costa, P. T., Jr., & McCrae, R. R. (1988). Personality in adulthood: A six-year longitudinal study of self-reports and spouse ratings on the NEO Personality Inventory. *Journal of Personality and Social Psychology, 54,* 853–863.

Costa, P. T., Jr., McCrae, R. R., Zonderman, A. B., Barbano, H. E., Lebowitz, B., & Larson, D. (1986). Cross-sectional studies of personality in a national sample: 2. Stability in neuroticism, extraversion, and openness. *Psychology and Aging, 1,* 144–149.

Cowan, N. (1984). On short and long auditory stores. *Psychological Bulletin, 96*, 341–370.

Cowan, N. (1988). Evolving conceptions of memory storage, selective attention, and their mutual constraints within the human information processing system. *Psychological Bulletin, 104*, 163–191.

Coyne, A. C. (1985). Adult age, presentation time, and memory performance. *Experimental Aging Research, 11*, 147–149.

Coyne, A. C., Allen, P. A., & Wickens, D. D. (1986). Influence of adult age on primary and secondary memory search. *Psychology and Aging, 1*, 187–194.

Coyne, A. C., Burger, M. C., Berry, J. M., & Botwinick, J. (1987). Adult age, information processing, and partial report performance. *Journal of Genetic Psychology, 148*, 219–224.

Coyne, A. C., Herman, J. F., & Botwinick, J. (1980). Age differences in acoustic and semantic recognition memory. *Perceptual and Motor Skills, 51*, 439–445.

Craik, F. I. M. (1968a). Short-term memory and the aging process. In G. A. Talland (Ed.), *Human aging and behavior.* New York: Academic Press.

Craik, F. I. M. (1968b). Two components in free recall. *Journal of Verbal Learning and Verbal Behavior, 7*, 996–1004.

Craik, F. I. M. (1971). Age differences in recognition memory. *Quarterly Journal of Experimental Psychology, 23*, 316–323.

Craik, F. I. M. (1977). Age differences in human memory. In J. E. Birren & K. W. Schaie (Eds.), *Handbook of the psychology of aging (1st ed.).* New York: Van Nostrand Reinhold.

Craik, F. I. M. (1983). On the transfer of information from temporary to permanent memory. *Philosophical Transactions of the Royal Society of London, 302*, 341–359.

Craik, F. I. M. (1985). Paradigms in human memory research. In L. -G. Nilsson & T. Archer (Eds.), *Perspectives on learning and memory.* Hillsdale, NJ: Erlbaum.

Craik, F. I. M. (1986). A functional account of age differences in memory. In F. Klix & H. Hagendorf (Eds.), *Human memory and cognitive capabilities: Mechanisms and performances.* Amsterdam: North Holland.

Craik, F. I. M., & Byrd, M. (1982). Aging and cognitive deficits: The role of attentional resources. In F. I. M. Craik & S. E. Trehub (Eds.), *Advances in the study of communication and affect: Vol. 8. Aging and Cognitive processes.* New York: Plenum Press.

Craik, F. I. M., Byrd, M., & Swanson, J. M. (1987). Patterns of memory loss in three elderly samples. *Psychology and Aging, 2*, 79–86.

Craik, F. I. M., & Dirkx, E. (1992). Age-related differences in three tests of visual imagery. *Psychology and Aging, 7*, 661–665.

Craik, F. I. M., & Jennings, J. M. (1992). Human memory. In F. I. M. Craik & T. A. Salthouse (Eds.), *The handbook of aging and cognition.* Hillsdale, NJ: Erlbaum.

Craik, F. I. M., & Lockhart, R. S. (1972). Levels of processing: A framework for memory research. *Journal of Verbal Learning and Verbal Behavior, 11*, 671–684.

Craik, F. I. M., & Masani, P. A. (1967). Age differences in the temporal integration of language. *British Journal of Psychology, 58*, 291–299.

Craik, F. I. M., & Masani, P. A. (1969). Age and intelligence differences in coding and retrieval of word lists. *British Journal of Psychology, 60*, 315–319.

Craik, F. I. M., & McDowd, J. M. (1987). Age differences in recall and recognition. *Journal of Experimental Psychology: Learning, Memory, and Cognition, 13*, 474–479.

Craik, F. I. M., Morris, L. W., Morris, R. G., & Loewen, E. R. (1990). Relations between source amnesia and frontal lobe functioning in a normal elderly sample. *Psychology and Aging, 5*, 148–151.

Craik, F. I. M., & Rabinowitz, J. C. (1984). Age differences in the acquisition and use of verbal information: A tutorial review. In H. Bouma & D. G. Bouwhuis (Eds.), *Attention and Performance X: Control of language processes*. London: Erlbaum.

Craik, F. I. M., & Rabinowitz, J. C. (1985). The effects of presentation rate and encoding task on age-related memory deficits. *Journal of Gerontology, 40*, 309–315.

Craik, F. I. M., & Simon, E. (1980). Age differences in memory: The roles of attention and depth of processing. In L. W. Poon, J. L. Fozard, L. S. Cermak, D. Arenberg, & L. W. Thompson (Eds.), *New directions in memory and aging: Proceedings of the George A. Talland Memorial Conference*. Hillsdale, NJ: Erlbaum.

Craik, F. I. M., & Tulving, E. (1975). Depth of processing and the retention of words in episodic memory. *Journal of Experimental Psychology: General, 104*, 268–294.

Crook, T. H., Bartus, R. T., Ferris, S. H., Whitehouse, P., Cohen, G. D., & Gershon, S. (1986). Age-associated memory impairment: Proposed diagnostic criteria and measures of clinical change—Report of a National Institute of Mental Health Work Group. *Developmental Neuropsychology, 2*, 261–276.

Crook, T. H., Ferris, S., McCarthy, M., & Rae, D. (1980). Utility of digit recall tasks for assessing memory in the aged. *Journal of Consulting and Clinical Psychology, 48*, 228–233.

Crook, T. H., & Larrabee, G. J. (1988). Interrelationships among everyday memory tests: Stability of factor structure with age. *Neuropsychology, 2*, 1–12.

Crook, T. H., & Larrabee, G. J. (1990). A self-rating scale for evaluating memory in everyday life. *Psychology and Aging, 5*, 48–47.

Crook, T. H., & Larrabee, G. J. (1992). Changes in facial recognition memory across the adult lifespan. *The Journals of Gerontology: Psychological Sciences, 47*, P138–141.

Crook, T. H., Larrabee, G. J., & Youngjohn, J. R. (1993). Age and incidental recall for a simulated everyday memory task. *The Journals of Gerontology: Psychological Sciences, 48*, P45–47.

Crook, T. H., & West, R. L. (1990). Name recall performance across the adult life-span. *British Journal of Psychology, 81*, 335–349.

Crossley, M., & Hiscock, M. (1992). Age-related differences in concurrent task performance of normal adults: Evidence for a decline in processing resources. *Psychology and Aging, 7*, 499–506.

Crossman, E. R. F. W., & Szafran, J. (1956). Changes with age in the speed of information-intake and discrimination. *Experimentia Supplementum IV*. Basel, Switzerland: Birkhauser.

Crovitz, H. F., & Quina-Holland, K. (1976). Proportion of episodic memories from early childhood by years of age. *Bulletin of the Psychonomic Society, 7*, 61–62.

Crovitz, H. F., & Schiffman, H. (1974). Frequency of episodic memories as a function of their age. *Bulletin of the Psychonomic Society, 4*, 517–518.

Crowder, R. G. (1976). *Principles of learning and memory*. Hillsdale, NJ: Erlbaum.

Crowder, R. G. (1980). Echoic memory and the study of aging memory systems. In L. W. Poon, J. L. Fozard, L. S. Cermak, D. Arenberg, & L. W. Thompson (Eds.), *New directions in memory and aging: Proceedings of the George A. Talland Memorial Conference*. Hillsdale, NJ: Erlbaum.

Crowder, R. G., & Morton, J. (1969). Precategorical acoustic storage (PAS). *Perception and Psychophysics, 5*, 365–373.

Czaja, S. J., Hammond, K., Blascovich, J., & Swede, H. (1989). Age-related differences in learning to use a text editing system. *Behavior and Information Technology, 8*, 309–319.

Czaja, S. J., & Sharit, J. (1993). Age differences in performance of computer-based work. *Psychology and Aging, 8*, 59–67.

Daneman, M., & Carpenter, P. A. (1980). Individual differences in working memory and reading. *Journal of Verbal Learning and Verbal Behavior, 19*, 450–466.

Darley, C. F., & Murdock, B. B., Jr. (1971). Effects of free recall testing on final recall and recognition. *Journal of Experimental Psychology, 91*, 66–73.

Darwin, C. J., Turvey, M. T., & Crowder, R. G. (1972). An auditory analogue of the Sperling partial-report procedure: Evidence for brief auditory storage. *Cognitive Psychology, 3*, 255–267.

Davies, A. D. M. (1967). Age and Memory for Designs Test. *British Journal of Social and Clinical Psychology, 6*, 228–233.

Davis, G. A., & Ball, H. E. (1989). Effects of age on comprehension of complex sentences in adulthood. *Journal of Speech and Hearing Research, 32*, 143–150.

Davis, H. P., Cohen, A., Gandy, M., Colombo, P., Van Dusseldorp, G., Simolke, N., & Romano, J. (1990). Lexical priming as a function of age. *Behavioral Neuroscience, 104*, 288–297.

Davis, S. H., & Obrist, W. D. (1966). Age differences in learning and retention of verbal material. *Cornell Journal of Social Relations, 1*, 95–103.

Dawson, M. E., & Schell, A. M. (1987). Human automatic and skeletal classical conditioning: The role of conscious cognitive factors. In G. Davey (Ed.), *Cognitive processes and Pavlovian conditioning in humans*. Chichester: Wiley.

Delbecq-Derouesne, J., & Beauvois, M. F. (1989). Memory processes and aging: A defect of automatic rather than controlled processes? *Archives of Gerontology and Geriatrics, Supplement 1*, 121–150.

Denney, N. W. (1974). Clustering in middle and old age. *Developmental Psychology, 10*, 471–475.

Denney, N. W., Dew, J. R., & Kihlstrom, J. F. (1992). An adult developmental study of the encoding of spatial location. *Experimental Aging Research, 18*, 25–32.

Denney, N. W., Miller, B. V., Dew, J. R., & Levav, A. L. (1991). An adult developmental study of contextual memory. *The Journals of Gerontology: Psychological Sciences, 46*, P44–50.

Desroches, H. F., Kaiman, B. D., & Ballard, H. I. (1966). Relationships between age and recall of meaningful material. *Psychological Reports, 18*, 920–922.

Devolder, P. A., Brigham, M. C., & Pressley, M. (1990). Memory performance awareness in younger and older adults. *Psychology and Aging, 5*, 291–303.

Dick, M. B., & Kean, M. L. (1989). Memory for internally generated words in Alzheimer-Type Dementia: Breakdown in encoding and semantic memory. *Brain and Cognition, 9*, 88–108.

Dick, M. B., Kean, M. L., & Sands, D. C. (1988). The preselection effect on the recall facilitation of motor movements in Alzheimer-Type Dementia. *The Journals of Gerontology: Psychological Sciences, 43*, P127–135.

Dick, M. B., Kean, M., & Sands, D. C. (1989). Memory for action events in Alzheimer-

Type Dementia: Further evidence of an encoding failure. *Brain and Cognition, 9*, 71–87.

Dillingham, A. E. (1981). Age and workplace injuries. *Aging and Work, 4*, 1–10.

Dirken, J. M. (1972). *Functional age of construction industrial workers. A transversal survey and a method of assessing functional age.* Groningen: Wolters-Nooordhoff.

Dirkx, E., & Craik, F. I. M. (1992). Age-related differences in memory as a function of imagery processing. *Psychology and Aging, 7*, 352–358.

Dixon, R. A. (1989). Questionnaire research on metamemory and aging: Issues of structure and function. In L. W. Poon, D. C. Rubin, & B. A. Wilson (Eds.), *Everyday cognition in adulthood and late life.* New York: Cambridge University Press.

Dixon, R. A., & Hultsch, D. F. (1983a). Metamemory and memory for text relationships in adulthood: A cross-validation study. *Journal of Gerontology, 38*, 689–694.

Dixon, R. A., & Hultsch, D. F. (1983b). Structure and development of metamemory in adulthood. *Journal of Gerontology, 38*, 682–688.

Dixon, R. A., Hultsch, D. F., Simon, E. W., & Von Eye, A. (1984). Verbal ability and text structure effects on adult age differences in text recall. *Journal of Verbal Learning and Verbal Behavior, 23*, 569–578.

Dixon, R. A., Simon, E. W., Nowak, C. A., & Hultsch, D. F. (1982). Text recall in adulthood as a function of level of information, input modality, and delay interval. *Journal of Gerontology, 37*, 358–364.

Dobbs, A. R., & Rule, B. G. (1987). Prospective memory and self-reports of memory abilities in older adults. *Canadian Journal of Psychology, 41*, 209–222.

Dobbs, A. R., & Rule, B. G. (1990). Adult age differences in working memory. *Psychology and Aging, 4*, 500–503.

Dorfman, D., Glanzer, M., & Kaufman, J. (1988). Aging effects on recognition memory when encoding and strategy are controlled. *Bulletin of the Psychonomic Society, 24*, 172–174.

Doty, B. A. (1966a). Age and avoidance conditioning in rats. *Journal of Gerontology, 21*, 287–290.

Doty, B. A. (1966b). Age differences in avoidance conditioning as a function of distribution of trials and task difficulty. *Journal of Genetic Psychology, 109*, 249–254.

Doty, B. A., & Doty, L. A. (1964). Effect of age and chlorpromazine on memory consolidation. *Journal of Comparative and Physiological Psychology, 57*, 331–334.

Doty, B. A., & Johnston, M. M. (1966). Effects of post-trial eserine administration, age and task difficulty on avoidance conditioning in rats. *Psychonomic Science, 6*, 101–102.

Drachman, D., & Leavitt, L. (1972). Memory impairment in the aged: Storage versus retrieval deficit. *Journal of Experimental Psychology, 93*, 302–308.

Drevenstedt, J., & Bellezza, F. S. (1993). Memory for self-generated narration in the elderly. *Psychology and Aging, 8*, 187–196.

Duchek, J. M. (1984). Encoding and retrieval differences between young and old: The impact of attentional capacity usage. *Developmental Psychology, 20*, 1173–1180.

Duke, L. W., Haley, W. E., & Bergquist, T. F. (1990). Behavioral interventions for age-related memory decline. In P. A. Wisocki (Ed.), *Handbook of clinical behavior therapy with the elderly client.* New York: Plenum Press.

Dunn, J. C., & Kirsner, K. (1989). Implicit memory: Task or process. In S. Lewandowsky,

J. C. Dunn, & K. Kirsner (Eds.), *Implicit Memory: Theoretical Issues*. Hillsdale, NJ: Erlbaum.

Durkin, M., Prescott, L., Furchtgott, E., Cantor, J., & Powell, D. A. (in preparation). Skill learning in the elderly: Relationship to verbal learning and classical conditioning.

Dywan, J., & Jacoby, L. (1990). Effects of aging on source monitoring differences in susceptibility to false fame. *Psychology and Aging, 5*, 379–397.

Earles, J. L., & Coon, V. E. (1994). Adult age differences in long term memory for performed activities. *The Journals of Gerontology: Psychological Sciences, 49*, 32–34.

Ebbinghaus, H. (1885). *Uber das gedactnis: Untersuchungen zur experimentellen psycholgie*. Leipzig: Duncker and Humbolt.

Effron, R. (1970). Effects of stimulus duration on perceptual onset and offset latencies. *Perception and Psychophysics, 8*, 231–234.

Egan, D. E., & Gomez, I. M. (1985). Assaying, isolating, and accommodating individual differences in learning a complex skill. In R. F. Dillon (Ed.), *Individual differences in cognition. Vol. 2*. San Diego: Academic Press.

Eich, J. E., Weingartner, H., Stillman, R. C., & Gillin, J. C. (1975). State-dependent accessibility of retrieval cues in the retention of a categorized list. *Journal of Verbal Learning and Verbal Behavior, 14*, 408–417.

Einstein, G. O., & Hunt, R. R. (1980). Levels of processing and integration: Additive effects of individual item and relational processing. *Journal of Experimental Psychology: Human Learning and Memory, 6*, 588–598.

Einstein, G. O., Holland, L. J., McDaniel, M. A., & Guynn, M. J. (1992). Age-related deficits in prospective memory: The influence of task complexity. *Psychology and Aging, 7*, 471–478.

Einstein, G. O., & McDaniel, M. A. (1990). Normal aging and prospective memory. *Journal of Experimental Psychology: Learning, Memory, and Cognition, 16*, 717–726.

Einstein, G. O., & McDaniel, M. A. (1991, November). *Aging and time- vs. event-based prospective memory*. Paper presented at the annual meeting of the Psychonomic Society, San Francisco, CA.

Eisdorfer, C. (1965). Verbal learning and response time in the aged. *Journal of Genetic Psychology, 107*, 15–22.

Eisdorfer, C., Axelrod, S., & Wilkie, F. L. (1963). Stimulus exposure time as a factor in serial learning in an aged sample. *Journal of Abnormal and Social Psychology, 67*, 594–600.

Eisdorfer, C., & Service, C. (1967). Verbal rote learning and superior intelligence in the aged. *Journal of Gerontology, 22*, 158–161.

Ekstrand, B. R., Wallace, W. P., & Underwood, B. J. (1966). A frequency theory of verbal discrimination learning. *Psychological Review, 73*, 566–578.

Elias, C. S., & Hirasuna, N. (1976). Age and semantic and phonological encoding. *Developmental Psychology, 12*, 497–503.

Elias, P. K., Elias, M. F., Robbins, M. A., & Gage, P. (1987). Acquisition of word-processing skills by younger, middle-age, and older adults. *Psychology and Aging, 2*, 340–348.

Ellis, H. C. (1972). *Fundamentals of human learning and cognition (1st ed.)*. Dubuque, IA: William C. Brown.

Ellis, H. C. (1978). *Fundamentals of human learning, memory, and cognition (2nd. ed.)*. Dubuque, IA: William C. Brown.

Ellis, N. R. (1990). Is memory for spatial location automatically encoded? *Memory &* *Cognition, 18*, 584–592.

Ellis, N. R. (1991). Automatic and effortful processes in memory for spatial location. *Bulletin of the Psychonomic Society, 29*, 28–30.

Ellis, N. R., Palmer, R. L., & Reeves, C. L. (1988). Developmental and intellectual differences in frequency processing. *Developmental Psychology, 24*, 38–45.

Ellis, N. R., & Rickard, T. C. (1989). The retention of automatically and effortfully encoded stimulus attributes. *Bulletin of the Psychonomic Society, 27*, 299–302.

Emery, O. (1985). Language and aging. *Experimental Aging Research, 11*, 3–60.

Engelkamp, J. E., & Cohen, R. L. (1991). Current issues in memory of action events. *Psychological Research, 53*, 175–182.

Era, P., & Heikkinen, E. (1985). Postural sway during standing and unexpected disturbance of balance in random samples of men of different ages. *Journal of Gerontology, 40*, 287–295.

Erber, J. T. (1974). Age differences in recognition memory. *Journal of Gerontology, 29*, 177–181.

Erber, J. T. (1978). Age differences in a controlled-lag recognition. *Experimental Aging Research, 4*, 195–206.

Erber, J. T. (1979, November). *The effect of encoding instructions on recall and recognition memory.* Paper presented at the annual meeting of the Gerontological Society, Washington, D.C.

Erber, J. T. (1981). Remote memory and age: A review. *Experimental Aging Research, 7*, 189–200.

Erber, J. T. (1984). Age differences in the effect of encoding congruence on incidental and cued recall. *Experimental Aging Research, 10*, 221–223.

Erber, J. T. (1987). Remote memory. In G. L. Maddox (Ed.), *The encyclopedia of aging.* New York: Springer.

Erber, J. T. (1989). Young and older adults' appraisal of memory failures in young and older adult target persons. *The Journals of Gerontology: Psychological Sciences, 44*, P170–175.

Erber, J. T., Abello, S., & Moniger, C. (1988). Age and individual differences in immediate and delayed effectiveness of mnemonic instructions. *Experimental Aging Research, 14*, 119–124.

Erber, J. T., Galt, D., Jr., & Botwinick, J. (1985). Age differences in the effects of contextual framework and word-familiarity on episodic memory. *Experimental Aging Research, 11*, 101–103.

Erber, J. T., Herman, T. G., & Botwinick, J. (1980). Age differences in memory as a function of depth of processing. *Experimental Aging Research, 6*, 341–348.

Erber, J. T., & Rothberg, S. T. (1991). Here's looking at you: The relative effects of age and attractiveness on judgments about memory. *The Journals of Gerontology: Psychological Sciences, 46*, P116–123.

Erber, J. T., Rothberg, S. T., Szuchman, L. T., & Etheart, M. E. (1993). How physicians appraise everyday memory failures of patients across the adult life span. *Experimental Aging Research, 19*, 195–208.

Erber, J. T., Szuchman, L. T., & Rothberg, S. T. (1990a). Everyday memory failure: Age differences in appraisal and attribution. *Psychology and Aging, 5*, 236–241.

Erber, J. T., Szuchman, L. T., & Rothberg, S. T. (1990b). Age, gender, and individual differences in memory failure appraisal. *Psychology and Aging, 5,* 600–603.

Eriksen, C. W., & Collins, J. F. (1967). Some temporal characteristics of visual pattern perception. *Journal of Experimental Psychology, 74,* 476–484.

Eriksen, C. W., Hamlin, R. M., & Daye, C. (1973). Aging adults and rate of memory scan. *Bulletin of the Psychonomic Society, 1,* 259–260.

Estes, W. K. (1955). Statistical theory of spontaneous recovery and regression. *Psychological Review, 62,* 145–154.

Estes, W. K. (1959). The statistical approach to learning theory. In S. Koch (Ed.), *Psychology: A study of a science.* New York: McGraw-Hill.

Evans, G. W., Brennan, P. L., Skorpanich, M. A., & Held, D. (1984). Cognitive mapping and elderly adults: Verbal and location memory for urban landmarks. *Journal of Gerontology, 39,* 452–457.

Eysenck, M. W. (1974). Age differences in incidental learning. *Developmental Psychology, 10,* 936–941.

Eysenck, M. W. (1975). Retrieval from semantic memory as a function of age. *Journal of Gerontology, 30,* 174–180.

Farrimond, T. (1967). Visual and auditory performance variations with age: Some implications. *Australian Journal of Psychology, 19,* 193–202.

Farrimond, T. (1968). Retention and recall: Incidental learning of visual and auditory material. *Journal of Genetic Psychology, 113,* 155–165.

Ferguson, S. A., Hashtroudi, S., & Johnson, M. K. (1992). Age differences in using source-relevant cues. *Psychology and Aging, 7,* 443–452.

Fernandez, A., & Glenberg, A. M. (1985). Changing environmental context does not reliably affect memory. *Memory & Cognition, 13,* 333–345.

Ferraro, F. R., & Kellas, G. (1992). Age-related changes in the effects of target orientation on word recognition. *The Journals of Gerontology: Psychological Sciences, 47,* P279–280.

Ferris, S. H., Crook, T., Clark, E., McCarthy, M., & Rae, D. (1980). Facial recognition memory deficits in normal aging and senile dementia. *Journal of Gerontology, 35,* 707–714.

Finkbinder, R. G., & Woodruff-Pak, D. S. (1991). Classical eyeblink conditioning in adulthood: Effects of age and interstimulus interval on acquisition in the trace paradigm. *Psychology and Aging, 6,* 109–117.

Finkel, S. J., & Yesavage, J. A. (1989). Learning mnemonics: A preliminary evaluation of a computer-aided instruction package for the elderly. *Experimental Aging Research, 15,* 199–201.

Finley, G. E., & Sharp, T. (1989). Name retrieval by the elderly in the tip-of-the-tongue paradigm: Demonstrable success in overcoming initial failure. *Educational Gerontology, 15,* 259–265.

Fisher, L. M. & McDowd, J. M. (1993). Item and relational processing in young and older adults. *The Journals of Gerontology: Psychological Sciences, 48,* P62–68.

Fisk, A. D., & Rogers, W. A. (1991). Toward an understanding of age-related memory and visual search effects. *Journal of Experimental Psychology: General, 120,* 131–149.

Fitts, P. M. (1964). Perceptual-motor skill learning. In A. W. Melton (Ed.), *Categories of human learning.* New York: Academic Press.

Fitzgerald, J. M. (1983). A developmental study of recall from natural categories. *Developmental Psychology, 19,* 9–14.

Fitzgerald, J. M. (1988). Vivid memories and the reminiscence phenomenon: The role of self-narrative. *Human Development, 31*, 261–273.

Fitzgerald, J. M., & Lawrence, R. (1984). Autobiographical memory across the life-span. *Journal of Gerontology, 39*, 692–698.

Flavell, J. H., & Wellman, H. W. (1977). Metamemory. In R. V. Kail & J. W. Hagen (Eds.), *Perspectives on the development of memory and cognition.* Hillsdale, NJ: Erlbaum.

Flicker, C., Ferris, S. H., Crook, T., & Bartus, R. T. (1989). Age differences in the vulnerability of facial recognition memory to proactive interference. *Experimental Aging Research, 15*, 189–194.

Flynn, T. M., & Storandt, M. (1990). Supplemental group discussions in memory training for older adults. *Psychology and Aging, 5*, 178–181.

Folstein, M. F., Folstein, S. E., & McHugh, P. H. (1975). Mini-Mental State: A practical method for grading the cognitive state of patients for the clinician. *Journal of Psychiatric Research, 12*, 189–198.

Foos, P. W. (1989a). Adult age differences in working memory. *Psychology and Aging, 4*, 269–275.

Foos, P. W. (1989b). Age differences in memory for two common objects. *The Journals of Gerontology: Psychological Sciences, 44*, P178–180.

Foos, P. W., & Wright, L. (1992). Adult age differences in the storage of information in working memory. *Experimental Aging Research, 18*, 51–57.

Foos, P. W., Sabol, M. A., Corral, G., & Mobley, L. (1987). Age differences in primary and secondary memory. *Bulletin of the Psychonomic Society, 25*, 159–160.

Fozard, J. L., & Waugh, N. C. (1969). Proactive inhibition of prompted items. *Psychonomic Science, 17*, 67–68.

Franklin, H. C., & Holding, D. H. (1977). Personal memories at different ages. *Quarterly Journal of Experimental Psychology, 29*, 527–532.

Fraser, D. C. (1958). Decay of immediate memory with age. *Nature, 182*, 1163.

Freedman, J. L., & Loftus, E. F. (1971). The retrieval of words from long-term memory. *Journal of Verbal Learning and Verbal Behavior, 10*, 107–115.

Freund, J. S., & Witte, K. L. (1976). Paired-associate transfer: Age of subjects, anticipation interval, association value, and paradigm. *American Journal of Psychology, 89*, 695–705.

Freund, J. S., & Witte, K. L. (1978, November). *Recognition and frequency judgments in young and elderly adults.* Paper presented at the annual meeting of the Psychonomic Society, San Antonio, Texas.

Freund, J. S., & Witte, K. L. (1979, November). *Learning-to-learn paired associates in young and elderly adults.* Paper presented at the annual meeting of the Gerontological Society, Washington, D.C.

Freund, J. S., & Witte, K. L. (1986). Recognition and frequency judgments in young and elderly adults. *American Journal of Psychology, 99*, 81–102.

Friedman, H. (1966). Memory organization in the aged. *Journal of Genetic Psychology, 109*, 3–8.

Friedman, H. (1974). Interrelation of two types of immediate memory in the aged. *Journal of Psychology, 87*, 177–181.

Frieske, D. A., & Park, D. C. (1993). Effects of organization and working memory on age differences in memory for scene information. *Experimental Aging Research, 19*, 321–332.

Fromholt, P., & Larsen, S. F. (1991). Autobiographical memory in normal aging and primary degenerative dementia (dementia of Alzheimer type). *The Journals of Gerontology: Psychological Sciences, 46,* 85–91.

Fuld, P. A., Katzman, R., Davies, P., & Terry, R. D. (1982). Intrusions as a sign of Alzheimer dementia: Chemical and pathological verification. *Archives of Neurology, 11,* 155–159.

Fullerton, A. M. (1988). Age differences in solving series problems requiring integration of new and old information. *International Journal of Aging and Human Development, 26,* 147–154.

Fulton, A., & Bartlett, J. C. (1991). Young and old faces in young and old heads: The factor of age in face recognition. *Psychology and Aging, 6,* 623–630.

Furchtgott, E., & Busemeyer, J. K. (1979). Heartrate and skin conductance during cognitive processes as a function of age. *Journal of Gerontology, 34,* 183–190.

Furry, C. A., & Baltes, P. B. (1973). The effect of age differences in ability-extraneous variables on the assessment of intelligence in children, adults, and the elderly. *Journal of Gerontology, 28,* 73–80.

Galton, F. (1911). *Inquiries into human faculty and its development (2nd Ed.).* New York: Dutton.

Gardiner, J. M. (1988). Functional aspects of recollective experience. *Memory & Cognition, 16,* 309–313.

Gardiner, J. M., & Parkin, A. J. (1990). Attention and recollective experience in recognition memory. *Memory & Cognition, 18,* 579–583.

Gatz, M., & Hurwicz, M-L. (1990). Are old people more depressed? Cross-sectional data on Center for Epidemiological Studies Depression Scale factors. *Psychology and Aging, 5,* 284–290.

Gaylord, S. A., & Marsh, G. R. (1975). Age differences in the speed of a spatial cognitive process. *Journal of Gerontology, 30,* 674–678.

Geiselman, R. E., & Bellezza, F. S. (1976). Long-term memory for speaker's voice and source location. *Memory & Cognition, 4,* 483–489.

Gerard, G., & Weisberg, L. A. (1986). MRI periventricular lesions in adults. *Neurology, 36,* 998–10001.

Gerard, L., Zacks, R. T., Hasher, L., & Radvansky, G. A. (1991). Age deficits in retrieval: The fan effect. *The Journals of Gerontology: Psychological Sciences, 46,* P131–136.

Giambra, L. M. (1989). Task-unrelated thought frequency as a function of age: A laboratory study. *Psychology & Aging, 4,* 136–143.

Giambra, L. M., & Arenberg, D. (1993). Adult age differences in forgetting sentences. *Psychology and Aging, 8,* 451–462.

Gick, M. L., Craik, F. I. M., & Morris, R. G. (1988). Task complexity and age differences in working memory. *Memory & Cognition, 16,* 353–361.

Gilbert, J. G. (1935). Mental efficiency in senescence. *Archives of Psychology, 27,* No. 188.

Gilbert, J. G. (1941). Memory loss in senescence. *Journal of Abnormal and Social Psychology, 36,* 73–86.

Gilbert, J. G. (1973). Thirty-five year follow-up study of intellectual functioning. *Journal of Gerontology, 28,* 68–72.

Gilbert, J. G., & Levee, R. F. (1971). Patterns of declining memory. *Journal of Gerontology, 26,* 70–75.

Gilewski, M. J., & Zelinski, E. M. (1986). Questionnaire assessment of memory complaints. In L. W. Poon (Ed.), *Handbook for clinical memory assessments of older adults*. Washington, D.C.: American Psychological Association.

Gilewski, M. J., Zelinski, E. M., & Schaie, K. W. (1990). The Memory Functioning Questionnaire for assessment of memory complaints in adulthood and old age. *Psychology and Aging, 5*, 482–490.

Gilewski, M. J., Zelinski, E. M., Schaie, K. W., & Thompson, L. W. (1983, August). *Abbreviating the Metamemory Questionnaire: Factor structure and norms for adults*. Paper presented at the annual meeting of the American Psychological Association, Anaheim, CA.

Gilmore, G. C., Allan, T. M., & Royer, F. L. (1986). Iconic memory and aging. *Journal of Gerontology, 41*, 183–190.

Gilson, E. Q., & Baddeley, A. D. (1969). Tactile short-term memory. *Quarterly Journal of Experimental Psychology, 21*, 180–184.

Gist, M., Rosen, B., & Schwoerer, C. (1988). The influence of training method and trainee on the acquisition of computer skills. *Personnel Psychology, 41*, 255–265.

Gladis, M., & Braun, H. (1958). Age differences in transfer and retroaction as a function of intertask response similarity. *Journal of Experimental Psychology, 55*, 25–30.

Glanzer, M., & Cunitz, A. (1966). Two storage mechanisms in free recall. *Journal of Verbal Learning and Verbal Behavior, 5*, 351–360.

Glenberg, A. M. (1976). Monotonic and nonmonotonic lag effects in paired-associate and recognition memory paradigms. *Journal of Verbal Learning and Verbal Behavior, 15*, 1–16.

Glenberg, A. M. (1979). Component-levels theory of the effects of spacing of repetitions on recall and recognition. *Memory & Cognition, 7*, 95–112.

Glenberg, A. M., & Adams, F. (1978). Type I rehearsal and recognition. *Journal of Verbal Learning and Verbal Behavior, 17*, 455–464.

Glenberg, A. M., & Bradley, M. M. (1979). Mental contiguity. *Journal of Experimental Psychology: Human Learning and Memory, 5*, 88–97.

Glenberg, A. M., Smith, S. M., & Green, C. (1977). Type I rehearsal: Maintenance and more. *Journal of Verbal Learning and Behavior, 16*, 339–352.

Glenberg, A. M., & Swanson, N. G. (1986). A temporal distinctiveness theory of recency and modality effects. *Journal of Experimental Psychology: Learning, Memory, and Cognition, 12*, 3–15.

Glynn, S. M., & Muth, K. D. (1979). Text-learning capabilities of older adults. *Educational Gerontology, 4*, 253–269.

Godden, D., & Baddeley, A. D. (1975). Context-dependent memory in two natural environments: On land and underwater. *British Journal of Psychology, 66*, 325–331.

Goggin, J. P. (1975, May). *The effects of aging on short-term memory*. Paper presented at the annual meeting of the Midwestern Psychological Association, Chicago.

Goggin, N. L., & Stelmach, G. E. (1990). Age-related deficits in cognitive-motor skills. In E. A. Lovelace (Ed.), *Aging and cognition: Mental processes, self-awareness, and interventions*. Amsterdam: North Holland.

Gold, D., Andres, D., Arbuckle, T., & Schwartzman, A. (1988). Measurement and correlates of verbosity in elderly people. *The Journals of Gerontology: Psychological Sciences, 43*, P27–33.

Gold, P. E., McGaugh, J. L., Hankins, L. L., Rose, R. P., & Vasquez, B. J. (1982). Age dependent changes in retention in rats. *Experimental Aging Research, 8,* 53–58.

Goldberg, Z., Syndulko, K., Lemon, J., Montan, B., Ulmer, R., & Tourtellotte, W. W. (1981, August). *Everyday memory problems in older adults.* Paper presented at the annual meeting of the American Psychological Association, Los Angeles, CA.

Goldfarb, W. (1941). An investigation of reaction time in older adults and its relationship to certain observed mental test patterns. *Contributions to Education* (No. 831). New York: Teachers College, Columbia University.

Goldstein, G., & Shelly, C. H. (1975). Similarities and differences between psychological deficit in aging and brain damage. *Journal of Gerontology, 30,* 448–455.

Goodrick, C. L. (1965). Operant level and light-contingent bar presses as a function of age and deprivation. *Psychological Reports, 17,* 283–288.

Goodrick, C. L. (1968). Learning, retention, and extinction of a complex maze habit for mature-young and senescent Wister albino rats. *Journal of Gerontology, 23,* 298–304.

Goodrick, C. L. (1969). Operant responding of nondeprived young and senescent male albino rats. *Journal of Genetic Psychology, 114,* 29–40.

Goodrick, C. L. (1970). Light- and dark-contingent bar pressing in the rat as a function of age and motivation. *Journal of Comparative and Physiological Psychology, 73,* 100–104.

Goodrick, C. L. (1972). Learning by mature-young and aged Wistar albino rats as a function of test complexity. *Journal of Gerontology, 27,* 353–357.

Goodrick, C. L. (1984). Effects of lifelong restricted feeding on complex maze performance in rats. *Age, 7,* 1–12.

Gordon, S. K. (1975). Organization and recall of related sentences by elderly and young adults. *Experimental Aging Research, 1,* 71–80.

Gordon, S. K., & Clark, W. C. (1974a). Adult age differences in word and nonsense syllable recognition memory and response criterion. *Journal of Gerontology, 29,* 659–665.

Gordon, S. K., & Clark, W. C. (1974b). Application of signal detection theory to prose recall and recognition in elderly and young adults. *Journal of Gerontology, 29,* 64–72.

Gorman, A. M. (1961). Recognition memory for nouns as a function of abstractness and frequency. *Journal of Experimental Psychology, 61,* 23–29.

Gottsdanker, R. (1980a). Aging and the use of advance probability information. *Journal of Motor Behavior, 12,* 133–143.

Gottsdanker, R. (1980b). Aging and the maintaining of preparation. *Experimental Aging Research, 15,* 13–27.

Gould, O. N., & Dixon, R. A. (1993). How we spent our vacation: Collaborative storytelling by young and old adults. *Psychology and Aging, 8,* 10–17.

Gould, O. N., Trevithick, L., & Dixon, R. A. (1991). Adult age differences in elaborations produced during prose recall. *Psychology and Aging, 6,* 93–99.

Goulet, L. R. (1972). New directions of research on aging and retention. *Journal of Gerontology, 27,* 52–60.

Graesser, A. C., Woll, S. B., Kowalski, D. J., & Smith, D. A. (1980). Memory for typical and atypical actions in scripted activities. *Journal of Experimental Psychology: Human Learning and Memory, 6,* 503–515.

Graf, P. (1990). Life-span changes in implicit and explicit memory. *Bulletin of the Psychonomic Society, 28,* 353–358.

Graf, P., & Schachter, D. L. (1985). Implicit and explicit memory for new associations in normal and amnesic subjects. *Journal of Experimental Psychology: Learning, Memory, and Cognition, 11*, 501–518.

Graf, P., Squire, L. R., & Mandler, G. (1984). The information amnesic patients do not forget. *Journal of Experimental Psychology: Learning, Memory, and Cognition, 10*, 164–178.

Grant, E. A., Storandt, M., & Botwinick, J. (1978). Incentive and practice in the psychomotor performance of the elderly. *Journal of Gerontology, 31*, 413–415.

Gratzinger, P., Sheikh, J. I., Friedman, L., & Tanke, E. (1990). Cognitive interventions to improve face-name recall: The role of personality trait differences. *Developmental Psychology, 26*, 889–893.

Greene, R. L. (1984). Incidental learning of event frequency. *Memory & Cognition, 12*, 90–95.

Greene, R. L. (1986). Sources of recency effects in free recall. *Psychological Bulletin, 99*, 221–228.

Greene, R. L. (1987). Effects of maintenance rehearsal on human memory. *Psychological Bulletin, 102*, 403–413.

Greene, R. L. (1989a). Immediate serial recall of mixed-modality lists. *Journal of Experimental Psychology: Learning, Memory, and Cognition, 15*, 266–274.

Greene, R. L. (1989b). Spacing effects in memory: Evidence for a two-process account. *Journal of Experimental Psychology: Learning, Memory, and Cognition, 15*, 371–377.

Greene, R. L. (1989c). Negative practice effects on frequency discriminations. *American Journal of Psychology, 102*, 225–230.

Greene, R. L., & Crowder, R. G. (1984). Modality and suffix effects in the absence of auditory stimulation. *Journal of Verbal Learning and Verbal Behavior, 23*, 371–382.

Greene, R. L., & Crowder, R. G. (1986). Recency effects in delayed recall of mouthed stimuli. *Memory & Cognition, 14*, 355–360.

Gregory, R. L. (1957). Increase in "neurological noise" as a factor in aging. In *Proceedings of the 4th Congress of the International Association of Gerontology, Merano, Italy*. Mearno, Italy: International Association of Gerontology.

Griew, S. (1959). Complexity of response and time of initiating responses in relation to age. *American Journal of Psychology, 72*, 83–86.

Gur, R. C., Mozley, P. D., Resnick, S. M., Gottlieb, G. E., Kohn, M., Zimmerman, R., Herman, G., Atlas, S., Grossman, R., Berretta, D., Erwin, R., & Gur, R. E. (1991). Gender differences in age effect on brain atrophy measured by magnetic resonance imagery. *Proceedings of the National Academy of Sciences, 88*, 2845–2849.

Gurland, B. J. (1976). The comparative frequency of depression in various adult age groups. *Journal of Gerontology, 31*, 283–292.

Gutman, M. A. (1965). The effects of age and extraversion on pursuit rotor reminiscence. *Journal of Gerontology, 20*, 346–350.

Guttentag, R. E. (1988). Processing relational and item-specific information: Effects of aging and division of attention. *Canadian Journal of Psychology, 42*, 414–423.

Guttentag, R. E. (1989). Age differences in dual-task performance: Procedures, assumptions, and results. *Developmental Review, 9*, 146–170.

Guttentag, R. E., & Hunt, R. R. (1988). Adult age differences in memory for imagined and performed actions. *The Journals of Gerontology: Psychological Sciences, 43*, P107–108.

Guttentag, R. E., & Madden, D. J. (1987). Adult age differences in the attentional capacity demands of letter matching. *Experimental Aging Research, 13*, 93–99.

Haaland, K. Y., Vranes, L. F., Goodwin, J. S., & Garry, P. J. (1987). Wisconsin Card Sort Test performance in a healthy elderly population. *Journal of Gerontology, 42*, 345–346.

Hall, T. C., Miller, K. H., & Corsellia, J. A. N. (1975). Variations in the human Pukinje cell population according to age and sex. *Neuropathology and Applied Neurobiology, 1*, 267–292.

Hamberger, M., & Friedman, D. (1992). Event-related potential correlates of repetition priming and stimulus classification in young, middle-aged, and older adults. *The Journals of Gerontology: Psychological Sciences, 47*, P395–406.

Hanley-Dunn, P., & McIntosh, J. L. (1984). Meaningfulness and recall of names by young and old adults. *Journal of Gerontology, 39*, 583–585.

Harker, J. O., & Riege, W. H. (1985). Aging and delay effects on recognition of words and designs. *Journal of Gerontology, 40*, 601–604.

Harkins, S. W., Chapman, C. R., & Eisdorfer, C. (1979). Memory loss and response bias in senescence. *Journal of Gerontology, 34*, 66–72.

Harrington, D. L., & Haaland, K. Y. (1992). Skill learning in the elderly: Diminished implicit and explicit memory for a motor sequence. *Psychology and Aging, 7*, 425–434.

Harris, J. E., & Wilkins, A. J. (1982). Remembering to do things: A theoretical framework and an illustrative experiment. *Human Learning, 1*, 123–136.

Hartley, A. A. (1992). Attention. In F. I. M. Craik & T. A. Salthouse (Eds.), *The handbook of aging and cognition*. Hillsdale, NJ: Erlbaum.

Hartley, A. A., Hartley, J. T., & Johnson, S. A. (1984). The older adult as computer user. In P. K. Robinson, J. Livingston, & J. E. Birren (Eds.), *Aging and technological advances*. New York: Plenum Press.

Hartley, J. T. (1986). Reader and text variables as determinants of discourse memory in adulthood. *Psychology and Aging, 1*, 150–158.

Hartley, J. T. (1989). Memory for prose: Perspectives on the reader. In L. W. Poon, D. C. Rubin, & B. A. Wilson (Eds.), *Everyday cognition in adulthood and late life*. New York: Cambridge University Press.

Hartley, J. T., Harker, J. O., & Walsh, D. A. (1980). Contemporary issues and new directions in adult development of learning and memory. In L. W. Poon (Ed.), *Aging in the 1980s: Some contemporary issues in the psychology of aging*. Washington, D.C.: American Psychological Association.

Hartley, J. T., & Walsh, D. A. (1980). The effect of monetary incentive on amount and rate of free recall in older and younger adults. *Journal of Gerontology, 35*, 899–905.

Hartman, M., & Hasher, L. (1991). Aging and suppression: memory for previously relevant information. *Psychology and Aging, 6*, 587–584.

Harwood, E., & Naylor, G. F. K. (1969). Recall and recognition in elderly and young subjects. *Australian Journal of Psychology, 21*, 251–257.

Hasher, L., & Chromiak, W. (1977). The processing of frequency information: An automatic mechanism? *Journal of Verbal Learning and Verbal Behavior, 16*, 173–184.

Hasher, L., Stoltzfus, E. R., Zacks, R. T., & Rypma, B. (1991). Age and inhibition. *Journal of Experimental Psychology: Learning, Memory, and Cognition, 17*, 163–169.

Hasher, L., & Zacks, R. T. (1979). Automatic and effortful processes in memory. *Journal of Experimental Psychology: General, 108*, 356–388.

Hasher, L., & Zacks, R. T. (1984). Automatic processing of fundamental information: The case of frequency of occurrence. *American Psychologist, 39*, 1372–1388.

Hasher, L., & Zacks, R. T. (1988). Working memory, comprehension, and aging: A review and a new view. In G. H. Bower (Ed.), *The psychology of learning and motivation: Advances in research and theory. Vol. 22*. San Diego: Academic Press.

Hashtroudi, L., Chrosniak, L. D., & Schwartz, B. L. (1991). Effects of aging on priming and skill learning. *Psychology and Aging, 6*, 605–615.

Hashtroudi, S., Johnson, M. K., & Chrosniak, L. D. (1989). Aging and source monitoring. *Psychology and Aging, 4*, 106–112.

Hashtroudi, S., Johnson, M. K., & Chrosniak, L. D. (1990). Aging and qualitative characteristics of memories for perceived and imagined complex events. *Psychology and Aging, 5*, 119–126.

Hashtroudi, S., Parker, E. S., Luis, J. D., & Reisen, C. A. (1989). Generation and elaboration in older adults. *Experimental Aging Research, 15*, 73–78.

Haug, H., Barmwater, U., Eggers, R., Fischer, D., Kuhl, S., & Sass, N. L. (1983). Anatomical changes in the aging brain: Morphometric analysis of the prosencephalon. In J. Cervos-Navarro & H. I. Sarkander (Eds.), *Aging: Vol. 21. Brain aging: Neuropathology and neuropharmacology*. New York: Raven Press.

Hauge, G. (1987). *Aging and memory for conversations*. Doctoral dissertation, University of Missouri-Columbia.

Hayslip, B., & Kennelly, K. J. (1982). Short-term memory and crystallized-fluid intelligence in adulthood. *Research on Aging, 4*, 314–332.

Haywood, K. M. (1980). Coincidence-anticipation accuracy across the life span. *Experimental Aging Research, 6*, 451–462.

Hebb, D. O. (1961). Distinctive features of learning in the higher animal. In J. F. Delafresnaye (Ed.), *Brain mechanisms and learning*. New York: Oxford University Press.

Hebb, D. O. (1978). On watching myself get old. *Psychology Today, 12*, 15–23.

Hellebusch, S. J. (1976). On improving learning and memory in the aged: The effects of mnemonic strategy, transfer, and generalization. *Dissertation Abstracta International*, 1459-B (University Microfilms No. 76-19, 496).

Heller, R. B., & Dobbs, A. R. (1993). Age differences in word finding in discourse and nondiscourse situations. *Psychology and Aging, 8*, 443–450.

Helstrup, T. (1986). Separate memory laws for recall of performed acts? *Scandinavian Journal of Psychology, 27*, 1–29.

Herman, J. F., & Bruce, P. R. (1981). Spatial knowledge of ambulatory and wheelchair-confined nursing home residents. *Experimental Aging Research, 7*, 491–496.

Heron, A., & Chown, S. M. (1967). *Age and function*. London: Churchill.

Heron, A., & Craik, F. I. M. (1964). Age differences in cumulative learning of meaningful and meaningless material. *Scandinavian Journal of Psychology, 5*, 209–217.

Herrmann, D. J. (1979, December). *The validity of memory questionnaires as related to a theory of memory introspection*. Paper presented at the annual meeting of the British Psychological Association, London.

Herrmann, D. J., & Neisser, U. (1978). An inventory of everyday memory experiences. In M. M. Gruneberg, P. E. Morris, & R. N. Sykes (Eds.), *Practical aspects of memory*. New York: Academic Press.

Hertzog, C. K., Dixon, R. A., & Hultsch, D. F. (1990). Relationships between metamemory, memory predictions, and memory task performance. *Psychology and Aging, 5*, 215–223.

Hertzog, C. K., Dixon, R. A., Schulenberg, J. E., & Hultsch, D. F. (1987). On the differentiation of memory beliefs from memory knowledge: The factor structure of the Metamemory in Adulthood Scale. *Experimental Aging Research*, *13*, 101–107.

Hertzog, C. K., Hultsch, D. F., & Dixon, R. A. (1987, August). *What do metamemory questionnaires measure? A construct validation study*. Paper presented at the annual meeting of the American Psychological Association, New York.

Hertzog, C. K., Hultsch, D. F., & Dixon, R. A. (1989). Evidence for the convergent validity of two self-report metamemory questionnaires. *Developmental Psychology*, *25*, 687–700.

Hertzog, C. K., Raskind, C. L., & Cannon, C. J. (1986). Age-related slowing in semantic information processing speed: An individual differences analysis. *Journal of Gerontology*, *41*, 500–502.

Hertzog, C. K., Williams, M. V., & Walsh, D. A. (1976). The effect of practice on age differences in central perceptual processing. *Journal of Gerontology*, *31*, 428–433.

Herzog, A. R., & Rodgers, W. L. (1989). Age differences in memory performance and memory ratings as measured in a sample survey. *Psychology and Aging*, *4*, 173–182.

Hess, T. M. (1984). Effects of semantically related and unrelated contexts on recognition memory of different-aged adults. *Journal of Gerontology*, *39*, 444–451.

Hess, T. M. (1985). Aging and context influences on recognition memory for typical and atypical script actions. *Developmental Psychology*, *21*, 1139–1151.

Hess, T. M. (1990). Aging and schematic influences on memory. In T. M. Hess (Ed.), *Aging and cognition: Knowledge utilization and organization*. Amsterdam: North Holland.

Hess, T. M., & Arnould, D. (1986). Adult age differences in memory for explicit and implicit sentence information. *Journal of Gerontology*, *41*, 191–194.

Hess, T. M., Donley, J., & Vandermaas, M. O. (1989). Aging-related changes in the processing and retention of script information. *Experimental Aging Research*, *15*, 89–96.

Hess, T. M., & Flannagan, D. A. (1992). Schema-based retrieval processes in young and older adults. *The Journals of Gerontology: Psychological Sciences*, *47*, P52–58.

Hess, T. M., Flannagan, D. A., & Tate, C. (1993). Aging and memory for schematically vs. taxonomically organized verbal materials. *The Journals of Gerontology: Psychological Sciences*, *48*, P37–44.

Hess, T. M., & Higgins, J. N. (1983). Context utilization in young and old adults. *Journal of Gerontology*, *38*, 65–71.

Hess, T. M., & Slaughter, S. J. (1986a). Aging effects on prototype abstraction and concept identification. *Journal of Gerontology*, *41*, 214–221.

Hess, T. M., & Slaughter, S. J. (1986b). Specific exemplar retention and prototype abstraction in young and old adults. *Psychology and Aging*, *1*, 202–207.

Hess, T. M., & Slaughter, S. J. (1990). Schematic knowledge influences on memory for scene information in young and older adults. *Developmental Psychology*, *26*, 855–865.

Hess, T. M., & Tate, C. S. (1991). Adult age differences in explanations and memory for behavioral information. *Psychology and Aging*, *6*, 86–90.

Hess, T. M., Vandermaas, M. O., Donley, J., & Snyder, S. S. (1987). Memory for sex-role consistent and inconsistent actions in young and old adults. *Journal of Gerontology*, *42*, 505–511.

Hill, L. B. (1957). A second quarter century of delayed recall or relearning at 80. *Journal of Educational Psychology*, *48*, 65–68.

Hill, R. D., Allen, C., & Gregory, K. (1990). Self-generated mnemonics for enhancing free-recall performance in older learners. *Experimental Aging Research, 16*, 141–145.

Hill, R. D., Allen, C., & McWhorter, P. (1991). Stories as a mnemonic aid for older learners. *Psychology and Aging, 6*, 484–486.

Hill, R. D., Crook, T. H., Zadek, A., Sheikh, J. I., & Yesavage, J. (1989). The effects of age on recall of information from a simulated television news broadcast. *Educational Gerontology, 15*, 607–613.

Hill, R. D., Evankovich, K. D., Sheikh, J. I., & Yesavage, J. (1987). Imagery mnemonic training in a patient with primary degenerative dementia. *Psychology and Aging, 2*, 204–205.

Hill, R. D., Sheikh, J. I., & Yesavage, J. (1987). The effect of mnemonic training on perceived recall confidence. *Experimental Aging Research, 13*, 185–188.

Hill, R. D., Sheikh, J. I., & Yesavage, J. (1988). Pretraining enhances mnemonic training in elderly adults. *Experimental Aging Research, 14*, 207–211.

Hill, R. D., Storandt, M., & Malley, M. (1993). The impact of long-term exercise training on psychological function in older adults. *The Journals of Gerontology: Psychological Sciences, 48*, P12–17.

Hill, R. D., Storandt, M., & Simeone, D. (1990). The effects of memory skills training and incentives on free recall in older learners. *The Journals of Gerontology: Psychological Sciences, 45*, P227–232.

Hill, R. D., & Vandervoort, D. (1992). The effects of state anxiety on recall performance in older learners. *Educational Gerontology, 18*, 597–605.

Hill, R. D., Yesavage, J., Sheikh, J. I., & Friedman, L. (1989). Mental status as a predictor of response to memory training in older adults. *Educational Gerontology, 15*, 633–639.

Hill, W. F. (1990). *Learning: A survey of psychological interpretations (5th ed.).* New York: Harper & Row.

Hinrichs, J. V. (1970). A two-process memory-strength theory for judgment of recency. *Psychological Review, 77*, 223–233.

Hintzman, D. L., & Block, R. A. (1971). Repetition and memory: Evidence for a multiple-trace hypothesis. *Journal of Experimental Psychology, 88*, 297–306.

Hintzman, D. L., & Stern, L. D. (1978). Contextual variability and memory for frequency. *Journal of Experimental Psychology: Human Learning and Memory, 4*, 539–549.

Hodgkins, J. (1962). Influence of age on the speed of reaction and movement in females. *Journal of Gerontology, 17*, 385–389.

Hogan, R. M., & Kintsch, W. (1971). Differential effects of study and test trials on long-term recognition and recall. *Journal of Verbal Learning and Verbal Behavior, 10*, 562–567.

Holding, D. H. (1975). Sensory storage reconsidered. *Memory & Cognition, 3*, 31–41.

Holding, D. H., Noonan, T. K., Pfau, H. D., & Holding, C. S. (1986). Data attribution, age, and the distribution of lifetime memories. *Journal of Gerontology, 41*, 481–485.

Holland, C. A., & Rabbitt, P. M. A. (1990). Autobiographical and text recall in the elderly: An investigation of a processing resource. *Quarterly Journal of Experimental Psychology, 42A*, 441–470.

Holland, C. A., & Rabbitt, P. M. A. (1992). Effect of age-related reductions in processing resources on text recall. *The Journals of Gerontology: Psychological Sciences, 47*, P129–137.

Hooper, F. M., Hooper, J. O., & Colbert, K. C. (1984). *Personality and memory correlates of intellectual functioning: Young adulthood to old age.* Basel: Karger.

Horn, J. L., Donaldson, G., & Engstrom, R. (1981). Apprehension, memory, and fluid intelligence decline in adulthood. *Research on Aging, 3,* 33–84.

Howard, D. V. (1980). Category norms: A comparison of the Battig and Montague (1969) norms with the responses of adults between the ages of 20 and 80. *Journal of Gerontology, 35,* 225–231.

Howard, D. V. (1983a). *Cognitive psychology.* New York: Macmillan.

Howard, D. V. (1983b). The effects of aging and degree of association on the semantic priming of lexical decisions. *Experimental Aging Research, 9,* 145–151.

Howard, D. V. (1988a). Implicit and explicit assessment of cognitive aging. In M. L. Howe & C. J. Brainerd (Eds.), *Cognitive development in adulthood: Progress in cognitive development research.* New York: Springer-Verlag.

Howard, D. V. (1988b). Aging and memory activation: The priming of semantic and episodic memories. In L. L. Light & D. M. Burke (Eds.), *Language memory and aging.* New York: Cambridge University Press.

Howard, D. V. (in press). Implicit memory: An expanding picture of cognitive aging. In K. W. Schaie (Ed.), *Annual review of gerontology and geriatrics.* New York: Springer.

Howard, D. V., Fry, A. F., & Brune, C. M. (1991). Aging and memory for new associations: Direct versus indirect measures. *Journal of Experimental Psychology: Learning, Memory, and Cognition, 17,* 779–792.

Howard, D. V., Heisey, J. G., & Shaw, R. J. (1986). Aging and the priming of newly learned associations. *Developmental Psychology, 22,* 78–85.

Howard, D. V., & Howard, J. H., Jr. (1989). Age differences in learning serial patterns: Direct versus indirect measures. *Psychology and Aging, 4,* 357–364.

Howard, D. V., & Howard, J. H., Jr. (1992). Adult age differences in the rate of learning serial patterns: Evidence from direct and indirect tests. *Psychology and Aging, 7,* 232–241.

Howard, D. V., Lasaga, M. L., & McAndrews, M. P. (1980). Semantic activation during memory encoding across the adult life span. *Journal of Gerontology, 35,* 884–890.

Howard, D. V., McAndrews, M. P., & Lasaga, M. I. (1981). Semantic priming of lexical decisions in young and old adults. *Journal of Gerontology, 36,* 707–714.

Howard, D. V., Shaw, R. J., & Heisey, J. G. (1986). Aging and the time course of semantic activation. *Journal of Gerontology, 41,* 195–203.

Howe, M. L. (1988). Measuring memory development in adulthood: A model-based approach to disentangling storage-retrieval contributions. In M. L. Howe & C. J. Brainerd (Eds.), *Cognitive development in adulthood: Progress in cognitive development research.* New York: Springer-Verlag.

Howe, M. L., & Hunter, M. A. (1986). Long-term memory in adulthood: An examination of the development of storage and retrieval processes at acquisition and retention. *Developmental Review, 6,* 334–364.

Howell, S. (1972). Familiarity and complexity in perceptual recognition. *Journal of Gerontology, 27,* 364–371.

Howes, J. L., & Katz, A. N. (1988). Assessing remote memory with an improved public events questionnaire. *Psychology and Aging, 3,* 142–150.

Hoyer, F. W., Hoyer, W. J., Treat, N. J., & Baltes, P. B. (1978). Training response speed in young and elderly women. *International Journal of Aging and Human Development, 9,* 247–253.

Hoyer, W. J. (1985). Aging and the development of expert cognition. In T. M. Shlecter & M. P. Toglia (Eds.), *New directions in cognitive science*. Norwood, NJ: Ablex.

Hubbert, H. B. (1915). The effect of age on habit formation in the albino rat. *Behavior Monographs, 2*.

Hulicka, I. M. (1965a, April). *Age group comparisons for the use of mediators*. Paper presented at the annual meeting of the Southwestern Psychological Association, Oklahoma City, Oklahoma.

Hulicka, I. M. (1965b). Age differences for intentional and incidental learning and recall scores. *Journal of the American Geriatric Society, 13*, 639–648.

Hulicka, I. M. (1966). Age differences in Wechsler Memory Scale scores. *Journal of Genetic Psychology, 109*, 134–145.

Hulicka, I. M. (1967a). Age differences in retention as a function of interference. *Journal of Gerontology, 22*, 180–184.

Hulicka, I. M. (1967b). Age changes and age differences in memory functioning. *The Gerontologist, 7*, 46–54.

Hulicka, I. M. (1967c). Short-term learning and memory proficiency as a function of age and health. *Journal of the American Geriatric Society, 15*, 285–294.

Hulicka, I. M. (1982). Memory functioning in late adulthood. In F. I. M. Craik & S. Trehub (Eds.), *Advances in the study of communication and affect: Vol. 8. Aging and cognitive processes*. New York: Plenum Press.

Hulicka, I. M., & Grossman, J. L. (1967). Age-group comparisons for the use of mediators in paired associate learning. *Journal of Gerontology, 22*, 46–51.

Hulicka, I. M., & Rust, I. D. (1964). Age-related retention deficit as a function of learning. *Journal of the American Geriatric Society, 11*, 1061–1065.

Hulicka, I. M., Sterns, H., & Grossman, J. L. (1967). Age-group comparisons of paired-associate learning as a function of paced and self-paced association and response times. *Journal of Gerontology, 22*, 274–280.

Hulicka, I. M., & Weiss, R. L. (1965). Age differences in retention as a function of learning. *Journal of Consulting Psychology, 29*, 125–129.

Hull, C. L. (1943). *Principles of behavior*. New York: Appleton-Century-Crofts.

Hultsch, D. F. (1969). Adult age differences in the organization of free recall. *Developmental Psychology, 1*, 673–678.

Hultsch, D. F. (1971a). Organization and memory in adulthood. *Human Development, 14*, 16–29.

Hultsch, D. F. (1971b). Adult age differences in free classification and free recall. *Developmental Psychology, 4*, 338–342.

Hultsch, D. F. (1974). Learning to learn in adulthood. *Journal of Gerontology, 29*, 302–308.

Hultsch, D. F. (1975). Adult age differences in retrieval: Trace-dependent and cue-dependent forgetting. *Developmental Psychology, 11*, 197–201.

Hultsch, D. F., & Craig, E. R. (1976). Adult age differences in the inhibition of recall as a function of retrieval cues. *Developmental Psychology, 12*, 83–84.

Hultsch, D. F., & Dixon, R. A. (1983). The role of pre-experimental knowledge in text processing in adulthood. *Experimental Aging Research, 9*, 17–22.

Hultsch, D. F., & Dixon, R. A. (1984). Memory for text materials in adulthood. In P. B. Baltes & O. G. Brim, Jr. (Eds.), *Life-span development and behavior. Vol. 6*. New York: Academic Press.

Hultsch, D. F., & Dixon, R. A. (1989). Learning and memory and aging. In J. E. Birren & K. W. Schaie (Eds.), *Handbook of the psychology of aging. 3rd. ed..* New York: Van Nostrand Reinhold.

Hultsch, D. F., Hammer, M., & Small, B. (1993). Age differences in cognitive performance in later life: Relationships to self-reported health and activity lifestyle. *The Journal of Gerontology: Psychological Sciences, 48,* P1–11.

Hultsch, D. F., Hertzog, C., & Dixon, R. A. (1984). Text recall in adulthood: The role of intellectual abilities. *Developmental Psychology, 20,* 1193–1208.

Hultsch, D. F., Hertzog, C., & Dixon, R. A. (1987). Age differences in metamemory: Resolving the inconsistencies. *Canadian Journal of Psychology, 41,* 193–208.

Hultsch, D. F., Hertzog, C., & Dixon, R. A. (1990). Ability correlates of memory performance in adulthood and aging. *Psychology and Aging, 5,* 356–368.

Hultsch, D. F., Hertzog, C., Small, B., McDonald-Miszczak, L. & Dixon, R. A. (1992). Short-term longitudinal change in cognitive performance in later life. *Psychology and Aging, 7,* 546–550.

Hultsch, D. F., Masson, M., & Small, B. (1991). Adult age differences in direct and indirect tests of memory. *The Journals of Gerontology: Psychological Sciences, 46,* P22–30.

Hunt, M. E., & Roll, M. K. (1987). Simulation in familiarizing older people with an unknown building. *The Gerontologist, 27,* 169–175.

Hunt, R. R., & Einstein, G. O. (1981). Relational and item specific information in memory. *Journal of Verbal Learning and Verbal Behavior, 20,* 497–514.

Hunt, R. R., & Elliott, J. M. (1980). The role of nonsemantic information in memory: Orthographic distinctiveness effects on retention. *Journal of Experimental Psychology: General, 109,* 49–74.

Huppert, F. A., & Kopelman, M. D. (1989). Rates of forgetting in normal aging: A comparison with dementia. *Neupsychologia, 27,* 849–860.

Husband, R. W. (1930). Certain age effects on maze performance. *Journal of Genetic Psychology, 37,* 325–328.

Hyde, T. S., & Jenkins, J. J. (1969). Differential effects of incidental tasks on the organization of recall of a list of highly associated words. *Journal of Experimental Psychology, 82,* 472–481.

Hyland, D. T., & Ackerman, A. M. (1988). Reminiscence and autobiographical memory in the study of the personal past. *The Journals of Gerontology: Psychological Sciences, 41,* P35–39.

Inglis, J., & Ankus, M. N. (1965). Effects of age on short-term storage and serial rote learning. *British Journal of Psychology, 56,* 183–195.

Ingram, D. K., Weindruch, R., Spangler, E. L., Freeman, J. R., & Walford, R. L. (1987). Dietary restriction benefits learning and motor performance of aged mice. *Journal of Gerontology, 42,* 78–81.

Inman, V. W., & Parkinson, S. R. (1983). Differences in Brown-Peterson recall as a function of age and retention interval. *Journal of Gerontology, 38,* 58–64.

Jackson, D. K., & Schneider, H. G. (1982). Age differences in organization and recall: An analysis of rehearsal processes. *Psychological Reports, 50,* 919–924.

Jackson, J. D., & Kemper, S. (1993). Age differences in summarizing descriptive and procedural texts. *Experimental Aging Research, 19,* 39–52.

Jacoby, L. L. (1983). Remembering the data: Analyzing interactive processes in reading. *Journal of Verbal Learning and Verbal Behavior, 22*, 485–508.

Jacoby, L. L. (1992, November). *Strategic versus automatic influences of memory: Attention, awareness, and control.* Paper presented at the annual meeting of the Psychonomic Society, St. Louis, MO.

Jacoby, L. L., & Dallas, M. (1981). On the relationship between autobiographical memory and perceptual learning. *Journal of Experimental Psychology: General, 110*, 306–340.

Jacoby, L. L., Kelley, C. M., Brown, J., & Jasechko, J. (1989). Becoming famous over night: Limits on the ability to avoid unconscious influences of the past. *Journal of Personality and Social Psychology, 56*, 326–338.

Jacoby, L. L., Toth, J. P., & Yonelinas, A. P. (1993). Separating conscious and unconscious influences of memory: Measuring recollection. *Journal of Experimental Psychology: General, 122*, 139–154.

Jacoby, L. L., & Witherspoon, D. (1982). Remembering without awareness. *Canadian Journal of Psychology, 36*, 300–324.

Jahnke, J. C., Davis, S. T., & Bower, R. E. (1989). Position and order information in recognition memory. *Journal of Experimental Psychology: Learning, Memory, and Cognition, 15*, 859–867.

Jakubczak, L. F. (1973). Age and animal behavior. In C. Eisdorfer & M. P. Lawton (Eds.), *The psychology of adult development and aging.* Washington, D.C.: American Psychological Association.

James, W. (1890). *Principles of psychology.* New York: Henry Holt.

Jenkins, J. J. (1974). Remember that old theory of memory? Well forget it. *American Psychologist, 29*, 785–795.

Jenkins, J. J. (1979). Four points to remember: A tetrahedral model of memory experiments. In J. C. Cermak & F. I. M. Craik (Eds.), *Levels of processing in human memory.* Hillsdale, NJ: Erlbaum.

Jennings, J. M., & Jacoby, L. L. (1993). Automatic versus intentional uses of memory: Aging, attention, and control. *Psychology and Aging, 8*, 283–293.

Jensen, A. R. (1962a). An empirical theory of the serial-position effect. *Journal of Psychology, 53*, 127–142.

Jensen, A. R. (1962b). Transfer between paired-associate and serial learning. *Journal of Verbal Learning and Verbal Behavior, 1*, 269–280.

Jerome, E. A. (1959). Age and learning—experimental studies. In J. E. Birren (Ed.), *Handbook of aging and the individual.* Chicago: University of Chicago Press.

Johnson, L. K. (1973). *Changes in memory as a function of age.* Doctoral Dissertation, University of Southern California.

Johnson, M. K., & Raye, C. L. (1981). Reality monitoring. *Psychological Review, 88*, 67–85.

Johnson, M. K., Peterson, M. A., Yap, E. C., & Rose, P. M. (1989). Frequency judgments: The problem of defining a perceptual event. *Journal of Experimental Psychology: Learning, Memory, and Cognition, 15*, 126–136.

Johnson, M. M. S., Schmitt, F. A., & Pietrukowicz, M. (1989). The memory advantages of the generation effect: Age and process differences. *The Journals of Gerontology: Psychological Sciences, 44*, P91–94.

Johnson, N. F. (1978). The memorial structure of organized sequences. *Memory & Cognition, 6*, 233–239.

Johnson, P. J. (1967). Nature of mediational processes in concept-identification problems. *Journal of Experimental Psychology, 73*, 391–393.

Jones, D. M., & Macken, W. J. (1993). Irrelevant tones produce an irrelevant speech effect: Implications for phonological coding in working memory. *Journal of Experimental Psychology: Learning, Memory, and Cognition, 19*, 369–381.

Jones, H. E., Conrad, H. S., & Horn, A. (1928). Psychological studies of motion pictures: II. Observation and recall as a function of age. *California Publications in Psychology, 3*, 225–243.

Jonides, J., & Naveh-Benjamin, M. (1987). Estimating frequency of occurrence. *Journal of Experimental Psychology: Learning, Memory, and Cognition, 13*, 230–240.

Jordan, T. (1978). Age differences in visual and kinesthetic short-term memory. *Perceptual and Motor Skills, 46*, 667–674.

Jordan, T. C., & Rabbitt, P. M. A. (1977). Response times to stimuli of increasing complexity as a function of aging. *British Journal of Psychology, 68*, 189–201.

Kahn, H. L., Zarit, S. H., Hilbert, N. M., & Niederehe, G. A. (1975). Memory complaint and impairment in the aged: The effect of depression and altered brain function. *Archives of General Psychiatry, 32*, 1560–1573.

Kaufman, A. S. (1990). *Assessing adolescent and adult IQ*. Boston: Allyn & Bacon.

Kausler, D. H. (1963). Comparison of anticipation and recall methods for geriatric subjects. *Psychological Reports, 13*, 702.

Kausler, D. H. (1970). Retention-forgetting as a nomological network for developmental research. In L. R. Goulet & P. B. Baltes (Eds.), *Life-span developmental psychology: Research and theory*. New York: Academic Press.

Kausler, D. H. (1974). *Psychology of verbal learning and memory*. New York: Academic Press.

Kausler, D. H. (1978). Comments on Winn and Elias: Testing the rehearsal deficit hypothesis. *Experimental Aging Research, 4*, 343–347.

Kausler, D. H. (1980). Imagery ratings for young and elderly adults. *Experimental Aging Research, 6*, 185–188.

Kausler, D. H. (1985). Episodic memory: Memorizing performance. In N. Charness (Ed.), *Aging and human performance*. Chichester: John Wiley.

Kausler, D. H. (1989a). Comments on aging memory and its everyday operations. In L. W. Poon, D. C. Rubin, & B. A. Wilson (Eds.), *Everyday cognition in adulthood and late life*. New York: Cambridge University Press.

Kausler, D. H. (1989b). Impairment in normal memory aging: Implications of laboratory evidence. In G. C. Gilmore, P. J. Whitehouse, & M. L. Wykle (Eds.), *Memory and Aging*. New York: Springer.

Kausler, D. H. (1990a). Motivation, human aging, and cognitive performance. In J. E. Birren & K. W. Schaie (Eds.), *Handbook of the psychology of aging (3rd. ed.)*. San Diego: Academic Press.

Kausler, D. H. (1990b). Automaticity of encoding and episodic memory processes. In E. A. Lovelace (Ed.), *Aging and cognition: Mental processes, self awareness and interventions*. Amsterdam: North Holland.

Kausler, D. H. (1991). *Experimental psychology, cognition, and human aging*. New York: Springer-Verlag.

Kausler, D. H., & Hakami, M. K. (1982). Frequency judgments by young and elderly adults for relevant stimuli with simultaneously present irrelevant stimuli. *Journal of Gerontology, 37*, 438–442.

Kausler, D. H., & Hakami, M. K. (1983a). Memory for activities: Adult age differences and intentionality. *Developmental Psychology, 19*, 889–894.

Kausler, D. H., & Hakami, M. K. (1983b). Memory for topics of conversation: Adult age differences and intentionality. *Experimental Aging Research, 9*, 153–157.

Kausler, D. H., Hakami, M. K., & Wright, R. E. (1982). Adult age differences in frequency judgments of categorical representations. *Journal of Gerontology, 37*, 365–371.

Kausler, D. H., & Kanoti, G. A. (1963). R-S learning and negative transfer effects with a mixed list. *Journal of Experimental Psychology, 65*, 201–205.

Kausler, D. H., & Kleim, D. M. (1978). Age differences in processing relevant versus irrelevant stimuli in multiple item recognition learning. *Journal of Gerontology, 33*, 87–93.

Kausler, D. H., Kleim, D. M., & Overcast, T. D. (1975). Item recognition following a multiple-item study trial for young and middle-aged adults. *Experimental Aging Research, 2*, 243–250.

Kausler, D. H., & Lair, C. V. (1965). R-S ("backward") paired-associate learning in elderly subjects. *Journal of Gerontology, 20*, 29–31.

Kausler, D. H., & Lair, C. V. (1966). Associative strength and paired-associate learning in elderly subjects. *Journal of Gerontology, 21*, 278–280.

Kausler, D. H., & Lichty, W. (1988). Memory for activities: Rehearsal-independence and aging. In M. L. Howe & C. J. Brainerd (Eds.), *Cognitive development in adulthood: Progress in cognitive development research.* New York: Springer-Verlag.

Kausler, D. H., Lichty, W., & Davis, R. T. (1985). Temporal memory for performed activities: Intentionality and adult age differences. *Developmental Psychology, 21*, 1132–1138.

Kausler, D. H., Lichty, W., & Freund, J. S. (1985). Adult age differences in recognition memory and frequency judgments for planned activities. *Developmental Psychology, 21*, 647–654.

Kausler, D. H., Lichty, W., & Hakami, M. K. (1984). Frequency judgments for distractor items in a short-term memory task: Instructional variation and adult age differences. *Journal of Verbal Learning and Verbal Behavior, 23*, 660–668.

Kausler, D. H., Lichty, W., Hakami, M. K., & Freund, J. S. (1986). Activity duration and adult age differences in memory for activity performance. *Psychology and Aging, 1*, 80–81.

Kausler, D. H., Pavur, E. J., Jr., & Yadrick, R. M. (1975). Single-item recognition following a verbal discrimination study trial. *Memory & Cognition, 3*, 135–139.

Kausler, D. H., & Phillips, P. L. (1988). Instructional variation and adult age differences in activity memory. *Experimental Aging Research, 14*, 195–199.

Kausler, D. H., & Puckett, J. M. (1979). Effects of word frequency on adult age differences in word memory span. *Experimental Aging Research, 5*, 161–169.

Kausler, D. H., & Puckett, J. M. (1980a). Frequency judgments and correlated cognitive abilities in young and elderly adults. *Journal of Gerontology, 35*, 376–382.

Kausler, D. H., & Puckett, J. M. (1980b). Adult age differences in recognition memory for a nonsemantic attribute. *Experimental Aging Research, 6*, 349–355.

Kausler, D. H., & Puckett, J. M. (1981a). Adult age differences in memory for sex of voice. *Journal of Gerontology, 36*, 44–50.

Kausler, D. H., & Puckett, J. M. (1981b). Adult age differences in memory for modality attributes. *Experimental Aging Research, 7*, 117–125.

Kausler, D. H., Salthouse, T. A., & Saults, J. S. (1987). Frequency-of-occurrence memory over the adult lifespan. *Experimental Aging Research, 13*, 159–161.

Kausler, D. H., Salthouse, T. A., & Saults, J. S. (1988). Temporal memory over the adult lifespan. *American Journal of Psychology, 101*, 207–215.

Kausler, D. H., Trapp, E. P. (1960). Motivation and cue utilization in intentional and incidental learning. *Psychological Review, 67*, 373–379.

Kausler, D. H., & Wiley, J. G. (1990a). Effects of prior retrieval on adult age differences in long-term recall of activities. *Experimental Aging Research, 16*, 185–189.

Kausler, D. H., & Wiley, J. G. (1990b). Temporal memory and content memory for actions: Adult age differences in acquisition and retention, *Experimental Aging Research, 16*, 147–150.

Kausler, D. H., & Wiley, J. G. (1991). Effects of short-term retrieval on adult age differences in long-term recall of actions. *Psychology and Aging, 6*, 661–665.

Kausler, D. H., Wiley, J. G., & Lieberwitz, K. J. (1992). Adult age differences in short-term memory and subsequent long-term memory for actions. *Psychology and Aging, 7*, 309–316.

Kausler, D. H., Wiley, J. G., & Phillips, P. L. (1990). Adult age differences in memory for massed versus distributed repeated actions. *Psychology and Aging, 5*, 530–534.

Kausler, D. H., Wright, R. E., & Hakami, M. K. (1981). Variation in task complexity and adult age differences in frequency-of-occurrence judgments. *Bulletin of the Psychonomic Society, 18*, 196–197.

Kay, H. (1951). Learning of a serial task by different age groups. *Quarterly Journal of Experimental Psychology, 3*, 166–183.

Kay, H. (1954). The effects of position in a display upon problem solving. *Quarterly Journal of Experimental Psychology, 6*, 155–169.

Kay, H. (1955). Some experiments on adult learning. In *Old age in the modern world*. Edinburgh, Scotland: Livingstone.

Kear-Calwell, J. J., & Heller, M. (1978). A normative study of the Wechsler Memory Scale. *Journal of Clinical Psychology, 34*, 437–442.

Keele, S. W. (1968). Movement control in skilled motor performance. *Psychological Bulletin, 70*, 387–403.

Keevil-Rogers, P., & Schnore, M. M. (1969). Short-term memory as a function of age in persons of above average intelligence. *Journal of Gerontology, 24*, 184–188.

Keitz, S. M., & Gounard, B. R. (1976). Age differences in adults' free recall of pictorial and word stimuli. *Educational Gerontology, 1*, 237–241.

Kellas, G., McCauley, C., & McFarland, C. E. (1975). Re-examination of externalized rehearsal. *Journal of Experimental Psychology: Human Learning and Memory, 104*, 84–90.

Kemper, S. (1986). Initiation of complex syntactic constructions by elderly adults. *Applied Psycholinguistics, 7*, 277–288.

Kemper, S. (1987a). Syntactic complexity and elderly adults' prose recall. *Experimental Aging Research, 13*, 47–52.

Kemper, S. (1987b). Life-span changes in syntactic complexity. *Journal of Gerontology, 42*, 323–328.

Kemper, S. (1988). Geriatric psycholinguistics. In L. L. Light & D. M. Burke (Eds.),

Language, memory, and aging. New York: Cambridge University Press.

Kemper, S. (1992). Language and aging. In F. I. M. Craik & T. A. Salthouse (Eds.), *Handbook of aging and cognition.* Hillsdale, NJ: Erlbaum.

Kemper, S., Kynette, D., Rash, S., Sprott, R., & O'Brien, K. (1989). Life-span changes to adults' language: Effects of memory and genre. *Applied Psycholinguistics, 10,* 49–66.

Kendall, B. S. (1962). Memory for designs performance in the seventh and eighth decades of life. *Perceptual and Motor Skills, 14,* 399–405.

Kendler, H. H., & Kendler, T. S. (1962). Vertical and horizontal processes in human problem solving. *Psychological Review, 69,* 1–18.

Keppel, G., & Mallory, W. A. (1969). Presentation rate and instruction to guess in free recall. *Journal of Experimental Psychology, 79,* 269–275.

Keppel, G., & Underwood, B. J. (1962). Proactive inhibition in short-term retention of single items. *Journal of Verbal Learning and Verbal Behavior, 1,* 153–161.

Kerr, B. (1978). Task factors that influence selection and preparation for voluntary movements. In G. E. Stelmach (Ed.), *Information processing in motor control and learning.* New York: Academic Press.

Kimble, G. A., & Pennypacker, H. W. (1963). Eyelid conditioning in young and aged subjects. *Journal of Genetic Psychology, 103,* 283–289.

King, H. F. (1955). An age-analysis of some agricultural accidents. *Occupational Psychology, 29,* 245–255.

Kinsbourne, M. (1973). Age effects on letter span related to rate and sequential dependency. *Journal of Gerontology, 28,* 317–319.

Kinsbourne, M., & Berryhill, J. L. (1972). The nature of the interaction between pacing and the age decrement in learning. *Journal of Gerontology, 27,* 471–477.

Kintsch, W. (1974). *The representation of meaning in memory.* Hillsdale, NJ: Erlbaum.

Kintsch, W., & van Dijk, T. A. (1978). Toward a model of text comprehension and production. *Psychological Review, 85,* 363–394.

Kirasic, K. C. (1989). Acquisition and utilization of spatial information by elderly adults: Implications for day-to-day situations. In L. W. Poon, D. C. Rubin, & B. A. Wilson (Eds.), *Everyday cognition in adulthood and late life.* New York: Cambridge University Press.

Kirasic, K. C. (1991). Spatial cognition and behavior in young and elderly adults: Implications for learning new environments. *Psychology and Aging, 6,* 10–18.

Kirasic, K. C., & Allen, G. L. (1985). Aging, spatial performance, and spatial competence. In N. Charness (Ed.), *Aging and human performance.* Chichester: John Wiley.

Kirasic, K. C., Allen, G. L., & Haggerty, D. (1992). Age-related differences in adults' macrospatial processes. *Experimental Aging Research, 18,* 33–40.

Kirasic, K. C., & Bernicki, M. R. (1990). Acquisition of spatial knowledge under conditions of temporospatial discontinuity in young and elderly adults. *Psychological Record, 52,* 76–79.

Kirsner, K. (1972). Developmental changes in short-term recognition memory. *British Journal of Psychology, 63,* 109–117.

Kliegl, R., & Lindenberger, U. (1988, April). *Age related intrusion errors in cued recall.* Paper presented at the Second Cognitive Aging Conference, Atlanta, GA.

Kliegl, R., Smith, J., & Baltes, P. B. (1989). Testing-the-limits and the study of adult age differences in cognitive plasticity of a mnemonic skill. *Developmental Psychology, 25,*

247–256.

Kliegl, R., Smith, J., & Baltes, P. B. (1990). On the locus of magnification of age differences during mnemonic training. *Developmental Psychology, 26*, 894–904.

Kline, D. W., Culler, M. P., & Sucec, J. (1977). Differences in inconspicuous word identification as a function of age and reversible-figure training. *Experimental Aging Research, 3*, 203–213.

Knill, F. B. (1966). *The effect of visual and verbal mnemonic devices on the paired-associate learning of an aged population.* Master's Thesis, University of Richmond.

Knopf, M. (1992). The age decline in memory: Can it be eliminated? In N. Fabris, D. Harman, D. L. Knook, E. Steinhagen-Thiessen, & I. Za-Nagy (Eds.), *Pathological processes of aging: Towards a multicausal interpretation.* New York: Annals of the New York Academy of Sciences.

Knopf, M., & Neidhardt, E. (1989a). Aging and memory for action events: The role of familiarity. *Developmental Psychology, 25*, 780–786.

Knopf, M., & Neidhardt, E. (1989b). Gedactnis fur Handlungerf unterschiedlicher Vertrautheir-Hineweise aus entwicklungspsychologischen Studien. *Sprache & Kognition, 8*, 203–215.

Knopman, D. S., & Nissen, M. J. (1987). Implicit learning in patients with probable Alzheimer's disease. *Neurology, 37*, 784–788.

Korchin, S. J., & Basowitz, H. (1957). Age differences in verbal learning. *Journal of Abnormal and Social Psychology, 54*, 64–69.

Koriat, A., Ben-Zur, H., & Sheffer, D. (1988). Telling the same story twice: Output monitoring and age. *Journal of Memory and Language, 27*, 23–39.

Kral, A. V. (1962). Senescent forgetfulness: Benign and malignant. *Journal of the Canadian Medical Association, 86*, 257–260.

Krauss, I. K., Florini, B., & Bellos, N. S. (1985, March). *Microcomputer applications for the elderly.* Paper presented at the annual meeting of the Association of Gerontologists in Higher Education, Washington, D.C.

Kriauciunas, R. (1968). The relationship of age and retention interval activity in short term memory. *Journal of Gerontology, 23*, 169–173.

Kroll, N. E. A., Parks, T., Parkinson, S. P., Bieber, S. L., & Johnson, A. L. (1970). Short-term memory while shadowing: Recall of visually and aurally presented letters. *Journal of Experimental Psychology, 85*, 220–224.

Kynette, D., & Kemper, S. (1986). Aging and the loss of grammatical forms: A cross-sectional study of language performance. *Language and Communication, 6*, 65–72.

Kynette, D., Kemper, S., Norman, S., & Cheung, H. (1990). Adults' word recall and word repetition. *Experimental Aging Research, 16*, 117–122.

Labouvie, G. (1988, November). *Mind and self in life-span development.* Paper presented at the annual meeting of the Gerontological Society of America, Chicago, IL.

Labouvie-Vief, G., & Blanchard-Fields, F. (1982). Cognitive aging and psychological growth. *Aging and Society, 2*, 183–209.

Labouvie-Vief, G., & Schell, D. (1982). Learning and memory in later life. In B. Wolman & G. Stricker (Eds.), *Handbook of developmental psychology.* Englewood Cliffs, NJ: Prentice Hall.

Labouvie-Vief, G., Schell, D., & Weaverdyck, S. (1982). *Recall deficit in the aged: A fable recalled.* Unpublished manuscript, Wayne State University.

Lachman, J. L., Lachman, R., & Thronesbery, C. (1979). Metamemory through the adult life span. *Developmental Psychology, 15,* 543–551.

Lachman, M. E., Weaver, S. L., Bandura, E., & Lewkowicz, C. J. (1992). Improving memory and control beliefs through cognitive restructuring and self-generated strategies. *The Journals of Gerontology: Psychological Sciences, 47,* P293–299.

Lachman, R., & Lachman, J. L. (1980). Age and the actualization of knowledge. In L. W. Poon, J. L. Fozard, L. S. Cermak, D. Arenberg, & L. W. Thompson (Eds.), *New directions in memory and aging.* Hillsdale, NJ: Erlbaum.

Lachman, R., Lachman, J. L., & Taylor, D. W. (1982). Reallocation of mental resources over the productive lifespan: Assumptions and task analysis. In F. I. M. Craik & S. Trehub (Eds.), *Aging and cognitive processes.* New York: Plenum.

Lachman, R., Lachman, J. L., & Butterfield, E. C. (1979). *Cognitive psychology and information processing.* Hillsdale, NJ: Erlbaum.

Lair, C. V., Moon, W. H., & Kausler, D. H. (1969). Associative interference in the paired-associate learning of middle-aged and old subjects. *Developmental Psychology, 1,* 548–552.

Landauer, T. K., & Freedman, J. L. (1968). Information retrieval from long-term memory: Category size and recognition time. *Journal of Verbal Learning and Verbal Behavior, 7,* 291–295.

Lapidot, M. B. (1987). Does the brain age uniformly? Evidence from effects of smooth pursuit eye movements on verbal and visual tasks. *Journal of Gerontology, 42,* 329–331.

Larrabee, G. J., & Crook, T. H. (1993). Do men show more rapid age-associated decline in simulated everyday verbal memory than do women? *Psychology and Aging, 8,* 68–71.

Larrabee, G. J., & Levin, H. S. (1986). Memory self-ratings and objective test performance in a normal elderly sample. *Journal of Clinical and Experimental Neuropsychology, 8,* 275–284.

Larish, D. D., & Stelmach, G. E. (1982). Preprogramming, programming, and reprogramming as a function of age. *Journal of Motor Behavior, 14,* 322–340.

Lashley, K. S. (1915). The acquisition of skill in archery. *Papers from the Tortugas Laboratory of the Carnegie Institution of Washington, 7,* 105–128.

Lashley, K. S. (1951). The problem of serial order in behavior. In L. A. Jeffress (Ed.), *Cerebral mechanisms in behavior: The Hixon Symposium.* New York: John Wiley.

Lauer, P. A. (1976). *The effects of different types of word processing on memory performance in young and elderly adults.* Doctoral dissertation, University of Colorado, 1975). *Dissertation Abstracts International, 36,* 5833-B.

Laurence, M. W. (1966). Age differences in performance and subjective organization in the free recall of pictorial material. *Canadian Journal of Psychology, 20,* 388–399.

Laurence, M. W. (1967). Memory loss with age: A test of two strategies for its retardation. *Psychonomic Science, 9,* 209–210.

Laurence, M. W., & Trotter, M. (1971). Effect of acoustic factors and list organization in multitrial free recall learning of college and elderly adults. *Developmental Psychology, 5,* 202–210.

LeBreck, D., & Baron, A. (1987). Age and practice effects in continuous recognition memory. *Journal of Gerontology, 42,* 89–91.

Lee, C. L., & Estes, W. K. (1977). Order and position in primary memory for letter strings. *Journal of Verbal Learning and Verbal Behavior, 16,* 395–418.

Leech, S., & Witte, K. L. (1971). Paired-associate learning in elderly adults as related to pacing and incentive conditions. *Developmental Psychology, 5*, 180.

Lehman, E. B., & Mellinger, J. C. (1984). Effects of aging on memory for presentation modality. *Developmental Psychology, 20*, 1210–1217.

Lehman, E. B., & Mellinger, J. C. (1986). Forgetting rates in modality memory for young, midlife, and older women. *Psychology and Aging, 1*, 178–179.

Leirer, V. O., Morrow, D. G., Pariante, G., & Doksum, T. (1989). Increasing influence of vaccination through voice mail. *Journal of the American Geriatric Society, 37*, 1147–1150.

Leirer, V. O., Morrow, D. G., Sheikh, J. I., & Pariante, G. (1990). Memory skills elders want to improve. *Experimental Aging Research, 17*, 155–158.

Leon, G. R., Gillum, B., Gillum, R., & Gouze, M. (1979). Personality stability and change over a 30 year period—middle age to old age. *Journal of Counseling and Clinical Psychology, 47*, 517–524.

Leonard, J. A. (1953). Advance information in sensorimotor skills. *Quarterly Journal of Experimental Psychology, 5*, 141–149.

Leonard, J. A., & Newman, R. C. (1965). On the acquisition and maintenance of high speed and high accuracy in a key board task. *Ergonomics, 8*, 281–304.

Levin, S. R., Petros, T. V., & Filippi, K. (1980, September). *Memory for television content by young and old adults*. Paper presented at the annual meeting of the American Psychological Association, Montreal.

Lewandowski, L. J., Kobus, D. A., Flood, M. M., & Hoyer, W. J. (1988, August). *Effects of age and experience on sonar performance*. Paper presented at the annual meeting of the American Psychological Association, Atlanta, Georgia.

Ley, P. (1978). Memory for medical information. In M. M. Gruneberg, P. E. Morris, & R. N. Sykes (Eds.), *Everyday memory, actions and absentmindedness*. London: Academic Press.

Ley, P. (1979). Memory for medical information. *British Journal of Social and Clinical Psychology, 18*, 245–255.

Ley, P., Whitworth, M. A., Skillbeck, C. E., Woodward, R., Pinsent, R. J., Pike, L. A., Clarkson, M. E., & Clark, P. B. (1976). Improving doctor-patient communication in general practice. *Journal of Royal College of General Practitioners, 26*, 720–724.

Lichty, W. (1986). *Aging and memory for activities*. Doctoral dissertation, University of Missouri-Columbia.

Lichty, W., Kausler, D. H., & Martinez, D. R. (1986). Adult age differences in memory for motor versus cognitive activities. *Experimental Aging Research, 12*, 227–230.

Lichty, W., Bressie, S., & Krell, R. (1988). When a fork is not a fork: Recall of performed activities as a function of age, generation, and bizarreness. In M. M. Gruneberg, P. E. Morris, & R. N. Sykes (Eds.), *Practical aspects of memory: Current research and issues. Vol. 2.* Toronto: John Wiley.

Light, K. E., & Spirduso, W. W. (1990). Effects of adult aging on the movement complexity factor of response programming. *The Journals of Gerontology: Psychological Sciences, 45*, P107–109.

Light, L. L. (1988a). Language and aging: Competence versus performance. In J. E. Birren & V. L. Bengston (Eds.), *Emergent theories of aging*. New York: Springer.

Light, L. L. (1988b). Preserved implicit memory in old age. In M. M. Gruneberg, P. E.

Morris, & R. N. Sykes (Eds.), *Practical aspects of memory: Current research and issues. Vol. 2.* New York: John Wiley.

Light, L. L. (1991). Memory and aging: Four hypotheses in search of data. *Annual review of psychology, 42,* 333–376.

Light, L. L. (1992). The organization of memory in old age. In F. I. M. Craik & T. A. Salthouse (Eds.), *The handbook of aging and cognition.* Hillsdale, NJ: Erlbaum.

Light, L. L., & Albertson, S. A. (1988). Comprehension of pragmatic implications in young and older adults. In L. L. Light & D. M. Burke (Eds.), *Language, memory, and aging.* New York: Cambridge University Press.

Light, L. L., & Albertson, S. A. (1989). Direct and indirect tests of memory for category exemplars in young and older adults. *Psychology and Aging, 4,* 487–492.

Light, L. L., & Anderson, P. A. (1983). Memory for scripts in young and older adults. *Memory & Cognition, 11,* 435–444.

Light, L. L., & Anderson, P. A. (1985). Working-memory capacity, age, and memory for discourse. *Journal of Gerontology, 40,* 737–747.

Light, L. L., Berger, D. E., & Bardales, M. (1975). Trade-off between memory for verbal items and their visual attributes. *Journal of Experimental Psychology: Human Learning and Memory, 104,* 188–193.

Light, L. L., & Burke, D. M. (1988). Patterns of language and memory in old age. In L. L. Light & D. M. Burke (Eds.), *Language, memory, and aging.* New York: Cambridge University Press.

Light, L. L., & Capps, J. L. (1986). Comprehension of pronouns in young and older adults. *Developmental Psychology, 22,* 580–585.

Light, L. L., LaVoie, D., Valencia-Laver, D., Owens, S. A. A., & Mead, G. (1992). Direct and indirect measures of memory for modality in young and older adults. *Journal of Experimental Psychology: Learning, Memory, and Cognition, 18,* 1284–1297.

Light, L. L., & Singh, A. (1987). Implicit and explicit memory in young and older adults. *Journal of Experimental Psychology: Learning, Memory, and Cognition, 13,* 531–541.

Light, L. L., Singh, A., & Capps, J. L. (1986). The dissociation of memory and awareness in young and older adults. *Journal of Clinical Neuropsychology, 8,* 62–74.

Light, L. L., & Zelinski, E. M. (1983). Memory for spatial information in young and old adults. *Developmental Psychology, 19,* 901–906.

Light, L. L., Zelinski, E. M., & Moore, M. (1982). Adult age differences in reasoning from new information. *Journal of Experimental Psychology: Learning, Memory, and Cognition, 8,* 435–447.

Lima, S. D., Hale, S., & Myerson, J. (1991). How general is general slowing? Evidence from the lexical domain. *Psychology and Aging, 6,* 416–425.

Lindenberger, U., Kleigl, R., & Baltes, P. B. (1992). Professional expertise does not eliminate age differences in imagery-based memory performance during adulthood. *Psychology and Aging, 7,* 585–593.

Linton, M. (1975). Memory for real-world events. In D. A. Norman & D. E. Rumelhart (Eds.), *Explorations in cognition.* San Francisco: W. H. Freeman.

Lipman, P. D. (1991). Age and exposure differences in the acquisition of route information. *Psychology and Aging, 6,* 128–133.

Lipman, P. D., & Caplan, L. J. (1992). Adult age differences in memory for routes: Effects of instructions and spatial diagram. *Psychology and Aging, 7,* 435–442.

Liss, J. M., Weismer, G., & Rosenbek, J. C. (1990). Selected acoustic characteristics of speech production in very old males. *The Journals of Gerontology: Psychological Sciences*, 45, P35–45.

List, J. A. (1986). Age and schematic differences in the reliability of eyewitness testimony. *Developmental Psychology, 22*, 50–67.

Liu, Z., & Kausler, D. H. (1993). Adult age differences in acquisition and retention of frequency-of-occurrence information for actions. *Bulletin of the Psychonomic Society, 31*, 69–71.

Lockhart, R. S. (1988). Conceptual specificity in thinking and remembering. In G. M. Davies & D. M. Thomson (Eds.), *Memory in context: Context in memory*. New York: John Wiley.

Loewen, E. R., Shaw, R. J., & Craik, F. I. M. (1990). Age differences in components of metamemory. *Experimental Aging Research, 16*, 43–48.

Loftus, E. F., Freedman, J. L., & Loftus, G. R. (1970). Retrieval of words from subordinate hierarchies. *Psychonomic Science, 21*, 235–236.

Loftus, G. R. (1985). Evaluating forgetting curves. *Journal of Experimental Psychology: Learning, Memory, and Cognition, 11*, 397–406.

Logan, F. A. (1977). Hybrid theory of classical conditioning. In G. H. Bower (Ed.), *The psychology of learning and memory: Advances in theory and research (Vol. 11)*. New York: Academic Press.

Lorsbach, T. C. (1990). The buildup of PI as a function of temporal spacing and adult age. *American Journal of Psychology, 103*, 26–31.

Lorsbach, T. C., & Simpson, G. B. (1984). Age differences in the rate of processing in short-term memory. *Journal of Gerontology, 39*, 315–321.

Lovelace, E. A., & Cooley, S. (1982). Free associations of older adults to single words and conceptually related word triads. *Journal of Gerontology, 37*, 432–437.

Lovelace, E. A., & Marsh, G. R. (1985). Prediction and evaluation of memory performance by young and old adults. *Journal of Gerontology, 40*, 192–197.

Loveless, N. E., & Sanford, A. J. (1974). Effects of age on the contingent negative variation and preparatory set in a reaction-time task. *Journal of Gerontology, 29*, 52–63.

Lowenthal, M. F., Berkman, P. L., Beuhler, J. A., Pierce, R. C., Robinson, B. C., & Trier, M. L. (1967). *Aging and mental disorder in San Francisco*. San Francisco: Jossey-Bass.

Luszcz, M. A. (1993). Orienting tasks as moderators of narrative and expository text recall in adulthood. *Psychology and Aging, 8*, 56–58.

Luszcz, M. A., Roberts, T. H., & Mattiske, J. K. (1990). Use of relational and item-specific information in remembering by younger and older adults. *Psychology and Aging, 5*, 242–249.

Macht, M. L., & Buschke, H. (1983). Age differences in cognitive effort in recall. *Journal of Gerontology, 38*, 695–700.

Macht, M. L., & Buschke, H. (1984). Speed of recall in aging. *Journal of Gerontology, 39*, 439–443.

MacKinnon, D. F., & Squire, L. R. (1989). Autobiographical memory and amnesia. *Psychobiology, 17*, 247–256.

Madden, D. J. (1985). Age-related slowing in the retrieval of information from long-term memory. *Journal of Gerontology, 40*, 208–210.

Madden, D. J. (1986). Adult age differences in visual word recognition: Semantic encoding and episodic retention. *Experimental Aging Research, 12,* 71–78.

Madden, D. J. (1988). Adult age differences in the effects of sentence context and stimulus degradation during visual word recognition. *Psychology and Aging, 3,* 167–172.

Madden, D. J. (1989). Visual word identification and age-related slowing. *Cognitive Development, 4,* 1–29.

Madden, D. J. (1992). Four to ten milliseconds per year: Age-related slowing of visual word identification. *The Journals of Gerontology: Psychological Sciences, 47,* P59–68.

Madden, D. J., Blumenthal, J. A., Allen, P. A., & Emery, C. F. (1989). Improving aerobic capacity in healthy older adults does not necessarily lead to improved cognitive performance. *Psychology and Aging, 4,* 307–320.

Madden, D. J., & Greene, H. A. (1987). From retina to response: Contrast sensitivity and memory retrieval during visual word recognition. *Experimental Aging Research, 13,* 15–21.

Madden, D. J., & Nebes, R. D. (1980). Aging and the development of automaticity in visual search. *Developmental Psychology, 16,* 377–384.

Madigan, S. A. (1971). Modality and order interactions in short-term memory for serial order. *Journal of Experimental Psychology, 87,* 294–296.

Maisto, A. A., & Queen, D. E. (1992). Memory for pictorial information and the picture superiority effect. *Educational Gerontology, 18,* 213–223.

Maki, R. H., & Ostby, R. S. (1987). Effects of level of processing and rehearsal on frequency judgments. *Journal of Experimental Psychology: Learning, Memory, and Cognition, 13,* 151–163.

Mandel, R. G., & Johnson, N. S. (1984). A developmental analysis of story recall and comprehension in adulthood. *Journal of Verbal Learning and Verbal Behavior, 23,* 643–659.

Mandler, G. (1967). Verbal learning. In G. Mandler, P. Mussen, N. Kogan, & M. A. Wallach (Eds.), *New directions in psychology III.* New York: Holt, Rinehart, & Winston.

Mandler, G. (1979). Organization, memory, and mental structures. In C. R. Puff (Ed.), *Memory, organization and structure.* New York: Academic Press.

Mandler, G. (1980). Recognizing: The judgment of previous occurrence. *Psychological Review, 87,* 252–271.

Mandler, G., & Pearlstone, Z. (1966). Free and constrained concept learning and subsequent recall. *Journal of Verbal Learning and Verbal Behavior, 5,* 126–131.

Manning, S. K., & Greenhut-Wertz, J. (1990). Visual and auditory modality and suffix effects in young and elderly adults. *Experimental Aging Research, 16,* 3–10.

Mäntylä, T. (1993). Knowing but not remembering: Adult age differences in recollective experience. *Memory & Cognition, 21,* 379–388.

Mäntylä, T. (in press a). Priming effects in prospective memory. *Memory, 1.*

Mäntylä, T. (in press, b). Remembering to remember: Adult age differences in prospective memory. *The Journals of Gerontology: Psychological Sciences.*

Mäntylä, T., & Bäckman, L. (1990). Encoding variability and age-related retrieval failures. *Psychology and Aging, 5,* 545–550.

Mäntylä, T., & Bäckman, L. (1992). Aging and memory for expected and unexpected objects in real-world settings. *Journal of Experimental Psychology: Learning, Memory, and Cognition, 18,* 1298–1309.

Marinesco, G., & Kreindler, A. (1934). Des réflexes conditionnels, troisième partie: Application des réflexes conditionnels à certains problèmes cliniques. *Journal Psychologie, 31*, 722–791.

Marks, L. E., & Miller, G. A. (1964). The role of semantic and syntactic constraints in the memorization of English sentences. *Journal of Verbal Learning and Verbal Behavior, 3*, 1–5.

Marshall, P. H., Elias, J. W., Webber, S. M., Gist, B. A., Winn, F. J., King, P., & Moore, S. A. (1978). Age differences in verbal mediation: A structural and functional analysis. *Experimental Aging Research, 4*, 175–193.

Marshall, P. H., Elias, J. W., & Wright, J. (1985). Age related factors in motor error detection and correction. *Experimental Aging Research, 11*, 201–206.

Martin, A. (1987). Representation of semantic and spatial knowledge in Alzheimer's patients: Implications for models of preserved learning in amnesia. *Journal of Clinical and Experimental Neuropsychology, 9*, 191–224.

Martin, M. (1986). Aging and patterns of change in everyday memory. *Human Learning, 5*, 63–74.

Maskarinec, A. S., & Brown, S. C. (1974). Positive and negative recency effects in free recall learning. *Journal of Verbal Learning and Verbal Behavior, 16*, 328–334.

Mason, S. E. (1979). Effects of orienting tasks on the recall and recognition performance of subjects differing in age. *Developmental Psychology, 15*, 467–469.

Mason, S. E. (1986). Age and gender as factors in facial recognition and identification. *Experimental Aging Research, 12*, 151–154.

Mason, S. E., & Smith, A. D. (1977). Imagery in the aged. *Experimental Aging Research, 3*, 17–32.

May, C. P., Hasher, L., & Stoltzfus, E. R. (1993). Optimal time of day and the magnitude of age differences in memory. *Psychological Science, 4*, 326–330.

Maylor, E. A. (1990a). Age and prospective memory. *Quarterly Journal of Experimental Psychology, 42A*, 471–493.

Maylor, E. A. (1990b). Recognizing and naming faces: Aging, memory retrieval, and the tip of the tongue state. *The Journals of Gerontology: Psychological Sciences, 45*, P215–226.

Maylor, E. A. (1990c). Age, blocking, and the tip of the tongue state. *British Journal of Psychology, 81*, 123–134.

Maylor, E. A. (1991). Remembering and naming tunes: Memory impairment in the elderly. *The Journals of Gerontology: Psychological Sciences, 46*, P207–217.

Maylor, E. A. (1993). Aging and forgetting in prospective and retrospective memory tasks. *Psychology and Aging, 8*, 420–428.

McCarthy, M., Ferris, S. H., Clark, E., & Crook, T. M. (1981). Acquisition and retention of categorized material in normal aging and senile dementia. *Experimental Aging Research, 7*, 127–136.

McCarty, D. L. (1980). Investigation of a visual imagery mnemonic device for acquiring face-name associations. *Journal of Experimental Psychology: Human Learning and Memory, 6*, 145–155.

McClelland, J. L., & Rumelhart, D. E. (1985). Distributed memory and the representation of general and specific information. *Journal of Experimental Psychology: General, 114*, 158–188.

McCormack, P. D. (1979). Autobiographical memory in the aged. *Canadian Journal of Psychology, 33*, 118–124.

McCormack, P. D. (1981). Temporal coding by young and elderly adults: A test of the Hasher-Zacks model. *Developmental Psychology, 17*, 509–515.

McCormack, P. D. (1982a). Temporal coding and study-phase retrieval in young and elderly adults. *Bulletin of the Psychonomic Society, 20*, 242–244.

McCormack, P. D. (1982b). Coding of spatial information by young and elderly adults. *Journal of Gerontology, 37*, 80–86.

McCormack, P. D. (1984). Aging and recognition memory: Methodological and interpretive problems. *Experimental Aging Research, 10*, 215–219.

McCrae, R. R., Arenberg, D., & Costa, P. T., Jr. (1987). Declines in divergent thinking with age: Cross-sectional, longitudinal and cross-sequential analyses. *Psychology and Aging, 2*, 130–137.

McDaniel, M. A., Einstein, G. O., Dunay, P. K., & Cobb, R. E. (1986). Encoding difficulty and memory: Toward a unifying theory. *Journal of Memory and Language, 25*, 645–656.

McDaniel, M. A., Ryan, E. B., & Cunningham, C. J. (1989). Encoding difficulty and memory enhancement for young and older readers. *Psychology and Aging, 4*, 333–338.

McDowd, J. M. (1986). The effects of age and extended practice on divided attention performance. *Journal of Gerontology, 41*, 764–769.

McDowd, J. M., & Botwinick, J. (1984). Rote and gist memory in relation to type of information, sensory mode, and age. *Journal of Genetic Psychology, 145*, 167–178.

McElroy, L. A., & Slamecka, N. J. (1982). Memorial consequences of generating nonwords: Implications for semantic memory interpretations of the generation effect. *Journal of Verbal Learning and Verbal Behavior, 21*, 249–259.

McEvoy, C. L., & Holley, P. E. (1990). Aging and the stability of activation and sampling in cued recall. *Psychology and Aging, 5*, 589–596.

McEvoy, C. L., & Moon, J. N. (1988). Assessment and treatment of everyday memory problems in the elderly. In M. M. Gruneberg, P. E. Morris, & R. N. Sykes (Eds.), *Practical aspects of memory: Current research and issues. Vol. 1.* Chichester: John Wiley.

McEvoy, C. L., Nelson, D. L., Holley, P. E., & Stelnicki, G. S. (1992). Implicit processing in the cued recall of young and old adults. *Psychology and Aging, 7*, 401–408.

McFarland, C. E., Jr., Frey, T. J., & Rhodes, D. D. (1980). Retrieval of internally versus externally generated words. *Journal of Verbal Learning and Verbal Behavior, 19*, 21–225.

McFarland, C. E., Jr., Warren, L. R., & Crockard, J. (1985). Memory for self-generated stimuli in young and old adults. *Journal of Gerontology, 40*, 206–207.

McFarland, R. A., & O'Doherty, B. M. (1959). Work and occupational skills. In J. E. Birren (Ed.), *Handbook of aging and the individual.* Chicago: University of Chicago Press.

McGhie, A. N., Chapman, J., & Lawson, J. S. (1965). Changes in immediate memory with age. *British Journal of Psychology, 56*, 69–75.

McGuire, L. C. (1993, June). *What the patient really remembers: The effect of information organization on recall.* Poster presented at the annual meeting of the American Psychological Society, Chicago, IL.

McIntyre, J. S., & Craik, F. I. M. (1987). Age differences in memory for item and source information. *Canadian Journal of Psychology, 41*, 175–192.

McKoon, G., & Ratcliff, R. (1979). Priming in episodic and semantic memory. *Journal of Verbal Learning and Verbal Behavior, 18*, 463–480.

McKoon, G., & Ratcliff, R. (1980). Priming in item recognition: The organization of propositions in memory for text. *Journal of Verbal Learning and Verbal Behavior, 19,* 369–386.

McKoon, G., Ratcliff, R., & Dell, G. S. (1986). A critical evaluation of the semantic-episodic distinction. *Journal of Experimental Psychology: Learning, Memory, and Cognition, 12,* 295–306.

McNulty, J. A., & Caird, W. (1966). Memory loss with age: Retrieval or storage? *Psychological Reports, 19,* 229–230.

Meacham, J. A., Leiman, B. (1975, September). *Remembering to perform future actions.* Paper presented at the annual meeting of the American Psychological Association, Chicago.

Mellinger, J. C., Lehman, E. B., Happ, L. K., & Grout, L. A. (1990). Cognitive effort in modality retrieval by young and older adults. *Experimental Aging Research, 16,* 35–42.

Melton, A. W. (1970). The situation with respect to the spacing of repetitions and memory. *Journal of Verbal Learning and Verbal Behavior, 9,* 596–606.

Melton, A. W., & Irwin, J. McD. (1940). The influence of degree of interpolated learning on retroactive inhibition and the overt transfer of specific responses. *American Journal of Psychology, 53,* 173–203.

Menich, S. R., & Baron, A. (1990). Age-related effects of reinforced practice on recognition memory: Consistent versus varied stimulus-response relations. *The Journals of Gerontology: Psychological Sciences, 45,* P88–93.

Mergler, N. L., Dusek, J. B., & Hoyer, W. J. (1977). Central/incidental recall and selective attention in young and elderly adults. *Experimental Aging Research, 3,* 49–60.

Mergler, N. L., & Goldstein, M. D. (1983). Why are there old people? Senescence as biological and cultural preparedness for the transmission of information. *Human Development, 26,* 72–90.

Merikle, P. M. (1980). Selection from visual persistence by perceptual groups and category membership. *Journal of Experimental Psychology: General, 109,* 279–295.

Meyer, B. J. F., & Rice, G. E. (1981). Information recalled from prose by young, middle and old readers. *Experimental Aging Research, 7,* 253–268.

Meyer, B. J. F., & Rice, G. E. (1983). Learning and memory from text across the adult life span. In J. Fine & R. O. Freedle (Eds.), *Developmental studies in discourse.* Norwood, NJ: Albex.

Meyer, B. J. F., & Rice, G. E. (1989). Prose processing in adulthood: The text, the reader, and the task. In L. W. Poon, D. C. Rubin, & B. A. Wilson (Eds.), *Everyday cognition in adulthood and late life.* New York: Cambridge University Press.

Meyer, B. J. F., Rice, G. E., Knight, C. C., & Jessen, J. L. (1979). Effects of comparative and descriptive types on the reading performance of young, middle, and old adults. *Research Report No. 7, Prose Learning Series.* Tempe, AZ: Department of Educational Psychology, Arizona State University.

Meyer, D., & Schvaneveldt, R. W. (1971). Facilitation in recognizing pairs of words: Evidence of a dependence between retrieval operations. *Journal of Experimental Psychology, 90,* 227–234.

Miles, W. R. (1931a). Measures of certain human abilities throughout the life span. *Proceedings of the National Academy of Science, U.S.A., 17,* 627–633.

Miles, W. R. (1931b). Correlation of reaction and coordination speed with age in adults. *American Journal of Psychology, 43,* 377–391.

Milgram, S., Greenwald, J., Kessler, S., McKenna, W., & Walters, J. (1972). A psychological map of New York City. *American Scientist, 60,* 194–200.

Miller, G. A. (1956). The magical number seven plus or minus two. Some limits on our capacity for processing information. *Psychological Review, 63,* 81–97.

Miller, G. A., Galanter, E., & Pribram, K. H. (1960). *Plans and the structure of behavior.* New York: Holt, Rinehart, & Winston.

Miller, G. A., & Selfridge, J. A. (1950). Verbal context and the recall of meaningful material. *American Journal of Psychology, 63,* 176–185.

Milligan, W. L., Powell, D. A., Harley, C., & Furchtgott, E. (1984). A comparison of physical health and psychosocial variables as predictors of reaction time and serial learning. *Journal of Gerontology, 39,* 704–710.

Milner, B. (1962). Les troubles des lésions hippocampiques bilatérales. In *Physiologie de Hippocampe.* Centre National de la Recherche Scientifique, Paris.

Mistler-Lachman, J. L. (1977). Spontaneous shift in encoding dimensions among elderly subjects. *Journal of Gerontology, 32,* 68–72.

Mitchell, D. B. (1989). How many memory systems? Evidence from aging. *Journal of Experimental Psychology: Learning, Memory, and Cognition, 15,* 31–49.

Mitchell, D. B., Brown, A. S., & Murphy, D. R. (1990). Dissociations between procedural and episodic memory: Effects of time and aging. *Psychology and Aging, 5,* 264–276.

Mitchell, D. B., Hunt, R. R., & Schmitt, F. A. (1986). The generation effect and reality monitoring: Evidence from dementia and normal aging. *Journal of Gerontology, 41,* 79–84.

Mitchell, D. B., & Perlmutter, M. (1986). Semantic activation and episodic memory: Age similarities and differences. *Developmental Psychology, 22,* 86–94.

Mittenberg, W., Seidenberg, M., O'Leary, D. S., & DiGuilo, D. V. (1989). Changes in cerebral functioning associated with normal aging. *Journal of Clinical and Experimental Neuropsychology, 11,* 918–932.

Modigliani, V., & Hedges, D. G. (1987). Distributed rehearsals and the primacy effect in single-trial free recall. *Journal of Experimental Psychology: Learning, Memory, and Cognition, 13,* 426–436.

Moenster, P. A. (1972). Learning and memory in relation to age. *Journal of Gerontology, 27,* 361–363.

Molander, B., & Bäckman, L. (1990). Age differences in the effects of background noise on motor and memory performance in a precision sport. *Experimental Aging Research, 16,* 55–60.

Monge, R. H. (1969). Learning in the adult years: Set or rigidity? *Human Development, 12,* 131–140.

Monge, R. H. (1971). Studies of verbal learning from the college years through middle age. *Journal of Gerontology, 26,* 324–329.

Monge, R. H., & Hultsch, D. F. (1971). Paired-associate learning as a function of adult age and the length of the anticipation and inspection intervals. *Journal of Gerontology, 26,* 157–162.

Mook, D. D. (1989). The myth of external validity. In L. W. Poon, D. C. Rubin, & B. A. Wilson (Eds.), *Everyday cognition in adulthood and late life.* New York: Cambridge University Press.

Moore, T. E., Richards, B., & Hood, J. (1984). Aging and the coding of spatial information. *Journal of Gerontology, 39*, 210–212.

Moray, N., Bates, A., & Barnett, T. (1965). Experiments on the four-eared man. *Journal of the Acoustical Society of America, 38*, 196–201.

Morrell, R. W., Park, D. C., & Poon, L. W. (1989). Quality of instructions on prescription drug labels: Effects on memory and comprehension in young and old adults. *The Gerontologist, 29*, 345–354.

Morrell, R. W., Park, D. C., & Poon, L. W. (1990). Effects of labelling techniques on memory and comprehension on prescription information in young and older adults. *The Journals of Gerontology: Psychological Sciences, 45*, P166–172.

Morris, C. D., Bransford, J. D., & Franks, J. J. (1977). Levels of processing versus transfer appropriate processing. *Journal of Verbal Learning and Verbal Behavior, 16*, 519–533.

Morris, R. G., Gick, M. L., & Craik, F. I. M. (1988). Processing resources and age differences in working memory. *Memory & Cognition, 16*, 362–366.

Morrow, D. G., Altieri, P., & Leirer, von O. (1992). Aging, narrative organization, presentation mode, and reference choice strategies. *Experimental Aging Research, 18*, 75–84.

Morrow, D. G., Leirer, von O., & Altieri, P. A. (1992). Aging, expertise, and narrative processing. *Psychology and Aging, 7*, 376–388.

Morrow, D. G., Leirer, von O., & Sheikh, J. (1988). Adherence and medication instructions: Review and recommendations. *Journal of the American Geriatric Society, 36*, 1147–1160.

Morrow, D. G., Leirer, von O., & Tanke, E. (1991). Elders' scheme for taking medication: Implications for instruction design. *The Journals of Gerontology: Psychological Sciences, 46*, P378–385.

Morrow, D. G., Leirer, von O., & Yesavage, J. (1990). The influence of alcohol and aging on radio communication during flight. *Aviation, Space, & Environmental Medicine, 61*, 12–20.

Morrow, D. G., Yesavage, J., Leirer, von O., & Tinklenberg, J. (1993). Influence of aging and practice on piloting tasks. *Experimental Aging Research, 19*, 53–70.

Mortimer, J. A., Pirozzolo, F. J., & Maletta, G. J. (1982). *The aging motor system.* New York: Praeger.

Morton, J. (1969). Interaction of information in word recognition. *Psychological Review, 76*, 165–178.

Moscovitch, M. (1982). A neuropsychological approach to perception and memory in normal and pathological aging. In F. I. M. Craik & S. Trehub (Eds.), *Aging and cognitive processes.* New York: Plenum Press.

Moscovitch, M., & Winocur, G. (1983). Contextual cues and release from proactive inhibition in old and young people. *Canadian Journal of Psychology, 37*, 331–344.

Moscovitch, M., Winocur, G., & McLachlan, D. (1986). Memory as assessed by recognition and reading time in normal and memory-impaired people with Alzheimer's Disease and other neurological disorders. *Journal of Experimental Psychology: General, 115*, 331–347.

Mueller, D. J., & Atlas, L. (1972). Resocialization of regressed elderly residents: A behavioral management approach. *Journal of Gerontology, 27*, 390–392.

Mueller, J. H., Kausler, D. H., & Faherty, A. (1980). Age and access time for different memory codes. *Experimental Aging Research, 6*, 445–450.

Mueller, J. H., Kausler, D. H., Faherty, A., & Oliveri, M. (1980). Reaction time as a function of age, anxiety and typicality. *Bulletin of the Psychonomic Society*, 16, 473–476.

Mueller, J. H., Rankin, J. L., & Carlomusto, M. (1979). Adult age differences in free recall as a function of basis of organization and method of presentation. *Journal of Gerontology*, 34, 375–380.

Müller, G. E., & Pilzecker, A. (1900). Experimentelle Beitrage zur lehre vom gedactnisses. *Zeitschrift fur Psychologie*, Erganzungsband.

Murphy, M. D., Sanders, R. E., Gabriesheski, A. S., & Schmitt, F. A. (1981). Metamemory in the aged. *Journal of Gerontology*, 25, 268–274.

Murphy, M. D., Schmitt, F. A., Caruso, M. J., & Sanders, R. E. (1987). Metamemory in older adults: The role of monitoring in serial recall. *Psychology and Aging*, 2, 331–339.

Murrell, F. H. (1970). The effect of extensive practice on age differences in reaction time. *Journal of Gerontology*, 25, 268–274.

Myerson, J., Ferraro, F. R., Hale, S., & Lima, S. D. (1992). General slowing in semantic priming and word recognition. *Psychology and Aging*, 7, 257–270.

Myerson, J., Hale, S., Wagstaff, D., Poon, L. W., & Smith, G. A. (1990). The information loss model: A mathematical theory of age-related cognitive slowing. *Psychological Review*, 97, 475–487.

Nappe, G. W., & Wollen, K. A. (1973). Effects of instructions to form common and bizarre mental images on retention. *Journal of Experimental Psychology*, 100, 6–8.

Naveh-Benjamin, M. (1987). Coding of spatial location: An automatic process? *Journal of Experimental Psychology: Learning, Memory, and Cognition*, 13, 595–605.

Naveh-Benjamin, M. (1988). Recognition memory of spatial location: Another failure to support automaticity. *Memory & Cognition*, 16, 437–445.

Naveh-Benjamin, M. (1990). Coding of temporal order information. *Journal of Experimental Psychology: Learning, Memory, and Cognition*, 16, 117–126.

Naveh-Benjamin, M., & Jonides, J. (1984). Maintenance rehearsal: A two-component analysis. *Journal of Experimental Psychology: Learning, Memory, and Cognition*, 10, 369–385.

Naveh-Benjamin, M., & Jonides, J. (1986). On the automaticity of frequency coding: Effects of competing task load, encoding strategy, and intention. *Journal of Experimental Psychology: Learning, Memory, and Cognition*, 12, 378–386.

Nebes, R. D. (1978). Vocal versus manual responses as a determinant of age differences in simple reaction time. *Journal of Gerontology*, 33, 884–889.

Nebes, R. D., & Andrews-Kulis, M. E. (1976). The effect of age on the speed of sentence formation and incidental-learning. *Experimental Aging Research*, 2, 315–331.

Neely, A. S., & Bäckman, L. (1993a). Maintenance of gains following multifactorial and unifactorial memory training in late adulthood. *Educational Gerontology*, 19, 105–117.

Neely, A. S., & Bäckman, L. (1993b). Long-term maintenance of gains from memory training in older adults: Two 3½ year follow-up studies. *The Journals of Gerontology: Psychological Sciences*, 48, P233–237.

Neely, J. H. (1977). Semantic priming and retrieval from lexical memory: Roles of inhibitionless spreading activation and limited capacity attention. *Journal of Experimental Psychology: General*, 106, 226–254.

Nehrke, M. F. (1973). Age and sex differences in discrimination learning and transfer of training. *Journal of Gerontology*, 28, 320–327.

Nehrke, M. F., & Coppinger, N. W. (1971). The effect of task dimensionality on discrimination learning and transfer of training in the aged. *Journal of Gerontology, 26,* 151–156.

Nehrke, M. F., & Sutterer, J. R. (1978). The effects of overtraining on mediational processes in elderly males. *Experimental Aging Research, 4,* 207–221.

Neisser, U. (1967). *Cognitive psychology.* New York: Appleton-Century-Crofts.

Nelson, D. L., Keelean, P. D., & Negrao, M. (1989). Word-fragment cuing: The lexical search hypothesis. *Journal of Experimental Psychology: Learning, Memory, and Cognition, 15,* 388–397.

Nelson, D. L., Schreiber, T. A., & McEvoy, C. L. (1992). Processing implicit and explicit representations. *Psychological Review, 99,* 322–348.

Nelson, T. O. (1977). Repetition and depth of processing. *Journal of Verbal Learning and Verbal Behavior, 16,* 151–172.

Newman, C. W., & Spitzer, J. B. (1983). Prolonged auditory processing time in the elderly: Evidence from a backward recognition-masking paradigm. *Audiology, 22,* 241–252.

Niederehe, G., & Camp, C. J. (1985). Signal detection analysis of recognition memory in depressed elderly. *Experimental Aging Research, 11,* 207–213.

Niederehe, G., Nielsen-Collins, K. E., Volpendesta, D., & Woods, A. M. (1981, November). *Metamemory processes and perceptions: Depression and age effects.* Paper presented at the annual meeting of the Gerontological Society of America, Toronto.

Nissen, M. J., & Bullemer, P. (1987). Attentional requirements of learning: Evidence from performance measures. *Cognitive Psychology, 19,* 1–32.

Noble, C. E., Baker, B. L., & Jones, T. A. (1964). Age and sex parameters in psychomotor learning. *Perceptual and Motor Skills, 19,* 935–945.

Noble, S. G. (1922). The acquisition of skill in the throwing of basket goals. *School and Society, 16,* 640–644.

Norman, D. A., & Wickelgren, W. A. (1965). Short-term recognition memory for single digits and pairs of digits. *Journal of Experimental Psychology, 70,* 479–489.

Norman, S., Kemper, S. Kynette, D. (1992). Adults' reading comprehension: Effects of syntactic complexity and working memory. *The Journals of Gerontology: Psychological Sciences, 47,* P258–265.

Norman, S., Kemper, S., Kynette, D. Cheung, H., & Anagnopoulos, C. (1991). Syntactic complexity and adults' running memory span. *The Journals of Gerontology: Psychological Sciences, 46,* P346–351.

Norris, M. P., & West, R. L. (1988, August). *Age differences in activity memory.* Poster presented at the annual meeting of the American Psychological Association, Atlanta, GA.

Norris, M. P., & West, R. L. (1990). Adult age differences in activity memory. In T. M. Hess (Ed.), *Aging and cognition: Knowledge organization and utilization.* Amsterdam: North Holland.

Norris, M. P., & West, R. L. (1991). Age differences in the recall of actions and cognitive activities: The effects of presentation rate and object cues. *Psychological Research, 53,* 188–194.

Norris, M. P., & West, R. L. (1993). Activity memory and aging: The role of motor retrieval and strategic processing. *Psychology and Aging, 8,* 81–86.

Nyberg, L., Nilsson, L-G., & Bäckman, L. (1992). Recall of actions, sentences, and nouns: Influences of adult age and passage of time. *Acta Psychologia, 79,* 245–254.

O'Hara, M. W., Hinrichs, J. V., Kohout, F. J., Wallace, R. B., & Lemke, J. H. (1986). Memory complaint and memory performance in the depressed elderly. *Psychology and Aging, 1,* 208–214.

Ohta, R. J. (1981). Spatial orientation in the elderly: The current status of understanding. In H. L. Pick, Jr., & L. P. Acvedolo (Eds.), *Spatial orientation: Theory, research, and application.* New York: Plenum.

Ozekes, M., & Gilleard, C. (1989). Remembering faces and drawings: A test of Hasher and Zacks' model of automatic processing in a Turkish sample. *The Journals of Gerontology: Psychological Sciences, 44,* P122–123.

Padgett, R. J., & Ratner, H. H. (1987). Older and younger adults memory for structured and unstructured events. *Experimental Aging Research, 13,* 133–139.

Page, P., Versttraete, D., Robb, J., & Etzwiler, D. (1981). Patient recall of self-care recommendations in diabetes. *Diabetes Care, 4,* 96–98.

Paivio, A. (1967). Paired-associate learning and free recall of nouns as a function of concreteness, specificity, imagery, and meaningfulness. *Psychological Reports, 20,* 239–245.

Paivio, A. (1969). Mental imagery in associative learning and memory. *Psychological Review, 76,* 241–263.

Paivio, A. (1971). *Imagery and verbal processes.* New York: Holt, Rinehart, & Winston.

Paivio, A. (1978). Comparisons of mental clocks. *Journal of Experimental Psychology: Human Perception and Performance, 4,* 61–71.

Paivio, A., Yuille, J. C., & Madigan, S. (1968). Concreteness, imagery, and meaningfulness values for 925 nouns. *Journal of Experimental Psychology Monograph, 76* (1, Pt. 2).

Palermo, D. S., & Jenkins, J. J. (1964). *Word association norms.* Minneapolis: University of Minnesota Press.

Parasuraman, R., & Giambra, L. (1991). Skill development in vigilance: Effects of event rate and age. *Psychology and Aging, 6,* 155–169.

Park, D. C. (1992). Applied cognitive aging research. In F. I. M. Craik & T. A. Salthouse (Eds.), *The handbook of aging and cognition.* Hillsdale, NJ: Erlbaum.

Park, D. C., Cherry, K. E., Smith, A. D., & Lafronza, V. (1990). Effects of distinctive context on memory for objects and their locations in young and older adults. *Psychology and Aging, 5,* 250–255.

Park, D. C., Morrell, R. W., Frieske, D., Blackburn, B., & Birchmore, D. (1991). Cognitive factors and the use of over-the-counter medication organizers by arthritis patients. *Human Factors, 33,* 57–67.

Park, D. C., Morrell, R. W., Frieske, D., & Kincaid, D. (1992). Medication adherence behaviors in older adults: Effects of external cognitive supports. *Psychology and Aging, 7,* 252–256.

Park, D. C., & Puglisi, J. T. (1985). Older adults memory for the color of pictures. *Journal of Gerontology, 40,* 198–204.

Park, D. C., Puglisi, J. T., & Lutz, R. (1982). Spatial memory in older adults: Effects of intentionality. *Journal of Gerontology, 37,* 330–335.

Park, D. C., Puglisi, J. T., & Smith, A. D. (1986). Memory for pictures: Does an age-related decline exist? *Psychology and Aging, 1,* 11–17.

Park, D. C., Puglisi, J. T., Smith, A. D., & Dudley, W. N. (1987). Cue utilization and encoding specificity in picture recognition by older adults. *Journal of Gerontology*, *42*, 423–425.

Park, D. C., Puglisi, J. T., & Sovacool, M. (1983). Memory for pictures, words, and spatial location in older adults: Evidence for pictorial superiority. *Journal of Gerontology*, *38*, 582–588.

Park, D. C., Puglisi, J. T., & Sovacool, M. (1984). Picture memory in older adults: Effects of contextual detail at encoding and retrieval. *Journal of Gerontology*, *39*, 213–215.

Park, D. C., Royal, D., Dudley, W., & Morrell, R. W. (1988). Forgetting of pictures over a long retention interval in young and older adults. *Psychology and Aging*, *3*, 94–95.

Park, D. C., & Shaw, R. J. (1992). Effect of environmental support on implicit and explicit memory in younger and older adults. *Psychology and Aging*, *7*, 632–642.

Park, D. C., Smith, A. D., Dudley, W. N., & Lafronza, V. N. (1989). Effects of age and a divided attention task presented during encoding and retrieval on memory. *Journal of Experimental Psychology: Learning, Memory, and Cognition*, *15*, 1185–1191.

Park, D. C., Smith, A. D., & Cavanaugh, J. C. (1990). Metamemories of memory researchers. *Memory & Cognition*, *18*, 321–327.

Park, D. C., Smith, A. D., Morrell, R. W., Puglisi, J. T., & Dudley, W. N. (1990). Effects of contextual integration on recall of pictures by older adults. *The Journals of Gerontology: Psychological Sciences*, *45*, P52–57.

Parkin, A. J., & Walter, B. M. (1991). Aging, short-term memory and frontal dysfunction. *Psychobiology*, *19*, 175–179.

Parkin, A. J., & Walter, B. M. (1992). Recollective experience, normal aging, and frontal dysfunction. *Psychology and Aging*, *7*, 290–298.

Parkinson, S. R. (1980). Aging and amnesia: A running span analysis. *Bulletin of the Psychonomic Society*, *15*, 215–217.

Parkinson, S. R. (1982). Performance deficits in short-term memory tasks: A comparison of amnesiac Korsakoff patients and the aged. In L. S. Cermak (Ed.), *Human memory and amnesia*. Hillsdale, NJ: Erlbaum.

Parkinson, S. R., Inman, V. W., & Dannenbaum, S. E. (1985). Adult age differences in short-term forgetting. *Acta Psychologica*, *60*, 83–101.

Parkinson, S. R., Lindholm, J. M., & Inman, V. W. (1982). An analysis of age differences in immediate recall. *Journal of Gerontology*, *37*, 425–431.

Parkinson, S. R., & Perey, A. (1980). Aging, digit span, and the stimulus suffix effect. *Journal of Gerontology*, *35*, 736–742.

Parks, C. W., Jr., Mitchell, D. B., & Perlmutter, M. (1986). Cognitive and social functioning across adulthood: Age or student status differences? *Psychology and Aging*, *1*, 248–254.

Patton, G. W. R., & Meit, M. (1993). Effect of aging on prospective and incidental memory. *Experimental Aging Research*, *19*, 165–176.

Pavur, E. J., Jr., Comeaux, J. M., & Zeringue, J. A. (1984). Younger and older adults' attention to relevant and irrelevant stimuli in free recall. *Experimental Aging Research*, *10*, 59–60.

Peak, D. T. (1968). Changes in short-term memory in a group of aging community residents. *Journal of Gerontology*, *23*, 9–16.

Peak, D. T. (1970). A replication study of changes in short-term memory in a group of aging community residents. *Journal of Gerontology*, *25*, 316–319.

Perfect, T. J., & Stollery, B. (1993). Memory and metamemory performance in older adults: One deficit or two? *Quarterly Journal of Experimental Psychology, 46A,* 119–136.

Perlmutter, M. (1978a). What is memory the aging of? *Developmental Psychology, 14,* 330–345.

Perlmutter, M. (1978b, November). *Age differences in the consistency of adults' associative responses.* Paper presented at the annual meeting of the Psychonomic Society, San Antonio, Texas.

Perlmutter, M. (1979a). Age differences in adults' free recall, cued recall, and recognition. *Journal of Gerontology, 34,* 533–539.

Perlmutter, M. (1979b). Age differences in the consistency of adults' associative responses. *Experimental Aging Research, 5,* 549–553.

Perlmutter, M., Adams, C., Berry, J., Kaplan, M., Person, D., & Verdonik, F. (1987). Aging and memory. *Annual Review of Gerontology & Geriatrics, 7,* 57–92.

Perlmutter, M., Metzger, R., Miller, K., & Nezworski, T. (1980). Memory of historical events. *Experimental Aging Research, 6,* 47–60.

Perlmutter, M., Metzger, R., Nezworski, T., & Miller, K. (1981). Spatial and temporal memory in 20 and 60 year olds. *Journal of Gerontology, 36,* 59–65.

Perlmutter, M., & Nyquist, L. (1990). Self-reported physical and mental health and intelligence performance across adulthood. *The Journals of Gerontology: Psychological Sciences, 45,* P145–155.

Perone, M., & Baron, A. (1982). Age-related effects of pacing on acquisition and performance of response sequences: An operant analysis. *Journal of Gerontology, 37,* 443–449.

Perone, M., & Baron, A. (1983a). Age-related preferences for paced and unpaced tasks in chained schedules of reinforcement. *Experimental Aging Research, 9,* 165–168.

Perone, M., & Baron, A. (1983b). Reduced age differences in omission errors after prolonged exposure to response pacing contingencies. *Developmental Psychology, 19,* 915–923.

Peterson, L. R., & Peterson, M. J. (1959). Short-term retention of individual verbal items. *Journal of Experimental Psychology, 58,* 193–198.

Petros, T. V., Norgaard, L., Olson, K., & Tabor, L. (1989). Effects of genre and verbal ability on adult age differences in sensitivity to text structure. *Psychology and Aging, 4,* 247–250.

Petros, T. V., Tabor, L., Cooney, T., & Chabot, R. J. (1983). Adult age differences in sensitivity to semantic structure of prose. *Developmental Psychology, 19,* 907–914.

Petros, T. V., Zehr, D., & Chabot, R. (1983). Adult age differences in accessing and retrieving information from long-term memory. *Journal of Gerontology, 38,* 589–592.

Pezdek, K. (1980). Life-span differences in semantic integration of pictures and sentences in memory. *Child Development, 51,* 720–729.

Pezdek, K. (1983). Memory for items and their spatial locations by young and elderly adults. *Developmental Psychology, 19,* 895–900.

Pezdek, K. (1987). Memory for pictures: A lifespan study of memory for visual detail. *Child Development, 58,* 807–815.

Pezdek, K., Whetstone, T., Reynolds, K., Askari, N., & Dougherty, Y. (1989). Memory for real-world scenes: The role of consistency with expectation. *Journal of Experimental Psychology: Learning, Memory, and Cognition, 15,* 587–595.

Phillips, P. L., & Kausler, D. H. (1992). Variation in external context and adult age differences in action memory. *Experimental Aging Research, 18*, 41–44.

Pierce, K., & Storandt, M. (1987). Similarities in visual imagery ability in young and old women. *Experimental Aging Research, 13*, 209–211.

Plomp, R. (1964). Rate of decay of auditory sensation. *Journal of the Acoustical Society of America, 36*, 277–282.

Plude, D. J., Raye, D. E., Hoyer, W. J., Post, T. A., Saynisch, M. J., & Hahn, M. V. (1983). Adult age differences in visual search as a function of information load and target mapping. *Developmental Psychology, 19*, 508–512.

Poon, L. W. (1985). Differences in human memory with aging: Nature, causes, and clinical implications. In J. E. Birren & K. W. Schaie (Eds.), *Handbook of the psychology of aging (2nd. edition)*. New York: Van Nostrand Reinhold.

Poon, L. W. (1986). *Handbook for clinical memory assessment of older adults*. Washington, D.C.: American Psychological Association.

Poon, L. W., & Fozard, J. L. (1978). Speed of retrieval from long-term memory in relation to age, familiarity, and datedness of information. *Journal of Gerontology, 33*, 711–717.

Poon, L. W., Fozard, J. L., Paulshock, D. R., & Thomas, J. C. (1979). A questionnaire assessment of age differences in retention of recent and remote events. *Experimental Aging Research, 5*, 401–411.

Poon, L. W., Fozard, J. L., & Treat, N. J. (1978). From clinical and research findings on memory to intervention programs. *Experimental Aging Research, 4*, 235–254.

Poon, L. W., Fozard, J. L., Vierck, V., Dailey, B. F., Cerella, J., & Zeller, P. (1976, August). *The effects of practice and information in feedback on age-related differences in performance, speed, variability, and error rates in a two-choice decision task*. Paper presented at the annual meeting of the American Psychological Association, Washington, D.C.

Poon, L. W., & Schaffer, G. (1982, August). *Prospective memory in young and elderly adults*. Paper presented at the annual meeting of the American Psychological Association, Washington, D.C.

Poon, L. W., & Walsh-Sweeney, L. (1981). Effects of bizarre and interacting imagery on learning and retrieval of the aged. *Experimental Aging Research, 7*, 65–70.

Poon, L. W., Walsh-Sweeney, L., & Fozard, J. L. (1980). Memory skill training for the elderly: Salient issues on the use of imagery mnemonics. In L. W. Poon, J. L. Fozard, L. S. Cermak, D. Arenberg, & L. W. Thompson (Eds.), *New directions in memory and aging: Proceedings of the George A. Talland Memorial Conference*. Hillsdale, NJ: Erlbaum.

Popkin, S. J., Gallagher, D., Thompson, L. W., & Moore, M. (1982). Memory complaint and performance in normal and depressed older adults. *Experimental Aging Research, 8*, 141–145.

Porteus, S. D. (1959). *The maze test and clinical psychology*. Palo Alto, CA: Pacific Books.

Posner, M. I., Boies, S. J., Eichelman, W., & Taylor, R. L. (1969). Retention of visual and name codes of single letters. *Journal of Experimental Psychology Monograph, 79*, 1–16.

Posner, M. I., & Mitchell, R. F. (1967). Chronometric analysis of classification. *Psychological Review, 74*, 392–409.

Posner, M. I., & Snyder, C. R. (1975). Attention and cognitive control. In R. L. Solso (Ed.), *Information processing and cognition*. Hillsdale, NJ: Erlbaum.

Postman, L. (1961). The present status of interference theory. In C. N. Cofer (Ed.), *Verbal learning and verbal behavior*. New York: McGraw-hill.

Postman, L. (1969). Experimental analysis of learning to learn. In G. H. Bower & J. T. Spence (Eds.), *The psychology of learning and motivation. Vol 3.* New York: Academic Press.

Postman, L., & Greenbloom, R. (1967). Conditions of cue selection in the acquisition of paired-associate lists. *Journal of Experimental Psychology, 73,* 91–100.

Postman, L., & Underwood, B. J. (1973). Critical issues in interference theory. *Memory & Cognition, 1,* 19–40.

Potvin, A. R., Tourtellotte, W. W., Pew, R. W., Albers, J. W., Henderson, W. G., & Snyder, D. N. (1973). The importance of age effects on performance in the assessment of clinical trials. *Journal of Chronic Diseases, 26,* 699–717.

Powell, D. A., Buchanan, S. L., & Hernandez, L. L. (1981). Age-related changes in classical (Pavlovian) conditioning in the New Zealand albino rabbit. *Experimental Aging Research, 7,* 453–465.

Pratt, M. W., Boyes, C., Robins, S., & Manchester, J. (1989). Telling tales: Working memory and the narrative cohesion of story retellings. *Developmental Psychology, 25,* 628–635.

Puckett, J. M., & Lawson, W. M. (1989). Absence of adult age differences in forgetting in the Brown-Peterson task. *Acta Psychologica, 72,* 159–175.

Puckett, J. M., & Stockburger, D. W. (1988). Absence of age-related proneness to short-term retroactive interference in the absence of rehearsal. *Psychology and Aging, 3,* 342–347.

Puff, C. R. (1970). Role of clustering in free recall. *Journal of Experimental Psychology, 86,* 384–386.

Puglisi, J. T. (1980). Semantic encoding in older adults as evidenced by release from proactive inhibition. *Journal of Gerontology, 35,* 743–745.

Puglisi, J. T. (1986). Age-related slowing in memory search for three-dimensional objects. *Journal of Gerontology, 41,* 72–78.

Puglisi, J. T., & Park, D. C. (1987). Perceptual elaboration and memory in older adults. *Journal of Gerontology, 42,* 160–162.

Puglisi, J. T., Park, D. C., & Smith, A. D. (1987). Picture associations among old and young adults. *Experimental Aging Research, 13,* 115–116.

Puglisi, J. T., Park, D. C., Smith, A. D., & Dudley, W. N. (1988). Age differences in encoding specificity. *The Journals of Gerontology: Psychological Sciences, 43,* P145–150.

Query, W. T., & Megran, J. (1983). Age-related norms for AVLT in a male patient population. *Journal of Clinical Psychology, 39,* 136–138.

Rabbitt, P. M. A. (1965). An age decrement in the ability to ignore irrelevant information. *Journal of Gerontology, 20,* 233–238.

Rabbitt, P. M. A. & Abson, V. (1990). Lost and found: Some logical and methodological limitations of self-report questionnaires as tools to study cognitive aging. *British Journal of Psychology, 81,* 1–16.

Rabbitt, P. M. A., & Birren, J. E. (1967). Age and responses to sequences of repetitive and interruptive signals. *Journal of Gerontology, 22,* 143–150.

Rabbitt, P. M. A., & McInnis, L. (1988). Do clever old people have earlier and richer first memories? *Psychology and Aging, 3,* 338–341.

Rabinowitz, J. C. (1984). Aging and recognition failure. *Journal of Gerontology, 41,* 368–375.

Rabinowitz, J. C. (1986). Priming in episodic memory. *Journal of Gerontology, 41*, 204–213.

Rabinowitz, J. C. (1989a). Age deficits under optimal study conditions. *Psychology and Aging, 4*, 378–380.

Rabinowitz, J. C. (1989b). Judgments of origin and generation effects: Comparisons between young and elderly subjects. *Psychology and Aging, 4*, 259–268.

Rabinowitz, J. C., & Ackerman, B. P. (1982). General encoding of episodic events by elderly adults. In F. I. M. Craik & S. Trehub (Eds.), *Aging and cognitive processes*. New York: Plenum Press.

Rabinowitz, J. C., Ackerman, B. P., Craik, F. I. M., & Hinchley, J. L. (1982). Aging and metamemory: The roles of relatedness and imagery. *Journal of Gerontology, 37*, 688–695.

Rabinowitz, J. C., & Craik, F. I. M. (1986). Prior retrieval effects in young and old adults. *Journal of Gerontology, 41*, 368–375.

Rabinowitz, J. C., Craik, F. I. M., & Ackerman, B. P. (1982). A processing resource account of age differences in recall. *Canadian Journal of Psychology, 36*, 325–344.

Rabinowitz, M., & Mandler, J. M. (1983). Organization and information retrieval. *Journal of Experimental Psychology: Learning, Memory, and Cognition, 9*, 430–439.

Radtke, R. C., McHewitt, E., & Jacoby, L. (1970). Number of alternatives and rate of presentation in verbal discrimination learning. *Journal of Experimental Psychology, 83*, 179–181.

Radvansky, G. A., Gerard, L., Zacks, R. T., & Hasher, L. (1990). Younger and older adults use of mental models as representations for text material. *Psychology and Aging, 5*, 209–214.

Rajaram, S., & Roediger, H. L., III. (1993). Direct comparisons of four implicit memory tests. *Journal of Experimental Psychology: Learning, Memory, and Cognition, 19*, 765–776.

Randt, C. T., Brown, E. R., & Osborne, D. P. (1980). A memory test for longitudinal measurement of mild to moderate deficits. *Clinical Neuropsychology, 2*, 184–194.

Rankin, J. L., & Collins, M. (1985). Adult age differences in memory elaborations. *Journal of Gerontology, 40*, 451–458.

Rankin, J. L., & Collins, M. (1986). The effects of memory elaboration on adult age differences in incidental recall. *Experimental Aging Research, 12*, 231–234.

Rankin, J. L. & Firnhaber, S. (1986). Adult age differences in memory: Effects of distinctiveness and common encodings. *Experimental Aging Research, 12*, 141–146.

Rankin, J. L., & Hinrichs, J. V. (1983). Age, presentation rate, and the effectiveness of structural and semantic recall cues. *Journal of Gerontology, 38*, 593–596.

Rankin, J. L., Hyland, T. P. (1983). The effects of orienting task on adult age differences in recall and recognition. *Experimental Aging Research, 9*, 159–164.

Rankin, J. L., Karol, R., & Tuten, C. (1984). Strategy use, recall, and recall organization in young, middle-aged, and elderly adults. *Experimental Aging Research, 10*, 193–196.

Rankin, J. L., & Kausler, D. H. (1979). Adult age differences in false recognitions. *Journal of Gerontology, 34*, 58–65.

Ratner, H. H., Schell, D. A., Crimmins, A., Mittelman, D., & Baldinelli, L. (1987). Changes in adults prose recall: Aging or cognitive demand? *Developmental Psychology, 23*, 521–525.

Raymond, B. J. (1971). Free recall among the aged. *Psychological Reports, 29*, 1179–1182.

Raz, N., Millman, D., & Moberg, P. J. (1989). Auditory memory and age-related differences in two-tone frquency discrimination: Trace decay and interference. *Experimental Aging Research, 15,* 43–47.

Read, D. E. (1987). Neuropsychological assessment of memory in the elderly. *Canadian Journal of Psychology, 41,* 158–174.

Rebok, G. W., & Balcerak, L. J. (1989). Memory self-efficacy and performance differences in young and old adults: The effect of mnemonic training. *Developmental Psychology, 25,* 714–721.

Rebok, G. W., Montaglione, G. J., & Bendlin, G. (1988). Effects of age and training on memory for pragmatic implications in advertising. *The Journals of Gerontology: Psychological Sciences, 43,* P75–78.

Reder, L. M., Wible, C., & Martin, J. (1986). Differential memory change with age: Exact retrieval versus plausible inference. *Journal of Experimental Psychology: Learning, Memory, and Cognition, 12,* 72–81.

Reitman, J. S. (1971). Mechanisms of forgetting in short-term memory. *Cognitive Psychology, 2,* 185–195.

Reitman, J. S. (1974). Without sureptitious rehearsal, information in short-term memory decays. *Journal of Verbal Learning and Verbal Behavior, 13,* 365–377.

Reno, R. (1979). Attribution of success and failure as a function of perceived age. *Journal of Gerontology, 34,* 709–715.

Rescorla, R. A. (1972). Informational variables in Pavlovian condition. In G. H. Bower (Ed.), *Psychology of learning and motivation: Advances in research and theory, Vol. 6.* New York: Academic Press.

Ribot, T. (1882). *Diseases of memory.* New York: Appleton.

Rice, D. M., Buchsbaum, M. S., Hardy, D., & Burgwald, L. (1991). Frontal left temporal slowing EEG activity is related to a verbal recent memory deficit in a non-demented elderly population. *The Journals of Gerontology: Psychological Sciences, 46,* P144–151.

Rice, G. E., & Meyer, B. J. F. (1986). Prose recall: Effects of aging, verbal ability, and reading behavior. *Journal of Gerontology, 41,* 469–480.

Rice, G. E., Meyer, B. J. F., & Miller, D. C. (1989). Using text structure to improve older adults recall of important medical information. *Educational Gerontology, 15,* 527–542.

Rice, G. E., & Okun, M. A. (1991). Older adults' memory for important medical information. *Experimental Aging Research, 17,* 90.

Richardson-Klavehn, A., & Bjork, R. A. (1988). Measures of memory. In M. R. Rosenzweig & L. W. Porter (Eds.), *Annual review of psychology. Vol. 39.* Palo Alto, CA: Annual Reviews, Inc.

Riege, W. H. (1982). Self-report and tests of memory aging. *Clinical Gerontologist, 1,* 23–36.

Riege, W. H., & Inman, V. (1981). Age differences in nonverbal memory tasks. *Journal of Gerontology, 36,* 51–58.

Riege, W. H., Kelly, K., & Klane, L. T. (1981). Age and error differences on memory for designs. *Perceptual and Motor Skills, 52,* 507–513.

Riegel, K. F., & Birren, J. E. (1965). Age differences in associative behavior. *Journal of Gerontology, 20,* 125–130.

Riegel, K. F., & Birren, J. E. (1966). Age differences in verbal associations. *Journal of Genetic Psychology, 108,* 153–170.

Riegel, K. F., & Riegel, R. M. (1964). Changes in associative behavior during later years of life: A cross-sectional analysis. *Vita Humana, 7,* 1–32.

Riggs, K. M., Wingfield, A., & Tun, P. A. (1993). Passage difficulty, speech rate, and age differences in memory for spoken text. *Experimental Aging Research, 19,* 111–128.

Rissenberg, M., & Glanzer, M. (1986). Picture superiority in free recall: The effects of normal aging and primary degenerative dementia. *Journal of Gerontology, 41,* 64–71.

Rissenberg, M., & Glanzer, M. (1987). Free recall and word finding ability in normal aging and Senile Dementia of the Alzheimer's type. *Journal of Gerontology, 42,* 318–322.

Robertson, E. A. (1973). *Age differences in primary and secondary memory processes.* Doctoral Dissertation, University of Southern California.

Robertson-Tchabo, E. A., & Arenberg, D. (1976). Age differences in cognition in healthy educated men: A factor analysis of experimental measures. *Experimental Aging Research, 2,* 75–89.

Robertson-Tchabo, E. A., & Arenberg, D. (1989). Assessment of memory in older adults. In T. Hunt & C. J. Lindley (Eds.), *Testing older adults.* Austin, TX: Pro-Ed.

Robertson-Tchabo, E. A., Hausman, C. P., & Arenberg, D. (1976). A classical mnemonic for older learners: A trip that works. *Educational Gerontology, 1,* 215–226.

Roediger, H. L., III, & Blaxton, T. A. (1987). Effects of varying modality, surface features, and retention interval on priming in word-fragment completion. *Memory & Cognition, 15,* 379–388.

Roenker, D. L., Thompson, C. P., & Brown, S. C. (1971). Comparison of measures for the estimation of clustering in free recall. *Psychological Bulletin, 76,* 45–48.

Rogers, C. J., Keyes, B. J., & Fuller, B. J. (1976). Solution shift performance in the elderly. *Journal of Gerontology, 31,* 670–675.

Rohling, M. L., & Scogin, F. R. (1993). Automatic and effortful memory processes in depressed persons. *The Journals of Gerontology: Psychological Sciences, 48,* P87–95.

Root, N. (1981). Injuries at work are fewer among older employees. *Monthly Labor Review, 104,* 30–34.

Rose, T. L., & Yesavage, J. A. (1983). Differential effects of a list-learning mnemonic in three age groups. *Gerontology, 29,* 293–298.

Rose, T. L., Yesavage, J. A., Hill, R. D., & Bower, G. H. (1986). Priming effects and recognition memory in young and elderly adults. *Experimental Aging Research, 12,* 31–37.

Ross, E. (1968). Effects of challenging and supportive instructions on verbal learning in older persons. *Journal of Educational Psychology, 59,* 261–266.

Rowe, E. J. (1974). Depth of processing in a frequency judgment task. *Journal of Verbal Learning and Verbal Behavior, 13,* 638–643.

Rowe, E. J., & Schnore, M. M. (1971). Item concreteness and reported strategies in paired-associate learning as a function of age. *Journal of Gerontology, 26,* 470–475.

Rubin, D. C. (1982). On the retention function for autobiographical memory. *Journal of Verbal Learning and Verbal Behavior, 21,* 21–38.

Rubin, D. C., Wetzler, S. E., & Nebes, R. D. (1986). Autobiographical memory across the lifespan. In D. C. Rubin (Ed.), *Autobiographical memory.* New York: Cambridge University Press.

Ruch, F. L. (1933). Adult learning. *Psychological Bulletin, 30,* 387–414.

Ruch, F. L. (1934). The differentiative effects of age upon human learning. *Journal of*

General Psychology, 11, 261–286.

Rugg, M. D., Furda, J., & Loriat, M. (1988). The effects of task on modulation of event-related potentials by word repetition. *Psychophysiology, 25,* 55–63.

Rundus, D. (1973). Negative effects of using list items as recall cues. *Journal of Verbal Learning and Verbal Behavior, 12,* 43–50.

Rundus, D., & Atkinson, R. C. (1970). Rehearsal processes in free recall: A procedure for direct observation. *Journal of Verbal Learning and Verbal Behavior, 9,* 99–105.

Russo, R., & Parkin, A. J. (1993). Age differences in implicit memory: More apparent than real. *Memory & Cognition, 21,* 73–80.

Ryan, E. B. (1992). Beliefs about memory changes across the adult life span. *The Journals of Gerontology: Psychological Sciences, 47,* P41–46.

Ryan, E. B., & See, S. K. (1983). Age-based beliefs about memory changes for self and others across adulthood. *The Journals of Gerontology: Psychological Sciences, 48,* P199–201.

Ryan, E. B., Szechtman, B., & Bodkin, J. (1992). Attitudes toward younger and older adults learning to use computers. *The Journals of Gerontology: Psychological Sciences, 47,* P95–101.

Rybarczyk, B. D., Hart, R. P., & Harkins, S. W. (1987). Age and forgetting rate with pictorial stimuli. *Psychology and Aging, 2,* 404–406.

Rybash, J. M., Hoyer, W. J., & Roodin, P. A. (1986). *Adult cognition and aging.* New York: Pergamon Press.

Sagar, H. J. (1990). Aging and age-related neurological diseases: Remote memory. In F. Boller & J. Grafman (Eds.), *Handbook of neuropsychology. Vol. 4: Aging and dementia.* Amsterdam: North Holland.

Sakitt, B. (1975). Locus of short-term visual storage. *Science, 190,* 1318–1319.

Sakitt, B., & Appleman, I. B. (1978). The effects of memory load and the contrast of the rod signal on partial-report superiority in a Sperling task. *Memory & Cognition, 6,* 562–567.

Salamé, P., & Baddeley, A. D. (1989). Effects of background music on phonological short-term memory. *Quarterly Journal of Experimental Psychology, 41A,* 197–122.

Salthouse, T. A. (1976). Age and tachhistoscopic perception. *Experimental Aging Research, 2,* 91–103.

Salthouse, T. A. (1980). Age and memory: Strategies for localizing the loss. In L. W. Poon, J. L. Fozard, L. S. Cermak, D. Arenberg, & L. W. Thompson (Eds.), *New directions in memory and aging: Proceedings of the George A. Talland Memorial Conference.* Hillsdale, NJ: Erlbaum.

Salthouse, T. A. (1982). *Adult cognition.* New York: Springer-Verlag.

Salthouse, T. A. (1984). Effects of age and skill in typing. *Journal of Experimental Psychology: General, 113,* 345–371.

Salthouse, T. A. (1985a). *A theory of cognitive aging.* Amsterdam: North-Holland.

Salthouse, T. A. (1985b). Speed of behavior and its implications for cognition. In J. E. Birren & K. W. Schaie (Eds.), *Handbook of the psychology of aging (2nd. ed).* New York: Van Nostrand Reinhold.

Salthouse, T. A. (1988a). The role of processing resources in cognitive aging. In M. L. Howe & C. J. Brainerd (Eds.), *Cognitive development in adulthood: Progress in cognitive development research.* New York: Springer-Verlag.

Salthouse, T. A. (1988b). Resource-reduction interpretations of cognitive aging. *Developmental Research*, 238–272.

Salthouse, T. A. (1988c). Initiating the formalization of theories of aging. *Psychology and Aging*, 3, 3–16.

Salthouse, T. A. (1990). Cognitive competence and expertise in aging. In J. E. Birren & K. W. Schaie (Eds.), *Handbook of the Psychology of Aging (3rd ed.)*. San Diego: Academic Press.

Salthouse, T. A. (1991). *Theoretical perspective on cognitive aging*. Hillsdale, NJ: Erlbaum.

Salthouse, T. A. (1992a). Reasoning and spatial abilities. In F.I.M. Craik & T. A. Salthouse (Eds.), *The handbook of aging and cognition*. Hillsdale, NJ: Erlbaum.

Salthouse, T. A. (1992b, November). *What type of speed mediates age differences in what type of cognition?* Paper presented at the annual meeting of the Psychonomic Society, St. Louis, MO.

Salthouse, T. A. (1993). Speed and knowledge as determinants of adult age differences in verbal tasks. *The Journals of Gerontology: Psychological Sciences*, 48, P29–36.

Salthouse, T. A. (in press). Speed mediation of adult age differences in cognition. *Developmental Psychology*.

Salthouse, T. A., & Babcock, R. L. (1991). Decomposing adult age differences in working memory. *Developmental Psychology*, 27, 763–776.

Salthouse, T. A., Babcock, R. L., & Shaw, R. J. (1991). Effects of adult age on structural and operational capacities in working memory. *Psychology and Aging*, 6, 118–127.

Salthouse, T. A., & Coon, V. E. (1993). Influence of task-specific processing speed on age differences in memory. *The Journals of Gerontology: Psychological Sciences*, 48, P245–255.

Salthouse, T. A., Kausler, D. H., & Saults, J. S. (1988a). Investigation of student status, background variables, and feasibility of standard tasks in cognitive aging research. *Psychology and Aging*, 3, 29–37.

Salthouse, T. A., Kausler, D. H., & Saults, J. S. (1988b). Utilization of path-analytic procedures to investigate the role of processing resources in cognitive aging. *Psychology and Aging*, 3, 158–166.

Salthouse, T. A., Kausler, D. H., & Saults, J. S. (1990). Age, self-assessed health status, and cognition. *The Journals of Gerontology: Psychological Sciences*, 45, P156–160.

Salthouse, T. A., & Lichty, W. (1985). Tests of the neural noise hypothesis of age-related cognitive change. *Journal of Gerontology*, 40, 443–450.

Salthouse, T. A., & Mitchell, D. R. D. (1989). Structural and operational capacities in integrative spatial ability. *Psychology and Aging*, 4, 18–25.

Salthouse, T. A., Mitchell, D. R. D., Skovronek, E., & Babcock, R. (1989). Effects of adult age and working memory on reasoning and spatial abilities. *Journal of Experimental Psychology: Learning, Memory, and Cognition*, 15, 507–516.

Salthouse, T. A., Rogan, J. D., & Prill, K. A. (1984). Division of attention: Age differences on a visually presented memory task. *Memory & Cognition*, 12, 613–620.

Salthouse, T. A., & Skovronek, E. (1992). Within-context assessment of working memory. *The Journals of Gerontology: Psychological Sciences*, 47, P110–129.

Salthouse, T. A., & Somberg, B. L. (1982). Skilled performance: Effects of adult age and experience on elementary processes. *Journal of Experimental Psychology: General, 111*, 176–207.

Saltzman, I. J. (1953). The orienting task in incidental and intentional learning. *American Journal of Psychology*, 66, 593–597.

Sanders, R. E., Gonzalez, E. G., Murphy, M. D., Liddle, C. L., & Vitina, J. R. (1987). Frequency of occurrence and the criteria for automatic processing. *Journal of Experimental Psychology: Learning, Memory, and Cognition*, 13, 241–250.

Sanders, R. E., Murphy, M. D., Schmitt, F. A., & Walsh, K. K. (1980). Age differences in free recall rehearsal strategies. *Journal of Gerontology*, 35, 550–558.

Sanders, R. E., Wise, J. L., Liddle, C. L., & Murphy, M. D. (1990). Adult age comparisons in the processing of event frequency information. *Psychology and Aging*, 5, 172–177.

Sands, L. P., & Meredith, W. (1992). Blood pressure and intellectual functioning in late midlife. *The Journals of Gerontology: Psychological Sciences*, 47, P81–84.

Scarborough, D. L., Cortese, C., & Scarborough, H. S. (1977). Frequency and repetition effects in lexical memory. *Journal of Experimental Psychology: Human Perception and Performance*, 3, 1–17.

Schacter, D. L. (1987). Memory, amnesia, and frontal lobe dysfunction. *Psychobiology*, 15, 21–36.

Schacter, D. L., Cooper, L. A., & Valdiserri, M. (1992). Implicit and explicit memory for novel visual objects in older and younger adults. *Psychology and Aging*, 7, 299–308.

Schacter, D. L., Harbluk, J. L., & McLachlan, D. (1984). Retrieval without recollection: An experimental analysis of source amnesia. *Journal of Verbal Learning and Verbal Behavior*, 23, 593–611.

Schacter, D. L., Kaszniak, A. W., Kihlstrom, J. F., & Valdiserri, M. (1991). The relation between source memory and aging. *Psychology and Aging*, 6, 559–568.

Schaie, K. W. (1983a). Age changes in adult intelligence. In D. S. Woodruff & J. E. Birren (Eds.), *Aging: Scientific perspectives and social issues*. Monterey, CA: Brooks/Cole.

Schaie, K. W. (1983b). The Seattle longitudinal study: A 21-year exploration of psychometric intelligence in adulthood. In K. W. Schaie (Ed.), *Longitudinal studies of adult psychological development*. New York: Guilford Press.

Schank, R. C., & Abelson, R. P. (1977). *Scripts, plans, goals, and understanding*. Hillsdale, NJ: Erlbaum.

Schear, J. M., & Nebes, R. D. (1980). Memory for verbal and spatial information as a function of age. *Experimental Aging Research*, 6, 271–281.

Schmitt, F. A., Murphy, M. D., & Sanders, R. E. (1981). Training older adult free recall rehearsal strategies. *Journal of Gerontology*, 36, 329–337.

Schneider, N. G., Gritz, E. R., & Jarvik, M. E. (1975). Age differences in learning, immediate, and one-week delayed recall. *Gerontolgia*, 21, 10–20.

Schneider, W., & Shiffrin, R. M. (1977). Controlled and automatic human information processing: I. Detection, search, and attention. *Psychological Review*, 84, 1–66.

Schonfield, A. E. D. (1965). Memory changes with age. *Nature*, 208, 918.

Schonfield, A. E. D. (1967). Memory loss with age: Acquisition and retrieval. *Psychological Reports*, 20, 223–226.

Schonfield, A. E. D. (1969a). Age and remembering. *Duke University Council on Aging and Human Development, Proceedings of Seminars*. Durham, NC: Duke University.

Schonfield, A. E. D. (1969b, July). *In search of early memories*. Paper presented at the Internatioinal Congress of Gerontology, Washington, D.C.

Schonfield, A. E. D., Davidson, H., & Jones, H. (1983). An example of age-associated interference in memorizing. *Journal of Gerontology, 38*, 204–210.

Schonfield, A. E. D., & Donaldson, W. (1966). Immediate memory as a function of intraseries variation. *Canadian Journal of Psychology, 20*, 218–227.

Schonfield, A. E. D., & Robertson, B. A. (1966). Memory storage and aging. *Canadian Journal of Aging, 20*, 228–236.

Schonfield, A. E. D., & Stones, M. J. (1979). Remembering and aging. In J. F. Kihlstrom & F. J. Evans (Eds.), *Functional disorders of memory*. Hillsdale, NJ: Erlbaum.

Schonfield, A. E. D., & Wenger, L. (1975). Age limitation of perceptual span. *Nature, 53*, 377–378.

Schulman, A. I. (1967). Word length and rarity in recognition memory. *Psychonomic Science, 9*, 211–212.

Schulz, R. W. (1955). Generalization of serial position effects in rote serial learning. *Journal of Experimental Psychology, 49*, 267–272.

Schweikert, R., & Boruff, B. (1985). Short-term memory capacity: Magic number or magic spell? *Journal of Experimental Psychology: Learning, Memory, and Cognition, 12*, 419–425.

Scialfa, C. T., & Margolis, R. B. (1986). Age differences in the commonality of free associations. *Experimental Aging Research, 12*, 95–98.

Scogin, F. R., & Bienas, J. L. (1988). A three-year follow-up of older adult participants in a memory-skills training program. *Psychology and Aging, 3*, 334–337.

Scogin, F. R., & Flynn, T. M. (1986). Manual for memory skills training. *Social and Behavioral Sciences Documents, 16*, 14.

Scogin, F., & Prohaska, M. (1992). The efficacy of self-taught memory training for community-dwelling older adults. *Educational Gerontology, 18*, 751–766.

Scogin, F. R., Storandt, M., & Lott, L. (1985). Memory-skills training, memory complaints, and depression in older adults. *Journal of Gerontology, 40*, 562–568.

Sczomak, J. (1989, November). *Prospective memory in the elderly: Efficacy of mnemonic strategies in naturalistic settings.* Paper presented at the annual meeting of the Gerontological Society of America, Minneapolis.

Severin, F. T., & Rigby, W. K. (1963). Influence of digit grouping on memory for telephone numbers. *Journal of Applied Psychology, 47*, 117–119.

Shaffer, L. H. (1973). Latency mechanisms in transcription. In S. Kornblum (Ed.), *Attention and performance, IV*. New York: Academic Press.

Shaffer, W. D., & LaBerge, D. (1979). Automatic semantic processing of unattended words. *Journal of Verbal Learning and Verbal Behavior, 18*, 413–426.

Shakow, D., Dolkart, M. B., & Goldman, R. (1941). The memory function in psychoses of the aged. *Diseases of the Nervous System, 2*, 43–48.

Shand, M. A. (1982). Sign-based short-term memory coding of American Sign Language signs and printed English words by congenitally deaf signers. *Cognitive Psychology, 14*, 1–12.

Shaps, L. P., & Nilsson, L-G. (1980). Encoding and retrieval operations in relation to age. *Developmental Psychology, 16*, 636–643.

Sharps, M. J. (1991). Spatial memory in young and elderly adults: Category structure of stimulus sets. *Psychology and Aging, 6*, 309–312.

Sharps, M. J., & Gollin, E. S. (1987). Memory for object locations in young and elderly adults. *Journal of Gerontology, 42*, 336–341.

Sharps, M. J., & Gollin, E. S. (1988). Aging and free recall for objects located in space. *Journal of Gerontology, 43*, P8–11.

Shaw, R. J. (1991). Age-related increases in the effects of automatic semantic activation. *Psychology and Aging, 6*, 595–604.

Shaw, R. J., & Craik, F. I. M. (1989). Age differences in predictions and performance on a cued recall task. *Psychology and Aging, 4*, 131–135.

Shepard, R. N. (1967). Recognition memory for words, sentences, and pictures. *Journal of Verbal Learning and Verbal Behavior, 6*, 156–163.

Shepard, R. N., & Metzler, J. (1971). Mental rotation of three-dimensional objects. *Science, 171*, 701–703.

Sherman, R. A. (1973). *Behavior modification: Theory and practice.* Monterey, CA: Brooks/ Cole.

Shichita, K., Hatano, S., Ohashi, Y., Shibata, H., & Matuzaki, T. (1986). Memory changes in the Benton Visual Retention Test between ages 70 and 75. *Journal of Gerontology, 41*, 385–386.

Shmavonian, B. M., Miller, L. H., & Cohen, S. I. (1968). Differences among age and sex groups in electro-dermal conditioning. *Psychophysiology, 5*, 119–131.

Shmavonian, B. M., Miller, L. H., & Cohen, S. I. (1970). Differences among age and sex groups with respect to cardiovascular conditioning and reactivity. *Journal of Gerontology, 25*, 87–94.

Shulman, H. G. (1970). Encoding and retention of semantic and phonemic information in short-term memory. *Journal of Verbal Learning and Verbal Behavior, 9*, 449–508.

Simon, E. (1979). Depth and elaboration of processing in relation to age. *Journal of Experimental Psychology: Human Learning and Memory, 5*, 115–124.

Simon, E. W., Dixon, R. A., Nowak, C. A., & Hultsch, D. F. (1982). Orienting task effects on text recall in adulthood. *Journal of Gerontology, 37*, 575–580.

Simon, J. R. (1960). Changes with age in the speed of performance on a dial setting task. *Ergonomics, 3*, 169–174.

Simon, J. R. (1967). Choice reaction time as a function of auditory S-R correspondence, age, and sex. *Ergonomics, 10*, 659–664.

Simon, S. L., Walsh, D. A., Regnier, V. A., & Krauss, I. K. (1992). Spatial cognition and neighborhood use: The relationship in older adults. *Psychology and Aging, 7*, 389–394.

Singleton, W. T. (1955). Age and performance timing on simple tasks. In *Old age in the modern world.* Edinburgh: Livingstone.

Sinnott, J. D. (1984, August). *Prospective and incidental everyday memory effects of age and passage of time.* Paper presented at the annual meeting of the American Psychological Association, Toronto, Canada.

Sinnott, J. D. (1986). Prospective/incidental and incidental everyday memory: Effects of age and passage of time. *Psychology and Aging, 1*, 110–116.

Sinnott, J. D. (1989). Prospective/intentional memory and aging: Memory as adaptive action. In L. W. Poon, D. C. Rubin, & B. A. Wilson (Eds.), *Everyday cognition in adulthood and late life.* New York: Cambridge University Press.

Slamecka, N. J. (1985). On comparing rates of forgetting: Comment on Loftus (1985). *Journal of Experimental Psychology: Learning, Memory, and Cognition, 11*, 812–816.

Slamecka, N. J., & Graf, P. (1978). The generation effect: Delineation of a phenomenon. *Journal of Experimental Psychology: Human Learning and Memory, 4*, 592–604.

Slamecka, N. J., & McElree, B. (1983). Normal forgetting of verbal lists as a function of their degree of learning. *Journal of Experimental Psychology: Learning, Memory, and Cognition, 9,* 384–397.

Sloman, S. A., Hayman, C. A. G., Ohta, N., Law, J., & Tulving, E. (1988). Forgetting in primed fragment completion. *Journal of Experimental Psychology: Learning, Memory, and Cognition, 14,* 223–239.

Smith, A. D. (1974). Response interference with organized recall in the aged. *Developmental Psychology, 10,* 867–880.

Smith, A. D. (1975a). Partial learning and recognition memory in the aged. *International Journal of Aging and Human Development, 6,* 359–365.

Smith, A. D. (1975b). Aging and interference with memory. *Journal of Gerontology, 30,* 319–325.

Smith, A. D. (1976). Aging and the total presentation time hypothesis. *Developmental Psychology, 12,* 87–88.

Smith, A. D. (1977). Adult age differences in cued recall. *Developmental Psychology, 13,* 326–331.

Smith, A. D. (1979a, November). *Age differences in memory as influenced by qualitatively different types of processing.* Paper presented at the annual meeting of the Gerontological Society, Washington, D.C.

Smith, A. D. (197b). The interaction between age and list length in free recall. *Journal of Gerontology, 34,* 381–387.

Smith, A. D. (1980). Age differences in encoding, storage, and retrieval. In L. W. Poon, J. L. Fozard, L. S. Cermak, D. Arenberg, & L. W. Thompson (Eds.), *New directions in memory and aging: Proceedings of the George A. Talland Memorial Conference.* Hillsdale, NJ: Erlbaum.

Smith, A. D., & Park, D. C. (1990). Adult age differences in memory for pictures and images. In E. A. Lovelace (Ed.), *Aging and cognition: Mental processes, self-awareness and interventions.* Amsterdam: North Holland.

Smith, A. D., Park, D. C., Cherry, K., & Berkovsky, K. (1990). Age differences in memory for concrete and abstract pictures. *The Journals of Gerontology: Psychological Sciences, 45,* P205–209.

Smith, A. D., & Winograd, E. (1978). Adult age differences in remembering faces. *Developmental Psychology, 14,* 443–444.

Smith, S. M., Glenberg, A. M., & Bjork, R. A. (1978). Environmental context and human memory. *Memory & Cognition, 6,* 342–253.

Smith, S. W., Rebok, G. W., Smith, W. R., Hall, S. E., & Alvin, M. (1983). Adult age differences in the use of story structure in delayed free recall. *Experimental Aging Research, 9,* 191–195.

Snoddy, G. S. (1926). Learning and stability. *Journal of Applied Psychology, 10,* 1–36.

Solomon, P. R., Blanchard, S., Levine, E., Velazquez, E., & Groccia-Ellison, M. (1991). Attenuation of age-related conditioning deficits in humans by extension of the interstimulus interval. *Psychology and Aging, 6,* 36–42.

Solomon, P. R., Pomerleau, D., Bennett, L., James, J., & Morse, D. L. (1989). Acquisition of the classically conditioned eyeblink response in humans over the lifespan. *Psychology and Aging, 4,* 34–41.

Solso, R. L. (1979). *Cognitive psychology (1st edition).* New York: Harcourt Brace Jovanovich.

Solso, R. L. (1988). *Cognitive psychology* (2nd edition). Boston: Allyn and Bacon.

Solyom, L., & Barik, H. C. (1965). Conditioning in senescence and senility. *Journal of Gerontology, 20,* 483–488.

Somberg, B. L., & Salthouse, T. A. (1982). Divided attention abilities in young and old adults. *Journal of Experimental Psychology: Human Perception and Performance, 8,* 651–663.

Spangler, E. L., & Ingram, D. K. (1986). Effects of inescapable shock on maze performance as a function of age in mice. *Experimental Aging Research, 12,* 39–42.

Speakman, D. C. (1954). The effect of age on the incidental relearning of stamp values. *Journal of Gerontology, 9,* 162–167.

Spear, N. E., Ekstrand, B. R., & Underwood, B. J. (1964). Association by contiguity. *Journal of Experimental Psychology, 67,* 151–161.

Spence, K. W. (1958). A theory of emotionally based drive (D) and its relation to performance in simple learning situations. *American Psychologist, 13,* 131–141.

Sperback, D. J., Whitbourne, S. K., & Hoyer, W. J. (1986). Age and openness to experience in autobiographical memory. *Experimental Aging Research, 12,* 169–172.

Sperling, G. (1960). The information available in brief visual presentations. *Psychological Monographs, 74* (11, Whole No.).

Spiker, C. C. (1977). Behaviorism, cognitive psychology, and the active organism. In N. Datan & H. W. Reese (Eds.), *Life-span developmental psychology: Dialectical perspectives on experimental research.* New York: Academic Press.

Spilich, G. J. (1983). Life span components of text processing: Structural and procedural changes. *Journal of Verbal Learning and Verbal Behavior, 22,* 231–244.

Spilich, G. J. (1985). Discourse comprehension across the span of life. In N. Charness (Ed.), *Aging and human performance.* Chichester: John Wiley.

Spilich, G. J., & Voss, J. F. (1982). Contextual effects upon text memory for young, aged-normal, and aged memory-impaired individuals. *Experimental Aging Research, 8,* 147–151.

Spirduso, W. W., & MacRae, P. G. (1990). Motor performance and aging. In J. E. Birren & K. W. Schaie (Eds.), *Handbook of the psychology of aging (3rd ed.).* San Diego: Academic Press.

Squire, L. R. (1974). Remote memory as affected by aging. *Neuropsychologia, 12,* 429–435.

Squire, L. R. (1986). Mechanisms of memory. *Science, 232,* 1612–1619.

Squire, L. R. (1989). On the course of forgetting in very long-term memory. *Journal of Experimental Psychology: Learning, Memory, and Cognition, 15,* 241–245.

Squire, L. R., & Butters, N. (1984). *Neuropsychology of memory.* New York: Guilford Press.

Squire, L. R., & Slater, P. C. (1975). Forgetting in very long-term memory as assessed by an improved questionnaire technique. *Journal of Experimental Psychology: Human Learning and Memory, 104,* 50–54.

Staats, A. W., & Staats, C. K. (1958). Attitudes established by classical conditioning. *Journal of Abnormal and Social Psychology, 57,* 37–40.

Stanovich, K. E. (1980). Toward an interactive-compensatory model of individual differences in the development of reading fluency. *Reading Research Quarterly, 16,* 32–71.

Stelmach, G. E., Amrhein, P. C., & Goggin, N. L. (1988). Age differences in bimanual coordination. *The Journals of Gerontology: Psychological Sciences, 43,* P18–23.

Stelmach, G. E., Goggin, N. L., & Amrhein, P. C. (1988). Aging and the restructuring of precued movements. *Psychology and Aging, 3,* 151–157.

Stelmach, G. E., Goggin, N. L., & Garcia-Colera, A. (1987). Movement specification time with age. *Experimental Aging Research, 13,* 39–46.

Sternberg, S. (1966). High speed scanning in human memory. *Science, 153,* 652–654.

Sternberg, S. (1969a). The discovery of processing stages: Extensions of Donders' method. *Acta Psychologica, 30,* 276–315.

Sternberg, S. (1969b). Memory scanning: Mental processes revealed by reaction time experiments. *American Scientist, 57,* 421–457.

Sterns, H. L., Barrett, G. V., & Alexander, R. A. (1985). Accidents and the aging individual. In J. E. Birren & K. W. Schaie (Eds.), *Handbook of the psychology of aging, 2nd. edition.* New York: Van Nostrand Reinhold.

Stigsdotter, A., & Bäckman, L. (1989). Multifactorial memory training with older adults: How to foster maintenance of improved performance. *Gerontology, 35,* 260–267.

Stine, E. L. (1986). Attribute-based similarity perception in younger and older adults. *Experimental Aging Research, 12,* 89–94.

Stine, E. L. (1990). Online processing of written text by younger and older adults. *Psychology and Aging, 5,* 68–78.

Stine, E. L., & Wingfield, A. (1987a). Process and strategy in memory for speech among younger and older adults. *Psychology and Aging, 2,* 272–279.

Stine, E. L., & Wingfield, A. (1987b). Levels upon levels: Predicting age differences in text recall. *Experimental Aging Research, 13,* 179–183.

Stine, E. L., & Wingfield, A. (1988). Memorability functions as an indicator of qualitative age differences in text recall. *Psychology and Aging, 3,* 179–183.

Stine, E. L., & Wingfield, A. (1990). The assessment of qualitative age differences in discourse processing. In T. M. Hess (Ed.), *Aging and cognition: Knowledge organization and utilization.* Amsterdam: North Holland.

Stine, E. L., Wingfield, A., & Myers, S. D. (1990). Age differences in processing information from television news: The effects of bisensory augmentation. *The Journals of Gerontology: Psychological Sciences, 45,* P1–8.

Stine, E. L., Wingfield, A., & Poon, L. W. (1986). How much and how fast: Rapid processing of spoken language in later adulthood. *Psychology and Aging, 1,* 303–311.

Stine, E. L., Wingfield, A., & Poon, L. W. (1989). Speech comprehension and memory through adulthood: The roles of time and strategy. In L. W. Poon, D. C. Rubin, & B. A. Wilson (Eds.), *Everyday cognition in adulthood and late life.* Cambridge: Cambridge University Press.

Stoltzfus, E. R., Hasher, L., Zacks, R. T., Ulivi, M. S., & Goldstein, D. (1993). Investigations of inhibition and interference in younger and older adults. *The Journals of Gerontology: Psychological Sciences, 48,* P179–188.

Stone, C. P. (1929). The age factor in animal learning: I. Rats in the problem box and the maze. *Genetic Psychology Monographs, 5.*

Storandt, M., Grant, E. A., & Gordon, B. C. (1978). Remote memory as a function of age and sex. *Experimental Aging Research, 4,* 365–375.

Strayer, D. L., Wickens, C. D., & Braune, R. (1987). Adult age differences in the speed and capacity of information processing: 2. An electrophysiological approach. *Psychology and Aging, 2,* 99–110.

Suci, G. H., Davidhoff, M. D., & Brown, J. C. (1962). Interference in short-term retention as a function of age. In C. Tibbitts & W. Donahue (Eds.), *Social and psychological aspects of aging*. New York: Columbia University Press.

Sunderland, A., Harris, J. E., & Baddeley, A. D. (1983). Do laboratory tests predict everyday memory? A neuropsychological study. *Journal of Verbal Learning and Verbal Behavior*, 22, 341–357.

Sunderland, A., Watts, K., Baddeley, A. D., & Harris, J. E. (1986). Subjective memory assessment and test performance in elderly adults. *Journal of Gerontology*, 41, 376–384.

Surber, J. R., Kowalski, A. H., & Pena-Paez, A. (1984). Effects of aging on the recall of extended expository prose. *Experimental Aging Research*, 10, 25–28.

Surwillo, W. W. (1963). The relation of simple response time to brain wave frequency and the effects of age. *Electroencephalography and Clinical Neurophysiology*, 15, 105–114.

Surwillow, W. W. (1968). Timing of behavior in senescence and the role of the central nervous system. In G. A. Talland (Ed.), *Human aging and behavior*. New York: Academic Press.

Swanson, L. W., & Lee, T. D. (1992). Effects of aging and schedules of knowledge of results on motor learning. *The Journals of Gerontology: Psychological Sciences*, 47, P406–411.

Szafran, J. (1953). *Some experiments on motor performance in relation to aging*. Thesis, Cambridge University.

Tachibana, K. (1927). On learning process of the aged. *Japanese Journal of Psychology*, 2, 635–653.

Talland, G. A. (1965a). Three estimates of the word span and their stability over the adult years. *Quarterly Journal of Experimental Psychology*, 17, 301–307.

Talland, G. A. (1965b). Initiation of response and reaction time in aging, and with brain damage. In A. T. Welford & J. E. Birren (Eds.), *Behavior, aging, and the nervous system*. Springfield, IL: Charles C. Thomas.

Talland, G. A. (1967). Age and the immediate memory span. *The Gerontologist*, 7, 4–9.

Talland, G. A. (1968). Age and the span of immediate recall. In G. A. Talland (Ed.), *Human aging and behavior*. New York: Academic Press.

Taub, H. A. (1966). Visual short-term memory as a function of age, rate, and schedule of presentation. *Journal of Gerontology*, 21, 388–391.

Taub, H. A. (1967). Paired-associate learning as a function of age, rate, and instructions. *Journal of Genetic Psychology*, 111, 41–46.

Taub, H. A. (1968). Aging and free recall. *Journal of Gerontology*, 23, 466–468.

Taub, H. A. (1972). A comparison of young adult and old groups on various digit span tasks. *Developmental Psychology*, 6, 60–65.

Taub, H. A. (1973). Memory span, practice, and aging. *Journal of Gerontology*, 28, 335–338.

Taub, H. A. (1974). Coding for short-term memory as a function of age. *Journal of Genetic Psychology*, 125, 309–314.

Taub, H. A. (1975). Mode of presentation, age, and short-term memory. *Journal of Gerontology*, 30, 56–59.

Taub, H. A. (1976). Method of presentation of meaningful prose to young and old adults. *Experimental Aging Research*, 2, 469–474.

Taub, H. A. (1979). Comprehension and memory of prose materials by young and old adults. *Experimental Aging Research*, 5, 3–13.

Taub, H. A. (1984). Underlining of prose material for elderly adults. *Educational Gerontology, 10*, 401–405.

Taub, H. A., & Kline, G. E. (1976). Modality effects and memory in the aged. *Educational Gerontology, 1*, 53–60.

Taub, H. A., & Kline, G. E. (1978). Recall of prose as a function of age and input modality. *Journal of Gerontology, 33*, 725–730.

Taub, H. A., & Long, M. K. (1972). The effects of practice on short-term memory of young and old subjects. *Journal of Gerontology, 27*, 494–499.

Taub, H. A., Sturr, J. F., & Monty, R. A. (1985). The effect of underlining cues upon memory of older adults. *Experimental Aging Research, 11*, 225–226.

Taub, H. A., & Walker, J. B. (1970). Short-term memory as a function of age and response interference. *Journal of Gerontology, 25*, 177–183.

Taylor, J. L., Miller, T. P., & Tinklenberg, J. (1992). Correlates of memory decline: A 4-year longitudinal study of older adults with memory complaints. *Psychology and Aging, 7*, 185–193.

Teasdale, N., Bard, C., LaRue, J., & Fleury, M. (1993). On the cognitive penetrability of posture control. *Experimental Aging Research, 19*, 1–13.

Theios, J. (1975). The components of response latency in simple human information tasks. In P. M. A. Rabbitt & S. Dornic (Eds.), *Attention and Performance, Vol. 5*. New York: Academic Press.

Thomas, J. C., Fozard, J. L., & Waugh, N. C. (1977). Age-related differences in naming latency. *American Journal of Psychology, 90*, 499–509.

Thomas, J. C., Waugh, N. C., & Fozard, J. L. (1978). Age and familiarity in memory scanning. *Journal of Gerontology, 33*, 528–533.

Thomas, J. L. (1985). Visual memory: Adult age differences in map recall and learning strategies. *Experimental Aging Research, 11*, 93–95.

Thompson, R. F. (1986). The neurobiology of learning and memory. *Science, 233*, 941–947.

Thomson, D. M., & Tulving, E. (1970). Associative encoding and retrieval: Weak and strong cues. *Journal of Experimental Psychology, 86*, 255–262.

Thorndike, E. L., Bregman, E. O., Tilton, J. W., & Woodyard, E. (1928). *Adult learning*. New York: Macmillan.

Thumin, F. (1962). Reminiscence as a function of chronological and mental age. *Journal of Gerontology, 17*, 392–396.

Till, R. E. (1985). Verbatim and inferential memory in young and elderly adults. *Journal of Gerontology, 40*, 316–323.

Till, R. E., Bartlett, J. C., & Doyle, A. H. (1982). Age differences in picture memory with resemblance and discrimination tasks. *Experimental Aging Research, 4*, 179–184.

Till, R. E., & Walsh, D. A. (1980). Encoding and retrieval factors in adult memory for implicational sentences. *Journal of Verbal Learning and Verbal Behavior, 19*, 1–16.

Time. (1980). People section. September 8.

Toglia, M. P., & Kimble, G. A. (1976). Recall and use of serial position information. *Journal of Experimental Psychology: Human Learning and Memory, 2*, 431–445.

Tolman, E. C. (1932). *Purposive behavior in animals and man*. New York: Appleton-Century-Crofts.

Toole, T., Pyne, A., & McTaraney, P. A. (1984). Age differences in memory for movement. *Experimental Aging Research, 10*, 205–210.

Trahan, D. E., Larrabee, G. J., & Levin, H. S. (1986). Age-related differences in recognition memory for pictures. *Experimental Aging Research, 12*, 147–150.

Traxler, A. J. (1973). Retroactive and proactive inhibition in young and elderly adults using an unpaced modified free recall task. *Psychological Reports, 32*, 215–222.

Traxler, A. J., & Britton, J. H. (1970). Age differences in retroaction as a function of anticipation interval and transfer paradigm. In *Proceedings of the 78th Annual Convention of the American Psychological Association*. Washington, D.C.: American Psychological Association.

Treat, N. J., Poon, L. W., & Fozard, J. L. (1981). Age, imagery, and practice in paired-associate learning. *Experimental Aging Research, 7*, 337–342.

Treat, N. J., Poon, L. W., Fozard, J. L., & Popkin, S. J. (1978). Toward applying cognitive skill training to memory problems. *Experimental Aging Research, 4*, 305–319.

Treat, N. J., & Reese, H. W. (1976). Age, imagery, and pacing in paired-associate learning. *Developmental Psychology, 12*, 119–124.

Trembly, D., & O'Connor, J. (1966). Growth and decline of natural and acquired intellectual characteristics. *Journal of Gerontology, 21*, 9–12.

Tresselt, M. E., & Mayzner, M. S. (1964). The Kent-Rosanoff norms as a function of age. *Psychonomic Science, 1*, 65–66.

Tubi, N., & Calev, A. (1989). Verbal and visuospatial recall by younger and older subjects: Use of matched tasks. *Psychology and Aging, 4*, 493–495.

Tulving, E. (1962). Subjective organization in free recall of "unrelated words." *Psychological Review, 69*, 344–354.

Tulving, E. (1964). Intratrial and intertrial retention: Notes toward a theory of free recall verbal learning. *Psychological Review, 71*, 219–237.

Tulving, E. (1968). Theoretical issues in free recall. In T. R. Dixon & D. L. Horton (Eds.), *Verbal behavior and general behavior theory*. Englewood Cliffs, NJ: Prentice Hall.

Tulving, E. (1972). Episodic and semantic memory. In E. Tulving & W. Donaldson (Eds.), *Organization of memory*. New York: Academic Press.

Tulving, E. (1979). Relation between encoding specificity and levels of processing. In L. S. Cermak & F. I. M. Craik (Eds.), *Levels of processing in human memory*. Hillsdale, NJ: Erlbaum.

Tulving, E. (1983). *Elements of episodic memory*. Oxford: Oxford University Press.

Tulving, E. (1985). How many memory systems are there? *American Psychologist, 40*, 385–398.

Tulving, E., & Arbuckle, T. Y. (1963). Sources of intratrial interference in immediate recall of paired associates. *Journal of Verbal Learning and Verbal Behavior, 1*, 321–334.

Tulving, E., & Colotla, V. A. (1970). Free recall of trilingual lists. *Cognitive Psychology, 1*, 86–98.

Tulving, E., & Gold, C. (1963). Stimulus information and contextual information as determinants of tachistoscopic recognition of words. *Journal of Experimental Psychology, 66*, 319–327.

Tulving, E., & Pearlstone, Z. (1966). Availability versus accessibility of information in memory for words. *Journal of Verbal Learning and Verbal Behavior, 5*, 381–391.

Tulving, E., Schacter, D. L., & Stark, H. A. (1982). Priming effects in word-fragment completion are independent of recognition memory. *Journal of Experimental Psychology: Learning, Memory, and Cognition, 8*, 336–342.

Tulving, E., & Thomson, D. M. (1973). Encoding specificity and retrieval processes in episodic memory. *Psychological Review, 80*, 352–373.

Tun, P. A. (1989). Age differences in processing expository and narrative text. *The Journals of Gerontology: Psychological Sciences, 44*, P9–15.

Tun, P. A., Wingfield, A., Stine, E. L., & Mecsas, C. (1992). Rapid speech processing and divided attention: Processing rate versus processing resources as an explanation of age effects. *Psychology and Aging, 7*, 546–550.

Tyler, S. W., Hertel, P. T., McCallum, M. C., & Ellis, H. C. (1979). Cognitive effort and memory. *Journal of Experimental Psychology: Learning, Memory, and Cognition, 5*, 607–617.

Tzeng, O. J. L., & Cotton, B. (1980). A study phase retrieval mode of temporal coding. *Journal of Experimental Psychology: Human Learning and Memory, 6*, 705–716.

Underwood, B. J. (1954). Speed of learning and amount retained. *Psychological Bulletin, 51*, 276–282.

Underwood, B. J. (1957). Interference and forgetting. *Psychological Review, 64*, 49–60.

Underwood, B. J. (1963). Stimulus selection in verbal learning. In C. N. Cofer & B. S. Musgrave (Eds.), *Verbal behavior and learning*. New York: McGraw-Hill.

Underwood, B. J. (1964). Degree of learning and the measurement of forgetting. *Journal of Verbal Learning and Verbal Behavior, 3*, 112–129.

Underwood, B. J. (1969). Attributes of memory. *Psychological Review, 76*, 559–573.

Underwood, B. J., & Postman, L. (1960). Extra-experimental sources of interference in forgetting. *Psychological Review, 67*, 73–95.

Underwood, B. J., & Schulz, R. W. (1960). *Meaningfulness and verbal learning*. Philadelphia: Lippincott.

Uttl, B., & Graf, P. (1993). Episodic spatial memory in adulthood. *Psychology and Aging, 8*, 257–273.

Verhaeghen, P., & Marcoen, A. (1993). More or less the same? A memorability analysis on episodic memory tasks in young and older adults. *The Journals of Gerontology: Psychological Sciences, 48*, P172–178.

Verhaeghen, P., Marcoen, A., & Goossens, L. (1992). Improving memory performance in the aged through mnemonic training: A meta-analytic study. *Psychology and Aging, 7*, 242–251.

Verhaeghen, P., Marcoen, A., & Goossens, L. (1993). Facts and fiction about memory aging: A quantitative integration of research findings. *The Journals of Gerontology: Psychological Sciences, 48*, P157–171.

Waddell, K. J., & Rogoff, B. (1981). Effect of contextual organization on spatial memory of middle-aged and older women. *Developmental Psychology, 17*, 877–885.

Wahlin, A., Backman, L., Mantyla, T., Herlitz, A., Vitanen, M., & Winblad, B. (1993). Prior knowledge and face recognition in a community-based sample of healthy very old adults. *The Journals of Gerontology: Psychological Sciences, 48*, P54–61.

Wallace, J. E., Krauter, E. E., & Campbell, B. (1980). Animal models of declining memory in the aged: Short-term and spatial memory in the aged rat. *Journal of Gerontology, 35*, 355–363.

Walsh, D. A. (1975). Age differences in learning and memory. In D. S. Woodruff & J. E.

Birren (Eds.), *Aging: Scientific perspectives and social issues.* New York: Van Nostrand Reinhold.

Walsh, D. A., & Baldwin, M. (1977). Age differences in integrated semantic memory. *Developmental Psychology, 13,* 509–514.

Walsh, D. A., Baldwin, M., & Finkle, T. J. (1980). Age differences in integrated semantic memory for abstract sentences. *Experimental Aging Research, 6,* 431–444.

Walsh, D. A., Krauss, I. K., & Regnier, V. A. (1981). Spatial ability, environmental knowledge, and environmental use: The elderly. In L. Liben, A. Patterson, & N. Newcombe (Eds.), *Spatial representation and behavior across the lifespan.* New York: Academic Press.

Walsh, D. A., & Prasse, M. J. (1980). Iconic memory and attentional processes in the aged. In L. W. Poon, J. L. Fozard, L. S. Cermak, D. Arenberg, & L. W. Thompson (Eds.), *New directions in memory and aging: Proceedings of the George A. Talland Memorial Conference.* Hillsdale, NJ: Erlbaum.

Warabi, T., Noda, H., & Kato, T. (1986). Effects of aging on sensorimotor functions of eye and hand movements. *Experimental Neurology, 92,* 686–697.

Warren, J. M. (1986). Appetitive learning by old mice. *Experimental Aging Research, 12,* 99–105.

Warren, L. R., & Mitchell, S. A. (1980). Age differences in judging the frequency of events. *Developmental Psychology, 16,* 116–120.

Warren, R. E. (1972). Stimulus encoding and memory. *Journal of Experimental Psychology, 94,* 90–100.

Warrington, E. K., & Sanders, H. I. (1971). The fate of old memories. *Quarterly Journal of Experimental Psychology, 23,* 432–442.

Warrington, E. K., & Silberstein, M. (1970). A questionnaire technique for investigating very long term memory. *Quarterly Journal of Experimental Psychology, 22,* 508–512.

Warrington, E. K., & Weiskrantz, L. (1968). New method of testing long-term retention with special reference to amnesic patients. *Nature, 217,* 972–974.

Warrington, E. K., & Weiskrantz, L. (1970). Amnesic syndrome: Consolidation or retrieval? *Nature, 228,* 629–630.

Watkins, M. J. (1977). The intricacy of memory span. *Memory & Cognition, 5,* 529–534.

Watkins, M. J., & Watkins, O. C. (1974). Processing of recency items for free recall. *Journal of Experimental Psychology, 101,* 488–493.

Watkins, O. C., & Watkins, M. J. (1975). Build-up of proactive inhibition as a cue-overload effect. *Journal of Experimental Psychology: Human Learning and Memory, 1,* 442–452.

Watkins, O. C., & Watkins, M. J. (1980). The modality effect and echoic persistence. *Journal of Experimental Psychology: General, 109,* 251–278.

Waugh, N. C. (1963). Immediate memory as a function of repetition. *Journal of Verbal Learning and Verbal Behavior, 2,* 107–112.

Waugh, N. C. (1980). Age-related differences in acquisition of a verbal habit. *Perceptual and Motor Skills, 50,* 435–438.

Waugh, N. C., & Anders, T. R. (1973). Searching through long-term verbal memory. In S. Kornblum (Ed.), *Attention and performance. IV.* New York: Academic Press.

Waugh, N. C., & Barr, R. A. (1980). Memory and mental tempo. In L. W. Poon, J. L.

Fozard, L. S. Cermak, D. Arenberg, & L. W. Thompson (Eds.), *New directions in memory and aging: Proceedings of the George A. Talland Memorial Conference*. Hillsdale, NJ: Erlbaum.

Waugh, N. C., & Barr, R. A. (1989). Does retention of word order require verbal labeling? *Experimental Aging Research, 15*, 111–112.

Waugh, N. C., & Norman, D. A. (1965). Primary memory. *Psychological Review, 72*, 89–104.

Waugh, N. C., & Vyas, S. (1980). Expectancy and choice reaction time in early and late adulthood. *Experimental Aging Research, 6*, 563–567.

Weber, R. J., Brown, L. T., & Weldon, J. K. (1978). Cognitive maps of environmental knowledge and preference in nursing home patients. *Experimental Aging Research, 3*, 157–174.

Wechsler, D. (1944). *The measurment of adult intelligence (3rd. ed.)*. Baltimore: Williams & Wilkins.

Wechsler, D. (1945). A standardized memory scale for clinical use. *Journal of Psychology, 19*, 87–95.

Wechsler, D. (1958). *The measurement and appraisal of adult intelligence (4th ed.)*. Baltimore: Williams & Wilkins.

Wechsler, D. (1981). *Wechsler Adult Intelligence Scale Revised*. New York: The Psychological Corporation.

Wechsler, D. (1987). *Manual for the Wechsler Memory Scale—Revised*. San Antonio, TX: The Psychological Corporation.

Weiskrantz, L., & Warrington, E. K. (1979). Conditioning in amnesic patients, *Neuropsychologica, 17*, 187–194.

Weiss, A. D. (1965). The locus of reaction time change with set, motivation, and age. *Journal of Gerontology, 20*, 60–64.

Welford, A. T. (1958). *Aging and human skill*. Oxford: Oxford University Press.

Welford, A. T. (1959). Psychomotor performance. In J. E. Birren (Ed.), *Handbook of aging and the individual*. Chicago: University of Chicago Press.

Welford, A. T. (1977). Motor performance. In J. E. Birren & K. W. Schaie (Eds.), *Handbook of the psychology of aging (1st ed.)*. New York: Van Nostrand Reinhold.

Welford, A. T. (1984a). Psychomotor performance. In C. Eisdorfer (Ed.), *Annual review of gerontology and geriatrics*. New York: Springer.

Welford, A. T. (1984b). Between bodily changes and performance: Some possible reasons for slowing with age. *Experimental Aging Research, 10*, 73–88.

Welford, A. T. (1987). Motor performance. In G. L. Maddox (Ed.), *The encyclopedia of aging*. New York: Springer.

Welford, A. T. (1989; S. Pacaud, edited and presented by A. T. Welford). Performance in relation to age and educational level: A monumental research. *Experimental Aging Research, 15*, 123–136.

Welford, A. T., Norris, A. H., & Shock, N. W. (1969). Speed and accuracy of movement and their changes. *Acta Psychologica, 30*, 3–15.

Wells, J. E. (1974). Strength theory and judgments of recency and frequency, *Journal of Verbal Learning and Verbal Behavior, 13*, 378–392.

West, R. L. (1984, August). *An analysis of prospective everyday memory*. Paper presented at the annual meeting of the American Psychological Association, Toronto, Canada.

West, R. L. (1986). Everyday memory and aging. *Developmental Neuropsychology, 2,* 323–344.

West, R. L. (1988). Prospective memory and aging. In M. M. Gruneberg, P. E. Morris, & R. N. Sykes (Eds.), *Practical aspects of memory: Current research and issues Vol. 2.* Chichester: John Wiley.

West, R. L. (1989). Planning practical memory training for the aged. In L. W. Poon, D. C. Rubin, & B. A. Wilson (Eds.), *Everyday cognition in adulthood and late life.* New York: Cambridge University Press.

West, R. L., & Boatwright, L. K. (1983). Age differences in cued recall and recognition under varying encoding and retrieval conditions. *Experimental Aging Research, 9,* 185–189.

West, R. L., Boatwright, L. K., & Schleser, R. (1984). The link between memory performance self-assessment and affective status. *Experimental Aging Research, 10,* 197–200.

West, R. L., & Cohen, S. L. (1985). The systematic use of semantic and acoustic processing by younger and older adults. *Experimental Aging Research, 11,* 81–86.

West, R. L., & Crook, T. H. (1990). Age differences in everyday memory: Laboratory analogues of telephone number recall. *Psychology and Aging, 5,* 520–529.

West, R. L., Crook, T. H., & Barron, K. L. (1992). Everyday memory performance across the life span: Effects of age and noncognitive individual differences. *Psychology and Aging, 7,* 72–82.

Whitbourne, S. K., & Slevin, A. E. (1978). Imagery and sentence retention in elderly and young adults. *Journal of Genetic Psychology, 133,* 287–298.

White, N. & Cunningham, W. R. (1982). What is the evidence for retrieval problems in the elderly? *Experimental Aging Research, 8,* 169–171.

Whitehead, W. E., Lurie, E., & Blackwell, B. (1976). Classical conditioning of decreases in human systolic blood pressure. *Journal of Applied Behavior Analysis, 9,* 153–157.

Wickelgren, W. A. (1975). Age and storage dynamics in continuous recognition memory. *Developmental Psychology, 11,* 165–169.

Wickens, D. D., Born, D. G., & Allen, C. K. (1963). Proactive inhibition and item similarity in short-term memory. *Journal of Verbal Learning and Verbal Behavior, 2,* 440–445.

Wickens, D. D., Moody, M. J., & Dow, R. (1981). The nature and timing of the retrieval process and of interference effects. *Journal of Experimental Psychology: General, 110,* 1–20.

Wiegersma, S., & Meertse, K. (1990). Subjective ordering, working memory, and aging. *Experimental Aging Research, 16,* 73–77.

Wiggs, C. L. (1993). Aging and memory for frequency of occurrence of novel visual stimuli: Direct and indirect measures. *Psychology and Aging, 8,* 400–410.

Wiggs, C. L., & Martin, A. (1993, June). *Age related changes on direct but not indirect measures of frequency monitoring.* Poster presented at the annual meeting of the American Psychological Society, Chicago, IL.

Wightman, F., Allen, P., Dolan, T., Kistler, D., & Jamieson, D. (1989). Temporal resolution in children. *Child Development, 60,* 611–624.

Wiley, J. G., & Kausler, D. H. (1993). Adult age differences in temporal memory for cyclic actions. *Experimental Aging Research, 19,* 351–365.

Wilkie, F., & Eisdorfer, C. (1977). Sex, verbal ability, and pacing differences in serial learning. *Journal of Gerontology, 32*, 63–67.

Wilkinson, A. C., & Koestler, R. (1983). Repeated recall: A new model and tests of its generalizability from childhood to old age. *Journal of Experimental Psychology: General, 112*, 423–449.

Willingham, D. B., Nissen, M. J., & Bullemer, P. (1989). On the development of procedural knowledge. *Journal of Experimental Psychology: Learning, Memory, and Cognition, 15*, 1047–1060.

Willoughby, R. R. (1927). Family similarities in mental test abilities. *Genetic Psychology Monographs, 2*, 235–277.

Willoughby, R. R. (1929). Incidental learning. *Journal of Educational Psychology, 20*, 671–682.

Wilson, B. A., Cockburn, J., & Baddeley, A. D. (1985). *The Rivermead Behavioural Memory Test.* Reading, Berkshire: Thames Valley Test Co.

Wilson, R. S., Bacon, L. D., Kramer, R. L., Fox, J. H., & Kaszniak, A. F. (1983). Word frequency effect and recognition memory in dementia of the Alzheimer's type, *Journal of Clinical Neuropsychology, 5*, 97–104.

Wimer, R. E. (1960). A supplementary report on age differences in retention over a twenty-four hour period. *Journal of Gerontology, 15*, 417–418.

Wimer, R. E., & Wigdor, B. T. (1958). Age differences in retention of learning. *Journal of Gerontology, 13*, 291–295.

Winchester, T., & Roy, E. (1991, November). *Visual aiming movements in young and older adults.* Paper presented at the annual meeting of the Canadian Society for Psychomotor Learning and Sport Psychology, London, Ontario, Canada.

Wingfield, A., Aberdeen, J. S., & Stine, E. A. L. (1991). Word onset gating and linguistic context in spoken word recognition by young and elderly adults. *The Journals of Gerontology: Psychological Sciences, 46*, P127–129.

Wingfield, A., Poon, L. W., Lombardi, L., & Lowe, D. (1985). Speed of processing in normal aging: Effects of speech rate, linguistic structure, and processing time. *Journal of Gerontology, 40*, 579–585.

Wingfield, A., & Stine, E. L. (1986). Organizational strategies in immediate recall of rapid speech by young and elderly adults. *Experimental Aging Research, 12*, 79–83.

Wingfield, A., Stine, E. L., Lahar, C. J., & Aberdeen, J. S. (1988). Does the capacity of working memory change with age? *Experimental Aging Research, 14*, 103–107.

Wingfield, A., Wayland, S. C., & Stine, E. A. L. (1992). Adult age differences in the use of prosody for syntactic parsing and recall of spoken sentences. *The Journals of Gerontology: Psychological Sciences, 47*, P350–356.

Winn, F. J., Jr., & Elias, J. W. (1978). Associative symmetry and item availability: Evidence for qualitative age differences in acquisition strategies. *Experimental Aging Research, 1*, 297–306.

Winn, F. J., Jr., Elias, J. W., & Marshall, P. H. (1976). Meaningfulness and interference as factors in paired-associate learning. *Educational Gerontology, 1*, 297–306.

Winocur, G., & Moscovitch, M. (1983). Paired-associate learning in institutionalized and noninstitutionalized old people: An analysis of interference and context effects. *Journal of Gerontology, 38*, 455–464.

Winograd, E., & Simon, E. W. (1980). Visual memory and imagery in the aged. In L. W. Poon, J. L. Fozard, L. S. Cermak, D. Arenberg, & L. W. Thompson (Eds.), *New direc-*

tions in aging: *Proceedings of the George A. Talland Memorial Conference*. Hillsdale, NJ: Erlbaum.

Winograd, E., Smith, A. D., & Simon, E. W. (1982). Aging and the picture superiority effect in recall. *Journal of Gerontology, 37*, 70–75.

Winograd, E., & Soloway, M. (1985). Reminding as a basis for temporal judgments. *Journal of Experimental Psychology: Learning, Memory, and Cognition, 11*, 262–271.

Winterling, D., Crook, T., Salama, M., & Gobert, J. (1986). A self-rating scale for assessing memory loss. In A. Bes, J. Cahn, S. Hoyer, J. P. Marc-Vergnes, & H. M. Wisniewski (Eds.), *Senile dementia: Early detection*. London-Paris: John Libbey Eurotext.

Witherspoon, D., & Moscovitch, M. (1989). Stochastic independence between two implicit memory tasks. *Journal of Experimental Psychology: Learning, Memory, and Cognition, 15*, 22–30.

Witte, K. L. (1971). Optional shift behavior in children and young and elderly adults. *Psychonomic Science, 25*, 329–330.

Witte, K. L. (1975). Paired-associate learning in young and elderly adults as related to presentation rate. *Psychological Bulletin, 82*, 975–985.

Witte, K. L., & Freund, J. S. (1976). Paired-associate learning in young and old adults as related to stimulus concreteness and presentation method. *Journal of Gerontology, 31*, 186–192.

Witte, K. L., Freund, J. S., & Brown-Whistler, S. (1993). Adult age differences in free recall and category clustering. *Experimental Aging Research, 19*, 15–28.

Witte, K. L., Freund, J. S., & Sebby, R. A. (1990). Age differences in free recall and subjective organization. *Psychology and Aging, 5*, 307–309.

Wood, I. E., & Pratt, J. D. (1987). Pegword mnemonic as an aid to memory in the elderly: A comparison of four age groups. *Educational Gerontology, 13*, 325–339.

Woodruff, D. S. (1975). Relationships among EEG alpha frequency, reaction time, and age: A biofeedback study. *Psychophysiology, 12*, 673–681.

Woodruff, D. S. (1982). Long-term biofeedback conditioning at two EEG frequencies in young and older subjects. *Psychophysiology, 19*, 593.

Woodruff, D. S., & Birren, J. E. (1972). Biofeedback conditioning of the EEG alpha rhythm in young and old subjects. *Proceedings of the 80th Annual Meeting of the American Psychological Association*, 673–674. Washington, D.C.: American Psychological Association.

Woodruff, D. S., & Kramer, D. A. (1979). EEG alpha slowing, refractory period, and reaction time in aging. *Experimental Aging Research, 5*, 279–292.

Woodruff-Pak, D. S. (1988). *Psychology and aging*. Englewood Cliffs, NJ: Prentice Hall.

Woodruf-Pak, D. S. (1990). Mammalian models of learning, memory, and aging. In J. E. Birren & K. W. Schaie (Eds.), *Handbook of the Psychology of Aging (3rd ed.)*. San Diego: Academic Press.

Woodruff-Pak, D. S., Lavond, D. G., Logan, C. G., & Thompson, R. F. (1987). Classical conditioning in 3-, 30-, and 45-month old rabbits: Behavioral learning and hippocampal unit activity. *Neurobiology of Aging, 8*, 101–108.

Woodruff-Pak, D. S., & Sheffield, J. B. (1987). Age differences in Purkinje cells and rate of classical conditioning in young and older rabbits. *Society for Neuroscience Abstracts, 13*, 41.

Woodruff-Pak, D. S., & Thompson, R. F. (1988). Classical conditioning of the eyeblink response in the delay paradigm in adults aged 18–83. *Psychology and Aging, 3,* 219–229.

Woodworth, R. S. (1938). *Experimental psychology.* New York: Henry Holt.

Worden, P. E., & Meggison, D. L. (1984). Aging and the category-recall relationship. *Journal of Gerontology, 39,* 322–324.

Worden, P. E., & Sherman-Brown, S. (1983). A word-frequency cohort effect in young versus elderly adults' memory for words. *Developmental Psychology, 19,* 521–530.

Wright, B. M., & Payne, R. B. (1985). Effects of aging on sex differences in psychomotor reminiscence and tracking proficiency. *Journal of Gerontology, 40,* 179–184.

Wright, J. M. von. (1957). An experimental study of human serial learning. *Societas scientiarum Fennica,* Commentations humanarum litterarum, *23,* No. 1.

Wright, R. E. (1981). Aging, divided attention, and processing capacity. *Journal of Gerontology, 36,* 605–614.

Wright, R. E. (1982). Adult age similarity in free recall output order and strategies. *Journal of Gerontology, 37,* 76–79.

Yarmey, A. D. (1984). Age as a factor in eyewitness memory. In G. L. Wells & E. F. Loftus (Eds.), *Eyewitness testimony: Psychological perspectives.* New York: Cambridge University Press.

Yarmey, A. D., & Bull, M. P. (1978). Where are you when President Kennedy was assassinated. *Bulletin of the Psychonomic Society, 11,* 133–135.

Yarmey, A. D., Jones, H. P. T., Rashid, S. (1984). Eyewitness memory of elderly and young adults. In D. J. Muller, D. E. Blackman, & A. J. Chapman (Eds.), *Psychology and law.* Chichester, England: John Wiley.

Yarmey, A. D., & Kent, J. (1980). Eyewitness identification by elderly and young adults. *Law and Human Behavior, 4,* 359–371.

Yesavage, J. A. (1983). Imagery pretraining and memory training in the elderly. *Gerontology, 29,* 271–275.

Yesavage, J. A., & Jacob, R. (1984). Effects of relaxation and mnemonics on memory attention and anxiety in the elderly. *Experimental Aging Research, 10,* 211–214.

Yesavage, J. A., Lapp, D., & Sheikh, J. I. Mnemonics as modified for use by the elderly. In L. W. Poon, D. C. Rubin, & B. A. Wilson (Eds.), *Everyday cognition in adulthood and late life.* New York: Cambridge University Press.

Yesavage, J. A., & Rose, T. L. (1984a). The effects of a face-name mnemonics in young, middle-aged, and elderly adults. *Experimental Aging Research, 10,* 55–57.

Yesavage, J. A., & Rose, T. L. (1984b). Semantic elaboration and the method of loci: A new trip for older learners. *Experimental Aging Research, 10,* 155–159.

Yesavage, J. A., Rose, T. L., & Bower, G. H. (1983). Interactive imagery and affective judgments improve face-name learning in the elderly. *Journal of Gerontology, 38,* 197–203.

Yesavage, J. A., Rose, T. L., & Spiegel, D. (1982). Relaxation training and memory improvement in elderly normals: Correlation of anxiety ratings and recall improvement. *Experimental Aging Research, 8,* 195–198.

Yesavage, J., Sheikh, J. I., Friedman, L., & Tanke, E. (1990). Learning mnemonics: Roles of aging and subtle cognitive impairment. *Psychology and Aging, 5,* 133–137.

Young, R. K. (1962). Tests of three hypotheses about the effective stimulus in serial learning. *Journal of Experimental Psychology, 63,* 307–313.

Zacks, R. T. (1982). Encoding strategies used by young and elderly adults in a keeping track task. *Journal of Gerontology*, *37*, 203–211.

Zacks, R. T., Hasher, L., Alba, J. W., Sanft, H., & Rose, K. C. (1984). Is temporal order encoded automatically? *Memory & Cognition*, *12*, 387–394.

Zacks, R. T., Hasher, L., Doren, B., Hamm, V., & Attig, M. S. (1987). Encoding and memory of explicit and implicit information. *Journal of Gerontology*, *42*, 418–422.

Zacks, R. T., Hasher, L., Sanft, H., & Rose, K. C. (1983). Encoding effort and recall: A cautionary note. *Journal of Experimental Psychology: Learning, Memory, and Cognition*, *9*, 747–756.

Zajonc, R. B. (1968). Attitudinal effects of mere exposure. *Journal of Personality and Social Psychology Monograph Supplement*, *9* (2, pt. 2), 1–27.

Zandri, E., & Charness, N. (1989). Training older and younger adults to use software. *Educational Gerontology*, *15*, 615–631.

Zaretsky, H., & Halberstam, J. (1968a). Age differences in paired-associate learning. *Journal of Gerontology*, *23*, 165–168.

Zaretsky, H., & Halberstam, J. (1968b). Effects of aging, brain damage, and associative strength on paired-associate learning and relearning. *Journal of Genetic Psychology*, *112*, 149–163.

Zarit, S. H., Cole, K. D., & Guider, R. L. (1981). Memory training strategies and subjective complaints of memory in the aged. *The Gerontologist*, *21*, 158–164.

Zarit, S. H., Gallagher, D., & Kramer, N. (1981). Memory training in the community aged: Effects of depression, memory complaint, and memory performance. *Educational Gerontology*, *6*, 11–27.

Zelinski, E. M., & Gilewski, M. J. (1988). Memory for prose and aging: A meta-analysis. In M. L. Howe & C. J. Brainerd (Eds.), *Cognitive development in adulthood: Progress in cognitive development research*. New York: Springer-Verlag.

Zelinski, E. M., Gilewski, M. J., & Anthony-Bergstone, C. R. (1990). The Memory Functioning Questionnaire: Concurrent validity with memory performance and self-reported memory failures. *Psychology and Aging*, *5*, 388–399.

Zelinski, E. M., Gilewski, M. J., & Schaie, K. W. (1993). Individual differences in cross-sectional and 3-year longitudinal memory performance across the adult life span. *Psychology and Aging*, *8*, 176–186.

Zelinski, E. M., Gilewski, M. J., & Thompson, L. W. (1980). Do laboratory tasks relate to self-assessment of memory ability in the young and old? In L. W. Poon, J. L. Fozard, L. S. Cermak, D. Arenberg, & L. W. Thompson (Eds.), *New directions in memory and aging: Proceedings of the George A. Talland Memorial Conference*. Hillsdale, NJ: Erlbaum.

Zelinski, E. M., & Light, L. L. (1988). Young and older adults' use of context in spatial memory. *Psychology and Aging*, *3*, 99–101.

Zelinski, E. M., Light, L. L., & Gilewski, M. J. (1984). Adult age differences in memory for prose: The question of sensitivity to passage structure. *Developmental Psychology*, *20*, 1181–1192.

Zelinski, E. M., & Miura, S. A. (1988). Effects of thematic information on script memory in young and old adults. *Psychology and Aging*, *3*, 292–299.

Zelinski, E. M., Walsh, D. A., & Thompson, L. W. (1978). Orienting task effects on EDR and free recall in three age groups. *Journal of Gerontology*, *33*, 239–245.

Zemore, R., & Eames, N. (1979). Psychic and somatic symptoms of depression among young adults, institutionalized aged and noninstitutionalized aged. *Journal of Gerontology, 34,* 716–722.

Zivian, M. T., & Darjes, R. W. (1983). Free recall by in-school and out-of-school adults: Performance and memory. *Developmental Psychology, 19,* 513–520.

Abello, S., 120, 122–123
Abelson, R. P., 300
Aberdeen, J. S., 152, 154, 216–218, 389
Alwin, U., 417
Ackerman, A. M., 353–354
Ackerman, B. P., 194–195, 264–266, 426
Adamowicz, J. K., 161
Adams, C., 133, 294–295, 423
Adams, F., 182
Adams, J. A., 45, 356
Adams-Price, C., 260
Adelson, E. H., 136
Alba, J. W., 313
Albers, J. W., 28, 152
Albert, M. L., 391
Albert, M. S., 92, 151, 251, 391
Albertson, S. A., 284, 379–380, 382
Alexander, R. A., 27
Allen, T. M., 140–141
Allard, F., 43
Allen, C., 115
Allen, C. K., 167
Allen, G. A., 268
Allen, G. L., 21, 23–24, 315
Allen, P., 142
Allen, P. A., 157, 172–173, 204, 206, 212, 225
Altiere, P., 287, 302–303
Alvin, M., 299
Amberson, J. L., 141
Amrhein, P. C., 31–32, 206
Anagnopoulos, C., 214, 305
Anders, T. R., 170–172
Anderson, D. C., 13, 18
Anderson, J. R., 23, 271, 276, 289
Anderson, M., 32
Anderson, P. A., 215–216
Andres, D., 224, 226, 228, 238, 295

Andrews-Kulis, M., 206
Ankus, M., 14, 152
Anooshian, I. J., 428
Anschutz, L., 108
Anshel, M. H., 34–36
Anthony-Bergstone, C. R., 419
Appelman, I. B., 136
Arbuckle, T. Y., 223–224, 226, 228, 238, 267, 295, 297, 307
Arenberg, D., 19, 28, 70–72, 89, 99–103, 107, 122, 124, 128, 146–148, 159, 161, 290–291, 362, 404
Arnould, D., 286, 287
Atkeson, B. M., 141
Atkinson, R. C., 108–109, 150, 172, 175, 177–179, 181, 253
Atlas, L., 14
Atlas, S., 72
Attig, M. S., 287, 308
Auday, B. C., 313
Axelrod, S., 36, 99–100
Ayllon, T., 14
Azari, N. P., 313
Azrin, N. H., 14

Babcock, R. L., 152, 154, 214–215, 218–219
Bäckman, L., 44, 114–116, 187, 193, 235–236, 248–249, 252–253, 259–260, 299, 333, 351, 368, 395, 432
Bacon, L. D., 171, 252
Baddeley, A. D., 19, 149, 155, 193, 203, 209–210, 214, 263, 418, 422–423
Bahrick, H. P., 260–261, 347–348
Bahrick, P. O., 347
Baker, B. L., 29, 48
Balcerak, J., 428–431

Baldinelli, L., 227, 304
Baldwin, M., 290–291
Ball, H. E., 288
Ballard, H. I., 363
Balota, D. A., 247–248, 400, 407–410
Baltes, M. M., 14
Baltes, P. B., 15, 73, 107–108, 224
Banaji, M. R., 200
Bandura, A., 428
Bandura, E., 111
Barbano, H. E., 228
Bard, C., 203
Bardales, M., 324
Barik, H. C., 8
Barmwater, U., 251
Barnett, T., 142
Baron, A., 15–16, 18, 56–58, 172, 250
Baron, R. A., 7
Barr, R. A., 179, 211, 257
Barrett, G. V., 27
Barrett, T. R., 187, 225
Barron, K. L., 227
Bartlett, F. C., 276, 290
Bartlett, J. C., 258–260
Bartlett, K., 242–243
Bartus, R. T., 133, 259
Basden, B. H., 242–243
Basden, D. R., 242–243
Bashore, T. R., 206
Basowitz, H., 69–70, 73–75, 77–78, 86–87
Bates, A., 142
Battig, W. F., 75, 232
Beauvois, M. E., 160
Begg, I., 279
Belbin, E., 66, 363–364
Bell, B. D., 422
Bellezza, F. S., 115, 323
Bellos, N. S., 34
Belmore, S. M., 283–285
Bendlin, G., 287
Bennett, L., 10–13
Ben-Zur, H., 343
Beres, C. A., 57–58
Berger, D. E., 324
Bergquist, T. F., 116–117
Berkman, P. L., 131

Berkovsky, K., 258
Berkowitz, B., 152–153, 390
Bernbach, H. A., 177
Bernicki, M. R., 23
Berretta, D., 72
Berry, J., 133, 423
Berry, J. M., 140, 428
Berryhill, J. L., 91
Beuhler, J. A., 131
Bieber, S. L., 161
Bielby, D. D., 295
Bienas, J. L., 113
Binks, M. G., 165
Birchmore, D., 272
Birren, J. E., 13, 16, 27–29, 31, 203–204,
    391, 393, 404
Bjork, R. A., 263, 268
Blackburn, B., 277
Blackwell, B., 7
Blanchard, S., 12
Blanchard-Fields, F., 295
Blascovich, J., 33
Blaxton, T. A., 373–374, 380
Bleeker, M. L., 72
Block, R. A., 307
Blumenthal, J. A., 153, 225
Boatwright, L. K., 188, 422
Boden, D., 295
Bodkin, J., 422
Bogartz, R. S., 356
Boies, S. J., 161
Bolla-Wilson, K., 72
Bolles, R. C., 16
Boritz, G. M., 33
Borkan, G. A., 28
Borkowski, J. G., 13, 18
Born, D. G., 167
Borod, J. C., 92
Boruff, B., 155
Bosman, E. A., 42–43
Botwinick, J., 8–9, 14–15, 28–29, 31, 36,
    78, 140, 147, 151–153, 187, 189, 191,
    279–280, 282, 350, 391, 424–427, 430
Bousfield, W. A., 231, 239
Bower, G. H., 110, 115, 267, 276, 289, 378
Bower, R. E., 103

Bowles, N. L., 391, 395, 398, 400–401, 413–414
Boyarsky, R. E., 128
Boyes, C., 215–216
Bradley, M. M., 84
Brainerd, C. J., 253, 365
Bransford, J. D., 193, 290–291
Braun, H. W., 8–9, 70, 359
Braune, R., 206
Bregman, E. O., 33–34, 67
Brennan, P. L., 25
Bressie, S., 330–331
Brewer, W. F., 302
Brigham, M. C., 112, 425, 428
Brinley, J. F., 28–29, 31, 206
Britton, B. K., 298
Britton, J. H., 128
Bromley, D. B., 99–100, 327, 415
Bronfenbrenner, U., 200
Brooks, B. M., 333–334
Brooks, D. N., 19
Brown, A. S., 364, 378, 394, 404
Brown, E. R., 327
Brown, J., 322
Brown, J. A., 162–163
Brown, J. C., 312, 362
Brown, L. T., 22–23
Brown, R., 412
Brown, S. C., 197, 236
Brown-Whistler, S., 234, 236–237, 244
Bruce, D., 200
Bruce, P. R., 23, 318, 424–427, 430
Brune, C. M., 382
Bruning, R. H., 364
Buchanan, M., 155
Buchanan, S. L., 10
Buchsbaum, M. S., 204
Bugelski, B. R., 106, 356
Bull, M. P., 350
Bullemer, P., 63, 130
Bunce, D. J., 32
Burger, M. C., 140
Burgwald, L., 204
Burke, D. M., 262, 284, 393, 395, 401–402, 412
Burnett, N., 43

Buschke, H., 187, 210–211, 244, 254, 261
Busemeyer, J. K., 244
Butterfield, E. C., 132, 391, 432
Butterfield, G. B., 391
Butters, N., 19
Byrd, M., 92, 186, 198, 226, 253, 294, 353, 405
Byrne, D., 7

Caird, W. K., 151, 156, 253
Calev, A., 162
Cameron, D. E., 355–357
Camp, C. J., 108, 115–116, 227, 391, 431
Campbell, B., 18
Canestrari, R. E., Jr., 78, 85–89, 91, 94–95
Cannon, C. J., 406
Cantor, J., 13–14, 41
Caplan, L. J., 23–24
Capps, J. L., 287, 364, 374–375
Carlomusto, M., 235, 239, 244
Carpenter, P. A., 215–216, 304
Caruso, M. J., 430–431
Cavanaugh, J. C., 115, 131–132, 345, 422–423
Ceci, S. J., 232
Cerella, J., 48, 140, 203, 206, 396, 398
Cermak, L. S., 19
Chabot, R., 292, 407
Chaikelson, J., 224, 226, 228
Chapman, C. R., 250
Chapman, J., 147
Charness, N., 33–34, 43, 57, 227
Cheney, M., 400
Cherry, K. E., 191–192, 258, 317–318, 320–321
Cheung, H., 155, 214, 305
Chiarello, C., 376, 398
Chown, S. M., 151
Chromiak, W., 307
Chrosniak, L. D., 47, 61–62, 343
Church, K. L., 398
Clancy, S. M., 56
Claparede, E., 58
Clark, E., 200, 259
Clark, J. E., 29–30
Clark, M. C., 115

Clark, P. B., 289
Clark, W. C., 249–250, 282
Clarkson, M. E., 289
Clarkson-Smith, L., 226
Clifton, J., 43
Cobb, F. R., 153, 225
Cobb, R. E., 297
Cochrane, C. J., 32
Cockburn, J., 272–274, 423
Cohen, A., 376
Cohen, G., 216, 271, 284–285, 296,
    342–343, 353–354, 364, 401, 412
Cohen, G. D., 133
Cohen, N. J., 59–61
Cohen, R. L., 246, 328, 333–334, 337,
    425
Cohen, S. I., 9
Cohen, S. L., 188
Colbert, K. C., 151
Cole, K. D., 113, 416, 418
Coleman, R. E., 153, 225
Collin, C., 272
Collins, A. M., 373, 389, 396
Collins, J. F., 141
Collins, M., 187, 191
Colombo, P., 376
Colotla, V. A., 159
Comeaux, J. M., 221–222
Conrad, H. S., 344
Conrad, R., 161
Cooley, S., 393, 395
Coon, V. E., 210, 368–369
Cooney, T., 292
Cooper, L. A., 381
Coppinger, N. W., 51
Corkin, S., 59
Corral, G., 160
Corsellis, J. A. N., 14
Cortese, C., 401
Costa, P. T., Jr., 113, 228, 404
Cotton, B., 314
Cowan, N., 134, 143–144
Coyne, A. C., 140, 157, 172–173, 189,
    424–427, 430
Craig, E. R., 234

Craik, F. I. M., 4, 96, 133, 152–153,
    155–156, 159, 165, 176, 181–182,
    186–188, 190–191, 193–196,
    199–200, 211–212, 216–218, 226,
    249, 253–255, 262, 264–266,
    269–270, 276–278, 321–322, 332,
    420, 426–427
Crimmins, A., 227, 304
Crockard, J., 245
Crook, T. H., 72, 98, 133, 152, 200, 227,
    244, 259, 345, 417, 423
Cross, H. A., 313
Crossley, H., 21, 85–86
Crossman, E. R. F. W., 28, 203
Crovitz, H. K., 353
Crowder, R. C., 103, 140, 142–143, 177,
    200
Crozier, L. C., 157, 204, 206
Culler, M. P., 47
Cunitz, A., 157, 159, 177, 196
Cunningham, C. J., 297
Cunningham, W. R., 253
Czaja, S. J., 33–34

Dailey, B. F., 48
Dallas, M., 371, 374, 377–378
Daneman, M., 215–216, 304
Dannenbaum, S. E., 166
Darjes, R. W., 112–113, 227, 234–235
Darley, C. F., 268
Darwin, C. J., 142
Davidoff, M. D., 362
Davidson, H., 167
Davies, A. D. M., 161, 167
Davies, P., 223
Davis, G., 117
Davis, G. A., 288
Davis, H. P., 376
Davis, R. T., 313, 328, 339–340
Davis, S. H., 363
Davis, S. T., 103
Dawson, M. E., 14
Daye, C., 171–172
Delbecq-Derouesne, J., 160
Dell, G. S., 388
Dennehey, D. M., 428

Denney, N. W., 235, 239–240, 258, 317
Desroches, H. F., 363
Devolder, P. A., 425, 428
Dew, J. R., 258, 317
Diaz, D. L., 400, 402
Dick, M. B., 36, 245, 333
DiGuilo, D. V., 251
Dillingham, A. E., 27
Dirken, J. M., 151
Dirkx, E., 96, 255
Dixon, R. A., 133, 219–220, 292–298,
    303–305, 364, 417–418, 420,
    422–423, 425, 428
Dobbs, A. R., 166, 214, 273, 413
Doksun, T., 272
Dolan, T., 142
Dolkart, M. B., 346
Donaldson, G., 235, 317–318, 320
Donaldson, W., 163–164
Donley, J., 300–301
Doren, B., 287
Dorfman, D., 187
Dorosz, M., 295
Doty, B. A., 17
Doty, L. A., 17
Dow, R., 173
Downs, S., 66, 363–364
Doyle, A. H., 258
Drachman, D., 152, 188, 223
Drevenstedt, J., 115
Duchek, J. M., 187, 247–248, 264, 266,
    401, 407–410
Dudley, W. N., 213–214, 257, 262,
    264–266, 365–366
Duke, L. W., 116–117
Dunay, P. K., 297
Dunn, J. C., 383
Durkin, M., 13–14, 41
Dusek, J. B., 161
Dywan, J., 322

♦

Eames, N., 227
Earles, J. L., 368–369
Ebbinghaus, H., 98–99
Effron, R., 142
Egan, D. E., 34

Eggers, R., 251
Eich, J. E., 266
Eichelman, W., 161
Einstein, G. O., 235, 238, 273–274
Eisdorfer, C., 99–103, 128, 250
Ekstrand, B. R., 84, 221
Elias, C. S., 167–168
Elias, J. W., 35, 75–76, 78–79, 81, 92
Elias, M. F., 34
Elias, P. K., 34
Elliott, J. M., 194
Ellis, H. C., 34, 45, 192
Ellis, N. R., 310, 326
Emery, C. F., 153, 225
Emery, O., 414
Engelkamp, J. E., 328
Engstrom, R., 235
Era, P., 203
Erber, J. T., 120, 122–123, 187–188, 191,
    249–250, 253, 349, 420
Eriksen, C. W., 141, 171–172
Erngrund, R., 187
Erwin, R., 72
Estes, W. K., 103, 248, 268
Etheart, M. E., 420
Etzwiler, D., 289
Evankovich, K. D., 116
Evans, G. W., 25
Eysenck, M. W., 185–187, 235, 404, 407

♦

Faherty, A., 405–407, 409
Farrimond, T., 161, 258
Faulkner, D., 342, 353–354, 364, 401, 412
Ferguson, S. A., 323–325
Fernandez, A., 263
Ferraro, F. R., 400, 402–403
Ferris, S. H., 133, 152, 200, 259
Filippi, K., 345
Finkbinder, R. G., 13
Finkel, S. J., 107
Finkle, T. J., 290–291
Finley, G. E., 412
Firnhaber, S., 195, 244
Fischer, D., 251
Fisher, L. M., 236, 238
Fisk, A. D., 207

Fitts, P. M., 26
Fitzgerald, J. M., 353–354, 394
Flannagan, D. A., 238–239, 302
Flavell, J. H., 415
Fleury, M., 203
Flicker, C., 259
Flood, M. M., 57
Florini, B. I., 34
Flynn, T. M., 114
Folstein, M. F., 111
Folstein, S. E., 111
Foos, P. W., 160, 220, 252
Fox, J. H., 252
Fozard, J. L., 28, 48, 92, 95, 120, 122,
    140, 170–172, 174, 249, 350–351,
    391–392, 396, 398, 417
Franklin, H. C., 353
Franks, J. J., 193, 290–291
Fraser, D. C., 163–164
Freedman, J. L., 389, 404
Freeman, J. R., 19–20
Freund, J. S., 78–79, 123–125, 128–129,
    234, 236–237, 241, 244, 308–309,
    328–331, 339–340
Frey, T. J., 244
Friedman, D., 381, 383
Friedman, H., 151, 156, 238
Friedman, L., 110–113
Frieske, D. A., 191–192, 258–259, 272
Fromholt, P., 353
Fry, A. F., 382
Fuld, P., 223
Fuller, B. J., 50–51
Fullerton, A. M., 290–291
Fulton, A., 259–260
Furchtgott, E., 13–14, 41, 224, 244
Furda, J., 381
Furry, C. A., 73

Gabriesheski, A. S., 428–430
Gage, P., 34
Gakkel, L. B., 8
Galanter, E., 106
Gallagher, D., 113
Galt, D., Jr., 191
Galton, F., 353

Gandy, M., 376
Garcia-Colera, A., 31
Gardiner, J. M., 250, 253, 333–334, 384
Garry, P. J., 251
Gatz, M., 227
Gaylord, S. A., 39
Geiselhart, R., 8–9
Geiselman, R. E., 323
George, L. K., 153, 225
Gerard, G., 251
Gerard, L., 271, 287–288
Gernsbacher, M., 326
Gershon, S., 133
Giambra, L. M., 54, 223, 365
Gick, M. L., 216–218
Gilbert, J. G., 71, 151
Gilewski, M. J., 283, 292, 294, 300, 304,
    416–418, 422
Gilleard, C., 310, 317
Gillin, J. C., 266
Gillum, B., 227
Gillum, R., 227
Gilmore, G. C., 140–141
Gilson, E. Q., 149
Gist, B. A., 92
Gist, M., 34
Gladis, M., 70, 359
Glanzer, M., 157, 159–160, 177, 187, 196,
    255, 258, 413
Glenberg, A. M., 84, 182, 246–247, 263,
    309, 315
Glynn, S. M., 298–299
Gobert, J., 417
Godden, D., 263
Goggin, J., 168
Goggin, N. L., 29, 31–32
Gold, C., 395–396, 401
Gold, D. P., 223–224, 226, 228, 238, 295
Gold, P. E., 17–18
Goldberg, Z., 418
Goldfarb, R. W., 28, 151
Goldman, R., 346
Goldstein, D., 207
Goldstein, G., 29
Goldstein, M. D., 295
Gollin, E. S., 320–321

Gomez, I. M., 34
Gonzalez, E. G., 308
Goodglass, H., 19, 92
Goodrick, C. L., 14, 19–20
Goodwin, J. S., 251
Goossens, L., 86, 111, 113–114, 187, 255
Gordon, B. C., 350, 352
Gordon, S. K., 235, 249–250, 279, 282
Gorman, A. M., 252, 255
Gorman, W., 326
Gottlieb, G. E., 72
Gottsdanker, R., 29, 31
Gould, O. N., 294–295
Goulet, L. R., 119
Gounard, B. R., 244, 255
Gouze, M., 227
Grady, J. G., 131–132
Graesser, A. C., 298, 300
Graf, P., 244, 318–319, 371–372, 382–383
Grant, E. A., 14–15, 350, 352
Gratzinger, P., 110, 113
Green, C., 309
Greenbloom, R., 82
Greene, H. A., 395
Greene, R. L., 143, 149, 182, 246, 308
Greenhut-Wertz, J., 144, 147
Greenwald, J., 22
Gregory, K., 115
Gregory, R. L., 203
Griew, S., 28
Gritz, E. R., 282
Groccia-Ellison, M., 12
Grossman, J. L., 89–90, 92–95
Grossman, R., 72
Groth, K. E., 204, 206
Grout, L. A., 325–326
Guider, R. L., 113, 416, 418
Gur, R. C., 72
Gur, R. E., 72
Gurland, B. J., 227
Gutman, M. A., 41
Guttentag, R. E., 187, 235, 332–333, 342
Guynn, M. J., 274

Haaland, K. Y., 65, 251
Haggerty, D., 23

Hahn, M. V., 55
Hakami, M. K., 221, 308–312, 328, 331, 344–345
Halberstam, J., 85
Hale, S., 204, 400
Haley, W. E., 116
Hall, S. E., 299
Hall, T. C., 14
Hamberger, M., 381, 383
Hamilton, T., 298
Hamlin, R. M., 171–172
Hamm, V., 287
Hammer, M., 226
Hammond, K., 33
Hankins, L. L., 17–18
Hanley-Dunn, P., 428
Happ, L. K., 325–326
Harbluk, J. L., 321
Hardy, D., 204
Harker, J. O., 23, 292, 364
Harkins, S. W., 250, 364–366
Harley, C., 224
Harrington, D. L., 65
Harris, J. E., 273, 418, 422–423
Harsany, M., 297, 300
Hart, R. P., 364–366
Hartley, A. A., 34, 226
Hartley, J. T., 23, 34, 199, 215, 223, 227, 292, 299, 303–304
Hartman, M., 222–223
Harwood, E., 363
Hasher, L., 192, 207, 212, 227, 271, 287–288, 296, 306–308, 311–313, 315
Hashtroudi, S., 47, 61–62, 191, 323, 325, 343
Hatano, S., 226
Haug, H., 251
Hauge, G., 344
Hausman, C. P., 107
Hayman, C. A. G., 375
Hayslip, B., Jr., 151
Haywood, K. M., 31
Hebb, D. O., 155, 412
Hedges, D. G., 180
Heikkinen, E., 203

Heisey, J. G., 398–400, 402–403
Held, D., 25
Hellebusch, S. J., 106
Heller, H. S., 151, 391
Heller, M., 282
Heller, R. B., 413
Helstrup, T., 334
Henderson, W. G., 28, 152
Herlitz, A., 116–117, 193, 299, 351
Herman, G., 72
Herman, J. F., 23, 189, 318
Herman, T. G., 187
Hernandez, L. L., 10
Heron, A., 151–152, 156, 276
Herrmann, D. J., 418
Hertel, P. T., 192, 418, 428
Hertzog, C. K., 53–54, 219–220, 304–305,
    364, 406, 420, 425, 428
Herzog, A. R., 344
Hess, T. M., 46, 195–196, 238–239, 259,
    286–287, 300–302
Higginbotham, M. B., 153, 225
Higgins, J. N., 195–196
Hilbert, N. M., 113, 227
Hill, L. B., 42
Hill, R. D., 110–111, 115–116, 225, 345,
    378, 431
Hill, W. F., 207–208
Hinchley, J. L., 426
Hinrichs, J. V., 188, 314, 422
Hintzman, D. L., 307
Hirasuna, N., 167–169
Hiscock, M., 21, 85–86
Hitch, G., 155, 212, 214
Hodgkins, J., 28
Hogan, R. M., 268
Holding, C. S., 353
Holding, D. H., 136, 353
Holland, C. A., 304
Holland, L. J., 274
Holley, P. E., 269–270
Holzbauer, I., 364
Hood, J., 318
Hooper, F. M., 151
Hooper, J. O., 151
Horn, A., 344

Horn, J. L., 235
Howard, D. V., 63–65, 232, 235, 374, 378,
    382, 385, 389, 394, 396, 398–400,
    402–403, 407–409, 411
Howard, J. H., Jr., 63–65
Howe, M. L., 254, 364–365
Howell, S., 257
Howes, J. L., 350–351
Hoyer, F. W., 15
Hoyer, W. J., 15, 43, 53–57, 161, 353, 376,
    398
Hubbert, H. B., 19
Hudson, B. R., 161
Hulicka, I. M., 89–90, 92–95, 98, 122,
    124, 230, 232–234, 241–244, 276,
    281–282, 359–364
Hull, C. L., 10, 20
Hultsch, D. F., 89–90, 120, 133, 219–220,
    226, 241–244, 292–293, 296–298,
    300, 303–305, 364, 376–377, 418,
    420, 422–423, 425, 428
Hunt, M. E., 23
Hunt, R. R., 194, 235, 238, 245, 332–333,
    342
Hunter, M. A., 364–365
Huppert, F. A., 365
Hurwicz, M-L., 227
Husband, R. W., 18–19
Hyde, T. S., 183–185
Hyland, D. T., 187–188
Hyland, T. P., 353–354

Inglis, J., 152
Ingram, D. K., 19–20
Inman, V. W., 159, 165–166, 176, 252
Irwin, J. McD., 117, 357

Jackson, D. K., 241
Jackson, J. D., 295, 299
Jacob, R., 110
Jacoby, L. L., 221, 322, 371–374, 377–378,
    385
Jahnke, J. C., 103
Jakubczak, L. F., 14
James, J., 10–13
James, W., 149–150

Jamieson, D., 142
Jarvik, M. E., 282
Jasechko, J., 322
Jenkins, J. J., 85, 183–185, 224
Jennings, J. M., 133, 385
Jensen, A. R., 103, 159
Jerome, E. A., 8, 19, 73
Jessen, J. L., 292, 296
Johnson, A. L., 161
Johnson, L. K., 187
Johnson, M. K., 315, 323, 325, 342–343
Johnson, M. M. S., 245
Johnson, N. F., 157
Johnson, N. S., 299
Johnson, P. J., 51
Johnson, S. A., 34
Johnston, M. M., 17
Jones, D. M., 203
Jones, H., 167
Jones, H. E., 344
Jones, H. P. T., 260
Jones, T. A., 29, 48
Jonides, J., 308, 335
Jordan, T., 35
Jordan, T. C., 28
Josephsson, S., 116–117
Juola, J. F., 172

Kahn, H. L., 113, 227
Kaiman, L. J., 363
Kanoti, G. A., 127–128
Kaplan, E., 92, 251
Kaplan, J., 133
Kaplan, M., 423
Karlsson, T., 299, 432
Karol, R., 235–236, 241, 244
Kaszniak, A. W., 171, 252, 323, 325
Kato, T., 35
Katz, A. N., 350–351
Katzman, R., 223
Kaufman, A. S., 152
Kaufman, J., 187
Kausler, D. H., 4, 10, 36, 39, 53, 55,
	69–71, 74–76, 79, 80–81, 83, 85–87,
	89, 92, 95, 99–100, 103–104,
	117–119, 125–129, 133, 137,

153–155, 172, 200, 207, 209,
	220–221, 224–225, 227, 231, 239,
	250, 271–272, 280, 306, 308–318,
	323–332, 334–342, 344–345, 356,
	367–369, 390, 405–407, 409
Kay, H., 39, 276, 362
Kean, M. L., 36, 245, 333
Kear-Calwell, J. J., 282
Keele, S. W., 4646
Keelean, P. D., 373
Keevil-Rogers, P., 165
Keitz, S. M., 244, 255
Kellas, G., 179, 402–403
Kelly, C. M., 322
Kelly, K., 161
Kemper, S., 155, 214, 216, 283, 291, 295,
	305, 414–415
Kendall, B. S., 40, 50, 161
Kendler, H. H., 48, 50
Kendler, T. S., 48–50
Kennelly, K. J., 151
Kent, J., 260
Keppel, G. A., 163, 165, 197, 199
Kerr, B., 29
Kessler, S., 22
Keyes, B. J., 50–51
Kidd, E., 106
Kihlstrom, J. F., 317, 323, 325
Kimberlin, C., 364
Kimble, G. A., 8, 12, 313
Kincaid, D., 272
King, H. F., 27
King, P., 92
Kingma, J., 365
Kinsbourne, M., 91, 156, 164–165, 238,
	278
Kintsch, W., 268, 276, 283
Kirasic, K. C., 23–25, 315
Kirsner, K., 171–172, 383
Kistler, D., 142
Klane, L. T., 161
Kleim, D. M., 207, 220–221
Kliegl, R., 107–108, 126
Kline, D. W., 47
Kline, G. E., 282–283
Knight, C. C., 292, 296

Knill, F. B., 92, 94
Knopf, M., 332–334, 367
Knopman, D. S., 63
Kobus, D. A., 57
Koestler, R., 254
Kohn, M., 72
Kohout, F. J., 422
Kopelman, M. D., 365
Korchin, S. J., 69–70, 73–75, 77–78, 86–87
Koriat, A., 343
Kornetsky, C., 9
Kowalski, A. H., 299
Kowalski, D. J., 300
Kral, A. V., 133
Kramer, D. A., 16
Kramer, J. J., 108, 111
Kramer, N., 113
Kramer, R. L., 252
Krauss, I. K., 23–25, 34
Krauter, E. E., 18
Kreindler, A., 9, 47
Krell, R., 330–331
Kriauciunas, R., 152, 165
Kroll, N. E. A., 161
Kuhl, S., 251
Kynette, D., 155, 214, 305, 414–415

LaBerge, D., 189
Labouvie, G. V., 295
Labouvie-Vief, G., 295
Lachman, J. L., 132, 391, 432
Lachman, M. E., 111
Lachman, R., 132, 391, 432
Lafronza, V., 213–214, 320–321
Lahar, C. J., 152, 154, 216–218
Lair, C. V., 81, 85–87, 125–126
Landauer, T. K., 389, 401–402, 412
Lanphear, A. K., 29–30
Lapidot, M. B., 39, 92
Lapidus, S., 300
Lapp, D., 105
Larish, D. D., 31
Larrabee, G. J., 72, 98, 113, 257, 259, 417, 423
Larsen, S. F., 353

Larson, D., 228
Larsson, M., 235–236
LaRue, J., 203
Lasaga, M. L., 235, 396–397, 400
Lashley, K. S., 33, 46
Lauer, P. A., 187
Laurence, M. W., 232–233, 239–241
Laver, G. D., 412
LaVoie, D., 380–381
Lavond, D. G., 10
Law, J., 375
Lawrence, R., 353–354
Lawson, J. S., 147
Lawson, W. M., 166–167
Leavitt, J., 152, 188, 223
Lebowitz, B., 228
LeBreck, D., 250
Lee, C. L., 103
Lee, T. D., 40–41
Leech, S., 75
Lehman, E. B., 325–326
Leiman, B., 271
Leirer, V. O., 27, 105, 272, 287, 302–303
Lemke, J. H., 422
Lemon, J., 418
Leon, G. R., 227
Leonard, J. A., 28, 33
Leslie, J. E., 260
Levav, A. L., 258
Levee, R. F., 151
Levin, H. S., 113, 257
Levin, S. R., 345
Levine, E., 12
Lewandowski, L. J., 57
Lewis, R., 19
Lewkowicz, C. J., 111
Ley, P., 289, 344
Lichty, W., 204, 306, 309–310, 313, 326, 339–342
Liddle, C. L., 308, 310–311
Lieberwitz, K. J., 337–338
Light, K. E., 28–29
Light, L. L., 133, 187, 215–216, 262, 283–284, 287, 290–291, 300–301, 305, 318–320, 324, 364, 374–376, 379, 382

Lillyquist, T. D., 170–172
Lima, S. D., 400
Lindenberger, U., 108, 126
Lindholm, J. M., 159, 176
Linton, M., 321
Lipman, P. D., 23–24
Liss, J. M., 155
List, J. A., 260
Liu, Z., 339, 369
Lockhart, R. S., 181–182, 196, 262–263
Loewen, E. R., 322, 420
Loftus, E. F., 373, 396, 404
Loftus, G. R., 356, 364
Logan, C. G., 10
Logan, F. A., 13
Lombardi, L., 280
Long, M. K., 120
Loriat, M., 381
Lorsbach, T. C., 167, 189
Lott, L., 113, 416, 423
Lovelace, E. A., 393, 395, 424–425, 427
Loveless, N. E., 31
Lowe, D., 280
Lowenthal, M. F., 131
Luis, J. D., 191
Lurie, E., 7
Luszcz, M. A., 235, 238, 297–299
Lutz, R., 317

◆

Macht, M. L., 187, 210–211, 244, 254
MacKay, D., 412
Macken, W. J., 203
MacKinnon, D. F., 353
MacRae, P. G., 28
Madden, D. J., 153, 172, 296, 225, 395, 401–403, 405–406, 408
Madigan, S. A., 95, 144–145, 147
Mahler, W. A., 268
Maisto, A. A., 255, 257
Maki, R. H., 308
Malatesta, V. J., 141
Maletta, G. J., 28
Malley, M., 225
Mallory, W. A., 197, 199
Mammarella, S. L., 428
Manchester, J., 215–216, 295

Mandel, R. G., 299
Mandler, G., 229, 241, 253
Mandler, J. M., 238
Manning, S. K., 144, 147
Mäntylä, T., 187, 193, 248–249, 252–253, 274–275, 351, 371, 384–385, 395
Marcoen, A., 86, 111, 113–114, 187, 193, 255
Margolis, R. S., 393
Marinesco, G., 9, 47
Markley, R. P., 108, 115
Marka, L. E., 281
Marsh, G. R., 39, 424–425, 427
Marshall, P. H., 35, 75–76, 78–79, 92
Martin, A., 19, 386
Martin, J., 300, 412
Martin, M., 412
Martinez, D. R., 328–332
Masani, P. A., 188, 276–278
Maskarinec, A. S., 197
Mason, S. E., 106, 187, 259–260
Masson, M., 376–377
Mattila, W. R., 56
Mattiske, J. K., 235, 238
Matuzaki, T., 226
May, C. P., 296
Maylor, E. A., 252, 272–274, 412–413
Mayzner, M. S., 393
McAndrews, M. P., 235, 396–397, 400
McCallum, M. C., 192
McCarthy, M., 200, 259
McCarty, D. L., 109
McCauley, C., 179
McClelland, J. L., 208
McCormack, P. D., 250, 313, 317, 353
McCrae, R. R., 113, 228, 404
McDaniel, M. A., 273–274, 297
McDonald-Miszczak, L., 219–220
McDowd, J. M., 55–56, 236, 238, 249, 254, 430
McElree, B., 356
McElroy, L. A., 244
McEvoy, C. L., 269–270
McFarland, C. E., Jr., 179, 244–245
McFarland, R. A., 27
McGaugh, J. L., 17–18

McGhie, A. N., 147
McGuire, L. C., 345
McHewitt, E., 221
McHugh, P. H., 111
McInnis, L., 354
McIntosh, J. L., 428
McIntyre, J. S., 321–322
McKee, D. C., 153, 225
McKenna, W., 23
McKitrick, L. A., 116
McKoon, G., 388, 410
McLachlan, D., 61–62, 64, 321
McNeill, D., 412
McNulty, J. A., 253
McTarsney, P. A., 35–36
McWhorter, P., 115
Meacham, J. A., 271
Mead, G., 380
Meertse, K., 152, 215
Meggison, D. L., 241–243, 362
Megran, J., 244, 362
Meit, M., 272–273
Mellinger, J. C., 325–326
Melton, A. W., 117, 246–247, 357
Menich, S. R., 15–16, 172
Meredith, W., 152
Mergler, N. L., 161, 295
Merikle, P. M., 136
Metzger, R., 313, 318, 350
Metzler, J., 39
Meyer, B. J. F., 289, 292, 296, 299,
    303
Meyer, D., 400
Milberg, W., 151, 391
Miles, W. R., 28–29
Milgram, S., 22
Miller, B. V., 258
Miller, D. C., 289, 299
Miller, G. A., 106, 156, 277–278, 281
Miller, K., 313, 318, 350
Miller, K. H., 14
Miller, L. H., 9
Miller, T. P., 422
Milligan, W. L., 224
Millman, D., 142

Milner, B., 59
Mistler-Lachman, J. L., 167
Mitchell, D. B., 187, 189, 222, 227, 364,
    378, 382, 394, 404
Mitchell, D. R. D., 214–215, 218
Mitchell, R. F., 405
Mitchell, S. A., 308
Mittelman, D., 227, 304
Mittenberg, W., 251
Miura, S. A., 300–301
Moberg, P. J., 142
Mobley, L., 160
Modigliani, V., 180
Moenster, P. A., 282
Molander, B., 44
Monge, R. H., 75–76, 89–90, 120
Moniger, C., 120, 122–123
Montaglione, C. J., 287
Montague, W. E., 232, 356
Montan, B., 418
Monty, R. A., 299
Moody, M. J., 173
Mook, D. D., 200
Moon, J. N., 417, 423
Moon, W. H., 125–126
Moore, M., 113, 287
Moore, S. A., 92
Moore, T. E., 318
Moray, N., 142
Morrell, R. W., 257, 272, 289, 365–366
Morris, C. D., 193
Morris, J. C., 321
Morris, L. W., 322
Morris, R. G., 216–218, 322
Morrison, D. E., 391
Morrison, D. F., 29, 203
Morrow, D. G., 27, 195, 272, 287, 289,
    302–303
Morse, D. L., 10–13
Mortimer, J. A., 28
Morton, J., 143, 395
Morton, K. R., 423
Moscovitch, M., 61–62, 64, 92, 127,
    167–168, 187, 272, 383
Mozley, P. D., 72

Mueller, D. J., 14
Mueller, J. H., 235, 239, 244, 405–407, 409
Müller, G. E., 354
Murdock, B. B., Jr., 268
Murphy, D. R., 364, 378
Murphy, M. D., 179–180, 235, 308, 310–311, 326, 336, 428–431
Murrell, F. H., 48
Muth, K. D., 299
Myers, S. D., 345
Myerson, J., 204, 400

Nakamura, G. V., 302
Namazi, K. H., 204
Nappe, G. W., 92
Naveh-Benjamin, M., 308, 314–315, 335
Maylor, G. F. K., 363
Nebes, R. D., 172, 206, 315–316, 353
Neely, A. S., 114
Neely, J. H., 400
Negrao, M., 373
Nehrke, M. F., 51–52
Neidhardt, E., 332–334, 367
Neisser, U., 136, 141, 146, 418
Nelson, D. L., 269, 373
Nelson, T. O., 193, 199, 432
Newman, C. W., 142
Newman, R. C., 33
Nezworski, T., 313, 318, 350
Niederehe, G. A., 113, 227
Nielsen-Collins, K. E., 418
Niinikoski, J., 312
Nilsson, L-G., 235, 264, 333, 368
Nissen, M. J., 63, 130
Noble, C. E., 29, 48
Noble, S. G., 33
Noda, H., 35
Noonan, T. K., 353
Norgaard, L., 203–294, 299
Norman, D. A., 150–151, 175, 246
Norman, S., 155, 214, 305
Norris, A. H., 28
Norris, M. P., 328, 333, 339
Nowak, C. A., 294, 298

Nyberg, L., 368
Nyquist, L., 152, 224

Obler, L. K., 391, 413
O'Brien, K., 415
Obrist, W. D., 363
O'Connor, J., 161
O'Doherty, B. M., 27
O'Hara, M. W., 422
Ohashi, Y., 226
Ohta, N., 23, 375
Okun, M. A., 289
O'Leary, D. S., 251
Oliveri, M., 409
Olson, K., 293–296, 299
Osborne, D. P., 327
Osman, A., 206
Ostby, R. S., 308
Overcast, T., 220
Owens, S. A. A., 380–381
Ozekes, M., 310, 317

Pacaud, S., 39, 69
Padgett, R. J., 338
Paivio, A., 92, 95–96, 254–255, 258, 279
Palermo, D. D., 85
Palmer, R. L., 310
Parasuraman, R., 54
Pariante, G., 105, 272
Park, D. C., 115, 191–192, 213–214, 255–259, 262, 264–266, 272–273, 289, 317–318, 320–321, 326, 364–366, 377–378, 394
Parker, E. S., 191
Parkin, A. J., 53, 250–252, 313, 378–379
Parkinson, S. R., 144–145, 152, 159–161, 165–166, 176
Parks, C. W., Jr., 227
Parks, T., 161
Patterson, M. B., 204
Patton, G. W. R., 272–273
Paullin, R., 247–248
Paulshock, D. R., 350–351
Pavur, E. J., Jr., 220–222
Payne, R. B., 36–37, 41

Peak, D. T., 327
Pearlstone, 2, 187, 231, 241
Peck, V., 432
Pena-Paez, A., 299
Penland, M., 298
Pennypacker, H. W., 8, 12
Perey, A., 144–145
Perfect, J., 425
Perlmutter, M., 131–133, 152, 187,
     189, 222, 224, 227, 313, 318, 345,
     350, 391, 393, 418, 422–423,
     425, 430
Perone, M., 15, 18
Person, D., 133, 423
Peters, L., 393, 395
Peterson, L. R., 162–164
Peterson, M. A., 315
Peterson, M. J., 162–164
Petros, T. V., 292–296, 299, 345
Pew, R. W., 28, 152
Pezdek, K., 252, 258, 291, 317
Pfau, H. D., 353
Phillips, P. L., 335–336, 341, 367–368
Pierce, K., 96
Pierce, R. C., 131
Pietrukowicz, M., 245
Pignatiello, M. F., 431
Pike, L. A., 289
Pilzecker, A., 354
Pinsent, R. J., 289
Pirozzolo, F. J., 28
Plomp, R., 142
Plude, D., 55
Pollack, R. H., 141
Pomerleau, D., 10–13
Poon, L. W., 48, 92, 95, 120, 122, 133,
     140, 203–204, 206, 212, 272–273,
     280, 283–284, 289, 347, 350–351,
     391–392, 395, 398, 400–401,
     413–414, 422–423
Popkin, S. J., 92, 113
Porteus, S. D., 19
Posner, M. I., 161–162, 398, 405
Post, T. A., 55
Postman, L., 4, 82, 117, 119, 363
Potvin, A. R., 28, 152

Powell, D. A., 10, 13–14, 41, 224
Prasse, M. J., 139
Pratt, J. D., 106, 215–216
Pratt, M. W., 295
Prescott, L., 13–14, 41
Pressley, M., 112, 425, 428
Pribram, K. H., 106
Prill, K. A., 55
Prohaska, M., 114
Puckett, J. M., 70, 74–75, 154–155,
     166–167, 308, 323–325
Puff, C. R., 232
Puglisi, J. T., 167, 172, 192, 256–258, 262,
     264–266, 317, 326, 364, 394
Pyne, A., 35–36

                          ◆

Quarrington, B., 14
Queen, D. E., 255, 277
Query, W. T., 244, 362
Quillian, N. R., 389
Quina-Holland, K., 353

                          ◆

Rabbitt, P. M. A., 28, 31, 44, 207, 304,
     354, 417
Rabinowitz, J. C., 186, 194–195, 200,
     211–212, 216, 238, 245–246,
     264–266, 269–270, 332, 343,
     410–411, 426, 430
Radtke, R. C., 221
Radvansky, G. A., 271, 287–288
Rae, D., 152, 259
Rajaram, S., 383
Randt, C. T., 327
Rankin, J. L., 187–189, 191, 195,
     235–236, 239, 241, 244, 250
Rash, S., 415
Rashid, S., 260
Raskind, C. L., 406
Ratcliff, R., 388, 410
Ratner, H. H., 227, 304, 339
Raugh, M. R., 108–109
Raye, C. L., 342
Raye, D. E., 55
Raymond, B. J., 159, 196
Raz, N., 142
Read, D. E., 318

Rebok, G. W., 286, 299, 428–431
Reder, L. M., 300
Reese, H. W., 95
Reeves, C. L., 310
Regnier, V. A., 23–25
Reisen, C. A., 191
Reitman, J. S., 163, 166
Reno, R., 422
Rescorla, R. A., 13
Resnick, S. M., 72
Rhodes, D. D., 244
Ribot, T., 346
Rice, D. M., 204
Rice, G. E., 289, 292, 296, 299, 303
Richards, B., 318
Richardson-Klavehn, A., 372
Rickard, T. C., 326
Riddick, C. C., 29–30
Riege, W. H., 161, 252, 364
Riegel, K. F., 29, 203, 393, 416, 418
Riegel, R. M., 393
Rigby, M. K., 157
Riggs, K. M., 296
Rissenberg, M., 160, 255, 258, 413
Robb, J., 289
Robbin, J. S., 28, 31
Robbins, M. A., 34
Roberts, T. H., 235, 238
Robertson, B. A., 249
Robertson, E. A., 147
Robertson-Tchabo, E. A., 19, 28, 71–72,
    99, 107, 128, 161, 290–291
Robins, S., 215–216, 295
Robinson, B. C., 131
Rodgers, W. L., 344
Roediger, H. L., III., 373–374, 380, 383
Roenker, D. L., 236
Rogan, J. D., 55
Rogers, C. J., 50–51
Rogers, W. A., 207
Rogoff, B., 320
Rohling, M. L., 227
Roll, N. K., 23
Romano, J., 376
Roodin, P. A., 43
Root, N., 27

Rose, K. C., 192, 313
Rose, P. M., 315
Rose, R. P., 17–18
Rose, T. L., 107, 109–111, 378
Rosen, B., 34
Rosenbak, J. C., 155
Rosinski, R. R., 21, 23
Ross, E., 85
Rothberg, S. T., 420
Rowe, E. J., 95–96, 308
Rowley, R. L., 191–192
Roy, E., 35
Royal, D., 365–366
Royer, F. L., 140–141
Rubin, D. C., 353
Ruch, F. L., 33–34, 37–38, 67–70, 72–73,
    77, 118, 125
Rugg, M. D., 381
Rule, B. G., 166, 214, 273
Rumelhart, D. E., 208
Rundus, D., 177–179, 234
Rusenbek, J. C., 155
Russo, R., 53, 313, 378–379
Rust, I. D., 364
Ryan, E. B., 297, 420, 422–423
Rybarczyk, B. D., 364–366
Rybash, J. M., 43
Rypma, B., 207

Sabol, M. A., 160
Sagar, H. J., 353
Sakitt, B., 136
Salama, M., 417
Salamé, P., 203
Salthouse, T. A., 28, 30, 41–44, 46–48,
    55–57, 70–71, 96–97, 104, 139–140,
    152–154, 159, 179, 185, 201–204,
    206, 208–212, 214–216, 218–219,
    223–225, 227, 310–311, 313–314,
    316–317, 339–341, 349, 404
Saltzman, I. J., 183
Sanders, H. I., 350–351
Sanders, R. E., 179–180, 235, 308,
    310–311, 326, 336, 428–431
Sandler, S. P., 246, 333–334
Sands, D. C., 36, 333

Sands, L. P., 152
Sanford, A. J., 31
Sanft, H., 192, 313
Sass, N. L., 251
Saults, J. S., 70–71, 104, 153–154,
    201–203, 224–225, 227, 310–311,
    313–314, 316–317, 339–341
Saynisch, M. J., 55
Scarborough, D. L., 401
Scarborough, H. S., 401
Schacter, D. L., 315, 321, 323, 325,
    371–375, 381
Schaffer, G., 272–273
Schaie, K. W., 224, 304, 418–419
Schank, R. C., 300
Schear, J. M., 316
Scheikert, R., 155
Schell, A. M., 14
Schell, D., 295
Schell, D. A., 227, 304
Schiebolk, S., 153, 225
Schiffman, H., 353
Schleser, R., 422
Schmitt, F. A., 179–180, 235, 245,
    428–431
Schneider, H. G., 241
Schneider, W., 172
Schnore, M. M., 95–96, 165
Schonfield, A. E. D., 136, 163–167, 249,
    253, 261, 347, 352
Schreiber, T. A., 269
Schroeder, K., 246, 333–334
Schulenberg, J. E., 420
Schulman, A. I., 252
Schulz, R. W., 77, 91, 103, 315
Schumann, C. E., 33
Schvaneveldt, R. W., 400
Schwartz, B. L., 47, 61–62
Schwartzman, A. E., 224, 226, 228, 295
Schwoerer, C., 34
Scialfa, C. T., 393
Scogin, F. R., 113–114, 227, 416, 423
Sczomak, T., 272
Sebby, R. A., 241
See, S. K., 422
Segmen, J., 106

Seidenberg, M., 251
Selfridge, J. A., 277–278
Service, C., 99–103
Severin, F. T., 157
Shaffer, L. H., 46
Shaffer, W. D., 189
Shakow, D., 346
Shand, M. A., 162
Shaps, L. P., 264
Sharit, J., 34
Sharp, T., 412
Sharpa, M. J., 320–321
Shaw, R. J., 187, 189, 214–215, 222,
    377–378, 398–400, 402–403,
    408–411, 420, 426–427
Sheffer, D., 343
Sheffield, J. B., 14
Sheikh, J. I., 105, 110–113, 116, 289, 345,
    431
Shelly, C. H., 29
Shepard, R. N., 39, 254
Sherman, R. A., 7
Sherman-Brown, S., 244
Shibata, H., 226
Shichita, K., 226
Shiffrin, R. M., 150, 172, 175, 181, 253
Shmavonian, B. M., 9
Shock, N. W., 28
Shulman, H. G., 189
Siegel, A. W., 21, 23
Silberstein, M., 349–350
Simeone, C., 115
Simolke, N. V., 376
Simon, E., 187–188, 190–191, 262
Simon, E. W., 255–256, 260, 292–296,
    298
Simon, J. R., 28, 30
Simon, S. L., 23–24
Simpson, G. B., 189
Singh, A., 187, 364, 374–376
Singleton, W. T., 28
Sinnott, J. D., 272–273
Skillbeck, C. E., 289
Skorpanich, M. A., 25
Skovronek, E., 214–215, 218
Slamecka, N. J., 244, 356

Slater, P. C., 349
Slaughter, S. J., 46, 259
Slevin, A. E., 279
Sloman, S. A., 375
Small, B., 219–220, 226, 376–377
Smith, A. D., 106, 115, 133, 187–189, 211, 213–214, 241, 255–259, 262, 264–268, 320–321, 364, 394
Smith, D. A., 300
Smith, G. A., 204, 400
Smith, J., 107–108
Smith, P. T., 273–274
Smith, S. M., 263, 309
Smith, S. W., 299
Smith, W. R., 299
Snelus, P., 347
Snoddy, G. S., 34, 36
Snyder, C. R., 398
Snyder, D. N., 28, 152
Snyder, S. S., 300
Solomon, P. R., 10–13
Soloway, M., 314
Solso, R. L., 133, 136, 141–142
Solyom, L., 8
Somberg, B. L., 47–48, 55–57
Sovacool, M., 256–257
Spangler, E. L., 19–20
Speakman, D. C., 351
Spear, N. E., 84
Spence, K. W., 10, 73
Sperback, D. J., 353
Sperling, G., 137–139, 142–143
Spiegel, D., 111
Spiker, C. C., 82
Spilich, G. J., 280, 284, 292–293
Spirduso, W. W., 28–29
Spitzer, J. B., 142
Sprott, R., 415
Squire, L. R., 59–61, 349–350, 353, 372
Staats, A. W., 7
Staats, C. K., 7
Stanfield, G. G., 422
Stanovich, K. E., 402
Stark, H. A., 372–375
Stelmach, G. E., 29, 31–32

Stelnicki, 269
Stern, L. D., 307
Sternberg, S., 29, 169–172
Sterns, H. L., 27, 89–90
Stigsdotter, A., 116–117
Stillman, R. C., 266
Stine, E. L., 152, 154, 212, 216–218, 223, 280, 283–284, 287, 294–295, 305, 345, 389, 395
Stockburger, D. W., 166–167
Stollery, B., 425
Stoltzfus, E. R., 207, 296
Stone, C. P., 19
Stones, M. J., 352
Storandt, M., 14–15, 96, 113–115, 147, 151–153, 222, 279–280, 350, 352, 391, 416, 423
Strater, L., 259
Strayer, D. L., 206
Sturr, J. F., 299
Sucec, J., 47
Suci, G. H., 362
Sunderland, A. S., 418, 422–423
Surber, J. R., 299
Surwillow, W. W., 16
Sutcliffe, J., 165
Sutterer, N. J., 52
Swanson, J. M., 226, 253
Swanson, L. W., 40–41
Swanson, N. G., 315
Swede, H., 33
Syndulko, K., 418
Szafran, J., 28, 34–36, 204
Szechtmen, B., 422
Szuchman, L. T., 420

Tabor, L., 232, 292–296, 299
Tachibana, K., 33
Talland, G. A., 147, 152–154, 165, 212
Tanke, E., 111–113, 289
Tate, C., 238–239
Taub, H. A., 90, 147, 152, 156–157, 223, 267–268, 282–286, 299
Taylor, D. W., 432
Taylor, J. L., 422
Taylor, R. L., 161

Teasdale, N., 203
Terry, R. D., 223
Theios, J., 29, 206
Thomas, J. C., Jr., 28, 174, 350–351
Thomas, J. L., 318
Thomason, N., 155
Thompson, C. P., 236
Thompson, L. W., 29, 113, 139, 187, 292,
    294, 416–419
Thompson, R. F., 10–12, 14
Thomson, D. M., 262–264
Thorndike, E. L., 33–34, 67
Thronesbery, C., 391, 432
Thumin, F., 41
Till, R. E., 258, 284–286, 326
Tilse, C. S., 423
Tilton, J. W., 33–34, 67
Time, 347
Tinklenberg, J., 27, 422
Toglia, M. P., 313
Tolman, E. C., 20
Toole, T., 35–36
Toth, J. P., 385
Tourtellotte, W. W., 28, 152, 418
Trahan, D. E., 257
Trapp, E. P., 97
Traxler, A. J., 128, 362
Treat, N. J., 15, 92, 95, 120, 122, 417
Trembly, D., 161
Tresselt, M. E., 393
Trevithick, L., 294
Trier, M. L., 131
Trotter, M., 239
Tubbs, A., 260
Tubi, N., 162
Tulving, E., 133, 159, 187, 190–191, 231,
    240, 262–264, 267, 372–375,
    387–388, 395–396, 401, 409
Tun, P. A., 280, 296, 299, 305
Turvey, M. T., 142
Tuten, C., 235–236, 241, 244
Tyler, S. W., 192
Tzeng, O. J. L., 314

Ulivit, M. S., 207
Ulmer, R., 418

Underwood, B. J., 4, 77, 81, 84, 91, 117,
    163, 165, 221, 307, 356, 363
Uttl, B., 318–319

Valdiserri, M., 325
Valencia-Laver, D., 380
Vanderleck, V. F., 300
Vandermaas, M. O., 300–301
Vandervoort, D., 111
van Dijk, T. A., 283
Van Dusseldorp, 376
Vasquez, B. J., 17–18
Velazquez, E., 12
Verdonik, F., 133, 423
Verhaeghen, P., 86, 113–114, 187, 193,
    255
Versttraete, D., 289
Vierck, V., 48
Vitanen, M., 116–117, 351
Vitina, J. R., 308
Volpendeate, D., 418
Von Dras, D., 32
Von Eye, A., 303–304
Voss, J. F., 280
Vranes, L. F., 251
Vyas, S. M., 31

Waddell, K. J., 320
Wagstaff, D., 204, 400
Wahlin, A., 351
Walford, R., 19–20
Walker, J. B., 267–268
Wallace, J. E., 18
Wallace, R. B., 422
Wallace, W. P., 221
Walsh, D. A., 23–25, 53–54, 133, 139,
    187, 199, 223, 284–286, 290–292
Walsh, K. K., 179–180
Walsh-Riddle, M., 153, 225
Walsh-Sweeney, L., 92, 95
Walter, B. M., 250–252, 384–385
Walters, J., 22
Warabi, T., 35
Warr, P. B., 32
Warren, J. M., 19
Warren, L. R., 245, 308

Warren, R. E., 396
Warrington, E. K., 58, 349–351, 370–371
Watkins, M. J., 146, 149, 155
Watkins, O. C., 146, 149
Watkins, S. K., 225
Watts, K., 422
Waugh, N. C., 28, 31, 150–151, 172, 175, 179, 206, 211, 246, 249, 257
Wayland, S. C., 280
Weaver, S. L., 111
Weaverdyck, S., 295
Webber, S. N., 92
Weber, R. J., 22–23
Weber, T. A., 206
Wechsler, D., 14, 85, 152, 225, 281
Weindruch, R., 19–20
Weingartner, H., 266
Weisberg, L. A., 251
Weiskrantz, L., 58, 370–374
Weismer, G., 155
Weiss, A. D., 29
Weiss, R. L., 363
Weldon, J. K., 22–23
Welford, A. T., 28, 34–39, 69, 203, 212, 216, 352, 355
Wellman, H. W., 415
Wells, J. E., 246
Wenger, L., 136
West, R. L., 105, 152, 188, 227, 244, 272–273, 315, 328, 333, 339, 422, 428
Wetzler, S. E., 353
Whetstone, T., 252
Whitbourne, S. K., 279, 353
White, H., 400, 402
White, N., 253
Whitehead, W. E., 7
Whitehouse, P., 133
Whitworth, M. A., 289
Wible, C., 300
Wickelgren, W. A., 246, 250
Wickens, C. D., 206
Wickens, D. D., 167, 172–173
Wiergersma, S., 152
Wigdor, B. T., 359–361

Wiggs, C. L., 386
Wightman, F., 142
Wiley, J. G., 328, 332, 334–338, 341–42, 368–369
Wilkie, F., 99–100
Wilkins, A. J., 273
Wilkinson, A. C., 254
Williams, D., 395
Williams, D. M., 203
Williams, M. V., 53–54
Willingham, D. B., 130
Willoughby, R. R., 67
Wilson, B. A., 423
Wilson, R. S., 171, 252
Wimer, R. E., 359–361, 363
Winblad, B., 351
Winchester, T., 35
Wingfield, A., 152, 154, 212, 216–218, 223, 280, 283–284, 294–296, 305, 345, 389
Winn, F. J., 75–76, 78–79, 81, 92
Winocur, G., 61–62, 64, 127, 167–168
Winograd, E., 255–256, 259–260, 314
Winterling, D., 417
Wise, J. L., 310–311
Witherspoon, D., 383
Witte, K. L., 52, 75, 78–79, 87, 123–125, 128–129, 234, 236–237, 241, 244, 308–309
Wittlinger, R. P., 347
Woll, S. B., 300
Wollen, K. A., 92
Wood, I. E., 106
Woodruff, D. S., 16
Woodruff-Pak, D. S., 10–14, 16–17, 19
Woods, A. M., 418
Woodward, R., 289
Woodworth, R. S., 136
Woodyard, E., 33–34, 67
Worden, P. E., 241–242, 362
Worthley, J., 412
Wright, B. M., 36–37, 41
Wright, J., 35
Wright, J. M. von, 19
Wright, L., 220
Wright, M., 187

Wright, R. E., 159, 198–199, 212, 308, 311–312

Yadrick, R. M., 220
Yap, E. C., 315
Yarmey, A. D., 260, 350
Yee, P. L., 401–402
Yesavage, J., 27, 105, 107, 109–112, 116, 345, 378, 431
Yonelinas, A. P., 385
Young, R. K., 103
Youngjohn, J. R., 98
Yuille, J. C., 95

Zacks, R. T., 192, 207, 212, 227, 271, 287–288, 306, 308, 311–313, 315

Zadek, A., 345
Zajonc, R. B., 386
Zandri, E., 34
Zaretsky, H., 85
Zarit, S. H., 113, 227, 416, 418
Zehr, D., 407
Zelinski, E. M., 187, 283, 287, 290, 292, 294, 304, 318–320, 416–418, 422
Zeller, P., 48
Zemore, R., 227
Zerbe, M. B., 14
Zerinque, J. A., 221–222
Zimmerman, R., 72
Zinna, N. U., 8
Zivian, M. T., 112–113, 227, 234–235
Zonderman, A. B., 228

Accidents, age differences, 27
Action memory and activity memory, *see
also* Incidental learning/memory
versus intentional learning/memory,
Retention and long-term forgetting
cognitive versus motor activity, 329–330
clustering, 333
content, 327–335
cyclic actions, 341–342
definitions, 327–328
duration of an activity, 330–331
enactment during recall, 334
everyday memory, 326–327
familiarity of actions, 333
frequency-of-occurrence memory,
339
generation effect, 330–331
reality monitoring, 342–343
recognition memory, 332, 334
rehearsal independency, 327–328
repetition of actions, 333–334
retrieval processes, 334–335, 341
serial position effects, 328–330
short-term memory, 337–339
source memory, 342–343
subject-performed tasks (SPTs), 328
task variability in age differences,
331–332
temporal memory, 339–342
two-stage model of encoding, 335–339
Age-Associated Memory Impairment
(AAMI), 133
Alzheimer's Disease
detection of dementia, 416
discourse memory, 293
mnemonic training, 116–117
operant conditioning, 14

Amnesics
autobiographical memory, 353
implicit memory, 370–372
procedural learning, 57–61
source memory, 321
Anxiety
age differences, 10
effects on learning, 10, 73, 111
effects on memory, 228
effects on mnemonic training, 111
Articulatory loop, *see* Working memory
Associationism
classical learning theory, 2, 13, 77
stage analysis, 2, 77
Attention, *see* Divided attention,
Perceptual learning, Selective
attention, Vigilance
Autobiographical memory, *see* Retention
and long-term forgetting
Automaticity of encoding
continuum with effortful encoding, 326
criteria, 308
definition, 212, 306
in frequency-of-occurrence memory, 307
in other noncontent attributes, 326
in spatial memory, 307
in temporal memory, 307, 312–313
working memory by-pass, 212–213
Avoidance learning, *see* Operant
conditioning

◆

Behavior modification, *see* Classical
conditioning, Operant conditioning
Biofeedback, *see* Operant conditioning
Bridge, *see* Expertise
Brinley-plot, *see* Processing rate model of
episodic memory

◆

Case memory, *see* Incidental learning/
    memory versus intentional learning/
    memory
Categorical organization, *see*
    Organizational processes
Cautiousness, age differences, 250
Cerebellum, *see* Classical conditioning
Cerebral hemisphere asymmetry
    imaginal mediation, 92
    mirror tracing, 39
    verbal learning, 72
Chess, *see* Expertise
Chunking, *see* Digit span, Letter span
Classical conditioning
    age differences in acquisition and
        extinction, 8–13
    associative explanation, 13
    awareness, 14
    behavior modification, 7
    cerebellum, 14
    definition, 5–6
    delay procedure, 5
    differentiation (discrimination
        learning), 9–10
    extinction, 6
    habituation, 12–13
    information processing explanation, 14
    model for various learning phenomena,
        7–8
    nonassociative (nonlearning) factors, 10
    trace procedure, 13
Clustering, *see* Action memory and
    activity memory, Organizational
    processes in memory
Cognitive effort, *see* Levels of processing
    model of episodic memory
Cognitive maps, *see* Instrumental learning
Cognitive support, *see* Levels of processing
    model of episodic memory
Cohort effects, 70, 99
Complexity hypothesis, *see* Processing rate
    model of episodic memory
Comprehension, *see* Discourse memory
Computational span, *see* Working memory
Computer skills, *see* Motor-skill learning

Concreteness effect, *see* Picture memory
Consistency effect, *see* Recognition
    memory
Contextualism, 224
Conversations, memory of, *see* Incidental
    learning/memory versus intentional
    learning/memory
    age differences, 343–344
    rehearsal independence, 343
Cue overload principle, *see* Echoic
    memory, Organizational processes in
    memory

◆

Depression
    incidence, 227
    effects on learning, 113
    effects on memory, 227–228
    effects on mnemonic training, 113
Depth of processing, *see* Levels of
    processing model of episodic memory
Digit span, *see also* Intelligence
    assessment of working memory, 214, 218
    backward span, 153
    chunking, 156–157
    everyday memory, 151–152
    forward span, 151–153
    health, 152–153
    meaningfulness of items, 152, 277
    practice effects, 57
    presentation rate, 152
    secondary memory, 155, 157
Digit symbol test, *see also* Intelligence
    age differences, 57–58
    assessment of processing rate, 210
    definition, 67
    fluid intelligence, 108
    paired-associate learning analysis, 67
    practice effects, 57
Discourse memory, *see also* Incidental
    learning/memory versus intentional
    learning/memory
    annotative and denotative elaborations,
        294–295
    attributes of longer discourse, 298–299
    attributes of sentences, 283
    comprehension, 283–289, 305

everyday memory, 276
expertise, 302–303
hierarchical organization, 289
idea recall, 281–282
inferences, 284–286
longer discourse memory, 289–305
meaningful versus meaningless material,
    276–277
medical information, 289
mental representations of sentences,
    287–288
modality of sentence presentations,
    282–283
paragraph memory, 225, 281–289
prior knowledge, 299–300
procedural variables for longer discourse,
    294–298
propositions, 283, 289, 292–294
prosody, 280
qualitative changes in discourse
    memory, 294–295
rate of sentence presentation, 280
reading time, 287, 305
retrieval processes, 284, 286–287
schema abstraction, 290–291
schema utilization, 302
scripts, 300–301
sentence memory, 277–281
structural variables of longer discourse,
    298–299
syntactic and semantic constraints,
    277–278, 280
verbal ability, 303–304
working memory, 215–216, 304–305
Discrimination learning, see Classical
    conditioning, Perceptual learning
Dissociation, see Implicit memory,
    Procedural learning
Divided attention
    definition, 55
    effects of practice, 55–56
    effects on working memory, 213–214,
        257
Dual coding theory, see Picture memory
Dual-store models of episodic memory, see
    also Working memory

analysis of primacy effects, 176–181
analysis of recency effects, 157–160
description, 149–151, 175–176
distributed rehearsal, 180–181
elaborative rehearsal, 179–180
limited capacity of STS, 135, 175
number of rehearsals, 177–179
primary memory, 175
retrieval processes, 181
rote rehearsal, 177–181
secondary (long-term) episodic memory,
    175–181
short-term store, 134–135
transmission of traces to long-term store,
    177
                        ◆
Echoic memory
    adaptation to environment, 141
    age differences, 142–149
    cue overload, 149
    measurement of capacity and duration,
        142–144
    modality effect, 144–149
    preperceptual auditory store, 141–142
    short-term and long-term components,
        143–144
    suffix effect, 143–144
Ecological and external validity, 8, 75,
    199–201, 276, 292, 318
Educational level as a confounding
    variable, 69
Effortful processing, 213, 229, see also
    Levels of processing model of episodic
    memory
Elaborative rehearsal, see Levels of
    processing model of episodic memory
Encoding specificity, see Retrieval
    processes
Encoding variability, 246
Episodic memory, see also Dual-store
    models of episodic memory,
    Inhibition model of episodic memory,
    Secondary (long-term) episodic
    memory
    automatic versus effortful, 212–213
    definition, 132–133

Everyday learning and memory, *see* Action
    memory and activity memory, Digit
    span, Discourse memory, Face
    memory, Frequency-of-occurrence
    memory, Generic (semantic) memory,
    Incidental learning/memory versus
    intentional learning/memory,
    Instrumental learning, Learning,
    Levels of processing model of episodic
    memory, Mnemonics, Paired-associate
    learning, Temporal memory
Exercise, effects on memory performances,
    225
Expertise, *see also* Discourse memory
    athletics, 43
    bridge, 57
    chess, 57
    medical technicians, 56
    miniature golfers, 44
    musicians, 27, 43
    perceptual skills, 56–57
    schema-based, 302–303
    sonor operators, 57
    typists, 42–44
Explicit memory, 372
Eyewitness testimony, *see* Face memory
    ◆
Face memory
    age differences, 259–260
    age of faces, 259–260
    change of expression, 260
    everyday memory, 260–261
    eyewitness testimony, 260–262
Factual knowledge, *see* Lexicon,
    Metamemory
False fame effect, *see* Source memory
False recognition effect, *see* Face memory,
    Recognition memory
Flanker effect, 189, 222
Flashbulb memory, *see* Source memory
Forgetting, *see* Implicit memory, Retention
    and long-term forgetting, Short-term
    memory
Free-recall task
    definition, 157–158
    multitrial, 243–244

physical health, 225
Frequency-of-occurrence memory, *see also*
    Action memory and activity memory,
    Automaticity of encoding, Implicit
    memory, Incidental learning/memory
    versus intentional learning/memory,
    Retention and long-term forgetting
    age differences, 308–312
    categorical information, 311–312
    everyday memory, 307, 311
    generation effect, 312
    interpretative problems, 311
    irrelevant versus relevant stimuli, 312
    methods and procedures, 307–308
    nonoptimal model, 311
    prototypal role, 307
    rehearsal independence, 307
    retrieval processes, 311, 326
    working memory, 311
Frontal lobe dysfunctioning, 322, 404
    ◆
Gating theory, 16
General resources, *see also* Inhibition
    model of episodic memory, Motor-
    skill learning, Processing rate model
    of episodic memory, Working memory
    alternative conceptualizations, 202–203
    definition, 201–202
    generality of deficits, 223–228
    inhibition model overview, 207
    motor-skill learning, 39
    network theory, 207–208
    processing deficits, 200–201
    processing rate model of episodic
        memory overview, 203–207
    relationship to cognitive performances,
        201–203
    working memory model of episodic
        memory overview, 203–204
Generation effect in memory, 244–245, *see
    also* Action memory and activity
    memory, Frequency-of-occurrence
    memory
Generic (semantic) memory, *see also*
    Lexicon, Metamemory
    definition, 132–134, 387

everyday memory, 387
separate memory systems, 388, 409–412

♦

Health (physical), effects on performances,
    see Digit span, Free recall task, Paired-
    associate learning, Serial learning

♦

Iconic memory
    adaptation to environment, 136
    age differences, 139–141
    definition, 135–136
    measurement of capacity and duration,
        137–141
    partial report, 137
    whole report, 137
Imagery, see also Paired-associate learning
    age differences, 95–97
    ease of constructing image, 95–97
    vividness of images, 96
Imaginal mediation, see Paired-associate
    learning
Implicit memory
    age differences, 374–382
    category instances, 379–380
    conscious recollection, 371–372,
        383–385
    data-driven conceptualization, 373–374
    definition, 370–371
    dissociations, 372
    forgetting, 372–373, 375
    fragment-completion test, 370–371
    frequency-of-occurrence memory,
        385–386
    homophones, 378
    perceptual identification test, 370, 374
    priming, 378, 380
    process-dissociation procedure, 385
    semantic memory conceptualization,
        372–373
    stem-completion test, 370–371
    stochastic independence, 375, 383
    task interactions with age, 382–383
    three-dimensional objects, 381
Incidental learning/memory versus
    intentional learning/memory
    action memory, 334

activity memory, 328
case memory, 325
conversations, memory of, 343–344
discourse memory, 296–297
free recall, 183–186
frequency-of-occurrence memory,
    307–308
modality memory, 325–326
paired-associate learning, 81, 97–98
picture color memory, 326
sex of voice memory, 323–324
spatial memory, 317–319
temporal memory, 313
Information processing theory, 4, 13, 133,
    201, see also Classical conditioning
Inhibition model of episodic memory, see
    also General resources
    intrusion errors, 223
    irrelevant thoughts, 222–223
    irrelevant versus relevant stimuli, 207,
        220–223
    negative transfer, 223
    nonsearch paradigm, 221–222
    search paradigm, 220–221
Instrumental learning
    adaptation to environment, 2, 21
    age differences in maze learning, 18–19
    age differences in spatial learning, 21,
        25
    cognitive maps, 20
    everyday learning, 2, 21
    explanation of age differences, 20–21
    knowledge of novel environments,
        22–25
    maze learning, 18–21
    spatial learning, 21–25
Intelligence, relationship to
    digit span test, 152
    digit symbol test, 157
    discourse memory, 304
    mnemonic training, 108
Interference proneness
    interpair interference, 75–77
    long-term forgetting, 355
    paired-associate learning, 68
    transfer, 118

Interference theory, 357, 363
Irrelevant versus relevant stimuli, *see*
    Frequency-of-occurrence memory,
    Inhibition model of episodic memory,
    Selective attention
Item-specific processing, *see* Organizational
    processes in memory

◆

Knowledge of results, *see* Motor-skill
    learning

◆

Lag effect, 246–249
Learning, *see also* Classical conditioning,
    Instrumental learning, Motor-skill
    learning, Paired-associate learning,
    Perceptual learning, Serial learning,
    Verbal learning
    adaptation to environment, 1–3
    contrast with memory, 2–3
    curves of rate of learning, 8
    definition, 3
    everyday learning, 1–3
    monistic theory, 2
    performance-learning distinction, 72–73
    pluralistic theory, 2
Letter span
    age differences, 153–154
    chunking, 157
    length of series, 156
    secondary (long-term) memory,
        156–157
Levels of processing model of episodic
        memory, *see also* General resources
    analysis of recency effects, 196–199
    cognitive effort, 192
    cognitive support, 191–193
    cued recall versus noncued recall,
        187–192
    deep processing, 181
    depth of processing dimension, 181
    distinctiveness of memory traces,
        193–196
    durability of memory traces, 181–182
    elaboration deficits, 190–192
    elaborative rehearsal, 182–183
    everyday memory, 200

maintenance rehearsal, 182
mediational versus production deficits,
    186–187
orienting tasks, 183–186
overall evaluation, 199–201
retrieval processes, 187–188
semantic processing deficits, 186–189
sensory memory traces, 181
shallow processing, 181
Lexicon, *see also* Verbal ability, Vocabulary
        tests
    access to words, 395–396
    age differences in access to categorical
        information, 404–409
    age differences in factual knowledge,
        391
    age differences in structure, 388–395
    age differences in word access, 395–402
    attentional processes, 400–401
    definition of lexical memory, 387–388
    definition-to-word deficit, 413–414
    episodic memory priming effects,
        410–412
    everyday memory, 387
    generational differences, 391–392
    lexical decision, 397–398
    lexical priming effects, 395–396, 399
    mental dictionary, 135, 388
    pronunciation time, 396
    separate memory systems, 409–412
    spoken word onset, 389
    spreading activation, 396
    stimulus degradation, 402–403
    Stroop test, 396–397
    syntax, 414–415
    tip-of-the-tongue (TOT) state, 412–413
    verbal fluency, 404
    word associations, 392–395
Limited capacity, *see* Dual-store models of
        episodic memory, Working memory
Long-term episodic memory, *see* Secondary
        (long-term) episodic memory
Long-term store (LTS), 134, 176

◆

Maintenance rehearsal, *see* Levels of
        processing model of episodic memory

Maze learning, *see* Instrumental learning
Mediational deficit, *see* Paired-associate
    learning, Levels of processing model
    of episodic memory
Medical information, *see* Discourse
    memory
Medication compliance, *see* Prospective
    memory
Memory
    contrasted with learning, 2–3
    diary studies, 31–32
    episodic memory definition, 132
    everyday, 131–132
    generic (semantic) memory definition,
        132–133
    failures, 131–132
    overall model of the memory system,
        134–135
    sensory memory definition, 133–135
Memory complainers
    mnemonic training, 113
    performance on memory tasks, 113, 416
Memory span, *see* Digit span, Letter span,
    Word span, Working memory
Memory training, *see* Mnemonics
Mental activity, effects on memory
    performances, 226–227, 304
Mental rotation, 38–39, 92
Mental skill learning, 57
Metamemory
    components, 415–416
    definition, 415
    evaluating failures of memory, 420–421,
        423–424
    factual knowledge, 431–432
    Memory (Functioning) Questionnaire,
        418–420
    Metamemory in Adulthood
        questionnaire, 418, 420–421
    monitoring, 428–431
    off-line component, 416–424
    on-line component, 424–428
    postdiction of memory performance,
        428
    prediction of memory performance,
        427–428

    questionnaires, 417–418
    relationships of self-evaluations to
        memory performances, 422–423
    self-efficacy questionnaires, 428
Mini-Mental State Examination, 111–112
Mnemonics, *see also* Alzheimer's Disease,
    Anxiety, Depression, Memory
    complainers, Personality traits,
    Retention and long-term forgetting
    alternative methods, 113–117
    computer-assisted instruction, 107–110
    definition, 105
    everyday memory, 108
    fluid intelligence, 108
    keyword method, 105, 108–110
    method of loci, 105–108
    organizational training, 115
    pegword method, 105–106
    preference of method, 112
    problems in use, 114–115
    self-instruction, 114
    story construction, 115
Modality memory, age differences,
    325–326, *see also* Incidental learning/
    memory versus intentional learning/
    memory
Mood-dependent memory, *see* Retrieval
    processes
Motivation, *see also* Anxiety, Performance-
    learning distinction
    and paired-associate learning, 72–73
    and prospective memory, 273
Motor behaviors, attributes of, *see also*
    Reaction time
    change in direction of movement, 32
    coincidence–anticipation, 31–32
    coordination of bimanual movements,
        31
    mental blocks, 32
    response speed, 28
Motor-skill learning, *see also* General
    resources
    adaptation to environment, 26–27
    age differences, 32–41
    closed loop versus open loop, 45–46
    cognitive processes, 39

Motor-skill learning (*continued*)
  computer skills, 33–34
  continuous responses, 36–41
  discrete responses, 34–36
  early research, 32–33
  expertise, 42–44
  explanation of age differences, 44–46
  general resource decrement hypothesis, 39
  kinesthetic and proprioceptive stimuli, 35–36
  knowledge of results, 34–35, 40–41
  maintenance of skill, 26–27, 41–42
  mirror tracing task, 36
  movement of arm task, 35–36
  problem solving component, 39, 45
  programs for skilled activities, 46
  prototype abstraction, 45–46
  pursuit rotor task, 37
  realworld tasks, 32–34
  reminiscence, 41
  two-hand coordination, 39
  typing, 33, 42–44
Movies, memory of, 344

Network theory, *see* General resources
Neural noise hypothesis, *see* Processing rate model of episodic memory
Nonspecific transfer, *see* Transfer
Nursing home residents and institutionalized elderly people
  operant conditioning, 14
  spatial learning, 22–23
  transfer, 127

Operant conditioning
  age differences, 14–18
  avoidance learning, 17–18
  behavior modification, 14
  biofeedback and brain waves, 16
  definition and procedures, 5–6
  matching-to-sample task, 15–16
  negative reinforcement, 5
  positive reinforcement, 5–6
  punishment training, 5–6
  response speed, 14–16

Organizational processes in memory
  basic concepts, 229–230
  categorical, 230–238
  clustering, 231, 235–238
  cue overload, 234
  item-specific processing, 234–235, 238
  relational processing, 234–235
  rhymes, 239
  schema, 239
  scripts, 238–239
  seriation, 237–238
  subjective organization, 240–243
  synonyms, 239–240
Output interference, *see* Retrieval processes

Paired-associate learning
  age differences, cross-sectional, 69–71, 73–76
  age differences, longitudinal, 71
  anticipation method, 89
  associative analysis, 77, 83
  confounding by nonage attributes, 70
  definition, 66
  early studies, 67–69
  everyday learning, 66, 75, 79, 81–82, 105
  imaginal mediation, 82–84
  incidental learning versus intentional learning, 81, 97–98
  mediational training, 91–97
  methodological problems, 69–77
  physical health, 70–71
  production deficit, 92
  production inefficiency, 95
  rate of item presentation, 86–91
  recall method, 89
  rehearsal rate, 80, 83
  relationships to other tasks, 67, 98, 103, 106–109
  response learning, 77–79, 127
  rote rehearsal, 83–84
  R-S learning, 79–81, 128
  sex differences, 72
  S-R learning, 83–84
  stage analysis, 77–86

stimulus learning, 81–82, 118, 129–130
time-lag comparisons, 70
total time principle, 91
verbal mediation, 94–95
Pattern recognition, *see* Perceptual
    learning
Perceptual learning
    attentional learning, 54–56
    definition, 46–47
    discrimination learning, 47–53
    pattern recognition learning, 53–54
    reversal versus nonreversal shifts,
        48–53
    target detection learning, 47
Performance-learning distinction, 72–73,
    100, 102–103
Permastore, *see* Retention and long-term
    forgetting
Personality traits
    relatedness to memory performances,
        227–228
    relatedness to mnemonic training, 113
Picture memory, *see also* Working memory
    concreteness effect, 254–255
    dual coding theory, 254–255, 258
    objects versus words, 256–258
    picture superiority effect, 254
    scene memory, 258–259
    scripts, 259
Picture superiority effect, *see* Picture
    memory
Primacy effect, 157–158, *see also* Dual
    store models of episodic memory,
    Levels of processing model of episodic
    memory
Primary memory, *see* Dual-store models of
    episodic memory
Proactive inhibition, *see also* Short-term
    memory
    long-term forgetting, 354–355
    short-term forgetting, 163–165
Procedural learning, *see also* Amnesics
    age differences, 63–65
    dissociation, 57–63
    relatedness to nonspecific transfer, 64,
        130

Processing rate model of episodic memory,
    see also Digit symbol test, General
    resources
    assessment of processing rate, 210
    Brinley-plot, 206
    contradictory evidence, 210–212
    loss of information, 204
    neural noise hypothesis, 203–204
    neural transmission, 204
    relationship to working memory,
        218–220
    slowing down principle, 203–204
    slowing down/complexity hypothesis,
        204–206, 399–400, 403
    supportive evidence, 210
Production deficit, *see* Paired-associate
    learning, Levels of processing model
    of episodic memory
Production inefficiency, *see* Paired-
    associate learning
Prospective memory, *see also* Motivation
    contrast with retrospective memory,
        271–272
    event-based retrieval versus time-based
        retrieval, 274–275
    laboratory tests, 273–275
    medication compliance, 272–273
    nonlaboratory tests, 272–273
    self-initiated retrieval, 274–275
Prototype abstraction, *see* Motor-skill
    learning

                        ◆

Reaction time
    advance cues, 31
    premotor and motor components, 29
    response selection training, 29–30
    set, 31
    speed and response complexity,
        28–29
Reading span, *see* Working memory
Reality monitoring, *see* Action memory
    and activity memory
Recency effect, 157–160, *see also* Dual-
    store models of episodic memory,
    Levels of processing model of episodic
    memory

Recognition memory, *see also* Action
memory and activity memory
consistency effect, 252–253
continuous, 250
contrasted with recall, 253–254
false recognition effect, 189
multiple item, 220–221
recollection versus familiarity, 250–252
retrieval processes, 253–254
signal detection analysis, 250
single item, 249–253
word-frequency effect, 252
Rehearsal independency, 306, *see also*
Action memory and activity memory,
Conversations, memory of,
Frequency-of-occurrence memory,
Temporal memory
Release from proactive inhibition, *see*
Short-term memory
Reminiscence, *see* Motor-skill learning
Retention and long-term forgetting, *see
also* Implicit memory, Interference
proneness, Interference theory,
Proactive inhibition, Source memory
actions and activities, 367–369
autobiographical memory, 352–354
decay of information, 163–165
frequency-of-occurrence memory, 369
mnemonics, 106, 108
newsworthy events, 349–352
permastore, 347–349
real-life forgetting, 346–352
remote (very long-term) memory, 347
retroactive inhibition, 354–355
single list forgetting, 362–369
successive lists, 357–362
temporal memory, 369
Retrieval processes, *see also* Action
memory and activity memory,
Discourse memory, Dual-store models
of episodic memory, Frequency-of-
occurrence memory, Levels of
processing model of episodic memory,
Prospective memory, Recognition
memory
consistency of retrieval, 261

encoding specificity, 261–267
indirect retrieval, 269–270
mood-dependent memory, 267
output interference, 234, 267–268
recall exceeding recognition,
263–264
retrieval practice, 116, 268–269,
334–335
State dependent memory, 266–267
Retrospective memory, *see* Prospective
memory
Reversal versus nonreversal shifts, *see*
Perceptual learning
Rote rehearsal, *see* Paired-associate
learning

Schema, *see* Discourse memory,
Organizational processes in memory
Scripts, *see* Discourse memory,
Organizational processes in memory
Secondary (long-term) episodic memory,
149–150, *see also* Digit span, Dual-
store models of episodic memory,
Letter span, Word span
Selective attention, *see also* Inhibition
model of episodic memory
definition, 54–55
irrelevant stimuli versus relevant
stimuli, 54–55
practice effects, 55
Semantic memory, *see* Generic (semantic)
memory
Senile Dementia of the Alzheimer's Type
(SDAT), *see* Alzheimer's Disease
Sensory memory, *see also* Echoic memory,
Iconic memory
definition, 133–135
other senses, 149
sensory register, 134–135
Serial learning
age differences, 98–99
age-sensitive processes, 102–104
definition and procedure, 98–99
mediation, 103
physical health, 224
presentation rate, 100–101

serial position effects, 99–100
stimulus-response analysis, 103
temporal memory analysis, 103–104
Serial position effects, *see* Action
     memory and activity memory, Serial
     learning
Sex of voice memory, 323–325, *see also*
     Incidental learning/memory versus
     intentional learning/memory
Short-term memory, *see also* Action
     memory and activity memory,
     Memory span, Recency effect
Brown-Peterson procedure, 162–163
capacity of STS, 151–160
dual stores, 150
empirical phenomena, 165, 167
primary memory, 133–134, 149–150
rate of forgetting, 162–168
release from proactive inhibition,
     167–168
representation of information in STS,
     160–162
scanning/search of STS, 168–172
scanning/search of LTS, 172–174
short-term store (STS), 150–151
transmission of traces to LTS, 163, 177
Slowing down principle, *see* Processing
     rate model of episodic memory
Source memory, *see also* Amnesics
age differences, 321–323
false fame effect, 322
flashbulb memory, 321, 350
source amnesia, 321
source forgetting, 321
Span of apprehension, 136–137
Spatial learning, *see* Instrumental
     learning
Spatial memory, 315–321, *see also*
     Incidental learning/memory versus
     intentional learning/memory
Specific transfer, *see* Transfer
Spreading activation, *see* Lexicon
Stage analysis, *see* Associationism, Paired-
     associate learning
State dependent memory, *see* Retrieval
     processes

Stimulus persistence principle, 36,
     141–142
Stroop test, *see* Lexicon
Subject-performed tasks (SPTs), *see*
     Action memory and activity
     memory
Syntax, *see* Lexicon
                          ◆

Television programs, memory of,
     344–345
Temporal memory, *see also*, Action
     memory and activity memory
age differences, 313–315
conjointed features, 315
everyday memory, 312, 315
rehearsal independency, 312–313
Time-lag comparisons, *see* Paired-associate
     learning
Tip-of-the-tongue (TOT) state, *see*
     Lexicon
Total time principle, *see* Paired-associate
     learning
Transfer, *see also* Inhibition model of
     episodic memory, Interference
     proneness
A-B, A-B', 118–121, 130
A-B, A'-B, 129
A-B, A-Br, 125–126
A-B, A-C, 117–124, 127
A-B, C-B, 127–128, 130
A-B, C-D, 119–121, 123–124, 127
definition, 117
everyday learning, 117–118
interference proneness, 118
learning-to-learn, 119
mediation, 118, 129
negative transfer, 117, 122–128
nonspecific transfer, 107, 117–119, 120,
     122
positive transfer, 117, 128–129
research design, 117–118
specific transfer, 117–120, 122–129
theory and processes, 117–119,
     126–128
warm-up, 119
Typing, *see* Expertise, Motor-skill learning

•

Verbal ability, 69, 100–102, 393–394, *see also* Discourse memory
Verbal fluency, *see* Lexicon
Verbal learning, 2–3, 66, 105, *see also* Paired-associate learning, Serial learning
Verbosity, 223
Vigilance
  definition, 54
  effects of practice, 54
  irrelevant thoughts, 223
Vocabulary tests
  age differences, 390–391
  relationship to word associations, 393–394

•

Word associations, *see* Lexicon, Vocabulary tests
Word-frequency effect, *see* Recognition memory
Word span
  age differences, 153–156
  approximation to English words, 156
  assessment of working memory, 218
  free recall versus serial recall, 153–154
  secondary memory component, 155–156

word frequency, 154
Working memory, *see also* Automaticity of encoding, Digit span, Discourse memory, Divided attention, Frequency-of-occurrence memory, General resources, Processing rate model of episodic memory, Word span
  articulatory loop, 155, 212
  assessment of capacity, 214–220
  computational span, 214–215
  definition and alternative conceptualizations, 203–204
  limited capacity, 135, 203
  longitudinal decline, 219–220
  modified digit span, 214
  picture memory, 215
  processing efficiency, 219
  reading/listening span, 215–217
  relationship episodic memory, 193, 213–216
  relationship to dual-store models, 150–151
  spatial-line test, 215
  storage component versus processing component, 216, 218–220
  text-span, 214–216